# CONTENTS

Contents

Neuromuscular Disorders in Children:
A Multidisciplinary Approach to
Management

Clinics in Developmental Medicine

# Neuromuscular Disorders in Children: A Multidisciplinary Approach to Management

Edited by

NICOLAS DECONINCK
Department of Pediatric Neurology and Neuromuscular Reference
Centre, HUDERF, Université Libre de Bruxelles, Brussels, Belgium and
Department of Pediatric Neurology and Neuromuscular Reference
Centre, UZ Gent, Ghent, Belgium

NATHALIE GOEMANS
Department of Pediatric Neurology, Neuromuscular Reference Center
for Children, University Hospitals Leuven, University of Leuven, Leuven,
Belgium

2019
Mac Keith Press

Contents

*Contents*

## SECTION 8: PSYCHOSOCIAL ASPECTS

# AUTHOR APPOINTMENTS

**Boglárka Bánsági**   Centre for Metabolic Diseases, University Hospital Leuven, Leuven, Belgium

**Sandra Coppens**   Neuromuscular Reference Center, Université Libre de Bruxelles, Brussels, Belgium

**Stacy Cossette**   Congenital Muscle Disease Tissue Repository Manager, Medical College of Wisconsin, WI, USA

**Rudy van Coster**   Pediatric Neurology, Ghent University, Belgium

**Basil T Darras**   Joseph J. Volpe Professor of Neurology, Harvard Medical School; Associate Neurologist-in-Chief, Division of Clinical Neurology, Boston Children's Hospital, Boston, MA, USA

**Nicolas Deconinck**   Department of Pediatric Neurology and Neuromuscular Reference Center, HUDERF, Université Libre de Bruxelles, Brussels, Belgium

**Imelda de Groot**   Associate Professor, Consultant pediatric Rehabilitation, Department of Rehabilitation, Radboud University Medical Centre, Nijmegen, The Netherlands

**Liesbeth De Waele**   Department of Paediatric Neurology, University Hospitals Leuven, Leuven, Belguim

**Tina Duong**   Physical Therapist; Clinical Research Manager, Division of Neuromuscular Medicine, Stanford Health Care, Palo Alto, CA, USA

**Sam Geuens**   Clinical Neuropsychologist, University Hospitals Leuven, Leuven, Belgium

**Nathalie Goemans**   Department of Pediatric Neurology, Neuromuscular Reference Center for Children, University Hospitals Leuven, University of Leuven, Leuven, Belgium

**Laurence Goffin**      Department of Pediatrics HUDERF, Université
                         Libre de Bruxelles; Department of Pediatrics,
                         CHIREC Delta, Brussels, Belgium

**Anne Lennox**          Founding Parent and Chief Executive,
                         Myotubular Trust, UK

**Wendy K M Liew**       Clinical Fellow in Neurology, Boston Children's
                         Hospital and Harvard Medical School, Boston
                         MA; Consultant Pediatrician and Neurologist,
                         SBCC Baby & Child Clinic, Neurology Centre;
                         Visiting Consultant, Neurology Service,
                         Department of Pediatrics, KK Women's and
                         Children's Hospital, Singapore

**Oscar Mayer**          Medical Director, Pulmonary Function
                         Testing Laboratory, The Children's Hospital of
                         Philadelphia; Professor of Clinical Pediatrics,
                         Perelman School of Medicine at the University
                         of Pennsylvania, PA, USA

**Anna G Mayhew**        John Walton Muscular Dystrophy Research
                         Centre, Newcastle upon Tyne, UK

**Pierre Moens**         Surgeon-in-chief, Paediatric orthopaedics and
                         spinal deformities, University Hospitals Leuven,
                         Leuven, Belguim

**Maarten van Nuffel**   Assistant-Surgeon-in-chief, Hand Unit,
                         Department of Orthopaedics, University
                         Hospitals Leuven, Leuven, Belgium

**Hasan Özen**           Hacettepe University Children's Hospital,
                         Department of Paediatric Gastroenterology,
                         Hepatology and Nutrition, Ankara, Turkey

**Lionel Paternoster**   Department of Paediatric Neurology,
                         Queen Fabiola Children's University Hospital,
                         Université Libre de Bruxelles, Brussels, Belgium

**Ros Quinlivan**        Consultant in Neuromuscular Disorders,
                         MRC Centre for Neuromuscular Diseases,
                         National Hospital for Neurology and
                         Neurosurgery, London, UK

**Gauthier Remiche**     Head of the Neuromuscular Reference Center
                         Erasme-HUDERF, Department of Neurology,
                         Hôpital Erasme, Université Libre de Bruxelles,
                         Brussels, Belgium

| | |
|---|---|
| **Kristy Rose** | Paediatric Physiotherapist, Paediatric Gait Analysis Service of New South Wales, The Children's Hospital at Westmead, Sydney, Australia |
| **Anne Rutkowski** | Kaiser SCPMG, Los Angeles, CA, USA |
| **Hemant Sawnani** | Associate Professor, Department of Pediatrics, University of Cincinnati; Division of Pulmonology & Section of Sleep Medicine, Cincinnati Children's Hospital Medical Center, Cincinnati, OH, USA |
| **Ann F Schrooten** | Parent of a child with a congenital muscular dystrophy, founder and board member of The Willow Tree Foundation, Phoenix, AZ, USA |
| **Thomas Sejerson** | Professor, Senior Consultant, Pediatric Neurology, Department of Women's and Children's Health, Karolinska Institute, Stockholm, Sweden |
| **Laurent Servais** | Centre de Référence des Maladies Neuromusculaires, CHU de Liège, Liège, Belgium; Institute i-Motion, Hôpital Armand Trousseau, Paris, France |
| **Banu Sundar** | Assistant Professor in Neurology, University of Massachusetts Medical School, Worcester, MA, USA |
| **Haluk Topaloglu** | Hacettepe University Children's Hospital, Department of Child Neurology, Ankara, Turkey |
| **Michel Toussaint** | Head of Therapy and Research, Centre for Home Mechanical Ventilation and Neuromuscular Disorders, Department of Rehabilitation, Inkendaal Rehabilitation Hospital, Brussels, Belgium |
| **Karim Wahbi** | Cardiology Department, Cochin Hospital, Paris Descartes University, Paris, France |
| **Peter Witters** | Centre for Metabolic Diseases, University Hospitals Leuven, Leuven, Belgium |

# FOREWORD

Neuromuscular Disorders (NMDs) cover all diseases that affect one or more components of the "motor unit", composed of the alpha-motor neuron, spinal nerve roots, the peripheral nerves with their axons and myelin sheets, the neuromuscular junction, and last but not least, the muscle fibers. In peripheral neuropathies, sensory fibers and the spinal ganglia can also be affected. NMDs are rare diseases with an age-specific overall prevalence in children and adolescents of 60-70/100.000. Only 15% of cases are due to an acquired, mostly inflammatory aetiology, while most are due to a broad spectrum of rare inborn causes. Of those, Duchenne Muscular Dystrophy (DMD) and Spinal Muscular Atrophy (SMA) have by far the highest incidence (18 and 12/100.000, respectively). Unfortunately, the most prevalent of these genetic syndromes exhibits a rapidly progressive course resulting in severe disability and a significantly shortened life-span.

This is probably why until only a few decades ago, general society and many physicians were hardly aware of these diseases. They were considered ominous without treatment perspectives, and the patients and their families were left alone, frequently in deep desperation, to deal with the diseases' consequences. However, as the genetic cause of these diseases was gradually deciphered, beginning in the 1980s, the scientific community's interest in their aetiology, pathophysiology, natural history, and hopefully cure, rose, and persists with increasing speed and success. In parallel and in close collaboration with growing numbers of patient and family support groups, innovative measures of symptomatic treatment to improve quality of life and psychosocial well-being are being developed.

This book addresses the progress made in diagnosis and classification, and particularly in treatment of NMDs. It has been written by an international group of experts highly experienced in their respective diagnostic and therapeutic fields. It comprises their up-to-date views and experiences from differential diagnosis, and monitoring the clinical course to the treatment, development and application of best-practice strategies and psychosocial care for patients and their families.

The book starts with a description of the burdensome and psychologically stressful situation of the patients and their families after the diagnosis of a NMD and its significance over their entire life span. This is followed by an overview of methods and results in developing best-practice guidelines and standards-of-care for many of these diseases, based on analyses of the scientific literature and formal consensual processes of clinical experts. The need for interdisciplinary and inter-professional co-operation in caring for these patients is highlighted already in this first part of the book.

In the second part, the nosological groups of NMDs are discussed chapter by chapter, covering the presenting symptoms, diagnosis, and differential diagnosis, genetic aspects, best-practice treatment and clinical course, and recent and (hopefully) future therapeutic developments. This discussion addresses not only the most frequent DMD, SMA and

Charcot-Marie-Tooth neuropathies, but also rarer entities such as congenital myopathies, myasthenic syndromes and hereditary ion-channel dysfunctions. The less frequent acquired and usually treatable diseases such as juvenile dermatomyositis, inflammatory polyneuropathies, and myasthenia gravis are also fully covered along with their recent therapy recommendations.

The third part details the monitoring of symptoms and complications as well as treatment strategies for the different groups of patients in the fields and from the perspectives of physiotherapy, occupational therapy, technical aids, orthopaedics, orthopaedic surgery, gastrointestinal, respiratory and cardiac care, and last but not least, psychosocial care.

I congratulate the editors and authors on this comprehensive and up-to-date book which is the first on NMDs in children. It is consistently patient-centred, will help readers learn about the latest classification and treatment options for these diseases, and hopefully influence their attitudes and decisions when caring for patients with neuromuscular disorders. With broad distribution this book will help to improve the fate and quality of life of many patients suffering from NMDs, as well as their families.

**Rudolf Korinthenberg, M.D.**
Professor Emeritus of Neuropaediatrics and Muscular Disorders,
Center of Paediatrics and Adolescent Medicine,
University Medical Centre Freiburg, Germany

# PREFACE

Neuromuscular disorders are rare but often devastating for patients and their families. Their effects on the life-course trajectories of young people can be profound and long lasting. They are very often associated with dysfunction of a number of physiological systems, leading to complex symptoms and needs, e.g. impairments that require orthopaedic services, cause pain, respiratory, cardiac, and psychological distress. This increases the burden for patients, impacting participation and quality of life, and calls for complex and multidisciplinary management.

Over the last 20 years, the outlook has started to change drastically, both as a result of societal changes with respect to disability and advances in molecular genetics and histopathological technology. The latter have enabled the recognition and understanding of the underlying molecular mechanisms of many different neuromuscular conditions, highlighting therapeutic targets for the future or emerging applications, thus opening an era for new specific, sometimes gene tailored, treatment approaches.

Nowadays, clinicians undertaking training and a career in the neuromuscular disorders field very often have to "pick" their knowledge from informal contacts with more senior experts in their respective hospitals. Moreover, the knowledge and expertise in the management of some ultra rare neuromuscular disorders is often limited to a very few specialized centres that are scattered across the world and not always accessible for every student.

With this collaborative work on the management of neuromuscular disorders we aim to gather for the first time in one place the knowledge from recognized experts from various backgrounds, including clinicians, surgeons, geneticists, physiotherapists, psychologists, and parents.

On completing this writing odyssey, we are reminded of our first face-to-face meeting with Ann-Marie Halligan and Udoka Ohuonu from Mac Keith Press, at the congress of the World Muscle Society in Brighton. Ann-Marie and Udoka showed confidence in the merits of our approach for this project. Moreover it could not have become a reality without the benevolent support of Bernard Dan who helped us to structure its first steps.

An important milestone was also the decision to work together as editors, combining our personal experience and expertise in the field of neuromuscular disorders; each of us motivating the other to bring to its term a fantastic but very intensive project. We were very satisfied to build a common view on what should be the unifying idea of this work, and then to enlist contributors to build a book we hope will be new, appreciated, and useful in the field of neuromuscular disorders.

Important for us was to re-position "clinical evaluation" as key in this exciting era of high-level medicine. Thus, we included a description of the clinical features of neuromuscular disorders. The care and management of neuromuscular diseases start with a correct diagnosis. The recognition of clinical signs and symptoms will raise suspicion and prompt an early diagnosis. Modern genetics has drastically improved the diagnostic journey for neuromuscular disorders. However, a thorough insight in clinical features has become even more important, for example in clarifying the genotype-phenotype correlation when applying whole sequencing techniques in rare diseases.

As highlighted by Rudolf Korinthenberg in the foreword, this work has been driven by our conviction that a coordinated multidisciplinary approach of management is essential to improve the quality of life of children with neuromuscular diseases and their families. This should be based as much as possible on the application of guidelines throughout all stages of the disease. We hope that this work will contribute to this end.

We live in exciting times, with promising therapeutic strategies, in development or even yet approved by the regulatory authorities, that could impact on disease progression. Throughout the book, we aimed to provide the reader with the most recent update on therapeutic advances, both in preclinical and clinical development. In addition, we highlighted the importance of validated and harmonized outcome measures for the evaluation of disease progression and the impact of interventions.

This book is the result of an intensive collaborative process. We would like to thank all the contributors, all of whom are noted experts in their fields, who enthusiastically embarked on this project, and responded to our editorial requests. We are very grateful for their commitment to produce high quality information, which reflects our longstanding collaboration in sharing expertise in this domain.

The book could not have been completed without the support and energy of Ann-Marie Halligan, Udoka Ohuonu, Lucy White, Sally Wilkinson, Rosie Outred, Duncan Potter, Tiffany Bertrand and Elke De Vos.

Finally, we would like to express our gratitude to all the patients and families, whose lives and experiences were an inspiration for the writing of this book, but more generally, have long inspired our work in the neuromuscular field.

**Nicolas Deconinck and Nathalie Goemans**

# Section 1
## Introduction

# 1
# PARENT PERSPECTIVES ON NEUROMUSCULAR DISORDERS: FROM DIAGNOSIS, TO PARENTING AND LIVING WITH, TO ADVANCE CARE PLANNING AND PREPARING FOR DEATH

*Anne Rutkowski, Stacy Cossette, Anne Lennox and Ann F Schrooten*

## Introduction

When a neuromuscular disease diagnosis is made, parents may leave the clinic or hospital in shock. They may not have heard or processed any information relayed by the medical professional after receiving the diagnosis. Time may seem to stand still. There are extended family members waiting to hear the news, who must be called, messaged, or seen.

Acceptance can be difficult, and soon the parents realize that nothing will be the same again. The unknowns that lie ahead may feel overwhelming. There will be a steep learning curve to understand both the disease and how their lives will change. Most parents and extended family members will have no prior knowledge about genetics and be even less familiar with the specific neuromuscular disorder that now affects their family.

Perceptions about the disorder will evolve. Parents will need to learn by trial and error how to provide the required care, master sophisticated in-home medical equipment, and navigate both the social and medical environments to ensure optimal care and quality of life. The parent's and child's health and emotional well-being will impact quality of life. The ability to cope will matter more than disease severity.

This chapter will evaluate four milestones when parenting a child with a neuromuscular disorder: 1) obtaining a genetic diagnosis, 2) living with the chronic neuromuscular disorder, 3) advance care planning and 4) preparing for death. These milestones may occur in parallel or sequentially. While significant advances have been made in genetic testing technologies, access to testing, engagement of palliative and psychological support, and discussions regarding advance care are often lacking. Support through community and advocacy forums and the world wide web provide additional resources that are complementary to medical counsel.

## Diagnosis

Genetic testing can have a demonstrable impact on families and affected individuals (Smith et al. 2004). Testing may provide individual benefits, such as family planning, the end of a diagnostic odyssey and additional testing, the ability to connect with others similarly affected, and tailored medical management. The possible drawbacks of genetic testing may include the persistence of anxiety and depression in some individuals with positive or negative test results, and health discrimination (Vansenne et al. 2009; Kang 2011). Societal benefits of genetic testing include an improved understanding of a particular disease presentation, genotype to phenotype correlations, and overall disease prevalence.

While it is generally accepted that genetic testing provides potential individual and society benefits, not all clinicians endorse genetic testing in neuromuscular conditions without clinical trials or therapeutic intervention. This lack of endorsement can be a significant barrier as clinicians are the gatekeepers (Toiviainen et al. 2003).

Several studies have interrogated clinician attitudes towards presymptomatic or susceptibility testing. Clinicians report concerns that laypeople's attitudes towards genetic testing lead to high expectations with limited disease knowledge (Toiviainen et al. 2003; Hall et al. 2015). However, there are no studies that evaluate clinician attitudes and barriers to ordering genetic testing in symptomatic patients, including children and adults with presumed neuromuscular disorders.

Clinician barriers may include a bias against genetic testing, uncertainty about which genetic test to order, how to interpret genetic test results, and how to provide appropriate counseling once test results are obtained. A recent study of neurologists and psychiatrists showed that 49% of neurologists did not have a genetic professional to refer patients to and thought testing could harm the patient (Salm et al. 2014). Having access to a genetic counselor increased the likelihood that the neurologist would order genetic testing.

Additional barriers to genetic testing include lack of access to commercial or research-based testing, lack of financial ability to pay for testing, and lack of access to clinicians with neuromuscular expertise. A recent report on care of Duchenne muscular dystrophy patients in Mexico highlights the challenges in obtaining adequate care, starting with a delay in noticing first symptoms. Mean age at death in this cohort is $18.94 \pm 6.73$ years with a clear acknowledgement of the reduced life span of their cohort compared to developed countries (López-Hernández et al. 2014). The late diagnosis and low percentage of genetically confirmed cases may further impede proactive medical management and relate directly to lower survival. However, there are no randomized control trials to evaluate whether genetic testing has improved health outcomes or is cost effective.

### DELAY IN GENETIC DIAGNOSIS

There are multiple reports of documented delays in obtaining a genetic diagnosis in children and adults with neuromuscular disorders (Table 1.1). Diagnostic delays can lead to additional affected children within a family and extended and costly diagnostic workups. The length of delay may vary by severity with an urgency afforded to the more severe phenotypes (Table 1.1).

3

**TABLE 1.1**
**Delay in genetic diagnosis**

| Neuromuscular disorder | Adult/child population | Average time from symptoms to diagnosis (Country) | Reference |
|---|---|---|---|
| Duchenne muscular dystrophy | Child | 2.5 years (United States) | Ciafaloni 2009 |
| Duchenne muscular dystrophy | Child | 1.6 years (Europe) | Van Ruiten 2014 |
| Myotonic dystrophy (DM2) | Adult | 14 years | Hilbert 2013 |
| Spinal muscular atrophy (SMA) | Child/ Adult | 3.6 months (SMA1), 14.3 months (SMA2) and 43.6 months (SMA3) | Lin 2015 |
| Genetically confirmed muscular dystrophy | Adult | 4.3 years | Spuler 2011 |

FAMILY COPING ONCE A GENETIC DIAGNOSIS IS MADE

The majority of studies evaluating short and long-term psychological effects of genetic testing have been performed in presymptomatic individuals. A survey of presymptomatic individuals at risk for dominant neuromuscular disorders demonstrates a high acceptance of genetic testing, regardless of the results (Smith et al. 2004).

Genetic testing may lead to a range of feelings including, blame, guilt, and isolation for some individuals, while others report an improved quality of life. Anxiety and depression may persist in some presymptomatic individuals with positive or negative results. In a retrospective review, presymptomatic and symptomatic individuals differed in their perception of their health and levels of anxiety and depression before genetic testing, with no long-term psychological impairment in either group after testing (Vansenne et al. 2009).

ADVANCES IN GENETIC TESTING AND PHYSICIAN EDUCATION

Advances in genetic testing technology, including the use of next generation and whole exome sequencing, have improved the yield of a genetic diagnosis in presumed neuromuscular patients to as high as 40% (Savarese et al. 2016; Ghaoui et al. 2015). The use of these technologies may lead to a larger number of patients identified as having a variant of unknown significance with results that are difficult to interpret. Interpretation of variants can be challenging due to overlapping phenotypes, variability in disease transmission, and lack of inclusion of phenotypic patient data on commercial order forms. It can take years to reclassify a variant of unknown significance and there can be a significant burden to recontact patients and inform them of reclassification of their variant status (Pyeritz 2011; Hunter et al. 2001).

Lay people can have difficulty in understanding the difference between a pathologic mutation and a variant of unknown significance test result in the context of susceptibility testing (Hall et al. 2015; Lindor et al. 2013). It is unclear whether parents and affected individuals understand the difference in genetic technologies, the low yield of definitive testing for new phenotypes, and whether this knowledge is important in providing informed consent. It is recommended that neurologists and pediatricians work together with geneticists and genetic counselors to improve diagnostic yield and communicate diagnostic testing results. It is important to provide the family with realistic turnaround times for genetic testing, especially research-based testing, and a mechanism for the family to contact the testing laboratory.

When a diagnosis is not made, families may turn to direct-to-consumer commercial genetic testing. The lack of consultation with a clinician may preclude a lay person's understanding of the type of testing offered, the clinical validity of the test, and a thorough interpretation of positive and negative results in the context of their presumed diagnosis. While geneticists are reluctant to recommend direct to consumer testing for these reasons, there appears to be an increased interest by the lay public with an assumption that clinicians will help interpret results (Howard and Borry 2013; McGuire et al. 2009).

Access to preimplantation genetic diagnosis has improved. Parents of a child with a neuromuscular disorder may choose to undergo preimplantation genetic diagnosis to ensure additional unaffected children. Many neurologists and psychiatrists, however, do not feel comfortable discussing preimplantation genetic diagnosis with parents of an affected child (Klitzman et al. 2014).

Parents of children with neuromuscular disorders strongly support newborn screening, with 95.9% of parents of children with Duchenne muscular dystrophy, Becker muscular dystrophy, or spinal muscular atrophy and 92.6% among expectant parents supporting a screening program (Wood et al. 2014; Chung et al. 2016). No negative psychosocial impacts of newborn screening were identified among those families who received a diagnosis through newborn screening. However, ethical questions persist and include risks and benefits, whether it should require informed consent, be limited to boys, what is the ideal timing for screening (prenatal, newborn, or later in infancy), and what factors influence this determination.

Given the advances in genetic testing technology, preimplantation genetic testing, direct-to-consumer genetic testing, and newborn screening, these topics should be included as part of the medical school curriculum with a more in-depth evaluation of discrepancies between physician and lay person attitudes and knowledge gaps, including physician understanding of lay person priorities. A recent study demonstrated a significant improvement in medical student knowledge, attitudes, intended behavior, and self-efficacy related to genetic testing after completing a curriculum on genetic testing (Metcalf et al. 2010).

**Quality of life and the lived experience**

Most neuromuscular disorders are life-long, life-limiting, disabling conditions. Quality of life for those with neuromuscular disorders and their parents is lower than normative controls, but not always as low as one might predict due to the influence of coping strategies (Bach et al. 1991; Bann et al. 2015). Internal coping strategies, such as adjusting life goals and self-confidence, are critical to positive adjustment. External coping mechanisms, such as respite care and accessible transportation, lead to better adjustment. Standardized scales have identified individual, family, and community domains that may be impacted in neuromuscular disorders (Bann et al. 2015; Abresch et al. 2002) (Table 1.2).

Disease severity does not necessarily have a negative impact on an affected person's perception of quality of life (Bach et al. 1991). This is termed the disability paradox. While

**TABLE 1.2**
**Factors affecting quality of life for those with neuromuscular disease**

| Individual level | Family level | Community level |
|---|---|---|
| Age | Socio-economic status | Accessibility |
| Sex | Caregiver respite | NMD-related resources |
| Education level | NMD-related beliefs | Inclusion precepts |
| Health knowledge | Values | Attitudes |
| Employment opportunities | Expectations | |
| Income | | |
| Confidence | | |
| Affordable health insurance | | |

NMD: neuromuscular disease.

functional impairment has an admittedly negative impact on muscle strength, independence level, and activity level, an affected person's satisfaction with the frequency and quality of care given, alternate values, adjusted expectations, and acceptance of one's current condition may explain the paradox (Graham et al. 2014; Kohler et al. 2005; Chen and Clark 2007). The most severe neuromuscular disorders are also the most apparent and, therefore, difficulties experienced may be better appreciated by observers who may be more sympathetic towards the affected child and parents. The severely affected child and the family may have less difficulty obtaining needed accommodations, health aids, healthcare services, and financial assistance. Conversely, those mild-to-moderately affected can experience a relatively negative perception of quality of life. (Houwen-van Opstal et al. 2014). The expectations placed upon those mild-to-moderately affected may be unreasonably high, they might not qualify for assistance or services, and they may not identify with the abled members of their community, nor the disabled members, leading to loneliness and isolation.

A lower quality of life correlates significantly with loss of function and the rate at which function is lost. Those with congenital-onset disorders along the spectrum from mild-to-severe often do not perceive a dramatic loss in function and independence, therefore, they may have higher quality of life perceptions (Narayanaswami et al. 2000). However, some of those with late-onset disorders may experience significant losses as their condition worsens. Interestingly, there may be a loss-of-function effect that can result in positive feelings in those children who have a devoted caregiver and healthy home environment. As the ability to stand or transfer positions decreases, or if arm function reduces, boys with Duchenne muscular dystrophy have been found to perceive more understanding and love from parents and "feel happier at home" (Houwen-van Opstal et al. 2014).

Children with chronic disorders have up to a three-fold increase in psychosocial complications when compared to their healthy peers (Thompson et al. 1992). Depression, anxiety, and psychological maladjustment are some of the most common issues identified in children and adolescents with chronic conditions (Perrin et al. 2012). One study found that 59% of those with slowly progressive neuromuscular disorders had high depression scores and 90%

6

had high anxiety scores (Ozer et al. 2010). The unpredictable nature of a neuromuscular disorder often leads to anxiety for many (Ozer et al. 2010; Rose et al. 2012).

There sometimes can be a mismatch between how parents rate their child's physical and mental health and how the child would rate it. In one study, 22% of parents rated their son's physical and mental health lower than their sons did (Lim et al. 2014). Social acceptance of the child with Duchenne muscular dystrophy was viewed as higher when rated by the affected boys, but lower when rated by the parent. The parents may have a broader perspective of what acceptance means, and may be more aware of the ways their children are not being accepted that go unnoticed by the boys themselves. The mood of the boys with Duchenne muscular dystrophy was more likely to be viewed as happy by the affected children, while reported as less happy by the parent (Houwen-van Opstal et al. 2014). These discrepancies may be related to parents using their own values to interpret limitations experienced by their children.

Transitions from childhood to teenage years may be accompanied by changes in quality of life perceptions (Perrin et al. 2012; Rose et al. 2012). The teenage years bring concerns with individuation, rebellion against status quo, and socialization which includes fitting-in and mating-up (Perrin et al. 2012). When teens were asked what it is like to live with their neuromuscular disorder, responses were that it takes a lot of extra effort every day, and that it is restraining, painful, and worrisome (Woodgate 1998). The themes adolescents bring up consistently when asked about living with a chronic condition include: developing/maintaining friendships, having a normal life, family importance, attitude about treatment, school experiences, encounters with clinicians, and the future (Perrin et al. 2012; Taylor et al. 2008).

With better technological advancements and medical care, young people with chronic, life-threatening conditions are more often living into adulthood. Most teens with neuromuscular disorders have grown-up with limited duties and responsibilities, but as legal adults, they may now be expected to take charge of their own care. This phase can be overwhelming for young adults, and adherence to healthy practices and/or treatment may waver at this time. The complexities of managing their level of care are best learned gradually over years of time, so it is recommended to start early and to be patient with the learning process. The adult medical care system may be different from the pediatric system in ways that do not support the best interests of someone with a neuromuscular disease. Medical supplies and equipment will be designed for large adult bodies, for example, which may be inappropriate for an adult with a neuromuscular disorder. Also, adult care practitioners are often not trained in pediatric-onset conditions like these and they may not know how to best treat the adult patient. Parents are usually accustomed to acting as advocates for their child, a role that may benefit the young adult patient throughout the transition to adult care, and whenever there is a change in the type or level of care required. Achieving a balance between the young adult's need for independence, and the parent's need to have adequate information to support their child's best interests during the transition, prepares all parties for success and a greater likelihood of satisfaction. (DH/Child Health and Maternity Services Branch et al. 2006).

For adults with neuromuscular disorders, the loss or lack of ever achieving independence, along with increasing dependence upon others and technical aids, can be discouraging

(Nätterlund et al. 2000). A scientist with muscular dystrophy recounts his personal loss of ability: "It is falling, broken bones, struggling to breathe, watching one ability after another vanish" (Munn 2010). He describes falling in a snow bank in the darkness with only the hope that a kind, able person would come along soon to help him up. He summarizes his appraisal of his diminishing quality of life by saying, "What they and I need is hope that this whole horrible thing can be reversed" (Munn 2010).

Coping skills are a stronger predictor of emotional health outcomes for affected persons when compared to the disease perceptions they have (Dempster et al. 2015). Effective coping skills (i.e. acceptance, venting, doing something about it) were found to be the most important factor in quality of life for participants across many studies. The level of self-confidence was also predictive of how well someone copes with a neuromuscular disorder (Rose et al. 2012; Dempster et al. 2015; Davis 1993; Thomas et al. 2014).

Personal values and expectations play a significant role in perceptions of quality of life. Individuals that perceive misalignment between their aspirations and their actual abilities, especially as the disease progresses, experience a greater negative impact on quality of life (Bann et al. 2015).

PARENTAL QUALITY OF LIFE AND LIVED EXPERIENCE

When a family receives a neuromuscular diagnosis, it can be overwhelming. There will be many unpredictable challenges along the way and unfortunate circumstances that the entire family must adapt to in order to thrive. It can be a devastating blow for parents to realize there is little they can do, which may leave them feeling inadequate and hopeless (Davis 1993).

Parents are profoundly affected by their child's condition. Isolation, loneliness, stress, anxiety, anger, exhaustion, and depression are reported to impact quality of life for parents of children with Duchenne muscular dystrophy or other chronic health conditions (Perrin et al. 2012; Barlow and Ellard 2006; de Moura et al. 2015; Yilmaz et al. 2010). The caregiving activities are often physically demanding and require load-lifting, bending, pushing, and pulling many times each day (de Moura et al. 2015; Yilmaz et al. 2010). Parents often have little to no personal time, neglect hobbies and interests, limit family and social outings, and their relationships may suffer (Magliano et al. 2014; Perrin et al. 2012; Davis 1993; Davey et al. 2015).

The home is oftentimes not a haven, but a busy medical center, with service providers intruding upon family life (Davey et al. 2015). The home may need renovations to meet present and future needs. Families may decide to move to a more accessible home. Some may move closer to their family of origin to have ready access to willing helpers. The financial burden on the family can be tremendous and often includes special transportation, mobility equipment, communication aids, home medical equipment, hospital bills, expensive medications, therapies, and lost wages (Perrin et al. 2012; Davis 1993; Wolff et al. 2010).

Parents worry about their child being in pain, disfigured, rejected by peers, isolated, and unhappy (Davis 1993). Each acute illness is cause for great concern, an expansion of the already numerous cares, and any possible hospitalization represents a disruption to the lives of the entire family. Each health crisis may resurrect a fear that parents have suppressed in order to carry on.

Fathers experience psychosocial, family, and economic difficulties. Psychosocial problems include depressive and post-traumatic stress disorder symptoms upon learning of their child's diagnosis, tremendous guilt for having passed the disorder to the child, and the need to be strong for the family (Wolff et al. 2010). Family problems include marital disagreement about how to parent the child, conflicts with extended family, siblings who feel fathers are harder on them, and struggles between feeling overprotective and giving the right amount of discipline and independence. Fathers found that just knowing someone else was in it with them, such as a spouse, made them feel better, as did having help from extended family. For some fathers, access to public assistance helped them to cope better. One father interviewed had developed fortitude from his child's determination (Wolff et al. 2010).

Mothers in particular tend to leave the workforce in order to care for their child with a neuromuscular disorder. While this is often necessary for the level of care required, giving up a rewarding job or career can have negative consequences for the mother who no longer has this outlet as a means for boosting self-esteem, feeling independent, having status, expressing creativity/interest, companionship, or being productive in her community. These losses are even more detrimental when considering that they are many of the very activities and feelings that could help a parent to cope with the daily stressors, thereby further decreasing their ability to cope with the difficulties of caring for a child with a chronic condition (Davis 1993).

Spousal relationships suffer when there is a child with a neuromuscular disorder. This is often related to fewer needs being met in the relationship, having little time for each other, and no ability to get away as a couple. Increased stress, disagreement about how to parent the child, different coping styles, lack of communication, no child care options or respite, and the brunt of the responsibilities falling onto one parent all impact the relationship. The one parent who is doing most of the caregiving work may feel resentment, while the partner doing little of the work may feel neglected. Spouses sometimes blame the other for the heritable neuromuscular disorder (Davis 1993).

Disease severity negatively impacts quality of life for parent caregivers. Families with children that have more severe conditions requiring home medical equipment may experience a greater level of stress. Quality of life for parents of children with Duchenne muscular dystrophy is lower than normative controls. However, lower burden scores were noted in parents of ambulatory children that had higher levels of social support, as would be expected. The size and developmental stage of the child also impacts the caregiver's quality of life perceptions. For example, bowel dysfunction may be very manageable in a two-year-old, but difficult when the child becomes a teenager and adult (Perrin et al. 2012).

There is upheaval for siblings that often results in behavioral and psychological problems and resentment. Siblings may experience depression, anxiety, lower activity levels, fewer social opportunities, and effects on their cognitive development. They may become irritable, jealous, anxious, and socially withdrawn. Their academic performance may decline and they may miss out on opportunities due to a shifting of most resources to the child with a neuromuscular disorder. These factors can lead to lower self-esteem in siblings and guilt for feeling the way they do (Perrin et al. 2012).

Friendships may be lost because the parent can no longer find the time to maintain them or the friend was uncomfortable maintaining the friendship. Oftentimes the friends no longer have enough in common to continue a relationship. However, those friends could be replaced in virtual relationships via social media with other parents facing similar life circumstances. Social support is crucial to parents. It can provide practical help, diversion, and it positively impacts parental self-esteem (Davis 1993).

Fatal neuromuscular disorders bring greater amounts of psychological distress to parents and siblings (Davis 1993). True effects of the disorder on all family members are often masked by denial-like coping strategies when surveys and interviews are done. Clinicians must use observations and gather input from those outside the situation in order to obtain a more accurate evaluation of the psychological impact (Barlow and Ellard 2006).

COPING

Even though the family experiences considerable stress, some members may adapt well, while other members collapse. Coping styles that avoid social support and involve catastrophizing are associated with worse outcomes (Davis 1993; Perrin et al. 2012). Coping ability affects disease course, willingness to explore treatment options, and how effective treatment can be (Davis 1993). When affected children and family members can reset their goals and expectations, they may experience a better perception of quality of life (Rose et al. 2012).

Parental perceptions are the foundation for how the family will function and cope. Accordingly, parents are the ones to focus attention on in treatment settings (Davis 1993; Thomas et al. 2014). Most people do not want to admit psychological difficulties because they assume it reflects badly upon them. Framing the need as that of the entire family who can benefit from counseling helps encourage parents and children to productively engage in counseling. Knowing this, practitioners are best advised to include all family members in counseling efforts (Davis 1993).

Parents can develop new values, goals, and attitudes in light of the diagnosis. A positive reinterpretation of the situation and subsequent growth can lead to better adjustment (Thomas et al. 2014). Those that have hope and a positive outlook tend to experience better outcomes (Barlow and Ellard 2006). How parents construe the child now that they know about the diagnosis is directly related to how well the family will adapt and thrive (Thomas et al. 2014). It is best to see them as a child first, and then see the muscle disorder with all its consequences. When those affected and the parents realize that they are all in it together, they can learn to appreciate each other's feelings and empathize with what each is going through.

Parents and family members sometimes develop unhealthy coping strategies as they care for a child with a neuromuscular disorder. Some of the most commonly used dysfunctional coping strategies are overprotection of the child, denial of reality, and magical thinking. Protecting the child is natural, and overprotection is a gray area for some parents. For example, parents may not share distressing news with the child to spare him or her anguish, nor involve the child in communications with clinicians who often present the prognosis as grim. They may not insist upon age-and-ability-appropriate responsibility or may avoid disciplining the child. While discipline may seem like it adds to the gross unfairness of having the neuromuscular disorder, without it, the child may end up uncooperative, self-absorbed, and unable to share or relate kindly to others. These personal qualities would make for a very unattractive friend or mate which may put such a child at an even greater disadvantage socially. Furthermore, this results in major problems within the family and can affect parental and sibling expressions of love for the affected child (Thomas et al. 2014; Buchanan et al. 1979).

Some family members may fail to differentiate the child from the disease. This is problematic because the child may end up identifying himself or herself as the disease. Such a self-conception is not compatible with therapy, treatment, or a cure and may result in the child's refusal to engage in therapies that could alleviate discomfort, mitigate limitations, and prolong a higher-quality life (Davis 1993).

Factors that mitigate the burden of neuromuscular disease include internal coping strategies as well as external resources. Because functional impairment is natural for affected individuals, some are bothered less by what they cannot do. For those individuals experiencing deterioration of their condition, a positive reappraisal of their situation can make a difference in how well they cope (Nätterlund et al. 2000). Families need access to external resources, such as respite or financial aid, and greater participation in social activities that are meaningful to them in order to experience an improved quality of life (Davey et al. 2015; Dowling and Dolan 2001; Yantzi et al. 2007).

Parents have a natural inclination to cure their child as part of their desire to protect, provide, and problem-solve. Parental confidence in the ability to provide excellent care must be supported by clinicians and can lead to better outcomes for the child (Davis 1993).

SOCIETAL CHALLENGES OF LIVING WITH A NEUROMUSCULAR DISORDER

Social integration and community participation are enriching aspects of life. When a family member has a neuromuscular disorder, the entire family often is restricted in the level of community participation they can obtain. Leaving the residence may require additional assistance and added expense (Davey et al. 2015; Yilmaz et al. 2010). Community access requires curb cut-outs, ramps, elevators, lift systems, and accessible transportation. Barriers to community access can include attitudinal, communication, physical, policy, programmatic, social, and transportation (Center for Disease Control and Prevention et al. 2016). The lack of accessibility may be unanticipated, such as an elevator malfunction at the child's school, friends or relatives that cannot be visited due to steps or narrow doorways, and no accessible parking. Many vacation destinations and activities to be enjoyed while on vacation are not completely accessible to these families.

The economic burden of neuromuscular disorders is another consideration. In the United States (US), the liability over the course of the disease has been estimated at an average yearly cost for each patient (medical, non-medical, and indirect) of "$63 693 for ALS [amyotrophic lateral sclerosis], $50 952 for DMD [Duchenne muscular dystrophy], and $32 236 for DM [myotonic dystrophy]. Population-wide national costs were $1 023 million (ALS), $787 million (DMD) and $448 million (DM)" (Larkindale et al. 2014). In another study, a total of 770 participants from Germany, Italy, the United Kingdom (UK), and the US completed questionnaires to gauge costs incurred due to the muscle disease in their respective families. The results showed that, "the total societal burden was estimated at between \$80 120 and \$120 910 per patient and annum, and increased markedly with disease progression. The corresponding household burden was estimated at between \$58 440 and \$71 900" (Landfeldt et al. 2014).

Even with the best coping skills, resources, and care, neuromuscular disorders are life-limiting conditions. End-of-life discussions with those living with neuromuscular disorders and their parents are challenging yet critical for planning and assessing the ongoing health and well-being of the family unit.

**Advance care planning and preparing for death**
The increasing numbers, complexities, and technology dependencies of children and young adults with neuromuscular disorders calls for advance care planning to increase quality of life and promote patient autonomy (Horridge 2015; Lotz et al. 2015). Advance care planning is an ongoing process that guides patients and their families to an understanding of the diagnosis, prognosis, decisions, and treatment options they may consider (Edwards et al. 2012). The benefits of advance care planning, as perceived by clinicians, include providing a sense of security and control, improving quality of care, and ensuring that patients' and parents' wishes are respected (Lotz et al. 2015).

Parents who are less prepared for the death of a child suffer more bereavement complications. Parental grief when a child dies is poorly understood by professionals despite universal acceptance of the overwhelming pain and distress grieving parents experience. Parents often say they want to be a part of the care team, and they want their expertise as parent caregivers to be recognized. Parents want their child and their family values to be respected and their traditions accommodated during the time of advance care planning.

The importance of making memories within this limited time, and having no regrets after the child is gone, cannot be overstated. While witnessing the death of an infant or child is naturally distressing for everyone, parents often report that no matter how harrowing the time, they treasure every moment as a memory.

**Importance of advance care planning**
In advance, clinician-initiated discussions about the possibility of death may help families communicate among themselves what might otherwise remain unspoken. If these discussions are avoided, patients and families may not have an opportunity to state their wishes, such as the preferred place of care and of death. Such discussions may help with the grieving process, establishment of realistic hope, and effective coping (Horridge 2015). Studies have demonstrated that parents of children with chronic conditions find that advance care planning is, or would be, beneficial to them, and they wish to know all the options, including the option to forgo interventions (Edwards et al. 2012).

Advance care planning provides a sense of security and control for both medical professionals and parents, while clarifying goals of care and providing a clear direction. Advance care planning can improve quality of care by avoiding treatments that are not in the family's best interests and reduce unnecessary suffering. Having a written advance care directive in place can lead to a decreased number of emergency and intensive care interventions for the child and ensure that the care provided is consistent with the parent's and child's treatment goals (Lotz et al. 2015).

Ideally, discussions regarding goals of care should be initiated upon diagnosis and revisited during a period when the patient is stable (Durall et al. 2012; Hauer and Wolfe 2014). Unfortunately, the majority of clinicians find that advance care planning happens too late in the patient's clinical course (Edwards et al. 2012; Durall et al. 2012). Many of these discussions typically take place during an acute illness or deterioration and during a hospitalization, or when death is imminent (Edwards et al. 2012; Durall et al. 2012; Hauer and Wolfe 2014).

Identifying the potential barriers to advance care planning will allow the clinician to better engage families and encourage advance care planning before critical illness. The late timing of advance care planning indicates that many families are not open to discuss end-of-life issues at a time when their child is relatively stable. Therefore, clinicians should offer anticipatory guidance and proactively gauge family readiness for advance care planning discussions. Advance care planning is not a single discussion intended to elicit a particular decision. Rather, advance care planning involves ongoing discussions with an emphasis on informing the family about events that could occur, guiding them as they consider treatment options, and reassuring them that caring for their child will be the primary goal under all circumstances (Edwards et al. 2012).

BARRIERS TO ADVANCE CARE PLANNING

Although there is an increasing recognition of the benefits to advance care planning, there continue to be barriers to utilization (Hauer and Wolfe 2014). The challenges stem from both clinicians and families (Edwards et al. 2012).

Barriers reported by clinicians highlight their fear and discomfort with the topic. Clinicians are reluctant to address end-of-life issues with patients and parents because they fear taking away hope, and risk losing the trusting relationship with the family (Lotz et al. 2015). However, studies do not support these concerns. Greater information disclosure may actually support hope, even when the child's prognosis is poor. Higher levels of parental optimism were associated with increased likelihood of parental enactment of an order for limited intervention. On the other hand, withholding information may promote false hope, leading to feelings of betrayal, anger, and mistrust (Durall et al. 2012).

Clinician uncertainty about the patient's prognosis and not knowing how, or the right time, to address the issue of advance care planning creates barriers to advance care discussions (Horridge 2015; Lotz et al. 2015; Edwards et al. 2012; Durall et al. 2012; Hauer and Wolfe 2014). Clinicians' avoidance of raising sensitive, difficult issues with families and projecting their own lack of readiness to discuss these issues onto families also inhibit advance care planning. Clinicians may also be unable or unwilling to accept their patient's fate, and may make conscious and unconscious attempts to impose their own values on the family (Edwards et al. 2012).

The majority of clinicians view advance care planning as a multi-professional process that should include all relevant healthcare providers in the community. However, insufficient information sharing between clinicians and the lack of a continuous contact person are reported as barriers to the cooperation deemed indispensable for advance care planning (Lotz et al. 2015). Other reported factors limiting the implementation of advance care planning include shortage of time and lack of funds.

Clinicians perceive parental prognostic understanding and attitudes as the most common barriers to advance care planning (Durall et al. 2012). The top three parental barriers were reported to be unrealistic expectations, differences between clinician and patient/parent understanding of prognosis, and lack of parent readiness to have the discussion (Horridge 2015; Durall et al. 2012; Hauer and Wolfe 2014).

A study involving children on long-term assisted ventilation with life-limiting conditions recognized that a family may have an idealistic outlook on the child's prognosis because the child has survived a previous critical illness. In addition, the development of a mutually dependent relationship between the child and family members who have devoted so much energy to the child's care gives rise to parental resistance to end-of-life discussions (Edwards et al. 2012).

The burden of responsibility felt by parents when signing an advance care directive for their child is a factor of their resistance (Lotz et al. 2015). This can be especially difficult when the child suffers from a communication impairment and is unable to express his or her wishes.

Inadequate communication is often the source of barriers to advance care discussions. Patients and family members may be waiting for the clinical team to initiate the discussion, or may not be aware of the need for such discussions. The clinical team may assume the family is not ready for the discussion because they have not yet introduced the subject.

To better prepare clinicians for advance care discussions, physician trainee and continuing education programs should include topics on communication skills, managing prognostic uncertainty, and how to make decisions to forgo life-sustaining therapy (Durall et al. 2012).

DEATH OF A CHILD

For those parents whose infant is never well enough to leave the hospital, the hospital environment is the sole place they will parent their child. Medical professionals involved in the infant's care need to acknowledge that the family will experience their entire relationship with their child in a hospital environment which is a public place and a working environment. In this public environment, parents sometimes need help to feel comfortable with providing a natural, loving relationship (Meyer et al. 2006; McGraw et al. 2012).

Parents need to be parents even in the hospital. They should be respected as competent to carry out as much of their child's care as they wish. Parents want meaningful roles in providing love, comfort, and care for their child (McGraw et al. 2012).

> We ... didn't know how to comfort him. He was sedated. You know, the thing I remember the most was the one nurse who said that, "He likes to have his head rubbed". That was really important to us (McGraw et al. 2012).

Parents report a deep need for privacy and security for the whole family with more control over their child's environment. This includes limiting interruptions, the timing of routine observations, and having more quiet time (McGraw et al. 2012). Time spent as a family is very important (Tan et al. 2012). Every moment with their child is precious; therefore, asking parents to leave their child for lower priority reasons, such as meetings with clinicians, should be carefully considered (McGraw et al. 2012).

> And when the intensivist wanted to talk to us about what we were going to do next, we were always asked to go into this consult room. And so the whole time I was afraid we weren't going to be in the room with her. … If I had known then I would have said, "No. Can't we just talk about this right here? I want to talk about this right here," if I'd been a little more forceful. But I didn't know I was going to feel like this (McGraw 2012).

Parents want to be physically close to their dying child and will express regret about times they were not able to do this. Parents appreciate guidance to find ways they can be close to their child in a medical environment (McGraw et al. 2012).

> And I think she knew she was going to die because she said, "Will you get in the bed with me?" I couldn't do that with [pause] [crying] all the nurses …. Everybody in and out, you can't have those private moments. And I just wished I had got in bed with her one time and gave her that last hug before she became incoherent. I never got that chance because it's so damn busy in there (McGraw 2012).

Parents want to know that they pursued all reasonable treatment options and did everything possible for their child in the time they had (Caeymaex et al. 2011). They want to evaluate treatment options, not just the availability of those options, but in terms of their individual goals for their child. Clinicians should note that parents are generally able to distinguish between hope and wishful thinking (Xafis et al. 2015). Kindness, respect, and sympathy increase parental trust in clinicians' positive intentions (Caeymaex et al. 2011). After the death of a child, parents benefit from a continuation of kindness and respect, such as the gentle, unrushed handling of their child's body (Higgs et al. 2016).

LATER-LIFE LOSS

Advances in medical care, especially respiratory care, allow many children with neuromuscular disorders to live longer into their late teens and young adulthood. Death is a risk associated with any form of neuromuscular disorder, a fact that is sometimes lost to those that experience longer periods of relative stability. An acute episode, such as sudden illness or infection, can result in what parents perceive as an unexpected death of the child and not a foreseen outcome of the progression of their child's disorder (Edwards et al. 2012).

A parent whose child has a progressive neuromuscular disorder is often experienced with a hospital environment and particularly knowledgeable about the child's disorder. Many parents, however, report finding it difficult to advocate for their child, as their experience and knowledge is underestimated (McGraw et al. 2012). Clinicians should bear in mind that these parents may have had to prepare for their child's death on several occasions already.

A majority of parents spend a considerable amount of time trying to keep their children with a neuromuscular disorder stable at home to avoid hospital admissions. Keeping their child at home to die, and after death for a period of time, is a natural extension of this desire.

15

Eighty-nine percent of families who had time to make an advance plan about where their child would die chose home (Heath et al. 2010). Evidence that children and young people with a neuromuscular disorder would rather die at home than at a hospital setting has been extrapolated from work with adults and cancer patients (Bluebond-Langner et al. 2013). After a preferred location for the child's death is chosen, there should be continued flexibility as circumstances may change (Hauer and Wolfe 2014; Vickers et al. 2007). Some parents are very passionate about their child being cared for at home while also wanting the place of death to be elsewhere, such as a hospice (Vickers et al. 2007). It may be that the opportunity to plan where their child might die is more important to parents than the actual location it happens in the end.

Particularly in a short life, every single moment and interaction may take on special meaning:

> It sounds so strange but it was one of the most peaceful, beautiful things I've ever seen and ever been a part of. That sounds weird because it's your child. But that's how it started out. It was daddy and I and [my child]. That's how it started. And that's how it ended, with the three of us in a room together. There was something beautiful about that … I was able to get right in that bed with her (McGraw 2012).

A lack of privacy and autonomy in deciding how to be with their dying child is often reported as a source of deep and lasting regret for bereaved parents. Providing love and comfort, even in the most distressing of circumstances, becomes a memory that parents can draw on for peace during bereavement (Tan et al. 2012).

Studies show that parents who are less prepared for the death of their loved one are more prone to depression, anxiety, and complicated grief (Tan et al. 2012). Therefore, anything that can be done to support parents' plans for preparation of their child's death has a positive impact.

Hospice movement in the United Kingdom

A children's hospice is a publicly or charitably funded care home specifically designed to help children who are not expected to reach adulthood with the emotional and physical challenges they face, and also to provide respite care for their families. Until the 1980s, there was no provision anywhere in the world for respite and end-of-life care specifically for children with life-shortening conditions. The first hospice for children from birth to age 16, called Helen House, was founded in et al. 1982. There are now about 49 children's hospices around the world. Douglas House was opened in et al. 2004, the world's first specialist hospice for young adults aged 16 to 35 years (Helen & Douglas House et al. 2018). There are over 200 hospices in the UK supported by the national charity for hospice care, Hospice UK (Hospice UK, 2018).

Hospices should be respectful of individual family needs and customs, religious or secular. They can provide specialist doctors, nurses, and services such as family support and bereavement services for the entire family. Hospices generally offer short medically-supported breaks, as well as pain and symptom management, and end-of-life care. The family can stay on-site to enjoy being a parent and not a full-time carer; or they can leave their child in the experienced hands of medical care teams while they spend time as a couple or with their other children. Hospice care can be provided in the hospice, or sometimes services can be offered in the home (Together for short lives 2018).

**Role of the clinician**

Advances in genetic testing technology have improved the yield of a genetic diagnosis in presumed neuromuscular patients. Delays in obtaining a genetic diagnosis have been shown to impede medical management and lower survival. As the gatekeepers, it is imperative that clinicians endorse early and universal genetic testing for neuromuscular disorders. Genetic testing should be mandatory for all pediatric and adult neuromuscular disorders; and universal access to genetic testing, even for rare neuromuscular disorders, a priority. Genetic counselors are integral to implementation of universal genetic testing and should be part of every neuromuscular clinic. While families and affected individuals may have a limited grasp of genetic testing technology, disease knowledge, and interpretation of their own genetic testing results, this should not preclude offering genetic testing and counseling.

Living with a neuromuscular disorder impacts the quality of life of both the affected individual and their family. Parental quality of life perception forms the foundation of how the family will cope. Therefore, the clinician needs to give attention to parents in the treatment setting. Encouraging internal coping strategies and supporting access to external resources can mitigate the burden on affected individuals and their families, leading to better adjustment and an improved perception of quality of life.

The increased number of children living longer with neuromuscular disorders and technology dependency requires early, ongoing advance care planning discussions between the clinician, parents and, if appropriate, the affected child. The clinician should initiate discussions regarding the goals of care upon diagnosis or during a period when the child is stable, offering anticipatory guidance while gauging the family's readiness for advance care planning. Advance care planning discussions should involve a multidisciplinary team, which may include the primary care physician, palliative care, nursing, social work, and chaplaincy.

When a child nears death, it is important that the parent's role as caregiver and advocate be respected. Supporting the family's need for privacy, time and physical closeness with their dying child, and making memories is invaluable. Hospice care, if available, can provide the family with respite. In a hospital environment, interruptions to family time should be limited and asking parents to leave their child's side for lower priority reasons ought to be avoided. A parent's trust in a clinician's intentions is increased when kindness, respect, and sympathy are shown. Extending kindness and respect after the death of a child can have a positive and lasting impact on the family.

**Conclusion and key points**

Parenting a child with a neuromuscular disorder involves a multitude of emotions, responsibilities, and decisions from diagnosis to end of life. Obtaining a genetic diagnosis, living with a chronic neuromuscular disease, advance care planning, and preparing for death are significant milestones that parents may experience during their child's lifetime.

DIAGNOSIS: KEY POINTS

- There is a high acceptance of genetic testing by families and affected individuals regardless of the results.
- Universal access to genetic testing should be a priority regardless of whether there is a lack of treatment options.
- Genetic counselors are integral to the implementation of universal genetic testing and should be a part of every neuromuscular clinic.
- Developing either separate reports for the families or revising current language to make reports understandable to a lay person may facilitate understanding and ownership of results.
- Clinicians need to have knowledge of the diagnostic tools available and an understanding of the discrepancies between physician and lay person attitudes, including an understanding of the lay person's priorities.

QUALITY OF LIFE AND LIVED EXPERIENCE: KEY POINTS

- Quality of life for those with neuromuscular disorders and their parents is lower than normative controls, but not always as low as one may predict due to the influence of coping strategies.
- Internal coping strategies, like adjusting life goals and self-confidence, are critical to positive adjustment.
- External coping mechanisms, like respite care and accessible transportation, lead to better adjustment.
- Families need access to external resources, such as respite or financial aid, and greater participation in social activities that are meaningful to them in order to experience an improved quality of life.

ADVANCE CARE PLANNING AND PREPARING FOR DEATH: KEY POINTS

- Advance care planning is ideally initiated upon diagnosis and revisited during periods of stability.
- Advance care planning is not a single discussion, but rather ongoing discussions that inform families about events that could occur, guide them as they consider treatment options, and reassure them that caring for their child is the primary goal under all circumstances.
- Parents who are less prepared for the death of their child suffer more bereavement complications.
- Parents who live with a child's life-threatening condition are used to the duality of living with hope at the same time as preparing for the possibility of their child's death.
- Parents report feeling regret for what they were not able to do for their infant or child, but no regret for the things they were able to do, however small those actions seemed at the time.
- Parents want the loss of their child as an individual to be recognized as important and devastating, not simply "expected".

ROLE OF THE CLINICIAN: KEY POINTS

- Clinicians must endorse early and universal genetic testing for all pediatric and adult neuromuscular disorders, even for rare neuromuscular disorders.

- Clinicians can help mitigate the burden on affected individuals and their families by encouraging positive coping strategies and by supporting access to external resources in the form of referrals, letters of support, orders for supplies and equipment, and so forth.
- Clinicians should initiate advance care planning discussions early, have ongoing discussions during periods when the child is stable, and involve a multidisciplinary team in the advance care planning process.
- Respect for the parent's role as caregiver and advocate, as well as kindness and sympathy on the part of the clinician, before and after a child's death increases a parent's trust in the clinician, and can have a lasting and positive impact on the family.

## REFERENCES

Abresch RT, Carter GT, Jensen MP, Kilmer DD (2002) Assessment of pain and health-related quality of life in slowly progressive neuromuscular disease. *Am J Hosp Palliat Care* 19: 39–48.

Bach JR, Campagnolo DI, Hoeman S (1991) Life satisfaction of individuals with Duchenne muscular dystrophy using long-term mechanical ventilatory support. *Am J Phys Med Rehabil* 70: 129–135.

Bann CM, Abresch RT, Biesecker B, Conway KC, Heatwole C, Peay H et al. (2015) Measuring quality of life in muscular dystrophy. *Neurology* 84: 1034–1042.

Barlow JH, Ellard DR (2006) The psychosocial well-being of children with chronic disease, their parents and siblings: an overview of the research evidence base. *Child Care Health Dev* 32: 19–31.

Bluebond-Langner M, Beecham E, Candy B, Langner R, Jones L (2013) Preferred place of death for children and young people with life-limiting and life-threatening conditions: a systematic review of the literature and recommendations for future inquiry and policy. *Palliat Med* 27: 705–713.

Buchanan DC, LaBarbera CJ, Roelofs R, Olson W (1979) Reactions of families to children with Duchenne muscular dystrophy. *Gen Hosp Psychiatry* 1: 262–269.

Caeymaex L, Speranza M, Vasilescu C, Danan C, Bourrat MM, Garel M et al. (2011) Living with a crucial decision: a qualitative study of parental narratives three years after the loss of their newborn in the NICU. *PLoS One* 6:e28633.

Center for Disease Control and Prevention.(2016) *Common barriers to participation experienced by people with disabilities* [online]. http://www.cdc.gov/ncbddd/disabilityandhealth/disability-barriers.html#ref (accessed on 1 May 2016).

Chen JY, Clark MJ (2007) Family function in families of children with Duchenne muscular dystrophy. *Fam Community Health* 30: 296–304.

Chung J, Smith AL, Hughes SC, Niizawa G, Abdel-Hamid HZ, Naylor EW et al. (2016) Twenty-year follow-up of newborn screening for patients with muscular dystrophy. *Muscle Nerve* 53: 570–578.

Davey H, Imms C, Fossey E (2015) "Our child's significant disability shapes our lives": experiences of family social participation. *Disabil Rehabil* 37: 2264–2271.

Davis H (1993) *Counseling Parents of Children with Chronic Illness or Disability*. Oxford: Wiley-Blackwell.

de Moura MC, Wutzki HC, Voos MC, Resende MB, Reed UC, Hasue RH (2015) Is functional dependence of Duchenne muscular dystrophy patients determinant of the quality of life and burden of their caregivers? *Arq Neuropsiquiatr* 73: 52–57.

Dempster M, Howell D, McCorry NK (2015) Illness perceptions and coping in physical health conditions: A meta-analysis. *J Psychosom Res* 79: 506–513.

DH/Child Health and Maternity Services Branch (2006) *Transition: Getting it Right for Young People. Improving the Transition of Young People with Long Term Conditions from Children's to Adult Health Services*. Waterloo Road, London: Alcuin Edwards, Child Health and Maternity Services Branch. https://webarchive.nationalarchives.gov.uk (accessed on 1 May 2016).

Dowling M, Dolan L (2001) Families with children with disabilities – inequalities and the social model. *Disabil Soc* 16: 21–35.

Durall A, Zurakowski D, Wolfe J (2012) Barriers to conducting advance care discussions for children with life-threatening conditions. *Pediatrics* 129(4): e975–982. doi.10.1542/peds.2011–2695.

Edwards JD, Kun SS, Graham RJ, Keens TG (2012) End-of-life discussions and advance care planning for children on long-term assisted ventilation with life-limiting conditions. *J Palliat Care* 28: 21–27.

Ghaoui R, Cooper ST, Lek M, Jones K, Corbett A, Reddel SW et al. (2015) Use of whole-exome sequencing for diagnosis of limb-girdle muscular dystrophy: outcomes and lessons learned. *JAMA Neurol* 72: 1424–1432.

Graham CD, Weinman J, Sadjadi R, Chalder T, Petty R, Hanna MG et al. (2014) A multicentre postal survey investigating the contribution of illness perceptions, coping and optimism to quality of life and mood in adults with muscle disease. *Clin Rehabil* 28: 508–519.

Hall MJ, Forman AD, Montgomery SV, Rainey KL, Daly MB (2015) Understanding patient and provider perceptions and expectations of genomic medicine. *J Surg Oncol* 111: 9–17.

Hauer JM, Wolfe J (2014) Supportive and palliative care of children with metabolic and neurological diseases. *Curr Opin Support Palliat Care* 8: 296–302.

Heath JA, Clarke NE, Donath SM, McCarthy M, Anderson VA, Wolfe J (2010) Symptoms and suffering at the end of life in children with cancer: an Australian perspective. *Med J Aust* 192: 71–75.

Helen & Douglas House.(2018) Helen & Douglas House: Hospice care for children. https://www.helenand-douglas.org.uk (accessed on 2 April 2018).

Higgs EJ, McClaren BJ, Sahhar MA, Ryan MM, Forbes R (2016) "A short time but a lovely little short time": bereaved parents' experiences of having a child with spinal muscular atrophy type 1. *J Paediatr Child Health* 52: 40–46.

Hill DL, Miller VA, Hexem KR, Carroll KW, Faerber JA, Kang T et al. (2015) Problems and hopes perceived by mothers, fathers and physicians of children receiving palliative care. *Health Expect* 18: 1052–1065.

Horridge KA (2015) Advance Care Planning: practicalities, legalities, complexities and controversies. *Arch Dis Child* 100: 380–385.

Hospice UK (2018) Hospice UK. https://www.hospiceuk.org (accessed on 2 April 2018).

Houwen-van Opstal SLS, Jansen M, van Alfen N, de Groot IJM (2014) Health-related quality of life and its relation to disease severity in boys with Duchenne muscular dystrophy: satisfied boys, worrying parents – a case-control study. *J Child Neurol* 29: 1486–1495.

Howard HC, Borry P (2013) Survey of European clinical geneticists on awareness, experiences and attitudes towards direct-to-consumer genetic testing. *Genome Med* 5: 45.

Hunter AG, Sharpe N, Mullen M, Meschino WS (2001) Ethical, legal, and practical concerns about recontacting patients to inform them of new information: the case in medical genetics. *Am J Med Genet* 103: 265–276.

Kang PB (2011) Presymptomatic and early symptomatic genetic testing. *Continuum (Minneap Minn)* 17(2 Neurogenetics): 343–346.

Klitzman R, Abbate KJ, Chung WK, Ottman R, Leu CS, Appelbaum PS (2014) Views of preimplantation genetic diagnosis among psychiatrists and neurologists. *J Reprod Med* 59: 385–392.

Kohler M, Clarenbach CF, Böni L, Brack T, Russi EW, Bloch KE (2005) Quality of life, physical disability, and respiratory impairment in Duchenne muscular dystrophy. *Am J Respir Crit Care Med* 172: 1032–1036.

Landfeldt E, Lindgren P, Bell CF, Schmitt C, Guglieri M, Straub V et al. (2014) The burden of Duchenne muscular dystrophy: an international, cross-sectional study. *Neurology* 83: 529–536.

Larkindale J et al. (2014) *Cost of Illness for Neuromuscular Diseases in the U.S.* Tucson, AZ: Muscular Dystrophy Association. www.mda.org/sites/default/files/Report_Summary-Cost_of_Illness_0.pdf (accessed on 1 May 2016)

Lim Y, Velozo C, Bendixen RM (2014) The level of agreement between child self-reports and parent proxy-reports of health-related quality of life in boys with Duchenne muscular dystrophy. *Qual Life Res* 23: 1945–1952.

Lindor NM, Goldgar DE, Tavtigian SV, Plon SE, Couch FJ (2013) BRCA1/2 sequence variants of uncertain significance: a primer for providers to assist in discussions and in medical management. *Oncologist* 18: 518–524.

López-Hernández LB, Gómez-Díaz B, Escobar-Cedillo RE et al. (2014) Duchenne muscular dystrophy in a developing country: challenges in management and genetic counseling. *Genet Couns* 25(2): 129–41.

Lotz JD, Jox RJ, Borasio GD, Führer M (2015) Pediatric advance care planning from the perspective of health care professionals: a qualitative interview study. *Palliat Med* 29: 212–222.

Magliano L, D'Angelo MG, Vita G, Pane M, D'Amico A, Balottin U et al. (2014) Psychological and practical difficulties among parents and healthy siblings of children with Duchenne vs. Becker muscular dystrophy: an Italian comparative study. *Acta Myol* 33: 136–143.

McGraw SA, Truog RD, Solomon MZ, Cohen-Bearak A, Sellers DE, Meyer EC (2012) "I was able to still be her mom" parenting at end of life in the pediatric intensive care unit. *Pediatr Crit Care Med* 13:e350–e356.

McGuire AL, Diaz CM, Wang T, Hilsenbeck SG (2009) Social networkers' attitudes toward direct-to-consumer personal genome testing. *Am J Bioeth* 9: 3–10.

Metcalf MP, Tanner TB, Buchanan A (2010) Effectiveness of an online curriculum for medical students on genetics, genetic testing and counseling. *Med Educ Online* 15: 4856.

Meyer EC, Ritholz MD, Burns JP, Truog RD (2006) Improving the quality of end-of-life care in the pediatric intensive care unit: parents' priorities and recommendations. *Pediatrics* 117: 649–657.

Munn MW (2010) Living with muscular dystrophy: personal reflections. *Neuromuscul Disord* 20: 152–153.

Narayanaswami P, Bertorini TE, Pourmand R, Horner LH (2000) Long-term tracheostomy ventilation in neuromuscular diseases: patient acceptance and quality of life. *Neurorehabil Neural Repair* 14: 135–139.

Nätterlund B, Gunnarsson LG, Ahlström G (2000) Disability, coping and quality of life in individuals with muscular dystrophy: a prospective study over five years. *Disabil Rehabil* 22: 776–785.

Ozer S, Yildirim SA, Yilmaz O, Düger T, Yilmaz SA (2010) Assessment of health-related quality of life, depression, and anxiety in slowly and rapidly progressive neuromuscular disorders. *Neurosciences (Riyadh)* 15: 177–183.

Perrin JM, Gnanasekaran S, Delahaye J (2012) Psychological aspects of chronic health conditions. *Pediatr Rev* 33: 99–109.

Pyeritz RE (2011) The coming explosion in genetic testing – is there a duty to recontact? *N Engl J Med* 365: 1367–1369.

Rose MR, Sadjadi R, Weinman J, Akhtar T, Pandya S, Kissel JT et al. (2012) Role of disease severity, illness perceptions, and mood on quality of life in muscle disease. *Muscle Nerve* 46: 351–359.

Salm M, Abbate K, Appelbaum P, Ottman R, Chung W, Marder K et al. (2014) Use of genetic tests among neurologists and psychiatrists: knowledge, attitudes, behaviors, and needs for training. *J Genet Couns* 23: 156–163.

Savarese M et al. (2016) The genetic basis of undiagnosed muscular dystrophies and myopathies: results from 504 patients. *Neurology* 87: 71–76.

Smith CO, Lipe HP, Bird TD (2004) Impact of presymptomatic genetic testing for hereditary ataxia and neuromuscular disorders. Arch Neurol 61: 875–880.

Tan JS, Docherty SL, Barfield R, Brandon DH (2012) Addressing parental bereavement support needs at the end of life for infants with complex chronic conditions. *J Palliat Med* 15: 579–584.

Taylor RM, Gibson F, Franck LS (2008) The experience of living with a chronic illness during adolescence: a critical review of the literature. *J Clin Nurs* 17: 3083–3091.

Thomas PT, Rajaram P, Nalini A (2014) Psychosocial challenges in family caregiving with children suffering from Duchenne muscular dystrophy. *Health Soc Work* 39: 144–152.

Thompson RJJ Jr, Zeman JL, Fanurik D, Sirotkin-Roses M (1992) The role of parent stress and coping and family functioning in parent and child adjustment to Duchenne muscular dystrophy. *J Clin Psychol* 48: 11–19.

Together for short lives (2018) Together for short lives. http://www.togetherforshortlives.org.uk (accessed on 2 April 2018).

Toiviainen H, Jallinoja P, Aro AR, Hemminki E (2003) Medical and lay attitudes towards genetic screening and testing in Finland. *Eur J Hum Genet* 11: 565–572.

Vansenne F, Bossuyt PM, de Borgie CA (2009) Evaluating the psychological effects of genetic testing in symptomatic patients: a systematic review. *Genet Test Mol Biomarkers* 13: 555–563.

Vickers J, Thompson A, Collins GS, Childs M, Hain R, Paediatric Oncology Nurses' Forum/United Kingdom Children's Cancer Study Group Palliative Care Working Group (2007) Place and provision of palliative care for children with progressive cancer: a study by the Paediatric Oncology Nurses' Forum/United Kingdom Children's Cancer Study Group Palliative Care Working Group. *J Clin Oncol* 25: 4472–4476.

Wolff J, Pak J, Meeske K, Worden JW, Katz E (2010) Challenges and coping styles of fathers as primary medical caretakers: a multicultural qualitative study. *J Psychosoc Oncol* 28: 202–217.

Wood MF, Hughes SC, Hache LP, Naylor EW, Abdel-Hamid HZ, Barmada MM et al. (2014) Parental attitudes toward newborn screening for Duchenne/Becker muscular dystrophy and spinal muscular atrophy. *Muscle Nerve* 49: 822–828.

Woodgate RL (1998) Adolescents' perspectives of chronic illness: "it's hard". *J Pediatr Nurs* 13: 210–223.

Xafis V, Wilkinson D, Sullivan J (2015) What information do parents need when facing end-of-life decisions for their child? A meta-synthesis of parental feedback. *BMC Palliat Care* 14: 19.

Yantzi NM, Rosenberg MW, McKeever P (2007) Getting out of the house: the challenges mothers face when their children have long-term care needs. *Health Soc Care Community* 15: 45–55.

Yilmaz O, Yildirim SA, Oksüz C, Atay S, Turan E (2010) Mothers' depression and health-related quality of life in neuromuscular diseases: role of functional independence level of the children. *Pediatr Int* 52: 648–652.

# 2

# THE IMPORTANCE OF
# SETTING UP GUIDELINES FOR
# NEUROMUSCULAR DISORDERS

*Thomas Sejersen*

## Introduction

The intent of this chapter is to discuss the need for high-quality care guidelines for neuro-muscular disorders, the methods for producing such guidelines, the present status and future perspectives on the use of them.

## Historical perspectives

Increasingly, in several disease areas best practice guidelines for diagnosis and care have become useful tools for both patients and healthcare professionals (Burgers et al. 2013). The main reasons for developing best practice guidelines are that they allow (1) physicians and other healthcare professionals to make recommendations based on the best available evidence, (2) patients to ensure that their management follows recommendations based on the best available evidence, and (3) a common basis of diagnosis and clinical management in clinical multicentre trials. These advantages of best practice guidelines are essential for neuromuscular disorders. The scarcity of expertise in rare diseases, such as neuromuscular disorders, is a well-known and a far too common cause of late or wrong diagnosis and care (Eurordis 2009). Furthermore, clinical trials involving patients with rare diseases often rely on the recruitment of patients from multiple centres, so it is crucial that patients in the study are diagnosed in the same way, and have similar backgrounds of care to optimise the chance of elucidating the true effect of a certain therapy. However, in order for clinical guidelines to be useful and trustworthy, they must be carefully developed and updated, and based on best available evidence (Shaneyfelt and Centor 2009; Alonso-Coello et al. 2010; Graham et al. 2011; Sniderman and Furberg 2009). It should be emphasised that best available evidence for neuromuscular disorders is not often available from big randomised trials, but more frequently comes from smaller trials of varying quality, and on expert opinion when other evidence is lacking (Alonso-Coello et al. 2010). At present there is a lack of agreement on which principles should be employed in the development of care guidelines for neuromuscular disorders, and we lack an overview of which care guidelines for neuromuscular disorders exist and a common platform to locate and disseminate the guidelines that do exist.

We lack consensus on what methodological principles, common to all neuromuscular disorders, should be adhered to when developing new guidelines (Alonso-Coello et al. 2010; Graham et al. 2011; Burgers et al. 2003; Schünemann et al. 2014). However, in recent years several best care guidelines have been produced for neuromuscular disorders, adapting various acknowledged methodologies. The current chapter reviews the methodologies used for these, gives an overview of the existing best care guidelines for neuromuscular disorders, and perspectives on future development of care guidelines.

## Current situation

OVERVIEW OF METHODS USED FOR BEST PRACTICE GUIDELINE DEVELOPMENT

A general goal when establishing best care guidelines is that recommendations should be based on the best available evidence. The criterion standard for evidence-based medicine, i.e. randomised clinical trials, are often not available for neuromuscluar disorders or do not provide evidence at a sufficient level of detail to be useful as a basis for guideline recommendations. Even when robust scientific evidence about the benefits of assessments and interventions is lacking, physicians must nonetheless make decisions every day about whether or not to apply assessments and interventions. Consequently, in guideline development there is a need to combine the best available scientific evidence with the collective judgment of experts. This may be accomplished using different methods. For neuromuscular disorders the more commonly used methods include variations of the Delphi method, the RAND/UCLA Appropriateness Method (RAM), and the American Academy of Neurology (AAN) guideline methodology. In some instances the Appraisal of Guidelines for Research and Evaluation (AGREE) and the Grading of Recommendations Assessment, Development and Evaluation (GRADE) methods have also been employed. Below is a brief characterisation of each of these methods.

DELPHI TECHNIQUE

The Delphi technique is a method to solicit the opinions of experts through a series of appropriate questionnaires interspersed with additional information and opinion feedback in order to establish consensus. It was originally developed in 1953 to address military forecasting. Since then it has been used extensively as a forecasting instrument in industry and human services (Linstone et al. 1975). The Delphi technique has eventually also been frequently used in the medical field as means to establish consensus (Jones and Hunter 1995).

The basic idea behind the Delphi technique is to gather a group of experts, who may be geographically separated, to assess complex issues and reach consensus conclusions on these. Following the identification of participants, the process is typically composed of three or more rounds in which participants successively extract and reach consensus on (1) the most relevant problems, (2) how best to assess these problems, and (3) how best to manage these problems. In the original Delphi method the voting rounds are all anonymous, but in modifications of the Delphi technique, e.g. the RAM method (see the RAND/UCLA appropriateness methodology (RAM) section), one general open discussion may take place before the final voting round(s). The idea behind this approach is to combine the anonymity of participants with making contributions of ideas and voting "safe activities", while also giving participants the opportunity to reconsider their options in an open discussion.

RAND/UCLA APPROPRIATENESS METHODOLOGY

The RAND/UCLA appropriateness method (RAM) was originally developed in the mid-1980s with a primary aim of measuring overuse and underuse of medical and surgical procedures (Brook et al. 1986). It is based on the Delphi method, but importantly allows for an intervening open, non-anonymous discussion between voting rounds. The term "appropriateness" refers to the relative weight of the benefits and harms of a medical or surgical intervention. An appropriate procedure is one where "the expected health benefit (e.g., increased life expectancy, relief of pain, reduction in anxiety, improved functional capacity) exceeds the expected negative consequences (e.g., mortality, morbidity, anxiety, pain, time lost from work) by a sufficiently wide margin that the procedure is worth doing, exclusive of cost" (Brook et al. 1986; Kahan et al. 1994). The first step in developing recommendations based on the RAM method is to perform a detailed literature review to synthesise the best available scientific evidence on a procedure to be rated. At the same time, a list of specific clinical scenarios is produced in the form of a matrix, categorising patients who might present for the procedure in question in terms of their symptoms, medical history and/or results of diagnostic tests. These indications are grouped based on the primary presenting symptom leading to a patient being considered for further assessments or a particular intervention. A panel of experts is established, often based on recommendations from relevant medical societies. In the second step of the RAM method, the literature review and the list of indications, together with a list of definitions for all terms used in the indications list, are sent to the members of this expert panel. For each indication, panel members rate the benefit-to-harm ratio of the procedure on a scale of 1 to 9, where "1 means that the expected harms greatly outweigh the expected benefits, and 9 means that the expected benefits greatly outweigh the expected harms" (Brook et al. 1986; Kahan et al. 1994). Each panellist receives an individualised document showing the distribution of all the experts' first round ratings, together with his/her own specific ratings. During the meeting, panellists discuss the ratings, focusing on areas of disagreement, and are given the opportunity to modify the original list of indications and/or definitions, if desired. After discussing each chapter of the list of indications, they re-rate each indication individually. No attempt is made to force the panel to consensus. Instead, the two-round process is designed to sort out whether discrepant ratings are due to real clinical disagreement over the use of the procedure ("real" disagreement) or to fatigue or misunderstanding ("artefactual" disagreement). The panel members rate each of the indications twice, in a two-round "modified Delphi" process. In the first round, the ratings are made individually and anonymously, with no interaction among panellists. In the second round of the original RAM method, the panel members meet for 1–2 days under the leadership of a moderator experienced in using the method (Brook et al. 1986; Kahan et al. 1994). Each panel member receives a summary document showing the distribution of the first round ratings. During the meeting, panel members discuss the ratings, focusing on areas of disagreement. After discussions, they re-rate each indication, again anonymously and individually. Indications with median scores in the range 1–3 are classified as "inappropriate", those in the range 4–6 are rated as "uncertain", and those in the range 7–9 range as "appropriate" (Brook et al. 1986; Kahan et al. 1994).

The RAM method may include even a further round of voting for necessity criteria. The RAM definition of necessity is that:

- The procedure is appropriate, i.e., the health benefits exceed the risks by a sufficient margin to make it worth doing.
- It would be improper care not to offer the procedure to a patient.
- There is a reasonable chance that the procedure will benefit the patient.
- The magnitude of the expected benefit is not small (Kahan et al. 1994).

All four of these criteria must be met for a procedure to be considered as necessary for a particular indication. This rating is also done on a 1–9 scale, where 1 means that the procedure is clearly not necessary, and 9 means it is clearly necessary.

AMERICAN ACADEMY OF NEUROLOGY

In the clinical practice guidelines, the American Academy of Neurology (AAN) uses a strict evidence-based methodology that follows the Institute of Medicine's (IOM) standards for developing systematic reviews and Care Practice Guidelines (CPGs). The AAN guidelines are all based on a systematic review of the literature relevant to the specific clinical circumstances. The evidence derived from this literature review is presented to a panel of experts who develop the guideline conclusions and recommendations, achieved by a consensus building process. The first part of the process, finding and defining literature-based evidence, is an important step that is well described in the AAN guidelines (Gronseth et al. 2011). Apart from forming the basis for actual recommendations, the systematic literature review also has value in informing neurologists and patients of the limitations of the available evidence. The first goal of the process of making recommendations is to develop a recommendation that addresses a relevant clinical question. The second goal is to determine the confidence that adherence to the recommendation will improve outcomes. Confidence in the strength of recommendation is indicated by a level A (strongest level = "must" –this is rare), B (intermediate level ="should"), or C (lowest level = "may"). Reaching these final goals of recommendations first requires the confidence in the ability of the evidence to support practice recommendation to be rated, and, secondly, for the evidence to be placed into a clinical context by considering factors that could influence the recommendation. To to reach its goal of delivering so-called actionable recommendations, i.e. a specific action the clinician should perform, AAN has adopted a modified version of the Grading of Recommendations Assessment, Development and Evaluation (GRADE) process (see the GRADE section for further description). AAN care guidelines are developed in communication with the AAN Board of Directors and are supposed to be published in *Neurology*.

GRADE

The Grading of Recommendations Assessment, Development and Evaluation (GRADE) working group started in 2000 as an informal collaboration of people with an interest in addressing the shortcomings of grading systems in healthcare (www.gradeworkinggroup.org).

The working group has developed GRADE as an approach to grading quality (or certainty) of evidence and strength of recommendations. The basic idea behind GRADE is that systematic reviews and other methods for evidence-based recommendations are not sufficient for making well informed decisions or care guidelines. The GRADE instrument has been increasingly used by guideline developers in order to grade the importance and necessity of specific recommendations.

Criteria for the GRADE system include:

1. The certainty in the evidence (also known as quality of evidence or confidence in the estimates) should be defined consistently with the definitions used by the GRADE Working Group.
2. Explicit consideration should be given to each of the GRADE domains for assessing the certainty in the evidence (although different terminology may be used).
3. The overall certainty in the evidence should be assessed for each important outcome using four or three categories (such as high, moderate, low and/or very low) and definitions for each category that are consistent with the definitions used by the GRADE Working Group.
4. Evidence summaries and evidence to decision criteria should be used as the basis for judgments about the certainty in the evidence and the strength of recommendations. Ideally, evidence profiles should be used to assess the certainty in the evidence and these should be based on systematic reviews. At a minimum, the evidence that was assessed and the methods that were used to identify and appraise that evidence should be clearly described.
5. Explicit consideration should be given to each of the GRADE criteria for determining the direction and strength of a recommendation or decision. Ideally, GRADE evidence to decision frameworks should be used to document the considered research evidence, additional considerations and judgments transparently.
6. The strength of recommendations should be assessed using two categories (for or against an option) and definitions for each category such as strong and weak/conditional that are consistent with the definitions used by the GRADE Working Group (although different terminology may be used), such as strong (http://www.gradeworkinggroup.org).

### AGREE

The Appraisal of Guidelines for Research and Evaluation (AGREE) instrument was originally developed in 2003 (Grol et al. 2003), and updated (AGREE II) in 2010 (Brouwers et al. 2010). The purpose of the AGREE instrument is to assist clinical practice guideline developers to improve the quality and applicability of a guideline to be produced, and to provide a framework for assessing the quality of existing clinical practice guidelines. For this purpose, AGREE II consists of six domains covering 23 key items, each of which "captures a unique dimension of guideline quality" (Brouwers et al. 2010). The items within each domain are rated on a 7-point scale ("strongly disagree" to "strongly agree") (Table 2.1).

**TABLE 2.1**
**Items and content of AGREE II**

| Item | Content | Domain |
| --- | --- | --- |
| 1 | The overall objective(s) of the guideline is (are) specifically described. | Scope and Purpose |
| 2 | The health question(s) covered by the guideline is (are) specifically described. | |
| 3 | The population (patients, public, etc.) to whom the guideline is meant to apply is specifically described. | |
| 4 | The guideline development group includes individuals from all relevant professional groups. | Stakeholder Involvement |
| 5 | The views and preferences of the target population (patients, public, etc.) have been sought. | |
| 6 | The target users of the guideline are clearly defined. | |
| 7 | Systematic methods were used to search for evidence. | Rigour of Development |
| 8 | The criteria for selecting the evidence are clearly described. | |
| 9 | The strengths and limitations of the body of evidence are clearly described. | |
| 10 | The methods for formulating the recommendations are clearly described. | |
| 11 | The health benefits, side effects, and risks have been considered in formulating the recommendations. | |
| 12 | There is an explicit link between the recommendations and the supporting evidence. | |
| 13 | The guideline has been externally reviewed by experts prior to its publication. | |
| 14 | A procedure for updating the guideline is provided. | |
| 15 | The recommendations are specific and unambiguous. | Clarity of Presentation |
| 16 | The different options for management of the condition or health issue are clearly presented. | |
| 17 | Key recommendations are easily identifiable. | |
| 18 | The guideline describes facilitators and barriers to its application. | Applicability |
| 19 | The guideline provides advice and/or tools on how the recommendations can be put into practice. | |
| 20 | The potential resource implications of applying the recommendations have been considered. | |
| 21 | The guideline presents monitoring and/or auditing criteria. | |
| 22 | The views of the funding body have not influenced the content of the guideline. | Editorial Independence |
| 23 | Competing interests of guideline development group members have been recorded and addressed. | |

Hoffmann-Eßer et al. (2017)

For use of evaluating the quality of a clinical care guideline, AGREE II also includes two global rating items (overall assessments). In the first of these, the overall guideline quality is rated on a 7-point scale ("lowest possible quality" to "highest possible quality"). The second overall rating concludes on whether to use the guideline in practice or not. The AGREE instruments together are considered to be the most commonly used instruments for guideline appraisal (Hoffmann-Eßer et al. 2017).

## Overview of the current best practice guidelines for neuromuscular disorders

There are presently best practice care guidelines produced for more than 10 different neuromuscular diseases which aim to cover the multitude of areas and organ systems of importance in neuromuscular disorders (Table 2.2). These guidelines have been constructed using of different techniques, and with various level of rigour. What is common to them all is that they are based on a combination of literature-based evidence and an expert consensus building process. Several, but not all, have included patient or patient representatives in the process, and some have been produced also in a patient-friendly lay version (Table 2.2). Important to note is that several of the best practice guidelines for neuromuscular disorders have been produced on the initiative of patient organisations. Furthermore, a common feature of the available guidelines is to stress the importance for

**TABLE 2.2**
**Overview of best practice guidelines for neuromuscular diseases**

| Disease | Method | Family guide | Publication |
|---|---|---|---|
| Duchenne muscular dystrophy | RAM | Yes | Bushby et al. 2010a; 2010b<br>Birnkrant et al. 2018a; 2018b; 2018c |
| Spinal muscular dystrophy | Delphi | Yes<br>Planned | Wang et al. 2007<br>Mercuri et al. 2018<br>Finkel et al. 2018 |
| Congenital muscular dystrophies | Delphi<br>AAN | Yes | Wang et al. 2010<br>Kang et al. 2015 |
| Congenital myopathies | Delphi | Yes | Wang et al. 2012 |
| Limb-girdle muscular dystrophy | AAN | No | Narayanaswami et al. 2015 |
| Inclusion body myositis | Dephi | Planned | Jones et al. 2016 |
| Pompe disease (acid alpha-glucosidase deficiency) | Expert opinion | No | Cupler et al. 2012 |
| Glycogen storage disease III | Expert opinion | No | Kishnani et al. 2010 |
| Dermatomyositis | Nominal group technique | No | Huber et al. 2012 |
| Friedreich ataxia | Expert opinion | No | Corben et al. 2014 |
| Facioscapulohumeral muscular dystrophy | Expert opinion<br>AAN | No<br>Yes | Tawil et al. 2010; 2015 |
| Myasthenia gravis | RAM | No | Sanders et al. 2016 |

RAM: RAND/UCLA appropriateness method; AAN: American Academy of Neurology patients having access to a multidisciplinary team specialised in the particular disease/neuromuscular disorder.

The development of the best practice guideline for Duchenne muscular dystrophy (DMD) (published as two papers in *Lancet Neurology*, Bushby et al. 2010a; Bushby et al. 2010b) was facilitated by the US Centers for Disease Control and Prevention (CDC). The guideline was produced from the initiative of the patient organisation Parent Project Muscular Dystrophy (PPMD). The RAM method was chosen for guideline production, thus combining evidence with consensus of expert opinion. The panel consisted of 84 members divided into the areas of diagnosis, corticosteroid and other drug management, gastroenterology/speech/swallowing/nutrition, pulmonary management, cardiac management, psychosocial management, orthopaedic management and rehabilitation. Recommendations take into consideration the stage of the disease (presymptomatic, early ambulatory, late ambulatory, early non-ambulatory or late non-ambulatory). A total of 489 articles were selected in the literature search for best available evidence of management. Following ratings of most important signs and symptoms within each of the areas, ratings were also performed for suitable assessment tools and interventions for these symptoms. This was done by two anonymous ratings with in-person meetings in between. A user-friendly version of the guideline was produced, in collaboration with the TREAT-NMD Neuromuscular Network and patient advocacy groups, and this has been translated into approximately 20 languages (www.treat-nmd.eu/care/dmd). Updates of the guidelines have now been published (Birnkrant et al. 2018a; 2018b; 2018c).

The first comprehensive care guidelines for spinal muscular atrophy (SMA) were published in 2007 (Wang et al. 2007). They were produced using the Delphi technique, led by a 12-member Standard of Care Committee for SMA, as a standing committee for the International Coordinating Committee for Spinal Muscular Atrophy clinical trials (ICC). Eighty-six SMA experts from North America and Europe were invited to participate in the Delphi survey, focusing for each area on presenting signs and symptoms, diagnostic testing and intervention options. The intervention part was in turn divided into acute management and health maintenance. The resulting guidelines were divided into five areas: diagnostic/new interventions, pulmonary, gastro-intestinal/nutrition, orthopaedics/rehabilitation, and palliative care. Recommendations were grouped into present state of disease, i.e. whether the person with SMA is currently a non-sitter, sitter or ambulatory, rather than into SMA type. Similar to DMD, a lay friendly version has been produced and translated into several different languages (www.treat-nmd.eu/care/sma).

A two-part update of the SMA care guidelines was recently undertaken (Mercuri et al. 2018; Finkel et al. 2018). Similar to the previous guideline, a Delphi-like approach was used to combine evidence from the literature with a consensus of expert opinions. Part one presents an update on diagnosis, rehabilitation, orthopaedic and spinal management; and nutritional, swallowing and gastro-intestinal management. Part two includes recommendations related to pulmonary management, acute care, other organ involvement, ethical issues, medications, and the impact of new treatments for SMA. A patient-friendly version of the updated guideline is planned in a collaborative effort between patient organisations and the TREAT-NMD Neuromuscular Network.

CONGENITAL MUSCULAR DYSTROPHIES

In 2010, following the initiative of the patient organisation Cure CMD, best practice guidelines for congenital muscular dystrophy were published under the leadership of an International Standard of Care Committee for Congenital Muscular Dystrophy (Wang et al. 2010). The guidelines were established following the identification of relevant care issues, review of the literature for evidence-based practice, and a Delphi-based consensus among 33 participating experts, with an intervening workshop. The care recommendations were divided in seven areas: diagnosis, neurology, pulmonology, orthopaedics/ rehabilitation, gastroenterology/nutrition/speech/oral care, cardiology and palliative care. A family-friendly version of the guidelines was produced from the original publication in a collaborative effort between the patient organisation Cure CMD and the TREAT-NMD Neuromuscular Network, also supported by AFM and Telethon Italy (www.treat-nmd.eu/ care/cmd). More recently, guidelines on diagnosis and management have been produced using the AAN protocol for guideline development (Kang et al. 2015).

CONGENITAL MYOPATHIES

In 2009, a group of neuromuscular specialists initiated work to establish care guidelines for patients with congenital myopathy, in collaboration with the patient organisation Building Strength. Similar to the establishment of care guidelines for congenital muscular dystrophy, a Delphi-like approach was applied, including an in-person workshop. A focus was placed on topics applicable to several or all subtypes of congenital myopathy. A total of 59 experts participated in the production of the guideline, divided in five different working groups: diagnostics/genetics, neurology, pulmonology, orthopaedics/physical therapy and rehabilitation, and gastroenterology/nutrition/speech/oral care (Wang et al. 2012). A user-friendly version of the published guideline has been produced and is available at www.building-strength.org.

LIMB-GIRDLE MUSCULAR DYSTROPHY

In 2014 Narayanaswami et al. published a guideline which applied the AAN criteria for reviewing the current evidence and making practice recommendations for diagnosis and treatment of limb-girdle muscular dystrophies (LGMDs) (Narayanaswami et al. 2014). The guideline includes some other hereditary myopathies that may be considered forms of LGMD (e.g. Becker muscular dystrophy, hereditary inclusion body myositis and Emery–Dreifuss muscular dystrophy). The recommendations were based on literature searches for 1) frequency of genetically confirmed subtypes; 2) how often patients with LGMD subtypes have specific clinical features, including ethnic predilection, diagnostic patterns of weakness, respiratory and cardiac complications, laboratory abnormalities, specific patterns on imaging, and muscle biopsy features; and 3) evidence for effective therapies. A summary of the published guidelines for patients and their families was produced and is available at www.aan.com/Guidelines.

### INCLUSION BODY MYOSITIS

Following an European Neuromuscular Centre (ENMC) workshop on inclusion body myositis (IBM), work has been performed to produce best practice guidelines for IBM (Rose et al. 2013). A guideline development group was established of specialists in muscle disease from around the world, and a protocol was developed with the aim of establishing a consensus of opinion on questions relating to the diagnosis and management of IBM (Jones et al. 2016). An assessment of the quality of the evidence was achieved using the GRADE methodology for randomised controlled trials. This was combined with a three cycle Delphi-type consultation to formulate the best practice recommendations. Using this approach, a best care guideline covering aspects of diagnosis, drug treatment, physical and practical management, respiration, nutrition and cardiac management, psychosocial management, and multidisciplinary care is presently being summarised.

### POMPE DISEASE

A consensus report on treatment recommendations for late-onset Pompe disease (acid alpha-glucosidase deficiency) was published in 2012 (Cupler et al. 2012) by the American Association of Neuromuscular & Electrodiagnostic Medicine (AANEM). The guidelines were produced by a consensus committee of specialists with expertise in the diagnosis and treatment of Pompe disease. Using a modified consensus development conference method, the committee worked to create consensus-based treatment recommendations, where each panel member had major responsibility for a section to write and review.

### GLYCOGEN STORAGE DISEASE III

In 2010 an international group of 16 experts in diagnostic/genetic and management (cardiac, gastro-intestinal/dietary, neurologic, musculoskeletal, psychosocial, hepatic transplantation, general medical, and supportive and rehabilitative) aspects of glycogen storage disease III (GSD III) produced a diagnosis and management guideline (Kishnani et al. 2010). The work was based on literature review, followed by consensus building activity in the expert group. Consensus was defined as agreement among all members of the panel. For the most part, the published recommendations are to be considered as expert opinion.

### DERMATOMYOSITIS

In 2007 development of treatment recommendations for (moderate) juvenile dermatomyositis was initiated by the Childhood Arthritis and Rheumatology Research Alliance (CARRA), a north American organisation of paediatric rheumatologists. This eventually resulted in a consensus meeting in 2010 including 30 paediatric rheumatologists and four lay participants. Following a pre-meeting survey, to which 151 participants responded, a nominal group technique was adopted to reach a final consensus treatment plan. The resulting consensus document describes recommended therapy for moderate juvenile dermatomyositis throughout the treatment course, particularly regarding timing and rate of steroid tapering, duration of steroid therapy, and actions to be taken if patients were unchanged, worsening, experiencing medication side effects or disease complications (Huber et al. 2012).

FRIEDREICH ATAXIA

A very comprehensive consensus clinical management guideline for Friedreich ataxia (FRDA) was published in 2014 (Corben et al. 2014). Thirty-nine expert clinicians (Europe, Australia, Canada and USA) initially evaluated available published evidence related to FRDA clinical care. Where no published data specific to FRDA existed, recommendations were based on expert consensus or to data related to similar conditions. The guideline eventually presented 146 recommendations on best practice management for individuals with FRDA. Sixty-two per cent of the recommendations were based on expert opinion, indicating the lack of high-level quality clinical studies in the area.

FACIOSCAPULOHUMERAL MUSCULAR DYSTROPHY

A brief summary of recommended management and standards of care for facioscapulo-humeral muscular dystrophy (FSHD) was published in 2010 (Tawil et al. 2010). The recommendations were formulated based on evidence, when available, or on the consensus of opinion among 24 experts participating in a European Neuromuscular Centre (ENMC) workshop on standards of care for FSHD in January 2010.

A later effort to produce evidence-based care recommendations for FSHD was accomplished by a working group adopting the AAN method for best care guideline production (Tawil et al. 2015). A summary of this guideline for patients and their families is available at www.aan.com/Guidelines.

MYASTHENIA GRAVIS

In 2013, a task force of the Myasthenia Gravis Foundation of America (MGFA) convened a group of 15 international experts on myasthenia gravis to develop a treatment guideline. This resulted in the consensus guideline for the management of myasthenia gravis published in 2016 (Sanders et al. 2016). Following a non-systematic literature review, the RAM method was applied to quantify agreement and reach consensus on the appropriateness of an intervention. The final document includes guidance statements on: 1) symptomatic and immunosuppressive (IS) treatments, 2) IV immunoglobulin (IVIg) and plasma exchange (PLEX), 3) impending and manifest myasthenic crisis, 4) thymectomy, 5) juvenile myasthenia gravis (JMG). 6) myasthenia gravis with antibodies to muscle-specific tyrosine kinase (MuSK-MG), 7) myasthenia gravis in pregnancy.

**Future perspectives**

Over the next few years we are likely to see an increasing number of best practice guidelines being developed for neuromuscular disorders (NMDs). In order for these to be trustworthy and impact on the health of individuals with NMD, it is crucial not only that they are developed in a systematic way to present recommendations based on best available evidence, but also that they are properly disseminated and implemented. Guidelines, no matter how well

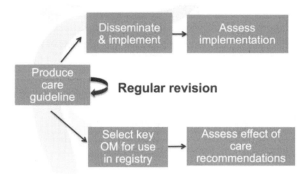

**Fig. 2.1.** Simplified scheme of the important steps after the development of best care guidelines for neuromuscular disorders.

they are based on evidence and well written, will not be better than the extent to which is it is implemented. The implementation of guidelines can, and should, be assessed to elucidate the impact of the guidelines (Bladen et al. 2014; Fig. 2.1). Collaborative efforts at national and international levels between healthcare professionals, networks of neuromuscular specialists, patient organisations, and learned societies are important and must use an array of methods to spread the knowledge on the availability of the guidelines and ensure that they are implemented.

To accomplish this, AGREE have set up recommendations for guideline development that serve well to summarise the most important steps for groups intending to set up guidelines for a specific neuromuscular disorder (Table 2.1).

It is worth emphasising the importance of incorporating "the views and preferences of the target populations" (Table 2.1, item 5). This has been part of both initiation of and development of several guidelines for NMDs (e.g. DMD, SMA, congenital muscular dystrophy, congenital myopathy) and will be important to consider for future guideline productions. Future guidelines are likely also to increasingly include the use of methods to grade the importance and necessity of recommendations, e.g. by use of GRADE. A dilemma here may be the feasibility of dealing with the large number of items in a care guideline that ideally should be graded. This may, at least partially, be overcome by initiating work on GRADE with a selection of a few of the most important topics/recommendations, with an intention and plan to subsequently grade the remaining items.

One crucial item for guideline development is that a contingency plan for how and when to update the newly developed guideline is often omitted. The time between updates of the care guidelines for DMD and SMA, for example, have been more than 7 years and 10 years, respectively.

Once the guidelines have been disseminated and implemented, we face another issue that should warrant more interest and action for improvement; namely, assessing, by way of selected key outcome measures in a registry, how interventions recommended in a best care guideline actually impact health (Fig. 2.1). This is true for the follow-up of care guidelines in any medical field, but is of particular importance for NMDs and other rare diseases where care recommendations, to a large extent, are built on expert consensus rather than high-level evidence such as large randomised trials. Such assessment would help the guideline developers, the users of the guidelines, and healthcare providers learn about the effectiveness of the recommendations. Furthermore, this knowledge would contain information that is useful for clinical trials as an up-to-date description of the effects of the best currently available care; for example, to be used for control purposes. It would be advantageous if such a follow-up registry on effectiveness of care recommendations were combined with work to develop a more generic post-marketing surveillance dataset of new drugs for NMDs; for example, as with ongoing work for SMA.

**Key points**
- The development of best practice care guidelines for NMDs allow:
  1. physicians and other healthcare professionals to make recommendations based on best available evidence;
  2. patients to ensure that their management follows recommendations based on best available evidence; and
  3. for a common basis of diagnosis and clinical management in clinical multicentre trials.

- Several methods exist to guide developers of such care guidelines to ensure high-quality work and to ensure recommendations are based on the best available evidence.
- The present chapter reviews methods of use for care guidelines for NMDs, an overview of existing guidelines for NMDs, and future perspectives on care guideline development in the area of NMDs.

## REFERENCES

Alonso-Coello P, Irfan A, Solà I, Gich I, Delgado-Noguera M, Rigau D et al. (2010) The quality of clinical practice guidelines over the last two decades: a systematic review of guideline appraisal studies. *Qual Saf Health Care* 19:e58.
Birnkrant DJ, Bushby K, Bann CM, Apkon SD, Blackwell A, Brumbaugh D et al. (2018a). Diagnosis and management of Duchenne muscular dystrophy, part 1: diagnosis, and neuromuscular, rehabilitation, endocrine, and gastrointestinal and nutritional management. *Lancet Neurol* 17: 251–267.
Birnkrant DJ, Bushby K, Bann CM, Alman BA, Apkon SD, Blackwell A et al. (2018b). Diagnosis and management of Duchenne muscular dystrophy, part 2: respiratory, cardiac, bone health, and orthopaedic management. *Lancet Neurol* 17: 347–361.
Birnkrant DJ, Bushby K, Bann CM, Apkon SD, Blackwell A, Colvin MK et al. (2018c). Diagnosis and management of Duchenne muscular dystrophy, part 3: primary care, emergency management, psychosocial care, and transitions of care across the lifespan. *Lancet Neurol* 17: 445–455.
Bladen CL, Thompson R, Jackson JM, Garland C, Wegel C, Ambrosini A et al. (2014) Mapping the differences in care for 5,000 spinal muscular atrophy patients, a survey of 24 national registries in North America, Australasia and Europe. *J Neurol* 261:152–163.
Brook RH, Chassin MR, Fink A et al. (1986) A method for the detailed assessment of the appropriateness of medical technologies. *Int J Technol Assess Health Care* 2: 53–63.
Brouwers MC et al. (2010) AGREE Next Steps Consortium. AGREE II: advancing guideline development, reporting, and evaluation in healthcare. *CMAJ* 182: E839–E842.
Burgers JS, Grol R, Klazinga NS, Mäkelä M, Zaat J, AGREE Collaboration (2003) Towards evidence-based clinical practice: an international survey of 18 clinical guideline programs. *Int J Qual Health Care* 15: 31–45.
Burgers J, Smolders M, Weijden T, Davis D, Grol R (2013) Clinical practice guidelines as a tool for improving patient care. *In* Grol R, Wensing M, Eccles M, Davis D (Eds), *Improving Patient Care: The Implementation of Change in Health Care*, 2nd ed. Oxford, UK: John Wiley & Sons, Ltd.

Bushby K, Finkel R, Birnkrant DJ, Case LE, Clemens PR, Cripe L et al. (2010a). Diagnosis and management of Duchenne muscular dystrophy, part 1: diagnosis, and pharmacological and psychosocial management. *Lancet Neurol* 9: 77–93.

Bushby K, Finkel R, Birnkrant DJ, Case LE, Clemens PR, Cripe L et al. (2010b). Diagnosis and management of Duchenne muscular dystrophy, part 2: implementation of multidisciplinary care. *Lancet Neurol* 9: 177–189.

Corben LA, Lynch D, Pandolfo M, Schulz JB, Delatycki MB, Clinical Management Guidelines Writing Group. (2014) Consensus clinical management guidelines for Friedreich ataxia. *Orphanet J Rare Dis* 9: 184.

Cupler EJ, Berger KI, Leshner RT, Wolfe GI, Han JJ, Barohn RJ et al. (2012) Consensus treatment recommendations for late-onset Pompe disease. *Muscle Nerve* 45: 319–333.

Eurordis (2009) *The Voice of 12 000 Patients, Experiences and Expectations of Rare Disease Patients on Diagnosis and Care in Europe*. www.eurordis.org.

Finkel RS, Mercuri E, Meyer OH, Simonds AK, Schroth MK, Graham RJ et al. (2018) Diagnosis and management of spinal muscular atrophy: Part 2: Pulmonary and acute care; medications, supplements and immunizations; other organ systems; and ethics. *Neuromuscul Disord* 28(3): 197–207. doi.10.1016/j.nmd.2017.11.004.

Graham R, Mancher M, Wolman DM (Eds) (2011) *Clinical Practice Guidelines We Can Trust*. Washington, DC: National Academies Press.

Grol R, Cluzeau FA, Burgers JS (2003) Clinical practice guidelines: towards better quality guidelines and increased international collaboration. *Br J Cancer* 89(Suppl 1): S4–S8.

Gronseth G, Woodroffe LM, Getchius TS (2011) *Clinical Practice Guideline Process Manual*. St. Paul, MN: American Academy of Neurology.

Hoffmann-Eßer W, Siering U, Neugebauer EA, Brockhaus AC, Lampert U, Eikermann M (2017) Guideline appraisal with AGREE II: Systematic review of the current evidence on how users handle the 2 overall assessments. *PLosOne* 12(3): e0174831. doi.10.1371/journal.pone.0174831.

Huber AM, Robinson AB, Reed AM, Abramson L, Bout-Tabaku S, Carrasco R et al. (2012) Consensus treatments for moderate juvenile dermatomyositis: beyond the first two months. Results of the second Childhood Arthritis and Rheumatology Research Alliance consensus conference. *Arthritis Care Res (Hoboken)* 64: 546–553.

Jones J, Hunter D (1995) Consensus methods for medical and health services research. *BMJ* 311: 376–380.

Jones KL, Sejersen T, Amato AA, Hilton-Jones D, Schmidt J, Wallace AC et al. (2016) A protocol to develop clinical guidelines for inclusion-body myositis. *Muscle Nerve* 53: 503–507.

Kahan JP, Bernstein SJ, Leape LL, Hilborne LH, Park RE, Parker L et al. (1994) Measuring the necessity of medical procedures. *Med Care* 32: 357–365.

Kang PB, Morrison L, Iannaccone ST, Graham RJ, Bönnemann CG, Rutkowski A et al. (2015) Evidence-based guideline summary: evaluation, diagnosis, and management of congenital muscular dystrophy: Report of the Guideline Development Subcommittee of the American Academy of Neurology and the Practice Issues Review Panel of the American Association of Neuromuscular & Electrodiagnostic Medicine. *Neurology* 84: 1369–1378.

Kishnani PS, Austin SL, Arn P, Bali DS, Boney A, Case LE et al. (2010) Glycogen storage disease type III diagnosis and management guidelines. *Genet Med* 12: 446–463.

Linstone HA, Turoff M (1975) *The Delphi Method: Techniques and Applications*. Reading, MA: Addison-Wesley Publishing Company.

Mercuri E, Finkel RS, Muntoni F, Wirth B, Montes J, Main M et al. (2018) Diagnosis and management of spinal muscular atrophy: Part 1: Recommendations for diagnosis, rehabilitation, orthopedic and nutritional care. *Neuromuscul Disord* 28(2): 103–115.

Narayanaswami P, Weiss M, Selcen D, David W, Raynor E, Carter G et al. (2014) Evidence-based guideline summary: diagnosis and treatment of limb-girdle and distal dystrophies: report of the guideline development subcommittee of the American Academy of Neurology and the practice issues review panel of the American Association of Neuromuscular & Electrodiagnostic Medicine. *Neurology* 83: 1453–1463.

Rose MR and ENMC IBM Working Group (2013) 188th ENMC International Workshop: Inclusion Body Myositis, 2–4 December 2011, Naarden, The Netherlands. *Neuromusc Dis* 23:1044–1055.

Sanders DB, Wolfe GI, Benatar M, Evoli A, Gilhus NE, Illa I et al. (2016) International consensus guidance for management of myasthenia gravis: executive summary. *Neurology* 87: 419–425.

Schünemann HJ, Wiercioch W, Etxeandia I, Falavigna M, Santesso N, Mustafa R et al. (2014) Guidelines 2.0: systematic development of a comprehensive checklist for a successful guideline enterprise. *CMAJ* 186: E123–E142.

Shaneyfelt TM, Centor RM (2009) Reassessment of clinical practice guidelines: go gently into that good night. *JAMA* 301: 868–869.

Sniderman AD, Furberg CD (2009) Why guideline-making requires reform. *JAMA* 301: 429–431.

Tawil R, van der Maarel S, Padberg GW, van Engelen BG (2010) 171st ENMC international workshop: standards of care and management of facioscapulohumeral muscular dystrophy. *Neuromuscul Disord* 20: 471–475.

Tawil R, Kissel JT, Heatwole C, Pandya S, Gronseth G, Benatar M et al. (2015) Evidence-based guideline summary: Evaluation, diagnosis, and management of facioscapulohumeral muscular dystrophy: Report of the Guideline Development, Dissemination, and Implementation Subcommittee of the American Academy of Neurology and the Practice Issues Review Panel of the American Association of Neuromuscular & Electrodiagnostic Medicine. *Neurology* 85: 357–364.

Wang CH, Finkel RS, Bertini ES, Schroth M, Simonds A, Wong B et al. (2007) Consensus statement for standard of care in spinal muscular atrophy. J Child Neurol 22: 1027–1049.

Wang CH, Bönnemann CG, Rutkowski A, Sejersen T, Bellini J, Battista V et al. (2010) Consensus statement on standard of care for congenital muscular dystrophies. *J Child Neurol* 25: 1559–1581.

Wang CH, Dowling JJ, North K, Schroth MK, Sejersen T, Shapiro F et al. (2012) Consensus statement on standard of care for congenital myopathies. *J Child Neurol* 27: 363–382.

# 3
# A MULTIDISCIPLINARY APPROACH AND MANAGEMENT AS BEST CARE MODEL IN NEUROMUSCULAR DISORDERS

*Nathalie Goemans*

Despite major advances in therapy development there is still no cure for the majority of neuromuscular disorders (NMD). However, a multidisciplinary medical, surgical and rehabilitative approach of symptoms have altered the natural course of these diseases, improving both quality of life and longevity (Eagle et al. 2007).

While nerve and muscles are primarily involved in NMD, the clinical features of this heterogeneous group of disorders encompass a multitude of extra muscular manifestation and secondary consequences of muscle weakness. The complexity of the problems of these patients require a coordinated care and management that should be provided in a multidisciplinary patient-centered approach to improve health and quality of life. This coordinated approach is recommended in a number of disease specific guidelines (Wang et al. 2007; Kang et al. 2015; Tawil et al. 2015; Narayanaswami et al. 2014) and has been shown effective in improving quality of life and survival (Rooney et al. 2015; Otto et al. 2017).

From a patient's perspective, centralizing and streamlining the access to expertise from different disciplines specialized in the management of NMD is perceived as a great value. This goes beyond a mere logistic and time saving perspective concerning the organization and attendance of different specialist clinics. The certitude that treatment decisions and care recommendation are decided, shared and endorsed by all the different healthcare experts involved in the management of their disease enhances confidence in medical care and the relationship with healthcare providers.

A multidisciplinary neuromuscular care center should provide a lifelong patient-centered accompaniment throughout the different stages of the disease, from diagnosis to end of life, addressing and anticipating the specific needs of the individual according to the stage of the disease. Multidisciplinary clinical teams consist of a core of physicians and healthcare professionals from many different disciplines, with expertise in the neuromuscular disorders-specific aspects of their specialty, under the lead of a (pediatric) neurologist, physiatrist or physician trained in diagnosis, care and rehabilitation of NMD.

Most often the team will include surgeons, physiotherapists, pneumologists, cardiologists, gastro enterologists, endocrinologists, and geneticists addressing the numerous aspects of neuromuscular diseases. In addition, physiotherapists, speech therapists and dieticians have a major impact in managing symptoms and preventing or delaying secondary complications. However, optimal care and management of these complex diseases should also address broader aspects of health and quality of life. Psychologists, social workers, nurses and occupational therapists should be part of the team to address psychosocial issues, to improve participation and provide support in achieving life goals. Communication and strong cohesion among care providers across the different disciplines, including the treating physician and the home care providers, is key. The multidisciplinary team should address age and stage specific issues in a timely manner, including a transition plan to adult care for children affected with a NMD and initiation of palliative care discussion in case of severe progressive disorders. The team's input is invaluable in providing information and sharing expertise with colleagues in specific situations such as emergencies and hospital admissions (Bushby et al. 2010; Wang et al. 2007; Kang et al. 2015; Tawil et al. 2015). Special care and expert input is needed to manage adequately specific situations such as myasthenic crises, (periodic) paralyzes, severely progressive Guillain–Barré. In addition, the intensive care providers should be aware of icreased peri-operative risks related to NMD such as malignant hyperthermia, adrenal crisis in steroid-treated Duchenne muscular dystrophy patients and increased risks of cardio-respiratory complications.

Most of the affected children worldwide live in low or middle income countries characterized by resource-limited settings, which challenges the organization of multidisciplinary care as proposed by published guidelines. However, these recommendations should not discourage the development of optimal care for NMD in remote and less privileged areas The key point is to identify a co-ordination physician with specific interest in NMD and their comorbidities, willing to instruct medical and paramedical colleagues in these specific domains. While sophisticated apparatus may not be available throughout all centers in the world, respiratory physiotherapy with positive pressure masks to enhance clearance of secretions, advice on adequate positioning/mobilization to avoid contractures, healthy eating habits, including adequate intake of nutrients, should be available even in resource-limited settings.

Most research on the value and cost-effectiveness of a multidisciplinary care setting for NMD has been conducted in amyotrophic lateral sclerosis (ALS), and has reported a better compliance to care guidelines and more efficient use of care resources (Chio et al. 2006; Cordesse et al. 2015; Boylan et al. 2015; Rooney et al. 2015). Moreover, a comprehensive multidisciplinary care has been associated to reduced hospitalizations and emergencies, increased survival and improved quality of life in ALS (Rooney et al. 2015; Van den Berg et al. 2005; Cordesse et al. 2015; Traynor et al. 2003).

Further assessment of the value of multidisciplinary care for NMD is warranted in the discussions with national or other health insurance systems to guarantee financial support for the sustainability of multidisciplinary teams as this require substantial commitment of staff time and resources (Paganoni et al. 2017). Measuring cost-effectiveness of multidisciplinary care is challenging due to the progressive course of many NMD and should include patient satisfaction and quality of life among other health indexes. Multidisciplinary care centers have an additional value from a research perspective by improving our insights in rare diseases and by centralizing expertise and patient numbers for clinical research. Patients advocacy groups are key partners in the negotiations with national or private health insurance systems to support multidisciplinary care by voicing their preferences and by contributing to the development of assessment tools that measure what really matters to patients with NMD.

**Key points**
- Multidisciplinary care is considered as the best care model for complex diseases such as NMD.
- Multidisciplinary care is a lifelong accompaniment of the patient and his/her family, addressing in a comprehensive approach all aspects of his/her disease and providing expert care and management throughout all stages of the disease.
- Further research is needed to assess value and cost-effectiveness of coordinated multidisciplinary care, to empower healthcare professionals in their negotiations with heath care payers to support this model for the benefit of the patients.

## REFERENCES

Boylan K, Levine T, Lomen-Hoerth C, Lyon M, Maginnis K, Callas P et al. (2015) Prospective study of cost of care at multidisciplinary ALS centers adhering to American Academy of Neurology (AAN) ALS practice parameters. *Amyotroph Lateral Scler Frontotemporal Degener* 17: 119–127.

Bushby K, Finkel R, Birnkrant DJ, Case LE, Clemens PR, Cripe L et al. (2010) Diagnosis and management of Duchenne muscular dystrophy, part 2: implementation of multidisciplinary care. *Lancet Neurol* 9: 177–189.

Chio A, Bottacchi E, Buffa C, Mutani R, Mora G & PARALS (2006) Positive effects of tertiary centres for amyotrophic lateral sclerosis on outcome and use of hospital facilities. *J Neurol Neurosurg Psychiatry* 77: 948–50.

Cordesse V, Sidorok F, Schimmel P, Holstein J, Meininger V (2015) Coordinated care affects hospitalization and prognosis in amyotrophic lateral sclerosis: a cohort study. *BMC Health Serv Res* 15: 134.

Eagle M, Bourke J, Bullock R, Gibson M, Mehta J, Giddings D et al. (2007) Managing Duchenne muscular dystrophy – the additive effect of spinal surgery and home nocturnal ventilation in improving survival. *Neuromuscul Disord* 17: 470–475.

Kang PB, Morrison L, Iannaccone ST, Graham RJ, Bönnemann CG, Rutkowski A et al. (2015) Evidence-based guideline summary: evaluation, diagnosis, and management of congenital muscular dystrophy: Report of the Guideline Development Subcommittee of the American Academy of Neurology and the Practice Issues Review Panel of the American Association of Neuromuscular & Electrodiagnostic Medicine. *Neurology* 84: 1369–1378.

Narayanaswami P, Weiss M, Selcen D, David W, Raynor E, Carter G et al. (2014) Evidence-based guideline summary: diagnosis and treatment of limb-girdle and distal dystrophies: report of the Guideline Development Subcommittee of the American Academy of Neurology and the Practice Issues Review Panel of the American Association of Neuromuscular & Electrodiagnostic Medicine. *Neurology* 83: 1453–1463.

Otto C, Steffensen BF, Højberg AL, Barkmann C, Rahbek J, Ravens-Sieberer U et al. (2017) Predictors of Health-Related Quality of Life in boys with Duchenne muscular dystrophy from six European countries. *J Neurol* 264: 709–723.

Paganoni S, Nicholson K, Leigh F, Swoboda K, Chad D, Drake K et al. (2017) Developing multidisciplinary clinics for neuromuscular care and research. *Muscle Nerve* 56: 848–858.

Rooney J, Byrne S, Heverin M, Tobin K, Dick A, Donaghy C et al. (2015) A multidisciplinary clinic approach improves survival in ALS: a comparative study of ALS in Ireland and Northern Ireland. *J Neurol Neurosurg Psychiatry* 86: 496–501.

Tawil R, Kissel JT, Heatwole C, Pandya S, Gronseth G, Benatar M et al. (2015) Evidence-based guideline summary: Evaluation, diagnosis, and management of facioscapulohumeral muscular dystrophy: Report of the Guideline Development, Dissemination, and Implementation Subcommittee of the American Academy of Neurology and the Practice Issues Review Panel of the American Association of Neuro-muscular & Electrodiagnostic Medicine. *Neurology* 85: 357–364.

Traynor BJ, Alexander M, Corr B, Frost E, Hardiman O (2003) Effect of a multidisciplinary amyotrophic lateral sclerosis (ALS) clinic on ALS survival: a population based study, 1996–2000. *J Neurol Neurosurg Psychiatry* 74: 1258–1261.

Van den Berg JP, Kalmijn S, Lindeman E, Veldink JH, de Visser M, Van der Graaff MM et al. (2005) Multi-disciplinary ALS care improves quality of life in patients with ALS. *Neurology* 65: 1264–1267.

Wang CH, Finkel RS, Bertini ES, Schroth M, Simonds A, Wong B et al. (2007) Consensus statement for standard of care in spinal muscular atrophy. *J Child Neurol* 22: 1027–1049.

# Section 2

## Assessment of a Child with a Neuromuscular Disorder: The Cornerstone for Management

# 4
# CLINICAL EVALUATION AND DIAGNOSTIC APPROACH

*Nicolas Deconinck, Sandra Coppens and Gauthier Remiche*

**Introduction**

This chapter is intended to refine the skills of clinicians and health professionals who are not already familiar with the diagnosis and management of neuromuscular disorders in children. It will provide a framework on how to conduct anamnesis, clinical examination and how to make first diagnostic hypothesis. In the second part of the chapter some key complementary investigations are described such as laboratory, and electrodiagnostics but also (gaining in importance over the years) muscle imaging and genetics, focusing on their ability to confirm initial clinical hypotheses. Muscle (and nerve) biopsy, a very important investigation in the field of neuromuscular disorders, will not be covered as it goes beyond the scope of this book.

The clinical approach to the evaluation of a neuromuscular patient requires as a starting point a very good comprehension of the physiological and pathophysiological principles that govern the functioning of the motor unit. The acquisition of this knowledge facilitates the practical application of the basic principles of the semiology but also a better understanding of the several exceptions and overlapping features of the symptoms.

Neuromuscular disorders are classified according to the anatomic structure of the motor unit. This classification is one of the corner stones helping the clinician in their diagnostic approach. Diseases of the anterior horn cell are referred to as neuronopathies; of the peripheral nerve as neuropathies; of the neuromuscular junction as neuromuscular transmission disorders or myasthenic syndromes, and of the myofiber as myopathies.

Classically, each of these subgroups presents with distinctive clinical features. So, it is crucial for young trainees in the field of pediatric medicine to combine the results of anamnesis, clinical observation and examination and orient them to one of these cardinal entities.

ANAMNESIS: ANSWERING KEY QUESTIONS

The clinical approach can be facilitated by systematically answering a set of key questions regarding the patient:

*What are the presenting complaints or symptoms of the patient?*

There are limited ways a neuromuscular disorder can manifest, and the complaints usually fall within one of the following categories: infantile floppiness or hypotonia, weakness, fatigue, delay in motor milestones, abnormal gait characteristics, muscle cramps, myalgias, respiratory difficulties. These complaints will be further discussed further in the First presenting symptoms section.

*At what age do symptoms appear and what is the temporal evolution?*

Asking patients, when possible, and their parents to describe the chronology of the clinical syndrome is critical. The temporary profile (the onset, duration, and evolution of the symptoms and signs) usually suggests one or more diagnostic possibilities and allows categorization.

Usually, neuropathies and muscular dystrophies of genetic origin are almost systematically progressive from the time of onset. However, in infants and young children, disease progression is often mitigated by normal childhood development. As a result, at certain points in early development, the parents may report that the child has stabilized or actually improved functionally. Other children have episodic or salutatory patterns to their clinical symptoms, which generally suggest an underlying ion channel disturbance or metabolic disease. In addition, inflammatory diseases of the neuromuscular system (for example dermatomyositis) may fluctuate symptomatically over time. In this case, the concomitant finding of elevated creatine kinase (CK) values, favors an inflammatory disease of muscle rather than a muscular dystrophy.

Perinatal severe weakness and respiratory distress in the delivery room may be seen in acute infantile spinal muscle atrophy (SMA) type I, myotubular myopathy, congenital hypomyelinating neuropathy, congenital infantile myasthenia, transitory neonatal myasthenia, and severe neurogenic arthrogryposis (Werdnig 1891; Hoffmann 1893; Batten 1903) (Fig. 4.1).

Weakness evident some days or weeks later during the newborn period raises other possibilities, such as spinal muscular atrophy, congenital muscular dystrophy, myotonic dystrophy, several congenital myopathies and myasthenic syndromes, but it is also important to recognize certain metabolic diseases such as acid maltase deficiency (Bönnemann et al. 2014; Oskoui et al. 2008, van Capelle et al. 2016).

*Are there particular events in the past medical history?*

Recapitulating past medical history of a neuromuscular disorder is crucial. A detailed history regarding pregnancy (e.g. quality of fetal movement or pregnancy complications, arthogryposis), and perinatal problems (evidence of fetal distress, respiratory difficulties in the delivery room, need for resuscitation or ventilation problems in early infancy, ongoing respiratory difficulties, swallowing/feeding difficulties and persistent hypotonia) should be obtained.

*Is there a family history of a neuromuscular disorder?*

Collecting consistent information regarding familial history may provide valuable insight through the diagnosis odyssey of a patient. Most disorders of the motor unit are genetically determined autosomal dominant, autosomal recessive, or X-linked disorders. Others are transmitted as maternal, non-Mendelian traits, pathognomonic of mitochondrial DNA mutations (Oskoui et al. 2008). So it is always recommended to examine the mother of a

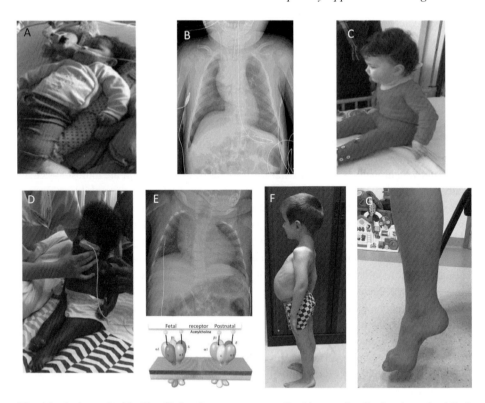

**Fig. 4.1. A**. 4 month-old girl suffering from severe generalized hypotonia, distal and proximal limb weakness, and requiring continuous non-invasive ventialtion. This pattern is typically observed in spinal muscular atrophy with respiratory distress type I (SMARD1). A pathogenic homozygous variant was found in the *IGHMBP2* gene. **B**. Same child as in A: Chest RX showing the typical image of diaphragmatic paralysis (predominating in the right hemidiaphragm of the patient). **C**. A 15 month-old SMA type I patient (bearing two *SMN2* copies) who was treated from the age of 3 months with a *SMN2* splicing modulator therapy, now achieving independent head control and sitting position. Notice the remaining axial hypotonia the weaknes of lower limbs. **D. & E**. A 4-month-old girl, born at term; transferred to NICU for development respiratory distress. The patient presented impressive arthrogryposis (hands, elbows, fingers, knees, ankles), right hip luxation, scoliosis; persistent axial hypotonia, and underdevelopped rib cage requiring intermittent non-invasive ventilatory support, feeding difficulties. Cognitive development is normal and familial history is negative. A mendeliome found a homozygous *c.117dupC* (p.Asn40fs) mutation in the gene coding for the fetal (gamma) subunit of the achetylcholine receptor (CHRNG), signing the diagnosis of Escobar syndrome, an intrauterine form of myasthenia; **F**. A 3-year-old child with a COL XII related congenital myopathy. Notice axial hypotonia with hyperlordosis, abdominal protrusion due to weak abdominal muscles and valgus flat feet. **G**. Typical image of a high foot arch with hammertoes in a patient with axonal form of Charcot–Marie–Tooth neuropathy.

weak newborn infant to determine whether she has evidence of myotonic dystrophy, myasthenia gravis, or another immune-mediated condition (Fig. 4.1).

*Are there precipitating factors?*

Identifying precipitating factors that may trigger the onset of symptoms is informative. The co-occurrence of particular elements/events associated with the onset of weakness may prove very useful. For example, when associated with fever or fasting, weakness, or gait disturbance leads to suspicion of a defect of fatty acid oxidation. Relating the specific inges- tion of meals (for example a high-carbohydrate meal) to weakness suggests the possibility of periodic paralysis. Patients with paramyotonia congenital may report frequent muscle stiffness and eyelid stiffness. A myasthenic crisis in the context of myasthenia gravis or an intermittent porphyria crisis may be precipitated by ingestion of specific drugs.

*Are there associated systemic symptoms or signs?*

One should pay attention during history collection to the involvement of other organs (central nervous system or other systems). For example, some congenital muscular dystro- phies may be accompanied by cerebellar and cerebral abnormal cortex development such as in alpha-dystroglycanopathies (Bönnemann et al. 2014) or Charcot–Marie–Tooth (CMT) by cerebellar or pyramidal tract signs in inherited and metabolic neuropathies (Reilly and Rossor 2014).

Cardiac disease often accompanies Duchenne muscular dystrophy (DMD), Becker muscular dystrophy, myotonic dystrophy, Emery–Dreifuss dystrophy, Lamin A/C (LMNA)- related congenital muscular dystrophy, Andersen Tawil syndrome, and various metabolic disorders, including mitochondrial diseases, acid maltase deficiency, and carnitine defi- ciency (Marian et al. 2016). In contrast, diseases affecting anterior horn cells, peripheral nerves and neuromuscular junctions spare the heart. Multisystemic involvement is common in mitochondrial disease; strokes or stroke-like episodes, migraine headaches, short stature, pigmentary retinopathy, sensorineural hearing loss, proximal limb weakness, and lactic aci- dosis are common findings in children with the MELAS (mitochondrial encephalopathy and lactic acidosis with stroke-like episodes) phenotype (Chinnery 2014).

Scoliosis is uncommon in ambulatory patients but is characteristic of Friedreich ataxia, and some forms of congenital myopathies or dystrophies, such as COL-6RD or selenopathies.

The observation of skin cheloids, or abnormal texture of the skin rises the possibility of COL-6RD (Foley et al. 2013). A typical face skin rash may indicate dermatopolymyositis.

History regarding cognitive development, type of school, and school performance may be important indicators of superimposed central nervous system (CNS) involvement.

*Which part of the motor unit is probably affected? Anatomical reasoning and symptom onset deciphering*

Neuronopathies classically involve the cell body, and neuropathies classically affect their extensions and the investing myelin sheath. Most important neuronopathies in the pediatric age group are the genetically determined spinal muscular atrophies. Their clinical picture varies to some degree, depending on the age at presentation. Infants with spinal muscu- lar atrophy are typically weak and areflexic. The alert infant lying quietly on the examin- ing table with a wide-eyed expression and tongue fasciculations, and predominantly distal movements of the limbs is easily recognized. The older child with the juvenile presentation has more obvious proximal weakness of the shoulder and pelvic girdle muscles and hypore- flexia, the clinical presentation of a dystrophinopathy. However, joint contractures are less common in children with juvenile spinal muscular atrophy, and serum creatine kinase values tend to be normal or only slightly elevated. Neurogenic disease causes more wasting than myopathic disease does, and the loss of muscle bulk is more distal.

Although sometimes difficult to evaluate in young children, associated sensory loss implicates the peripheral nerves and argues against motor neuron diseases, disorders of neuromuscular transmission, and myopathies. Loss of muscle stretch reflexes is also the hallmark of a peripheral neuropathy. Areflexia is the rule when sensory involvement is present. However, muscle stretch reflexes are often reduced or absent in patients with congenital non-progressive myopathies.

Disorders of the neuromuscular junction characteristically present with intermittent symptoms, including weakness and fatigue. In contrast, disorders of the anterior horn cell, peripheral nerve, and muscle generally present with fixed symptoms that are often progressive over time. Fatigue is also now more recognized as a symptom of denervating diseases, particularly spinal muscular atrophy (mainly SMA type III) (Montes et al. 2013).

Fatigue in the context of myasthenia very often begins during infancy, including symptoms such as hypotonia, ptosis, ocular motility disturbances and intermittent apnea. Disorders of the neuromuscular junction include genetic conditions such as congenital myasthenia, but also acquired disorders such as infant botulism, transient neonatal myasthenia gravis, fetal acetylcholine receptor inactivation syndrome, and juvenile myasthenia gravis. Each of these disorders is distinctive and often recognizable clinically by age at presentation and symptoms. As we will see further, electromyography (EMG) studies of the motor unit, particularly neuromuscular junction testing, as mentioned earlier, may be useful as an initial diagnostic study in these disorders.

Myopathies also are characterized by loss of strength, but the degree of weakness is disproportionate to the degree of muscular atrophy, particularly early in the clinical course. As mentioned previously, the extent of muscular atrophy appears disproportionate in neurogenic diseases. Patients with myopathies appear to be unduly weak, without significant loss of muscle bulk. DMD stands out as a striking example (see Chapter 10). A child with DMD appears remarkably weak, struggling to rise from the floor of walk up and down the stairs. The large proximal muscles are differentially affected, with relative preservation of the distal muscles.

In children there are exceptions to these generalizations, such as in myopathies affecting distal muscles such as in myotonic dystrophy type 1, some congenital myopathies, and Laing autosomal dominant distal myopathy (mutations in MYH7 ) (Laing et al. 1995).

Gowers' sign is a manifestation of pelvic girdle muscle weakness, most commonly seen in the setting of DMD (Gowers 1879; see Chapter 10), but it can also been seen in other neuromuscular disorders, such as juvenile spinal muscular atrophy, chronic inflammatory demyelinating polyneuropathy (CIDP) and mitochondrial diseases. Since the original description, however, clinicians have come to understand that this sign is present whenever there is significant weakness of the hip and knee extensors, regardless of whether the underlying disease process affects primarily nerve or muscle (Kugelberg and Welander,1956).

Muscle stretch reflexes tend to be relatively preserved with myopathic diseases and are roughly proportionate to the degree of atrophy. However, patients with congenital myopathies often have diminished reflexes or areflexia. Clinically, if the patient is notably weak with preserved muscle bulk and loss of muscle stretch reflexes, the condition is most likely a myopathy.

In children, the typical initial complaints from parents usually fall within one the following categories:

- infantile floppiness or hypotonia,
- weakness,
- delay in motor milestones,
- frequent falls, difficulty ascending stairs or arising from the floor,
- abnormal gait characteristics,
- muscle cramps, myalgias,
- respiratory difficulties.

We briefly discuss some key elements the clinician should bear in mind when considering, or "undigging", these complaints. They concern some typical aspects of the anamnesis but also the oriented clinical examination that accompanies the complaint.

*Hypotonia*

Hypotonia referred as a diminished resistance to passive movement is an important clinical examination finding in children with neuromuscular disorders. It is important to bear in mind that the most common etiology for infantile hypotonia is central, accounting for the vast majority of cases. The typical examples include Prader-Willi syndrome, Down syndrome, but also patients with an history of hypoxemia or toxic, infectious aggression during the perinatal period.

In the context of neuromuscular disorders, hypotonia is associated with true weakness (often generalized involving axial and limb muscles) which may be difficult to bring out. Even then weakness may exist without any primary pathology of the peripheral motor unit. Typical hypotonic infants with weakness may lie "frog-legged", with hips adducted and knees flexed. They have a marked head lag. A lack of spontaneous movement is also very suggestive of weakness.

Increased muscle stretch is a good indicator to the more common CNS mechanisms for hypotonia.

Evaluating hypotonia is often challenging in very young children and should take into account the evolving aspect of tonus through the first weeks after birth, the effect of fatigue on its evaluation, and its subjective component. It should then be observed consistently through several signs (the scarf sign, hypermobile joints, weak control of head) and over iterated examinations. In assessing tone, the child should be alert but not crying. Passive movements are used to evaluate the tonus of extremities. Truncal and nuchal tone may be best examined using tests of horizontal and vertical suspension. On vertical suspension, a healthy infant should maintain the head upright and midline without slipping through the examiner's hands. On horizontal suspension, the infant should maintain a straight back with the head upright and limbs flexed. In contrast, hypotonic infants may wrap over the examiner's arms.

The absent or markedly reduced antigravity movements has a very high sensitivity and specificity (0.97 and 0.75) to detect hypotonia from neuromuscular origin. In this context an history of reduced fetal movements and polyhydramnios and/or the presence of contractures is also very typical for neuromuscular disorders (Vasta et al. 2005; Harris 2008).

*Weakness*

Weakness is probably the most frequent reported complaint in children with neuromuscular disorders. In most neuromuscular disorders weakness is relatively symmetrical and involves a variable combination of limb and axial muscles. As a general rule in the case of myopathies, weakness is typically proximal and, when involving lower limbs, patients complain of difficulty arising from a low chair or toilet, getting up from a squatted position, or climbing stairs (Fig. 4.1). When the upper extremities are involved, patients notice trouble brushing their teeth, combing their hair or lifting objects overhead.

In the context of polyneuropathies, and some rare forms of distal myopathies, weakness will be distal and patients complain of gait instability due to foot drop or difficulties in hand manipulations.

Some neuromuscular disorders such as myasthenia, facioscapulohumeral muscular dystrophy (FSHD), mitochondrial diseases and Steinert muscular dystrophy, may also result in cranial muscle weakness resulting in complaints of slurred speech, difficulty swallowing or double vision, and palpebral ptosis.

Some neuromuscular disorders are however quite asymmetrical, such as FSHD, in which one might find prominent involvement of one side of the body or the congenital absence of a pectoral muscle (de Greef et al. 2010).

Determining the child's strength is central to the neuromuscular evaluation. The way to evaluate it is described in the Clinical examination section (p. 50).

*Delay in acquisition of motor milestones*

Children with neuromuscular disorders usually present with gross motor delays, although fine motor and cognitive delays may also be present. Identification starts with attention to caregiver concerns about the child's development, a concern that has been demonstrated to be right in the vast majority of cases (Lurio et al. 2015). In children, history regarding the acquisition of developmental milestones should be ascertained relating to head control, independent sitting (See Fig. 4.1), crawling, standing with and without support, walking with and without support, fine prehension, bimanual skill acquisition (bringing objects to midline, transfer of objects), and language acquisition. Some patients with a congenital myopathy, show a typical delay in milestone acquisition from early in infancy but nevertheless and unexpectedly finally acquire unassisted walking.

*Gait disturbance*

Information regarding gait characteristics (toe walking, excessive lordosis, etc.), running ability, transitions from floor to standing, stair climbing, falls, recreational/athletic performance, may be important clues to the presence of a neuromuscular disorder (see the Clinical examination section, p. 50).

*Muscle cramps, myalgias*

Cramps are the hallmark of denervating diseases. They are typically associated with intense muscle pain and may cause a palpable mass in the muscle. These symptoms typically occur with the muscle at rest and are brief in duration and sudden in onset. Cramps are typically associated with motor neurone discharges (for example when recorded with EMG).

Cramps are very common in children and may occur in the absence of definable disease, often happening at night and considered as benign.

On the pathological side, cramps usually indicate disease of the anterior horn cell, nerve roots, or peripheral nerve elements. Alternatively, cramping is seen with renal failure, hypothyroidism, hepatic failure, adrenal insufficiency, or disturbances of electrolyte balance, and its origin in this specific context is thought to be due to the presence of a metabolic derangement altering the neuronal microenvironment.

Myalgias and cramps may be brought to the front in some rare patients with a dystrophinopathy, and some limb-girdle dystrophies, such as in LGMD1C or metabolic myopathy (glycogen storage diseases, fatty acid oxidation defects, and mitochondrial disorders) (Foley et al. 2013; Berardo et al. 2010). In these cases the mechanism of cramping is less clear. Pain and cramping have also been described in inflammatory diseases such as dermatomyositis, and Guillain–Barré syndrome.

It is important to recognize several entities that may be confused with cramps. With disorders of muscle relaxation, as in myotonia and hypothyroidism, the patient may perceive an uncomfortable but painless muscle tightness or stiffness, often made worse in the cold. One can get a clue to myotonia if the patient admits to difficulty releasing a grip that improves with repeated contractions (Stern and Bernick 1990).

*Respiratory difficulties*

Respiratory failure is a very common symptom in the context of numerous acute and chronic neuromuscular disorders, but is often presenting as late course or as an acute complication of a generalized pre-existing weakness (for example Guillain–Barré syndrome).

As an initial presenting symptom in children it may have been seen in several contexts. In the context of the neonatal period (from birth to a few weeks after birth, often in an Neonatal Intensive Care Unit context), respiratory failure is almost systematically accompanied by a generalized weakness and should lead to the consideration of particular neuromuscular diseases that affect the diaphragmatic and intercostal muscles very early in life.

In ambulatory patients respiratory failure may be "on the front of the scene" in some conditions such as intermediary forms of COL6-RD, or titinopathies in the form of acute respiratory distress, or in some forms of congenital myasthenia or myasthenia gravis.

*Functional state mimicking neuromuscular conditions*

If symptoms of weakness, pain or sensory abnormalities are disproportionate or exist in the absence of signs, psychogenic issues such as conversion must be considered. Typically, symptoms do not follow an anatomical nerve distribution nor do the actions fit the symptoms. Although there is not always a clear psychiatric entity that can be established, difficulty with emotional expression and communication are commonly observed in the family of the affected child (Maloney 1980). It is now clear that children presenting with functional symptoms mimicking neuromuscular disorders need careful attention, and final outcome in the resolution of symptoms is better when child psychiatry and pediatric neurology work together in the evaluation and treatment of conversion. Treatment should emphasize health rather than disease (Maisami et al. 1987).

The diagnosis of conversion disorder can be a clinical challenge. Making the diagnosis early in the course of the presentation can reduce the child's and family's anxieties and reduce the need for costly and unnecessary tests and is associated with a better prognosis. A thorough physical examination and a careful psychiatric history are essential to screen for comorbid psychiatric illness. The therapeutic relationship between the clinician and the child and family will help them understand and better accept the diagnosis. It is not uncommon for children to be unable to verbally express the psychological factors that are stimulating their symptoms.

CLINICAL EXAMINATION

*The importance of observing children*

A particular aspect in clinical examination in young children is that very often reliable and consistent information will be captured when engaging a young child in natural play activities. Observation in natural contexts will surpass the information that can be obtained from formal examination, and this is very true for young children who may not easily respond to specific guidance. Concretely, observing the child's behavior and motor activities while taking a history from the parents often provides significant information. Moreover, the clinical examiner should propose play activities during which the child will spontaneously perform key activities: the way the child arises from the floor, climbs stairs or reaches over the head will be good markers of proximal strength; walking on the heels, or the toes, will evaluate distal strength, but also deep sensory proprioception. One can also note eye movements, the position of the upper eyelids, and the facial expression under these conditions, particularly if the child can be encouraged to smile or laugh, or if the child becomes distressed and demonstrates facial grimacing. By 2 years of age, the child is able to run quite well, kick a ball, and travel up and down stairs without hesitation. Standing on one leg and attempting to jump off a step is often accomplished by 3 years of age, and hopping on one foot is attempted by 4 years of age. By 5 years of age, the child is able to hop well on either leg (Fig. 4.1).

*Strength assessment*

Muscle testing can be accomplished with increasing detail with advancing age, although the functional measures of strength are often the most informative at any age. It is of course difficult to assess one particular muscle in isolation, one generally assesses some muscle groups in daily clinical practice. Nevertheless, a quick survey of major muscles is often informative and sufficient. The distribution of weakness should be noted (predominantly proximal versus distal; lower extremity versus upper extremity; focal versus generalized; isolated peripheral nerve distribution versus multiple peripheral nerves; or single versus multiple roots/myotomes). It is also very important to evaluate as accurately as possible axial musculature. For example, neck flexors are particularly important as they are preferentially affected in many myopathies. Careful assessment of scapular winging, scapular stabilization and scapular rotation is very helpful in the assessment of patients with FSHD and limb-girdle muscular dystrophy (LGMD). It should be noted whether extraocular, facial and bulbar muscles are involved or spared.

More formal assessment of all accessible muscle groups is done using the grading system originally developed by the Medical Research Council (MRC) (John et al. 1984). The MRC system has five grades: 0 for no movement of the muscle, 1 for a flicker or trace of movement, 2 for active movement with gravity eliminated, 3 for active movement against gravity, 4 for active movement against gravity and some applied resistance, and 5 for normal power. Strictly speaking, only the 0 grade is unequivocal.

When evaluating a patient with a suspected neuromuscular disorder one cannot omit the Gowers' maneuver. Gowers' sign is a manifestation of pelvic girdle muscle weakness, most commonly seen in patients with DMD but it definitely not specific and can be observed in many other neuromuscular disorders, such as juvenile spinal muscular atrophy (type III), CIDP, and mitochondrial diseases.

*Quantitative strength evaluation*
Quantitative strength measurements have been demonstrated to be far more sensitive than clinical strength testing for detecting weakness in children and adults with motor impairments. It is however rarely used in the context of routine clinical practice with children, but has been investigated as a marker of weakness evolution in the context of therapeutic clinical studies. Quantitative strength evaluation and functional assessment tools are detailed in Chapter 5.

*Sensory evaluation*
Sensory deficits are difficult to objectify at a young age. As a result, a sensorimotor neuropathy may be difficult to distinguish from a neuronopathy because the sensory loss may be difficult to define. The behavioral response is most valuable. A noxious stimulus elicits a prompt withdrawal of the limbs. If this reflex response is not accompanied by a grimace or cry, one should suspect a sensory disturbance. Deep sensory disturbances affecting proprioception may disturb the early motor milestones.

*Gait analysis*
With a patient presenting with gait disturbances, one may have to differentiate between cardinal components like muscle weakness and/or sensory deficit (these last being typically involved in neuromuscular disorders) and a cerebellar and/or coordination disorders typically of central origin. The stance and gait have to be investigated either by the observation of a child engaging in natural play conditions, during which the child will rise from the floor, climb stairs, and stand on one foot, or by testing specific elements during formal clinical examination, such as walking on the tips of the toes, the Romberg maneuver, and deep tendon reflexes evaluation.

More specifically regarding neuromuscular disorders, patients with proximal lower extremity weakness often exhibit a classic myopathic gait pattern (see Fig. 10.2). Initially, weakness of the hip extensors produces anterior pelvic tilt and a tendency for the trunk to be positioned anterior to the hip joint. Patients compensate for this by maintaining lumbar lordosis which positions their center of gravity/weight line posterior to the hip joints, thus stabilizing the hip in extension on the anterior capsule of the hip joint.

Patients with distal weakness involving ankle dorsiflexors and everters (for example as in CMT, Emery–Dreifuss muscular dystrophy, FSHD etc) often exhibit a foot slap at floor contact and a "steppage" gait pattern to facilitate swing phase clearance of the plantar-flexed ankle. Sometimes these patients may use circumduction at the hip as adaptation strategy to clear the plantar-flexed ankle. In this situation maintaining the ankle at neutral position with the use of ankle-foot orthoses (AFOs) is often very beneficial for the patient.

*Deep tendon Reflexes*

While deep tendon reflexes are generally depressed or absent (typically in neuropathies) in many neuromuscular diseases, they may be brisk in syndromes with superimposed upper motor neuron involvement, such as spastic paraplegic syndromes. It is important to remember that the presence of deep tendon reflexes (DTRs) does not necessarily exclude the presence of a neuromuscular disease.

*Myotonia*

The clinical finding common to all myotonic disorders is myotonia, which is a state of delayed relaxation or sustained contraction of skeletal muscle. Grip myotonia may be demonstrated by delayed opening of the hand with difficult extension of the fingers following a tight grip. Paradoxical myotonia is the situation where myotonia becomes worse with successive movements instead of improving with activity. Percussion myotonia may be elicited by percussion of the thenar eminence with a reflex hammer giving an adduction and flexion of the thumb with slow return. Other sites which may give a local contraction with percussion include the deltoid, brachioradialis and gluteal muscles. Occasionally, myotonia of the tongue draped over a tongue blade may be elicited with a midline tap of the finger, giving a bilateral contraction notch along the lateral portion of the tongue bilaterally with slow relaxation. Myotonic syndromes include myotonic muscular dystrophy type 1 (Steinert's disease), myotonia congenita (Thomsen disease), Becker-type myotonia congenita, paramyotonia congenita (Eulenburg disease), and Schwartz-Jampel syndrome (chondrodystrophic myotonia) (see Chapter 15).

*Contractures*

A more detailed description of the specific contractures most often present among the more common neuromuscular disorders conditions is presented in Chapter 21 (Skalsky and McDonald 2012). The presence of specific contractures can be helpful diagnostically, as in the clinical distinction between congenital muscular dystrophy which often presents with contractures versus other congenital structural myopathies which frequently present with hypotonia but no contractures. The presence of isolated elbow flexion contractures can be a diagnostic clue to Emery–Dreifuss muscular dystrophy (Muchir and Worman 2007).

In general, dystrophic myopathies have a greater predilection towards the development of contractures than other myopathies and neurogenic conditions.

*Serum laboratory studies*

A variety of neuromuscular diseases, particularly those characterized by sarcolemmal muscle membrane injury, show significant elevations in transaminases, aldolase, and creatine kinase. The creatine kinase enzyme catalyzes the release of high energy phosphates from creatine phosphate. It occurs mainly in muscle and leaks into the serum in large amounts in any disorder involving muscle fiber injury. The creatine kinase MM fraction is specific to skeletal muscle.

Before using this biomarker for guiding the clinician in the diagnosis of a neuromuscular disorders, what is considered as a normal value? Most laboratories use the central 95% of observations in white people as a reference range for serum creatine kinase, assuming that levels have a Gaussian (bell-shaped) distribution, which is usually about 0 to 200IU/L (Moghadam-Kia et al. 2016).

It is however important to keep in mind that an abnormal creatine kinase (>200IU/L) level was observed in 19% of men and 5% of women in a study of nearly 1 000 healthy young people, with potential risk of over-diagnosis. Creatine kinase values vary with sex and race (Lev et al. 1999).

Creatine kinase value elevation may be transient or chronic/long-lasting indicating different muscle etiologies. Having this in mind, a repeated creatine kinase measurement over time (for example after 7–14 days) is most of the time very informative regarding the possible etiology.

Transient elevations of creatine kinase are observed after exercise or heavy manual labor. Serum creatine kinase levels may increase to as much as 30 times the upper limit of normal within 24 hours of strenuous physical activity, then slowly decline over the next 7 days. The degree of creatine kinase elevation depends on the type and duration of exercise. It can be observed in the context of trauma, viral myositis, or in the context of after some moderate exercise in the context of some metabolic myopathies such as carnitine palmitoyltransferase II (CPT2) deficiency, McArdle disease and mitochondrial myopathies. In this context of early fatigue, painful cramps, and sometimes, when very severe, myoglobinuria are suggestive of the diagnosis.

The creatine kinase value is significantly and constantly elevated in the early stages of DMD and BMD with values up to 50–100 times normal, and a normal value typically excludes these diagnosis. Other forms of muscular dystrophy such as Emery–Dreifuss muscular dystrophy, limb-girdle muscular dystrophy, FSHD, and congenital muscular dystrophy, and acid maltase deficiency are typically associated with moderate elevations in creatine kinase (5 to 25 times normal). However, in congenital muscular dystrophy, the creatine kinase value may be extremely variable, ranging from normal values to a fairly marked elevation, and the severity of the disease cannot be inferred from the creatine kinase values. Creatine kinase values tend to decrease over time with increasing severity of the disease due to progressive loss of muscle fiber and irreversible cell death. Thus, a 3-year-old with DMD may have a creatine kinase value of 25 000 while a 10-year-old with DMD may show a creatine kinase value of 2 000 (Gospe et al. 1989).

Other conditions with significant elevations in creatine kinase may include polymyositis, dermatomyositis, acute rhabdomyolysis, and malignant hyperthermia.

Importantly, in a child with muscle weakness, a normal creatine kinase does not exclude a myopathy or other neuromuscular disorder. For example, in the context of congenital structural myopathies, creatine kinase is likely to be normal or only mildly elevated. In SMA type I, II and III patients creatine kinase levels have been found to be normal to elevated two- to four-fold (Eng et al. 1984). Normal creatine kinase values may be seen in the acute active phase of childhood dermatomyositis, even in the presence of severe weakness.

Myoglobinuria results from the breakdown of skeletal muscle known as rhabdomyolysis, a condition in which muscle cells breakdown, sending their contents into the bloodstream. Rhabdomyolysis is important to recognize as it can lead to acute renal failure, requiring a really specific medical management.

ELECTRODIAGNOSTICS

Despite recent evolutions of electroneuromyography (ENMG) in pediatrics, the misconception of an invasive and difficult ancillary test remains for numerous practitioners (Pitt 2011; Alshaikh et al. 2016; Pitt and Kang 2015). ENMG remains an essential tool to diagnose inherited and acquired neuromuscular disorders and was estimated to provide meaningful information at a rate of 94% (Pitt 2011; Pitt and Kang 2015; Preston and Shapiro 2013; Karakis et al. 2014; Rabie et al. 2007).

More specifically ENMG in pediatrics will provide essential information leading to diagnosis in many conditions such as motor neuron disease (e.g. spinal muscle atrophy), neuromuscular junction disorders (congenital myasthenic syndromes or myasthenia gravis), peripheral nerve disease (e.g. Charcot–Marie–Tooth) including its ability to distinguish axonal than demyelinating neuropathy. It also will provide essential information to orientate to a muscle disease or a myotonic syndrome (myogenic pattern and myotonic discharges respectively). However, several limitations should be underlined, such as a limited sensitivity to detect myogenic patterns or myotonic discharges in infants. Moreover the specificity of neuromuscular junction studies especially in neonates is also limited.

Several factors linked to the kind of diseases, the normative values and technical issues make using ENMG different in childhood than in adults (Pitt et al. 2015).

*Approach for the pediatric patient*

General approach

A time for reassurance and explanation should always be taken (avoiding words with negative connotation such as "needle" or "shock"). Parents should always be present and associated with the procedure. When possible the test should be done with the child on a parent's lap. Using additional tools to distract patient such as smartphone is also useful (Alshaikh et al. 2016; Pitt and Kang 2015; Oh 2003).

Material

For the nerve conduction velocity (NCV) study, recording surface electrodes are self-adhesive and pre-gelled that may be cut down for size-fitting purpose. It is preferred to use hand-held stimulation electrodes (with pads) to allow the limb to be encircled.

For needle electromyography, the most used disposable needle in pediatrics has a 0.30mm diameter. Recent electrodiagnostics software facilitates recording storages for collegial revision (Pitt and Kang 2015; Oh 2003).

Sedation and local anesthesia

Sedation may help the ENMG test to be performed but this has limitations. A slight sedation has the risk that the patient might wake up during the ENMG test. Deepest anesthesia (e.g. Propofol) may potentially lead to respiratory depression or inhalation and requires adequately trained staff and monitoring. Alternatively, mask-administrated nitrous oxide may be used. Sedation should be reserved for particular cases, especially in children between 2 and 6 years who are generally not able to understand but are able to be firmly opposed to the procedure (Preston and Shapiro 2013; Pereon 2012).

The use of anesthetic drugs may alter the quality of ENMG testing (e.g. F-waves modified by Propofol use) (Pitt and Kang 2015; Pereon 2012).

Local anesthetic cream such as amethocaine or xylocaine may be applied precisely where the needle will be placed roughly 30 minutes before needle electromyography (EMG) (Pitt et al. 2015).

*Normative values and interpretation*

Historical normative data are available in the literature (Oh 2003). One must remember that normative values vary depending on the patient's age, especially NCV. In consequence, to determine the demyelinating or axonal nature of a neuropathy based upon NCV analysis needs particular caution and use of the age-ranged reference table (Pitt and Kang 2015; Preston and Shapiro 2013; Oh 2003).

*General strategy of investigation*

The first requirement is to be experienced in pediatric ENMG and to use the appropriate materials. A recommended strategy is to initiate evaluation using the least uncomfortable tests and the more accessible nerves. For NCV, in order to increase tolerance, it is recommended to use non-recurrent mode, and the lowest possible current intensity, to favor increase of the duration of the stimulus rather than intensity, to increase intensity very progressively and to start with sensory studies. For needle EMG, one must select the lowest number of muscles (Pitt and Kang 2015; Preston and Shapiro 2013; Oh 2003).

In children the best reliability is found in the motor NCV study of the posterior tibial nerve for lower limbs and for sensory nerves, the median and ulnar are the easier to study (Pitt and Kang 2015; Oh 2003). The choice of the muscle to study should be oriented by the clinical question as well as by the possibility to obtain its activation. In this way the tibialis anterior has a place of choice since it may be easily activated by a stimulation of the plantar sole. Quadriceps femoris and iliopsoas are more difficult properly study. At upper limbs, generally biceps brachialis is preferred. In children it is recommended to study one muscle in detail rather than to proceed to a broad sampling (Pitt et al. 2015).

*Frequent clinical situations*

Generalized weakness

Differential diagnosis in this context is very broad. In a large propotion of cases, no diagnostic specific clinical sign is found. The first step is to exclude a peripheral neuropathy by performing sensory and motor NCV and a needle EMG of a distal muscle. If abnormalities orientates to a peripheral neuropathy, it is essential to determinate its axonal or demyelinating nature and whether some findings orientate to a genetically determined or acquired neuropathy (Pitt and Kang 2015; Potulska-Chromik et al. 2016; Nevo and Topaloglu 2002).

Several electrodiagnostic patterns for peripheral neuropathies have been defined. The main abnormalities found in demyelinating polyneuropathies are conduction blocks of motor fibers, reduced sensory nerves action potential, absence or prolonged F-waves latencies, and reduced conduction velocity (Polat et al. 2006) (Fig. 4.2A and 4.2B).

If one demonstrates neurogenic signs with needle EMG without sensory abnormalities on NVC study, the possibility of a motor neuron disease such as SMA should be considered (Fig. 4.2C). In this case a tongue EMG should be performed (genioglossus by the easily accessible submental route) (Pitt 2011; Pitt and Kang 2015). Since a negative investigation should not be conducted to exclude this diagnosis, SMN1 gene analysis is mandatory in all suspected SMA cases (Eng, Binder, and Koch 1984; Hwang, Lee et al. 2017; Cetin et al. 2009).

After excluding peripheral neuropathy and motor neuron disease, looking for a neuromuscular junction disorder or a myopathy is mandatory. To assess neuromuscular junction disorders in children, stimulated single fiber EMG (stimSFEMG) of the orbicular oculi is recommended. It is well tolerated, applicable without sedation, appropriate for children older than 3 months and has a high sensitivity. It may be combined with repetitive nerve stimulation (RNS) especially when stimSFEMG are equivocal (Fig. 4.2D). RNS should be performed after stimSFEMG because RNS may be not tolerated and is less sensitive than stimSFEMG (Pitt and Kang 2015; Pitt 2008, 2009; Rabie et al. 2007).

The possibility of a myogenic pattern should be assessed by needle EMG but its absence should not exclude the possibility of a myopathy. It typically includes shortening duration and amplitude decrease of the motor unit action potential, increased polyphasic potential number and early recruitment during slight contraction (Pitt and Kang 2015; Cetin et al. 2009; Rabie et al. 2007; Emeryk-Szajewska and Kopeć 2008).

Needle EMG may not detect myotonia in neonates and infants with type I myotonic dystrophy; however, when found, it may significantly reduce the differential diagnosis (Cetin et al. 2009; Shah et al. 2012; Ghosh and Sorenson 2015). In non-dystrophic myotonic syndromes the presence of electric myotonia may also help to orientate the diagnosis. However, since few studies have been published on this topic, data concerning sensitivity is not firmly established. In addition, it is important to remember that electric myotonia or myotonia-like discharges may be found in other myopathies such as central core disease or type II glycogenosis (Ghosh and Sorenson 2015; Shah et al. 2012).

Neonatal hypotonia

Neonatal hypotonia may be due to central or peripheral nervous system disease. ENMG helps to diagnose SMA or Charcot–Marie–Tooth but may remain normal especially in case

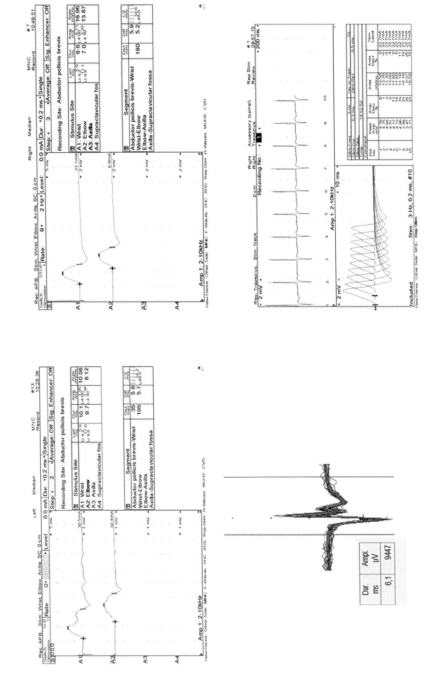

**Fig. 4.2. A** A 10-year-old boy presenting with Guillain–Barré syndrome having a motor nerve conduction velocity diminished at 71% of the lower normal value on the left median nerve. The amplitude of the compound motor action potential was also diminished. **B** A 9-year-old boy with a type 1A Charcot–Marie–Tooth disease. A decrease of the motor nerve conduction velocity is observed on the right median nerve (72%). The amplitude of the compound motor action potential is preserved. **C** A 17-year-old boy with spinal muscular atrophy type III. First symptoms were noticed at 5 years old and included lower limbs weakness. The EMG showed disseminated giant motor unit potentials as in the right extensor digitorum communis illustrated here (9 447 µV; normal < 4 000). **D** An 18-year-old girl with an autoimmune myasthenia gravis presenting her first symptoms at the age of 16. The 3Hz repetitive stimulation shows a maximal decrement of the compound motor action potential amplitude and area at the ninth stimulation (28% and 20% respectively). Anti-RACh antibodies were presents with high titers (6.7 nmol/L; normal < 0.1).

of congenital myopathy (Cetin et al. 2009). Due to the immaturity of the neuromuscular junction StimSFEMG is not considered as a reliable test in neonates younger than 3 months and little data is available on RNS in neonates (Pitt 2008).

Plexopathy

The most common plexopathy seen in childhood is the obstetric brachial plexus palsy. Despite the role of EMG having been questioned in this situation it should be useful for prognosis information (Pitt 2011; Pitt and Kang 2015; Gilbert and Tassin 1984).

In conclusion, electroneuromyography remains essential in the diagnostic work-up of many neuromuscular disorders in children. Despite one having to acknowledge that it requires some expertise, the misconceptions regarding its supposed lack of usefulness or accuracy and its excessive discomfort should be rectified by an improved communication based upon recent evidence.

MUSCLE IMAGING

Imaging techniques, such as computed tomography or resonance magnetic imaging, and ultrasound have assumed increasing importance in the diagnostic approach for patients with neuromuscular disorders and particularly muscle diseases, aiding clinical diagnosis and enriching pathological and genetic assessments. Among them, MRI has emerged as the most optimal one in its resolution capacity, discriminating with accuracy both individual muscles and muscle groups, important for establishing degree of involvement in general, as well as detailing internal muscle structure and intrinsic muscle patterns.

MRI is now being used for neuromuscular disease diagnosis and monitoring. This diagnostic method presents excellent soft-tissue characterization, especially when compared to older imaging techniques used for the study of muscle diseases, such as ultrasound or computed tomography.

Regarding the technique itself, the classic sequences that are used for myopathy evaluation in the upper and lower limbs are axial and coronal T1-weighted and T2-weighted images. With these two sequences MRI interpretation includes evaluation of muscle shape, volume and signal intensity. Expected general muscle volume and signal, adjusted according to age, are evaluated first, followed by volume and signal of each single muscle and muscle group, compared to surrounding and contralateral structures. For T2-weighted sequences, increased signal intensity is found when muscle edema is present, while increased signal intensity on T1-weighted images is observed in muscle undergoing fatty degeneration.

Use of whole-body MRI is steadily increasing. Fast spin echo (FSE) T1-weighted and T2-weighted as well as short-TI inversion recovery (STIR) images are acquired in the coronal plane (slice thickness is 5mm). Levels analyzed include: (1) head, neck and shoulder girdle, (2) chest, abdomen and pelvis (and upper limbs) and (3) thighs and calves. Images from different stations are processed and combined in the coronal plane to conform to produce whole-body magnetic resonance images (Fig. 4.3).

Hollingsworth et al. (2012) used a semi-quantitative grading scale describing degree of muscle involvement based on percentage of edema or fatty infiltration, in each mus-

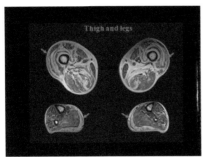
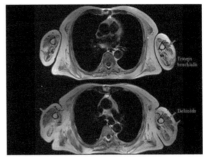
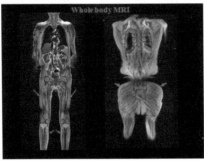

**Fig. 4.3.** Whole-body muscle MRI in COL VI-related myopathy. MRI T1 sequence: Systematic fatty infiltration progressing along fascias mainly in vastus lateralis muscles but also in paravertebral deltoids and triceps brachialis muscles. With courtesy: Dr. T. Stojkovic and Pr. R. Y. Carlier (IM, Paris).

cle group. Categories include: normal appearance (0), moth-eaten appearance with small scattered areas of high signal (1), moth-eaten appearance with confluent areas of high signal affecting less than 30% of total muscle volume (2a), moth-eaten appearance with confluent areas of high signal, compromising between 30–60% of muscle volume (2b), worn, blurred appearance due to confluence of focal areas (3) and a final stage of complete replacement of muscle by adipose tissue (4) (Hollingsworth et al. 2012).

Considering children specifically, MRI pattern recognition is particularly useful in the following clinical situations (Cejas et al. 2017; Leung 2017):

- Trying to differentiate genetic muscle entities such as in the context of congenital myopathies (CM), congenital dystrophies and limb-girdle dystrophies. In some forms of genetic forms congenital myopathies the pattern is almost pathognomonic.
- In RYR1 congenital myopathy for example, fatty infiltration and edema is observed predominantly in the pelvis at the level gluteus maximus, obturator externus and pectineus muscles, in thighs at the level sartorius, adductor magnus and quadriceps femoris and at the level of legs in soleus and peroneal muscles. In dynamin 2 myopathies, it is observed in pterygoid and thoracolumbar muscles.
- In COL6-CMD, muscle MRI (see figure 4.3) shows a characteristic pattern with diffuse involvement of fatty infiltration within thigh muscles with relative sparing of sartorius, gracilis, and adductor longus. Localization of fatty infiltration typically takes the form of a

rim of fat at the periphery of muscles particularly in vasti muscles, with a relative sparing of the central part indicative of endomysial fibrosis tracking along the muscle fascia. In the rectus femoris muscle fatty infiltration occurs along the central fascia specifically with a centrally located abnormal signal denoted as a "central shadow sign" on ultrasound (Mercuri and Muntoni 2012; Bönnemann et al. 2014). In selenoprotein 1-related myopathy (SEPN1-RM), selective involvement of the sartorius and great adductor muscles with sparing of the gracilis is very suggestive of the diagnosis.

- Magnetic resonance imaging has also been used to help differentiate between dystrophic myopathy and neurogenic atrophy due to spinal muscular atrophy. In the context of DMD it helps to show the initial pseudohypertrophy observed with disease progression.
- In dermatopolymyositis, focal or diffuse hyperintense lesions are observed in affected muscles on T2-weighted STIR images, suggesting edema due to inflammation. Distribution is usually bilateral, proximal, affecting initially pelvic girdle, then upper extremities, neck flexors, paravertebral and pharyngeal musculature. One can typically also identify soft-tissue and muscle calcifications.

Besides its growing role in helping clinicians achieving the right diagnosis, several characteristics of muscle MRI make it a promising a research tool for clinical trials and longitudinal studies (for example using 2- or 3-point Dixon techniques). MRI scans, based on a non-irradiating technique, are repeatable and non-invasive. Moreover images can be easily anonymized and registered for analysis by blinded reviewers. Compared to strength and function tests, MRI measurements may also be less vulnerable to confounding by the level of cooperation and effort on the part of the study subject. Several clinical trials of novel drugs in muscular dystrophy have reported using MRI as a secondary outcome measure, and at least one trial has reported using MRI as a primary outcome measure (Wagner et al. 2008; Campbell et al. 2016).

Finally, and very importantly, muscle imaging is also useful for the identification of appropriate muscle biopsy sites, determining distribution and extent of involvement, and for monitoring disease progression.

GENETIC APPROACH

Finally, modern diagnostics also requires working more and more in collaboration with other specialized neuromuscular disorders centers that are now forming networks, such as Treat-NMD and the recent initiative of EURO-NMD, which aim to standardize diagnostic and treatment approaches. Young clinicians should also master web-based tools such as Online Mendelian Inheritance in Man (OMIM) (https://www.omim.org), the gene table of neuromuscular diseases (www.musclegenetable.fr), and the DMD mutations database – UMD (www.umd.be/DMD/W_DMD/index.html).

Genetic diagnosis is essential for the patient with an inherited neuromuscular disorder and the patient's family. It is very helpful to target the screening of frequent complications associated with mutations in a specific gene (for example *SEPN1* and respiratory insufficiency) and to give an accurate long-term prognosis. Reaching a genetic diagnosis represents the end of a lengthy diagnostic odyssey and prevents the repetition of unnecessary invasive procedures (muscle or nerve biopsy, electromyography). At the family level, identification of the genetic etiology permits genetic and reproductive counselling, but also the screening of complications possibly associated with carrier status (for example DMD and cardiomyopathy, *RYR1* mutations and malignant hyperthermia susceptibility). Finally, an accurate genetic diagnosis allows the inclusion of the patient in targeted clinical trials and patient registries (Kassardjian et al. 2016).

Almost 500 genes have already been implicated in neuromuscular disorders. Genotype–phenotype correlations are not always straightforward. Some phenotypes can be caused by mutations located in several different genes (genotypic variability, for example alpha-dystroglycanopathies) and mutations in the same gene can cause different phenotypes (phenotypic variability). Genes implicated in neuromuscular disorders are among the largest genes of the human genome (*RYR1*, *DMD*, *NEB*, *TTN*). These factors can critically limit the efficacy of sequential gene testing.

Many recent studies have demonstrated the cost-effectiveness of next-generation sequencing (NGS) for the diagnosis of neuromuscular disorders (Schofield et al. 2017; Harris et al. 2017). NGS allows the sequencing of multiple genes in parallel (gene panels), of all the protein coding genes (whole exome sequencing or WES) or even of all the genome of an individual (whole genome sequencing or WGS). A very large number of variants can be found when the exome or genome of an individual is sequenced. Very large genes can present many rare single nucleotide variants (SNV) even in the general population. Distinguishing single nucleotide polymorphisms (SNP) from disease-causing mutations can be very tricky, particularly in huge genes such as *RYR1*, *NEB* or *TTN* (Ravenscroft et al. 2017). Knowing the frequency of the variant in "control" population databases (ExAC, 1000 Genomes, gnomAD) is very helpful for filtering the large amount of variants found by NGS techniques. In silico prediction tools (SIFT, Polyphen), which predict whether a missense variant is pathogenic for protein function, can also help the geneticist with pathogenicity assessment. Gene specific variation databases (for example, Leiden Open Variation Database or LOVD [www.lovd.nl]) are essential to collating disease-causing mutations around the world for rare diseases thus facilitating pathogenicity assessment of rare variants. However, false pathogenicity assessment in mutation databases occurs frequently and can have detrimental effects for the patient (MacArthur et al. 2014). Trio WES, in which the exome of the proband and the proband's two healthy parents is sequenced, has a significantly higher yield than sequencing the exome of the proband only. Indeed, trio WES is more sensitive for the detection of de novo and compound heterozygous variants (Lee et al. 2014). Recently, muscle RNA sequencing has demonstrated its efficacy at detecting a deep intronic mutation impacting splicing in the *COL6A1* gene of 27 patients (Cummings et al. 2017).

The clinician should always bear in mind that all the regions of the exome are not fully covered by WES and that targeted gene sequencing can be useful if the phenotype of the patient is strongly suggesting a mutation in a specific gene that is not fully covered by WES (Pena et al. 2017).

Targeted gene panels have the advantage of an increased depth of coverage, as well as the avoidance of incidental findings and their difficult management. WES has a lower coverage but allows the discovery of new genes for neuromuscular disorders and the expansion of the phenotypic spectrum associated with mutations in known genes.

NGS has some limitations that should be kept in mind when asking for genetic testing. Detection of gene deletions or duplications by NGS can be challenging. Gene deletions and duplications account for a considerable number of neuromuscular diseases that cannot be captured through NGS. 70% of the patients with DMD have single or multiple exon deletion or duplications. Multiplex ligation-dependent probe amplification (MLPA) remains the most widely used technique to accurately detect which exons are deleted or duplicated, a critical step for inclusion in exon-skipping clinical trials (Abbs et al. 2010). The diagnosis of SMA relies on the detection of an homozygous exon 7 deletion with or without exon 8 deletion in the *SMN1* gene. Evaluation of the number of *SMN2* copies is also useful for prognosis and inclusion in clinical trials. The criterion standard methods for a quantitative evaluation of *SMN1* and *SMN2* are MLPA and quantitative polymerase chain reaction (qPCR). New NGS approaches have been developed and can accurately detect *SMN1* deletions (Mercuri et al. 2017). Similarly, in myotubular myopathy (XLCNM), *MTM1* gene deletions or duplications represent 7% of the patients (Biancalana et al. 2017). Comparative genomic hybridization (CGH), which can accurately detect deletions or duplications, can thus be a very useful additional tool in the genetic workup of patients with a non-conclusive NGS analysis. Hopefully, in the near future, NGS techniques will allow a more accurate detection of gene deletions or duplications.

Similarly, NGS does not accurately detect triplet repeat expansions or deletions, which are found in several neuromuscular disorders such as myotonic dystrophy type 1 (CTG repeat expansion) or fascioscapulohumeral muscular dystrophy type 1 (D4Z4 repeat deletion). In myotonic dystrophy type 1, repeat-primed PCR is used to detect the presence of an expanded allele and southern blot is then use for the determination of the size of the expanded allele (Chakraborty et al. 2016).

## REFERENCES

Abbs S, Tuffery-Giraud S, Bakker E, Ferlini A, Sejersen T, Mueller CR (2010) Best practice guidelines on molecular diagnostics in Duchenne/Becker muscular dystrophies. *Neuromuscul Disord* 20: 422–427.

Alshaikh NM, Martinez JP, Pitt MC (2016) Perception of pain during electromyography in children: A prospective study. *Muscle Nerve* 54: 422–426.

Batten FE (1903) Three cases of myopathy, infantile type. *Brain* 27: 147–148.

Berardo A, DiMauro S, Hirano M (2010) A diagnostic algorithm for metabolic myopathies. *Curr Neurol Neurosci Rep* 10: 118–126.

Biancalana V, Scheidecker S, Miguet M, Laquerrière A, Romero NB, Stojkovic T et al. (2017) Affected female carriers of MTM1 mutations display a wide spectrum of clinical and pathological involvement: delineating diagnostic clues. *Acta Neuropathol* 134: 889–904.

Bönnemann CG, Wang CH, Quijano-Roy S, Deconinck N, Bertini E, Ferreiro A et al. (2014) Diagnostic approach to the congenital muscular dystrophies. *Neuromuscul Disord* 24: 289–311.

Campbell C, McMillan HJ, Mah JK, Tarnopolsky M, Selby K, McClure T et al. (2016) Myostatin inhibitor ACE-031 treatment of ambulatory boys with Duchenne muscular dystrophy: results of a randomized, placebo-controlled clinical trial. *Muscle Nerve* 55(4): 458–464. doi:10. 1002/mus.25268

Cejas CP, Serra MM, Galvez DFG, Cavassa EA, Taratuto AL, Vazquez GA et al. (2017) Muscle MRI in pediatrics: clinical, pathological and genetic correlation. *Pediatr Radiol* 47: 724–735.

Cetin E, Cuisset JM, Tiffreau V, Vallée L, Hurtevent JF, Thevenon A (2009) The value of electromyography in the aetiological diagnosis of hypotonia in infants and toddlers. *Ann Phys Rehabil Med* 52: 546–555.

Chakraborty S, Vatta M, Bachinski LL et al. (2016) Molecular diagnosis of myotonic dystrophy. *Curr Prot Hum Genet* 91(1): 9.29.1-9.29.19. doi.10.1002/cphg.22.

Chinnery PF (2014) Mitochondrial Disorders Overview, GeneReviews® [Internet]. Seattle (WA): University of Washington, Seattle; Last Update: 14 August 2014.

Clement E, Jungbluth H (2014) The congenital muscular dystrophies. In Hilton-Jones D, Turner MR (eds) *Oxford Textbook of Neuromuscular Disorders*, Oxford: Oxford University Press, pp. 229–242.

Cummings BB, Marshall JL, Tukiainen T, Lek M, Donkervoort S, Foley AR et al. (2017) Improving genetic diagnosis in Mendelian disease with transcriptome sequencing. *Sci Transl Med* 9: eaal5209.

de Greef JC, Lemmers RJLF, Camaño P, Day JW, Sacconi S, Dunand M et al. (2010) Clinical features of facioscapulohumeral muscular dystrophy 2. *Neurol* 75: 1548–1554.

Emeryk-Szajewska B, Kopeć J (2008) Electromyographic pattern in Duchenne and Becker muscular dystrophy. Part I: electromyographic pattern in subsequent stages of muscle lesion in Duchenne muscular dystrophy. *Electromyogr Clin Neurophysiol* 48: 265–277.

Eng GD, Binder H, Koch B (1984) Spinal muscular atrophy: experience in diagnosis and rehabilitation management of 60 patients. *Arch Phys Med Rehabil* 65: 549–553.

Foley AR, Quijano-Roy S, Collins J, Straub V, McCallum M, Deconinck N et al. (2013) Natural history of pulmonary function in collagen VI-related myopathies. *Brain* 136(Pt 12): 3625–3633.

Ghosh PS, Sorenson EJ (2015) Use of clinical and electrical myotonia to differentiate childhood myopathies. *J Child Neurol* 30: 1300–1306.

Gilbert A, Tassin JL (1984) [Surgical repair of the brachial plexus in obstetric paralysis]. *Chirurgie; memoires de l'Academie de chirurgie* 110: 70–5.

Ginsberg L (2014) Inherited metabolic neuropathies. In Hilton-Jones D, Turner MR (eds) *Oxford Textbook of Neuromuscular Disorders*, Oxford: Oxford University Press, pp. 85–90. doi.10.1093/med/9780199698073.003.0011.

Gospe SM Jr, Lazaro RP, Lava NS, Grootscholten PM, Scott MO, Fischbeck KH (1989) Familial X-linked myalgia and cramps: a nonprogressive myopathy associated with a deletion in the dystrophin gene. *Neurol* 39: 1277–1280.

Gowers WR (1879) Clinical lecture on pseudo-hypertrophic muscular paralysis. *Lancet* doi: 10.1016/S0140-6736(02)46375-1

Harris SR (2008) Congenital hypotonia: clinical and developmental assessment. *Dev Med Child Neurol* 50: 889–892.

Harris E, Topf A, Barresi R, Hudson J, Powell H, Tellez J et al. (2017) Exome sequences versus sequential gene testing in the UK highly specialised service for limb-girdle muscular dystrophy. *Orphanet J Rare Dis* 12: 151.

Hoffmann J (1893) Überchronische spinale Muskelatrophie im Kindesalter, auf familiärer Basis. *Dtsch Zeitschr Nervenheilk* 3: 427–470.

Hollingsworth KG, de Sousa PL, Straub V, Carlier PG (2012) Towards harmonization of protocols for MRI outcome measures in skeletal muscle studies: consensus recommendations from two TREAT-neuromuscular disorders NMR workshops, 2 May 2010, Stockholm, Sweden, 1–2 October 2009, Paris, France. *Neuromuscul Disord* 22(Suppl 2): S54–S67.

Hwang H, Lee JH, Choi YC (2017) Clinical characteristics of spinal muscular atrophy in Korea confirmed by genetic analysis. *yonsei Med J* 58: 1051–1054.

Jacob S, Viegas S, Hilton-Jones D (2014) Myasthenia gravis. In Hilton-Jones D, Turner MR (eds) *Oxford Textbook of Neuromuscular Disorders*, Oxford: Oxford University Press, pp. 184–194.

John J, John J, Medical Research Council (1984) Grading of muscle power: comparison of MRC and analogue scales by physiotherapists. *Int J Rehabil Res* 7: 173–181.

Karakis I, Liew W, Darras BT, Jones HR, Kang PB (2014) Referral and diagnostic trends in pediatric electromyography in the molecular era. *Muscle Nerve* 50: 244–249.

Kassardjian CD, Amato AA, Boon AJ, Childers MK, Klein CJ, AANEM Professional Practice Committee (2016) The utility of genetic testing in neuromuscular disease: A consensus statement from the AANEM on the clinical utility of genetic testing in diagnosis of neuromuscular disease. *Muscle Nerve* 54: 1007–1009.

Kugelberg E, Welander L (1956) Heredofamilial juvenile muscular atrophy simulating muscular dystrophy. *AMA Arch Neurol Psychiatry* 75: 500–509.

Laing NG, Laing BA, Meredith C, Wilton SD, Robbins P, Honeyman K et al. (1995) Autosomal dominant distal myopathy: linkage to chromosome 14. *Am J Hum Genet* 56: 422–427.

Lee H, Deignan JL, Dorrani N, Strom SP, Kantarci S, Quintero-Rivera F et al. (2014) Clinical exome sequencing for genetic identification of rare Mendelian disorders. *JAMA* 312: 1880–1887.

Leung DG (2017) Magnetic resonance imaging patterns of muscle involvement in genetic muscle diseases: a systematic review. *J Neurol* 264: 1320–1333.

Lev EI, Tur-Kaspa I, Ashkenazy I, Reiner A, Faraggi D, Shemer J et al. (1999) Distribution of serum creatine kinase activity in young healthy persons. *Clin Chim Acta* 279: 107–115.

Lurio JG, Peay HL, Mathews KD (2015) Recognition and management of motor delay and muscle weakness in children. *Am Fam Physician* 91: 38–44.

MacArthur DG, Manolio TA, Dimmock DP, Rehm HL, Shendure J, Abecasis GR et al. (2014) Guidelines for investigating causality of sequence variants in human disease. *Nature* 508: 469–476.

Maisami M, Freeman JM (1987) Conversion reactions in children as body language: a combined child psychiatry/neurology team approach to the management of functional neurologic disorders in children. *Pediatr* 80: 46–52.

Maloney MJ (1980) Diagnosing hysterical conversion reactions in children. *J Pediatr* 97: 1016–1020.

Marian AJ, van Rooij E, Roberts R (2016) Genetics and genomics of single-gene cardiovascular diseases: common hereditary cardiomyopathies as prototypes of single-gene disorders. *J Am Coll Cardiol* 68: 2831–2849.

Matthews E, Hanna M (2014) Skeletal muscle chanelopathies. In Hilton-Jones D, Turner MR (eds) *Oxford Textbook of Neuromuscular Disorders*, Oxford: Oxford University Press, pp. 316–325.

Mercuri E, Muntoni F (2012) The ever-expanding spectrum of congenital muscular dystrophies. *Ann Neurol* 72: 9–17.

Mercuri E, Finkel RS, Muntoni F, Wirth B, Montes J, Main M et al. (2017) Diagnosis and management of spinal muscular atrophy: Part 1: Recommendations for diagnosis, rehabilitation, orthopedic and nutritional care. *Neuromuscul Disord* 28(2): 103–115. doi: 10.1016/j.nmd.2017.11.005.

Moghadam-Kia S, Oddis CV, Aggarwal R (2016) Approach to asymptomatic creatine kinase elevation. *Cleve Clin J Med* 83: 37–42.

Montes J, Blumenschine M, Dunaway S, Alter AS, Engelstad K, Rao AK et al. (2013) Weakness and fatigue in diverse neuromuscular diseases. *J Child Neurol* 28: 1277–1283.

Muchir A, Worman HJ (2007) Emery-Dreifuss muscular dystrophy. *Curr Neurol Neurosci Rep* 7: 78–83.

Nevo Y, Topaloglu H (2002) 88th ENMC international workshop: childhood chronic inflammatory demyelinating polyneuropathy (including revised diagnostic criteria), Naarden, The Netherlands, December 8–10, 2000. *Neuromuscul Disord* 12: 195–200.

Oh SJ (2003) Pediatric nerve conduction studies. In Oh SJ (ed), *Clinical Electromyography, Nerve Conduction Studies*, 3rd edn. Philadelphia: Lippincott Williams and Wilkins.

Oskoui M, Jacobson L, Chung WK, Haddad J, Vincent A, Kaufmann P et al. (2008) Fetal acetylcholine receptor inactivation syndrome and maternal myasthenia gravis. *Neurol* 71: 2010–2012.

Pena LDM, Jiang YH, Schoch K, Spillmann RC, Walley N, Stong N et al. (2017) Undiagnosed Diseases Network Members, Goldstein DB, Shashi V Looking beyond the exome: a phenotype-first approach to molecular diagnostic resolution in rare and undiagnosed diseases. *Genet Med* 20: 464–469. doi.10.1038/gim.2017.128.

Pereon Y (2012) L'ENMG de l'enfant sans les pleurs. In Solal CV (ed) *XIIIemes Journées Francophones d'Electroneuromyographie*. Marseille: Sodal Editeur, pp. 93–125.

Pitt M (2008) Neurophysiological strategies for the diagnosis of disorders of the neuromuscular junction in children. *Dev Med Child Neurol* 50: 328–333.

Pitt M (2009) Workshop on the use of stimulation single fibre electromyography for the diagnosis of myasthenic syndromes in children held in the Institute of Child Health and Great Ormond Street Hospital for Children in London on April 24th, 2009. *Neuromuscul Disord* 19: 730–2.

Pitt M, Kang B (2015) Electromyography in Pediatrics. In Darras BT, Jones HR , Ryan MM, De Vivo DC (eds) *Neuromuscular Disorders of Infancy, Childhood and Adolescence, A Clinical Approach.* London: Elsevier. doi.10.1016/B978-0-12-417044-5.00003-2.

Pitt M (2011) Paediatric electromyography in the modern world: a personal view. *Dev Med Child Neurol* 53: 120–4.

Polat M, Tekgul H, Kilincer A, Tosun A, Terlemez S, Serdaroglu G et al. (2006) Electrodiagnostic pattern approach for childhood polyneuropathies. *Pediatr Neurol* 35: 11–17.

Potulska-Chromik A, Ryniewicz B, Aragon-Gawinska K, Kabzinska D, Seroka A, Lipowska M et al. (2016) Are electrophysiological criteria useful in distinguishing childhood demyelinating neuropathies? *J Peripher Nerv Syst* 21: 22–26.

Preston DC, Shapiro BE (2013) Approach to pediatric electromyography. In Preston DC, Shapiro BE (eds) *Electromyography and Neuromuscular Disorders Clinical–Electrophysiologic Correlations* 3rd edn. Philadephia: Elsevier.

Rabie M, Jossiphov J, Nevo Y (2007) Electromyography (EMG) accuracy compared to muscle biopsy in childhood. *J Child Neurol* 22: 803–808.

Ravenscroft G, Davis MR, Lamont P, Forrest A, Laing NG (2017) New era in genetics of early-onset muscle disease: breakthroughs and challenges. *Semin Cell Dev Biol* 64: 160–170.

Reilly MM, Rossor A (2014) Charcot–Marie–Tooth disease. In Hilton-Jones D, Turner MR (eds) *Oxford Textbook of Neuromuscular Disorders*, Oxford: Oxford University Press, pp. 61–74.

Schofield D, Alam K, Douglas L, Shrestha R, MacArthur DG, Davis M et al. (2017) Cost-effectiveness of massively parallel sequencing for diagnosis of paediatric muscle diseases. *NPJ Genom Med* 2: 4.

Shah DU, Darras BT, Markowitz JA, Jones HR Jr, Kang PB (2012) The spectrum of myotonic and myopathic disorders in a pediatric electromyography laboratory over 12 years. *Pediatr Neurol* 47: 97–100.

Skalsky AJ, McDonald CM (2012) Prevention and management of limb contractures in neuromuscular diseases. *Phys Med Rehabil Clin N Am* 23: 675–687.

Stern LZ, Bernick CS (1990) Muscle Cramps. In Walker HK, Dallas WH, Hurst JW *Clinical Methods: The History, Physical, and Laboratory Examinations*, 3rd edn. London: Butterworths, Chapter 53.

van Capelle CI, van der Meijden JC, van den Hout JMP, Jaeken J, Baethmann M, Voit T et al. (2016) Child-hood Pompe disease: clinical spectrum and genotype in 31 patients. *Orphanet J Rare Dis* 11: 65.

Vasta I, Kinali M, Messina S, Guzzetta A, Kapellou O, Manzur A, Cowan F, Muntoni F, Mercuri E (2005) Can clinical signs identify newborns with neuromuscular disorders? *J Pediatr* 146: 73–79.

Wagner KR, Fleckenstein JL, Amato AA, Barohn RJ, Bushby K, Escolar DM et al. (2008) A phase I/IItrial of MYO-029 in adult subjects with muscular dystrophy. *Ann Neurol* 63: 561–571.

Werdnig G (1891) Zwei früh infantile hereditare Fälle von progressiver Muskelatrophie unter dem Bilde der Dystrophie aber auf neurotischer Grundlage. *Arch Psych Nervenkrankh* 22: 437–480.

# 5
# THE IMPORTANCE OF EVALUATING FUNCTION IN NEUROMUSCULAR DISORDERS

*Anna G Mayhew*

## Introduction

Fundamental to a child's quality of life is the ability to participate in daily and social life within a given community. Participation, although not dependent on function, is certainly impacted by functional ability and for this reason assessment of motor performance/capacity is often included as part of a clinic visit. This is important for several reasons. Since timing is vital in planning management in children with neuromuscular diseases, it is beneficial to have instruments that can: (1) predict events such as loss of ambulation or inability to self-feed, (2) evaluate the effect of a given intervention such as orthotics or exercise, (3) assess change in functional ability over time in order to assess the rate of disease progression and particularly in clinical trials where novel therapies may impact functional ability. Understanding the context of any disability according to the International Classification of Function (ICF) (VanSant 2006) is also important. These domains (1) Body Functions and Structures; and (2) Activities and Participation, are often interdependent so that severe loss of muscle strength also means severe loss of activity and participation, but not always. For instance, a child with spinal muscular atrophy (SMA) II (able to sit but not walk) can have severe weakness and contractures but a high level of participation in school and socially, which means that to achieve a high level of "function" is not just dependent on physical elements but also includes a high level of cognition or motivation to function and adequate provision of equipment.

Functional ability in children with neuromuscular diseases (NMD) is an interaction of several physical components including muscle strength, contractures and hypermobility, growth, coordination of movements and the use of specific environments or aids to compensate for loss of muscle strength, or simply adaptation. Motivation to move is also important and is dependent on the child, family and the assessor to gain the best performance. This may be defined as pyschomodulation.

The ICF covers two areas: (1) Functioning and disability and (2) Contextual factors. This chapter primarily deals with the first area, which further describes three domains of function: Impairment, Activity and Participation (WHO, 2001). Participation, however, will be covered in greater depth in Chapter 20.

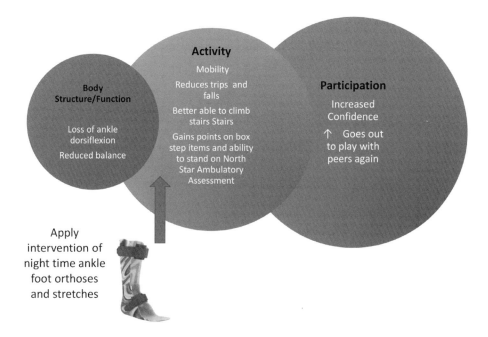

**Fig. 5.1.** Measuring impact of intervention according to the International Classification of Functioning, Disability and Health (ICF) classification on a young boy with duchenne muscular dystrophy. WHO (2001)

In neuromuscular disorders impairment is characterized by the loss of muscle strength (either pure loss of strength or change in weight or limb length where loss of strength becomes apparent) or range of motion (such as the ability to extend the knee or hyperextendable fingers), activity is defined as movements used to accomplish a task (such as rolling, walking or dressing) and participation is the ability to interact with peers and take part in social activities with other people (such as daily activities at home or in school) (Figure 5.1).

Assessment instruments are thus used for different purposes and different criteria of rigour may be applied when considering their suitability for a given situation. For example, in the clinical setting assessment needs to guide intervention. Loss of range of movement in the ankle joint as measured by a goniometer and functional ability such as ability to step off a step in an ambulant boy with Duchenne muscular dystrophy (DMD) may precipitate the prescription of night ankle foot orthoses (AFOs) and stretches. In a clinical trial reliable measurement of disease progression and the effect of therapeutic interventions requires not only clinically meaningful measures but also scientifically robust rating scales (Hobart et al. 2007) which must be able to capture meaningful change as a measurement tool (Walton et al. 2015). Rating scales often use response categories for a number of items to describe the underlying construct. For example the North Star Ambulatory Assessment (NSAA) has 17 items scored as 0, 1 or 2 to measure the construct of ambulatory performance in DMD. All 17 items should contribute to this measurement of ambulatory performance and the scores are defined as 0 – unable to perform the item, 1 – able but with some modification and 2 – able with no modification (Scott et al. 2012). The application of Rasch analysis to review this scale, however, revealed that the item "lifts head" did not fit this construct (a view supported by experts physiotherapists) so when the scale was linearized to create an accurate measurement tool – the item "lifts head" was deleted from the sum score (Mayhew et al. 2011; Mayhew et al. 2013). It remains in the scale, however, as clinically it has relevance to a boy's ability to rise from supine.

Psychometric methods help determine whether it is legitimate to produce a total scale score from a set of items and the extent to which this score is free from random error (reliability) and measure the construct they set out to measure (validity). Two main types of psychometric method exist often referred to as: traditional and modern (Hobart et al. 2007). Traditional methods are the most commonly used analyses for examining scale reliability and validity (Novick 1966). However, although traditional psychometric methods are widely used, they have several key limitations when evaluating a rating scales measurement properties. These include the following: (1) the data they generate are ordinal rather than interval; (2) scores for people and samples are scale dependent; and (3) scale properties such as reliability and validity are sample dependent. These limitations can be addressed by applying modern psychometric methods, such as Rasch analysis (Hobart and Cano 2009).

Importantly, modern methods focus on the relation between a person's measurement and their probability of responding to an item, rather than the relation between a person's measurement and their observed scale total score. Among the many benefits of this approach is that it leads to the legitimate summing of items to produce total scores and, in turn, total scores produce interval-level measures from ordinal-level rating scale data (Wright and Stone 1979; Wright 1989). This can help to improve the accuracy with which clinical change can be measured (Hobart and Cano 2009). These modern methods are becoming more frequently applied to patient centred outcome measures (PCOMs) – which includes clinical outcome assessments (COA) and clinician reported outcomes (ClinRO) – and are now likely to be applied to scales assessing performance in neuromuscular disorders (Cano et al. 2014; Klingels et al. 2016) and are helping our clinical tools gain greater validity and robustness (Ramsey et al. 2017).

It is also important when choosing an assessment for a given patient population, knowledge about floor and ceiling effects are known or explored to ensure that the instrument identifies changes regardless of level of ability. If a floor effect is present it means that the instrument cannot differentiate among the weaker patients and ceiling effect means the instrument does not identify differences among the stronger patients and would not pick up improvements if a child was already scoring the maximum number of "points". It is also possible that a scale measures a wide range of ability but "gaps" exist where measurement is poor because very few items measure at that level.

## Development of functional scales

Development of functional assessment instruments is a constantly evolving process, which began in the early 1960s. One of the first assessment instruments developed was a 10-stage classification of walking ability in children with DMD developed by Vignos, which is more commonly referred to as the Vignos Lower Extremity Functional Grade (Vignos et al. 1963). It is a practical clinical tool to determine the optimum time to manage boys with DMD using orthopedic surgery or long leg braces. It is still widely used clinically to broadly determine ambulatory function but was never validated using traditional or modern psychometrics. This is also the case for the Brooke Upper Extremity Functional Grade first published by Brooke in 1982 (Lord et al. 1987), which broadly describes arm function. These scales are examples of instruments which use ordinal categories to define broad function and can be useful in clinical practice or to determine the stage of a disease but generally are not sensitive enough to detect change in clinical trials. However, recent work has used a similar approach by combining broad but clinically meaningful categories, which has then been usefully mapped onto cost of illness and health-related quality of life data for DMD (Landfeldt et al. 2015).

## Disease specific measures

SPINAL MUSCULAR ATROPHY

- Hammersmith Functional Motor Scale Expanded (HFMSE) and Hammersmith Functional Motor Scale (HFMS) – ClinRO
- Hammersmith Functional Motor Scale Modified (HFMSM) – ClinRO
- Revised Hammersmith Scale for SMA (RHS) – ClinRO
- Upper Limb Module for SMA and Revised Upper Limb Module (RULM) – ClinRO
- Children's Hospital of Philadelphia Infant Test of Neuromuscular Disorders (CHOP INTEND) – ClinRO
- Test of Infant Motor Performance (TIMP), Test of Infant Motor Performance Screening Items (TIMPSI) – ClinRO.

DUCHENNE MUSCULAR DYSTROPHY

- North Star Ambulatory Assessment for DMD (NSAA) – ClinRO
- Performance of Upper Limb Module for DMD (Performance of Upper Limb (PUL) for DMD) – ClinRO
- Egen Klassifikation (EK) and Egen Klassifikation version 2 (EK2) – mixture of patient-reported outcome measure (PROM) and ClinRO
- PROM-Upper (PROM).

GENERIC SCALES

- Motor Function Measure for neuromuscular disease (MFM) – ClinRO
- Gross Motor Function Measure for Cerebral Palsy (GMFM) – ClinRO
- Activlim – PROM
- PEDI-CAT – PROM.

TIMED TESTS

- Time to run or walk 10m, climb four stairs and get to standing from lying supine
- Six-minute walk distance (6MWD)
- Timed up & go test (TUG).

In this section we focus on the different assessment instruments used to assess function in terms of impairment and activity in children with neuromuscular disease.

The assessment instruments are presented according to their relevance for two disorders, SMA and DMD as they capture a significant proportion of children with NMD. However, many of these scales and timed tests are relevant and clinically useful in other neuromuscular diseases. For example, the Hammersmith Functional Motor Scale Expanded can be used to assess motor performance in congenital muscular dystrophies providing contractures and their impact are also assessed, or sections of the GMFM may prove useful in capturing the ability of an undiagnosed neuromuscular disorder. Other disorders which result in loss of function perhaps later in life such as limb-girdle muscular dystrophies will require more demanding assessments which are currently under preparation. In the meantime – simple timed tests may be useful.

Each assessment/rating scale will be described according to:

- the underlying conceptual framework or measurement framework
- domain of ICF
- disease/disorder specificity
- level of function/age appropriate for
- methods and equipment required and any relevant training available
- evidence of psychometric robustness (validity, reliability) and ability to predict future loss of milestones, identify changes in relation to disease progression and responsiveness to treatment
- normal reference values
- clinical meaningfulness and relevance.

## Gross motor scales

VIGNOS LOWER EXTREMITY GRADE – CLINICIAN REPORTED OUTCOMES

*Measurement framework*: A 10 stage classification in DMD. It contains eight grades of walking and standing ability and two grades of non-ambulatory activity (Vignos et al. 1963).

*ICF domain*: Activity

*Disorder*: Developed for DMD, but also used in SMA

*Level of function*: *Ambulatory* and non-ambulatory

*Methods/Training*: None

*Psychometric evaluation*: None

*Normal reference values*: Natural history reference values in DMD (Henricson et al. 2013; McDonald et al. 1995)

*Clinical relevance*: It is useful for determining intervention (such as bracing, surgery or physiotherapy) in ambulatory boys with DMD (Vignos et al. 1963); however it is unlikely to be sensitive enough to guide intervention in the non-ambulatory stage of DMD, as it only has two functional grades.

BROOKE UPPER EXTREMITY GRADE – CLINICIAN REPORTED OUTCOMES

*Measurement framework*: A classification of upper extremity movements in 6 grades (1 = normal simultaneous abduction of both arms and 6 = no useful function of hands).

Was extended with 3 grades to increase differentiation among stronger patients (Mcdonald et al. 2013)

*ICF domain*: Activity

*Disorder*: Developed for DMD but also useful in SMA

*Level of function*: All ranges and ages

*Methods/Training*: None

*Psychometric evaluation*: None

*Normal reference values*: None. Natural history values in DMD (Henricson et al. 2013)

*Clinical relevance*: A useful but imprecise tool for assessing upper extremity function, which may also be applied in other NMD with proximal loss of muscle strength. However, it is hampered by ceiling effects in ambulatory patients and floor effects among very weak non-ambulatory patients with DMD or SMA. This limits is application. The Performance of Upper Limb (PUL) – see below – has included a modified Brooke scale.

THE DUCHENNE MUSCULAR DYSTROPHY FUNCTIONAL ABILITY SELF-ASSESSMENT TOOL (DMDSAT) VERSION 2.0 – PATIENT-REPORTED OUTCOME MEASURE

*Measurement framework*: A patient-reported outcome measure designed to measure functional ability in patients with DMD. It asked a boy or young man to grade walking ability (grades 0–5), arm function (grades 0–6), ability to transfer and need for respiratory support to produce a "global" measure of functional ability (Landfeldt et al. 2015)

*ICF domain*: Activity

*Disorder*: Developed for DMD specifically

*Level of function*: All ranges and ages

*Methods/Training*: None. Can be completed by family or individual

*Psychometric evaluation*: Modern psychometric evaluation conducted on UK sample and was used to map cost of illness and health-related quality of life data for DMD (Landfeldt et al. 2015).

*Normal reference values*: None.

*Clinical relevance*: Useful and simple method for assessing functional ability and easily completed by family or carer. Suitable for grading function for the breadth of the disease and will be more descriptive than those used in the standards of care document such as early non-ambulatory and late non-ambulatory (Bushby et al. 2010).

## Spinal muscular atrophy

HAMMERSMITH FUNCTIONAL MOTOR SCALE (HFMS) – CLINICIAN REPORTED OUTCOMES

*Measurement framework*: Motor performance scale as measured by a 20 items, with each item scored 0–2 with 0 defined as unable, 1 able with some adaptation and 2 – fully able with no modification. They are ordered in item difficulty and enable you to assess to a certain extent the level of ability seen in type II SMA from "just able to sit" to "standing and stepping".

*ICF domain*: Activity

*Disorder*: Spinal muscular atrophy (SMA)

*Level of function*: Non-ambulatory

*Methods/Training*: Requires manual and worksheets available. Training preferable. Equipment required:preferably plinth, floor mat is useful. Time to complete measurement tool: 10 to 15 minutes with a co-operative child.

*Psychometric evaluation*: In relation to disease (SMA), age (more than 29 months) and function in relation to disease (SMA), age (more than 29 months) and function level (limited mobility). Has well proven reliability inter-rater and inter-observer validity in content, and construct, predictive validity and sensitivity to change. Reliably used in children above the age of 30 months. Inter-observer reliability of the scale and stability of the scale over time in a cohort of 90 non-ambulant children with type II or III SMA (Mercuri et al. 2006; Main et al. 2003; Mazzone et al. 2014). Modern psychometric analysis reveals some weakness in the scale as a measurement tool (Cano et al. 2014) which is true of all associated scales in SMA.

*Measurement properties*: Ordinal scale, recorded by clinician

*Normal and reference values*: *Range of scores* from maximal to minimal function (40–0, 40 being the highest score).

*Clinical relevance*: Provides information on motor ability and clinical progression. Although it has issues with floor and ceiling effects: a floor effect in younger patients who are very weak (Werlauff et al. 2010) and a ceiling effect in ambulatory patients although it was not designed for this group (O'Hagen et al. 2007). This scale is validated in Spanish (Febrer et al. 2011). http://www.treat-nmd.eu/downloads/file/oms/ominfo/ROM7.2.OMP.0002.pdf

HAMMERSMITH FUNCTIONAL MOTOR SCALE EXPANDED (HFMSE) – CLINICIAN REPORTED OUTCOMES

*Measurement framework*: Items on the original HFMS were expanded to capture higher functioning SMA patients using 13 relevant additional items adapted from the Gross Motor Function Measure (GMFM), with their scoring adapted to a three-point scale as in the original version. A higher score indicates a higher level of function. This version includes items that capture kneeling and transition and ability on stairs.

*ICF domain*: Activity

*Disorder*: Spinal muscular atrophy type III and II with high functioning

*Level of function*: Ambulatory and non-ambulatory. Limited upper limb functional ability.

*Methods/Training*: Requires manual and worksheets,which are standardized and available. Training preferable.

Time of administration averaged 15–20 minutes. Equipment required four stairs and a bench is useful.

*Psychometric evaluation*: Traditional psychometric methods have been used to assess the HFMSE. Validated in relation to disease (SMA II and III with high functional level). Concurrent validity has been examined between the HFMSE and the GMFM (Glanzman et al. 2011) and HFMSE and MFM (Mazzone et al. 2014). Good test-retest (intra-rater) reliability. The HFMSE demonstrates significant associations with established measures of function, strength, and genotype, and discriminates patients based on function, diagnostic category, and bi-level positive airway pressure need. The HFMSE is a valid, time-efficient outcome measure for clinical trials in SMA types II and III and has been confirmed as a suitable clinical endpoint in this setting (Mercuri et al. 2017)

*Measurement properties*: Ordinal scale. Recorded by observer.

*Normal and reference values*: Range of scores from maximal to minimal function (66–0, 66 being the highest score)

*Clinical relevance*: Assessment with high level functioning in SMA II and III. Clinical meaningfulness has been demonstrated through focus groups (Pera et al. 2017) http://columbiasma.org/docs/cme-2010/Hammersmith%20Functional%20Motor%20Scale%20Expanded%20for%20SMA%20Type%20II%20and%20III%20-%20Manual%20of%20Procedures.pdf

HAMMERSMITH FUNCTIONAL MOTOR SCALE MODIFIED (MHFMS) – CLINICIAN REPORTED OUTCOMES

*Measurement framework*: This is only a slightly modified version of the original HFMS where the items were reordered to make administration easier and a manual more clearly defined administration. Item order was modified to minimize position changes and to decrease fatigue and undue stress on the children during testing (Krosschell et al. 2006)

*ICF domain*: Activity

*Disorder*: Spinal muscular atrophy type II

*Level of function*: non-ambulatory

*Psychometric evaluation*: Demonstrated reliability and validity in children with SMA older than 2 years of age (Krosschell et al. 2006). Test-retest reliability of the MHFMS in children with SMA type II who were less than 30 months of age was confirmed (Krosschell et al. 2011).

In addition the ability of typically developing children to successfully achieve all MHFMS skills by 12 months of age, suggests that after 12–15 months of age the MHFMS can be used with minimal risk being adversely influence by developmental progression (Krosschell et al. 2013).

*Measurement properties*: Ordinal scale. Recorded by observer.

*Normal and reference values*: Range of scores from 0–40

*Clinical relevance*: As HFMS. http://smaoutcomes.org/hammersmith_manual/manual_1.html

REVISED HAMMERSMITH SCALE (RHS) – CLINICIAN REPORTED OUTCOMES

*Measurement framework*: The development of this scale was to address some of the measurement issues of the HFMSE as identified by Rasch analysis (Cano et al. 2014) and improve the sensitivity of the scale to detect functional change observed with an evolving phenotype. It contains similar items to the original HFMSE as well as additional items from the NSAA. The scale consists of 36 item with most items scored as 0 (unable), 1 (able with adaptation) or 2 (able). A higher score denoting a higher level of function. It includes a timed rise from floor test and 10 metre walk/run test and also captures developmental milestones as outlined by WHO.

*ICF domain*: Activity

*Disorder*: SMA

*Level of function*: Ambulatory and non-ambulatory. Children and adults

*Methods/Training*: Requires stopwatch and box step and plinth/bed for assessment. Manual and worksheets available. Training preferable.

*Psychometric evaluation*: Modern psychometric methods have been used to assess the RHS for SMA in an international cohort as part of an iterative process and show the scale to be sufficiently robust (Ramsey et al. 2017) however, its ability to detect change over time needs to be confirmed.

*Normal reference values*: Not published

*Clinical relevance*: Items reflect many activities related to activities of daily life for children and young people.

CHILDREN'S HOSPITAL OF PHILADELPHIA INFANT TEST OF NEUROMUSCULAR DISORDERS – CLINICIAN REPORTED OUTCOMES

*Measurement framework*: Children's Hospital of Philadelphia Infant Test of Neuromuscular Disorders (CHOP INTEND) is a validated, 16-item scale with a score range of 0–64 which has been shown to be reliable in SMA type I patients (Glanzman et al. 2010; Finkel et al. 2014). CHOP INTEND was developed in part from the Test of Infant Motor Performance (TIMP; see Test of Infant Motor Performance section) and was designed to measure motor function in weak infants with neuromuscular disease. It includes both active movements, spontaneous or goal-directed, and elicited reflexive movements, and assesses head, neck, trunk, and proximal and distal limb strength. CHOP INTEND does not include respiratory or feeding assessments, but it has been structured to move from easiest to hardest. The grading includes lower scores (gravity eliminated) and higher scores (antigravity movements). It should be noted, however, that it does not include sitting or weight bearing, so it measures motor function below the sitting milestone.

*ICF domain*: Activity

*Disorder*: SMA type I and other infant presentations of very weak neuromuscular disorders

*Level of function*: Infants 0–2 years of age depending on how weak and how big they are.

*Methods/Training*: Firm surface for examination. It can be completed quite quickly depending on the behavioural state of the infant. They are only placed in prone for a short period of time and at the end of the testing procedure.

*Psychometric evaluation*: CHOP has been shown to be valid and reliable (Allan M. Glanzman et al. 2011; Glanzman et al. 2010). A CHOP INTEND score of approximately 20–22 points is seen in the typical symptomatic SMA type I infant. Two studies have confirmed that no infants with two copies of *SMN2* had a baseline value over 40 points (Finkel et al. aolb et al. 2016). There appears to be no correlation between CHOP INTEND scores and age in the SMA or control cohorts. It has been used as a clinical endpoint in SMA I trials which have demonstrated efficacy (Maharshi and Hasan 2017).

*Normal reference values*: Comparison of SMA infants with healthy controls has been conducted (Kolb et al. 2016).

*Clinical Relevance*: This is a useful and practical scale to perform in weak infants with neuromuscular disorders. It is short and therefore better tolerated than some scales.

*Proforma*: http://columbiasma.org/docs/cme-2010/CHOP%20INTEND%20for%20SMA%20Type%20I%20-%20Score%20Sheet.pdf

*Manual*: http://columbiasma.org/docs/cme-2010/CHOP-INTEND-for-SMA-Type-I-Manual-of-Procedures.pdf

TEST OF INFANT MOTOR PERFORMANCE (TIMP), TEST OF INFANT MOTOR PERFORMANCE SCREENING ITEMS (TIMPSI) – CLINICIAN REPORTED OUTCOMES

*Measurement framework*: Test of Infant Motor Performance (TIMP) is a motor performance scale validated for use in preterm infants less than 4 months of age and includes elicited and observed motor assessments. Because it is sensitive to age-related development and discriminates between those infants at low and high risk for motor problems, it predicts gross motor developmental delay in preterm infants. The TIMP has been shown to be a reliable test in type I SMA infants (Finkel et al. 2008); however, it takes a long time to perform and is quite fatiguing therefore the Test of Infant Motor Performance screening items (TIMPSI), which includes only the screening items, has also been used in SMA type 1. TIMPSI is a 29-item, 99-point scale. It tests rolling and crawling but does not test sitting.

*ICF domain*: Activity

*Disorder*: SMA type I and possible other infant presentations of neuromuscular disorders

*Level of function*: Infants

*Methods/Training*: Firm surface for examination. Requires quite a lot of position change/ strongly overlaps with items on the CHOP INTEND but scoring is not absolutely comparable. Training preferable.

*Psychometric evaluation*: TIMP and TIMPSI have been shown to be valid and reliable in type I SMA (Krosschell et al. 2013; Finkel et al. 2008). In the NeuroNEXT SMA infant biomarker study it was used to screen SMA and healthy infants' motor performance. Those who scored less than 41 on the TIMPSI were then evaluated using CHOP INTEND, and patients who scored 41 or greater on the TIMPSI were evaluated using the Alberta Infant Motor Scale (AIMS). SMA infants with two copies of *SMN2* had an average TIMPSI score of 27.2 (SD = 8.0, n = 16, range = 15–49). There was no correlation with age, and no SMA infant with two copies of *SMN2* had a TIMPSI score greater than 51. It was also part of the wider SMA scale evaluation (Cano et al. 2014).

*Normal reference values*: Comparison of SMA infants with healthy controls has been conducted for the TIMPSI (Kolb et al. 2016).

*Clinical relevance*: These are potential scales for assessing infants with neuromuscular disorders. However,they include many items tested in prone, which is not tolerated well by type I infants.

## Duchenne muscular dystrophy

NORTH STAR AMBULATORY ASSESSMENT (NSAA) – CLINICIAN REPORTED OUTCOMES

*Measurement framework*: This scale aims to measure the concept of ambulatory motor performance in DMD. It consists of 17 items with each item scored as 0 (unable), 1 (able with adaptation) or 2 (able). A higher score denoting a higher level of function. It includes a timed rise from floor test and 10 metre walk/run test. A revised order version now exists (NSAA-RO) which has exactly the same content but the items have been reordered so less position change is needed to conduct the test in the correct sequence. In addition its ability to assess those younger than fours years of age has been conducted and a revision produced to account for developmental progression (Mercuri et al. 2016).

*ICF domain*: Activity

*Disorder*: DMD – ambulatory

*Level of function*: Ambulatory. Children and young men

*Methods/Training*: Requires stopwatch and box step and plinth/bed for assessment. Manual and worksheets available. Training preferable. http://www.muscular-dystrophy.org/ assets/0002/5040/North_Star_Ambulatory_assessment.pdf

*Psychometric evaluation*: The development and reliability of this stage and disease specific scale are described (Scott et al. 2012) and validity in relationship to timed tests and 6 minute walk distance have been published as has reliability in a multicenter study (Mazzone et al. 2009). In addition modern psychometric evaluation, specifically Rasch analysis, has endorsed its suitability and robustness (Mayhew et al. 2011). Its responsiveness (in relation to steroid regime) has also been confirmed and a transformed, linearized version of the scale has been created which means that change scores are now comparable across the scale (10 points). A minimally important difference (MID) has been calculated on this linearized version of approximately 10 points (Mayhew et al. 2013). It has also been shown to detect change over time in a longitudinal study (Ricotti et al. 2016).

*Normal reference values*: By the age of 4 a maximum score should be achieved in typically developing children.

*Clinical relevance*: MID values are linked to functional gains or losses in motor ability. A change in 10 points on a transformed linearized scale equates to loss of ability to rise from the floor independently, to hop on one leg or stand still (Mayhew et al. 2013).

PERFORMANCE OF UPPER LIMB MODULE FOR DUCHENNE MUSCULAR DYSTROPHY (PUL FOR DMD) – CLINICIAN REPORTED OUTCOMES

*Measurement framework*: Following on from the development of the NSAA it was clear that a detailed module that would plot the progression of arm function was also required for late ambulatory and non-ambulatory boys and men with DMD. This test was specifically designed to measure motor performance in the upper limb. The scale was devised using items from several other sources as well as including novel items as current scales were considered inadequate for this population (Mazzone et al. 2012). It was created using patient and family group input (Mercuri et al. 2012) as well as exploratory Rasch analysis to explore item suitability (A. Mayhew et al. 2013). Ongoing development has further refined items to increase its reliability and validity in this population.

*ICF domain*: Activity

*Disorder*: DMD

*Level of function*: Late ambulatory to late stage non-ambulatory

*Methods/Training*: A small amount of standardized equipment is required. No formal training course currently exist

*Psychometric evaluation*: Reliability studies have been conducted (Pane et al. 2014). Further work needs to done on item scoring and responsiveness as well as natural history data but it has been used comparatively with the 6MWT (Pane et al. 2014)

*Normal reference values*: Full score in typically developing children achieved by age of 5 years (Pane et al. 2014)

*Clinical relevance*: The involvement of patient groups helped establish the clinical relevance of items. Some items such as bringing a cup to the mouth clearly have practical application to daily life.

E GEN K LASSIFIKATIONAND E GEN K LASSIFIKATION VERSION 2 – PATIENT-REPORTED OUTCOME MEASURES AND OBSERVATION

*Measurement framework*: The test has been developed to reflect the natural history of DMD in the non-ambulatory stage and aims to evaluate the overall physical function in non-ambulatory people with DMD or SMA. It focuses on particular changes that can benefit from intervention to preserve function (including respiratory support, the ability to drive a wheelchair). Egen Klassifikation (EK) consists of 10 items, each scored on four levels (0–3) with a higher score reflecting lower ability. The items cover activities with arms and trunk, the ability to cough and speak, physical well being related to symptoms of hypoventilation. Egen Klassifikation version 2 (EK2) consists of the same 10 items with the addition of seven new items focusing on problems with eating, using the hands, fatigue and holding the head up. EK2 has shown to be more discriminative than Egen Klassifikation among the weakest patients with DMD and SMA.

*ICF domain*: Egen Klassifikation and Egen Klassifikation 2 are composite scales including items from body – as well as activity/participation level.

*Disorder*: DMD and SMA

*Level of function*: Early non-ambulatory to late stage non-ambulatory

*Methods/Training*: Egen Klassifikationand Egen Klassifikation 2 are performed as a dialogue between evaluator and the patient and his relatives and an observation and assessment of the patient when sitting in his wheelchair.It takes approximately 10–15 minutes to discuss items with and observe the patient. A manual is available. EK, EK2 and manual are available in several other languages (Fagoaga et al. 2015; Alemdaroğlu et al. 2014).

*Psychometric evaluation*: Egen Klassifikation and Egen Klassifikation 2 have been tested for reliability (Steffensen et al. 2002) and different aspects of validity and sensitivity (Steffensen et al. 2001). It is strongly related to muscle strength (Steffensen et al. 2001) and in SMA it is also strongly related to FVC%. Sum of scores combined with FVC% predicted the need of assisted ventilation in DMD (Lyager, Steffensen and Juhl 1995). Exploratory Rasch analysis has been performed on EK2 in relation to SMA (Cano et al. 2014) and DMD to explore item robustness as a measurement tool. Preliminary results of that analysis indicate that reliability is acceptable and that EK2 covers more than one construct.

*Normal reference values*: None. Longitudinal data on DMD and SMA exist (Steffensen et al. 2001).

*Clinical relevance*: The scale is designed to reflect a person's own opinion of his functional ability, which is clarified by the evaluators observation. The scale can predict and help in evaluating management such as scoliosis surgery, respiratory support or changes to a wheelchair in non-ambulatory patients with DMD or SMA. It was developed in co-operation with patients.

PATIENT-REPORTED OUTCOME MEASURE – UPPER (PROM-UPPER)

*Measurement framework*: A patient-reported outcome measure (PROM) assessing upper limb function related to activities of daily living (ADL) that cannot be observed in a clinical setting. It includes a gross motor measure (DMD Functional Ability Self-Assessment Tool [DMD-SAT]) to capture the ability of the individual. It contains 32 items covering four domains of ADL (food, self-care, household and environment, leisure and communication). It was developed with the involvement of different stakeholders to ensure clinical relevance.

*ICF domain*: Activity

*Disorder*: DMD

*Level of function*: Ambulatory and non-ambulatory

*Methods/Training*: Simple questionnaire which includes the DMD-SAT. No training required.

*Psychometric evaluation*: The scale has demonstrated good reliability using traditional and modern methods. It shows good internal consistency and unidimensionality (Klingels et al. 2016)

*Measurement properties*: Ordinal scale completed by individual or carer.

*Normal and reference values*: Not published.

*Clinical relevance*: Useful tool that can better evaluate ability of boys and young men to perform ADL. Could be applied outside of the clinical setting to capture functional ability in the home setting.

MOTOR FUNCTION MEASURE FOR NEUROMUSCULAR DISEASE (MFM) – CLINICIAN REPORTED OUTCOMES

*Measurement framework*: The original Motor Function Measure (MFM) is a generic neuromuscular scale consisting of 32 items suitable for ambulatory and non-ambulatory individuals between the age of 6–62 years. There is a version with a reduced number of items (20) designed for use in children under six years of age (de Lattre et al. 2013). All items are scored on a four-point scale. 0 – cannot initiate the task, 1 – partially performs the task,

2 – performs the movement incompletely,or completely but imperfectly, 3 – performs the task fully and "normally". Individual item scoring are included in a detailed manual. Items belong to one of three different dimensions: standing and transfers (D1) axial and proximal motor ability (D2) distal motor ability (D3).

*ICF domain*: Activity

*Disorder*: Neuromuscular disease

*Level of function*: Ambulatory and non-ambulatory

*Methods/Training*: *It takes approximately* 30 to 50 minutes in total to complete. Equipment is specified in the user's manual. Some objects must be made available such as a tennis ball, coins, a CD. Training is required.

*Psychometric evaluation*: Validated with patients from 6 to 60 years old, diagnosed with a range of disorders including DMD, Becker muscular dystrophy, facio-scapulo-humeral dystrophy, limb-girdle muscular dystrophy, congenital muscular dystrophy, congenital myopathy, myotonic dystrophy, spinal muscular atrophy or hereditary motor and sensory neuropathy (Bérard et al. 2005). Responsiveness in SMA has also been evaluated (Vuillerot et al. 2013; Vuillerot et al. 2012) as well as in DMD (Vuillerot et al. 2010) and has been used longitudinally in a small sample (Vuillerot et al. 2013). The scale is generally reliable (Bérard et al. 2005) however its internal robustness as a measurement tool for SMA specifically has been raised as an issue along with all key scales used in this condition (Cano et al. 2014)

*Measurement properties*: Scale ordinal. Recorded by observer. Calculation of percentage score on dimension and total score sum as a percentage.

*Clinical relevance*: The MFM may also help to predict the lost of walk for patients with DMD. The MFM-20 appeared to be more sensitive in the very weak patients perhaps due to the inclusion of a distal domain. For particular disorders some items will not be relevant and may cause unnecessary fatigue. http://www.motor-function-measure.org/home.aspx

GROSS MOTOR FUNCTION MEASURE FOR CEREBRAL PALSY (GMFM) – CLINICIAN REPORTED OUTCOMES

*Measurement framework*: The original Gross Motor Function Measure (GMFM) consisted of an 88 item scale with a shortened version consisting of 66 items. All items are scored on a four-point scale. 0 – cannot initiate the task, 1 – partially performs the task, 2 – performs the movement incompletely, or completely but imperfectly, 3 – performs the task fully and "normally". Items belong to one of five different dimensions: A – lying and rolling, B – sitting, C – crawling and kneeling, D – standing, E – walking, running and jumping.

*ICF domain*: Activity

*Disorder*: Originally for Cerebral Palsy but has been applied in neuromuscular disorders including a clinical trial in SMA (Chen et al. 2010) and also in Pompe disease.

*Level of function*: Ambulatory and non-ambulatory

*Methods/Training*: The necessary equipment, specified in the user's manual, is usually found in a physiotherapy department. A small bench is useful for younger children. Standard stairs are also beneficial. A manual is available.

*Psychometric evaluation*: Mainly in Cerebral Palsy (Palisano et al. 2000; Russell et al. 2000) but also in SMA (Iannaccone and American Spinal Muscular Atrophy Randomized Trials 2002; Nelson et al. 2006).

*Measurement properties*: Scale ordinal

*Clinical relevance*: Lengthy to complete and some domains maybe inappropriate. Care must be made not to induce fatigue. Many of the items which measure right and left may not be necessary to capture clinically and others may be assumed (i.e. If they can walk up stairs no need to assess their ability to crawl up the stairs). Potentially useful if no disease specific tool is available but any sum scores should be treated with caution.

TIME TO RUN/WALK 10M (10M WALK, RUN), CLIMB FOUR STAIRS, DESCEND FOUR STAIRS AND TIME TO RISE FROM FLOOR

*Measurement framework*: The measurements are performed in seconds usually to one decimal place (i.e. 10.2 seconds) and used in children from the age of two years upwards.

*ICF domain*: Activity and participation

*Disorder*: DMD and SMA mainly but not exclusively.

*Level of function*: *Ambulatory* children

*Methods/Training*: No training is needed, but to ensure comparable data the standardization of starting and ending positions, clothing, footwear (usually barefoot) as well as instruction and encouragement of the child should be repeatable from test to test. A stopwatch should be used for all assessments and for clinical trials this should be a calibrated version. For the 10 metre walk/run test a free and quiet indoor area should be used preferably with a standard flooring and preferably not a carpet. For climbing stairs, four stairs of 14cm height and with rails in both sides are needed to get up as well as down the stairs. Getting to standing from supine needs a clean floor for the child to lie on.

*Psychometric evaluation*: Reliability and validity are tested in traditional ways. Modern analysis is not necessary as the measurement properties are on an interval scale and can be treated with parametric statistics.

*Normal reference values*: Natural history data available in DMD (McDonald et al. 2013b).

*Clinical relevance*: The assessments can assist in predicting the time for loss of major milestones such as loss of ambulation and therefore useful for planning treatment to preserve ambulation or the changes in the home for a child using wheelchair. This is particularly true of the rise from floor (RFF) test in DMD which can be a useful predictor of loss of ambulation (Mazzone et al. 2016).

SIX-MINUTE WALK DISTANCE FOR USE IN SPINAL MUSCULAR ATROPHY AND DUCHENNE MUSCULAR DYSTROPHY

*Measurement framework*: The Six-Minute Walk Distance (6MWT) aims to measure weakness (maximum distance walked without running or jogging) in DMD and SMA and fatigue (the ratio of distance walked in sixth minute to distance walked in first minute) in SMA (Montes et al. 2011; 2013). It has gained prominence as a primary outcome measure in clinical trials in DMD and is being applied in SMA trials also.

*ICF domain*: Activity/participation

*Disorder*: SMA and DMD

*Level of function*: Ambulant individuals

*Methods/Training*: A modified protocol exists based on original ATS guidelines (ATS 2002; McDonald et al. 2010). Usually a 25m course is used in NMD. Care should be taken that the correct protocol is applied as DMD studies often include full encouragement to be given throughout the test whereas the SMA protocol delivers feedback on a minute by minute basis with no additional encouragement (Montes et al. 2013).

*Psychometric evaluation*: The 6MWD has been shown to be safe and reliable in ambulatory boys with DMD (McDonald et al. 2010; Mcdonald, et al. 2013b). They walk much shorter distances relative to healthy boys and 6MWD can be correlated with age and height (Goemans et al. 2013). Longitudinal data in DMD show clinically meaningful change in 6MWD to be in the range of 20 to 30 metres, which can serve as a targeted treatment effect in 12-month trials in ambulatory DMD (McDonald et al. 2013b) and has been correlated with PROMs (Henricson et al. 2013). It has also been shown to be valid and reliable and sensitive to change in SMA (Mazzone et al. 2013; Dunaway Young et al. 2016).

*Normal reference values*: Total distance walked in 6 minutes has been standardized for age and sex in DMD and percent predicted values can summarize weakness (Goemans et al. 2013).

*Clinical relevance*: The ability to walk distances is relevant in many conditions but does not necessarily equate to that ability in the community. Not all clinical areas will have a suitable long corridor (requires a clear, quiet 30 metre corridor).

TIMED UP & GO TEST (TUG)

*Measurement framework*: The measurement is performed in seconds to the nearest tenth of a second (i.e. 7.8 seconds) and is particularly useful in older children who are more able.

*ICF domain*: Activity and participation

*Disorder*: SMA and others such as a Becker muscular dystrophy (BMD) or Limb-girdle muscular dystrophy (LGMD)

*Level of function*: Ambulatory children

*Methods/Training*: No training is needed, but to ensure comparable data the standardization of starting and ending positions, clothing, footwear as well as instruction and encouragement of the child should be identical from test to test. A stopwatch should be used for all assessments. The chair (standard with or without arms) has a maker line placed on the floor exactly 3 metres from the front legs of the chair. The child is asked to stand up, go as fast as they can and cross the marker, turn around and sit back down again.

*Psychometric evaluation*: The Timed Up & Go Test (TUG) has been shown to be useful in SMA (Dunaway et al. 2014)

*Normal reference values*: Not available.

*Clinical relevance*: The test is useful for high functioning ambulant children with NMD and as it includes a rise from chair and a turn has clinical relevance. It is also a good item for transitioning youngsters.

**Key points**

- Clinical outcome measures must be well defined and exhibit adequate measurement properties to assess change and potentially efficacy in NMDs.
- The importance of robust and meaningful patient centred outcome measures cannot be overstated in the current climate of advances in clinical trials and treatments, evolving phenotypes and greater expectations for standards of care around the globe.
- Making the most of our current measures and aspiring to more robust measure will require the involvement of multi-stakeholders with patient groups at the forefront (Morel and Cano 2017).

## REFERENCES

Alemdaroğlu İ et al. (2014) Turkish version of the Egen Klassifikation scale version 2: Validity and reliability in the Turkish population. *Turk Pediatr* 56(6): 643–650.

ATS Committee on Proficiency Standards for Clinical Pulmonary Function Laboratories (2002) ATS statement: Guidelines for the six-minute walk test. *Am J Respir Crit Care Med* 166(1): 111–117. doi: 10.1164/ajrccm.166.1.at1102.

Bérard C, Payan C, Hodgkinson I, Fermanian J, MFM Collaborative Study Group (2005) A motor function measure for neuromuscular diseases. Construction and validation study. *Neuromuscul Disord* 15: 463–470.

Bushby K, Finkel R, Birnkrant DJ, Case LE, Clemens PR, Cripe L et al. (2010) Diagnosis and management of Duchenne muscular dystrophy, part 2: implementation of multidisciplinary care. *Lancet Neurol* 9: 177–189.

Cano SJ, Mayhew A, Glanzman AM, Krosschell KJ, Swoboda KJ, Main M et al. (2014) Rasch analysis of clinical outcome measures in spinal muscular atrophy. *Muscle Nerve* 49: 422–430.

Chen T-H, Chang JG, Yang YH, Mai HH, Liang WC, Wu YC et al. (2010) Randomized, double-blind, placebo-controlled trial of hydroxyurea in spinal muscular atrophy. *Neurol* 75: 2190–2197.

Dunaway S, Montes J, Garber CE, Carr B, Kramer SS, Kamil-Rosenberg S et al. (2014) Performance of the timed "up & go" test in spinal muscular atrophy. *Muscle Nerve* 50: 273–277.

Dunaway Young S, Montes J, Kramer SS, Marra J, Salazar R, Cruz R et al. (2016) Six-minute walk test is reliable and valid in spinal muscular atrophy. *Muscle Nerve* 54: 836–842.

Fagoaga J, Girabent-Farrés M, Bagur-Calafat C, Febrer A, Steffensen BF (2015) [Functional assessment for people unable to walk due to spinal muscular atrophy and Duchenne muscular dystrophy. Translation and validation of the Egen Klassifikation 2 scale for the Spanish population]. *Revista de Neurologia* 60(10): 439–46.

Febrer A, Vigo M, Fagoaga J, Medina-Cantillo J, Rodríguez N, Tizzano E (2011) [Hammersmith functional rating scale for children with spinal muscular atrophy. Validation of the Spanish version]. *Revista de Neurologia* 53(11): 657–663.

Finkel RS, Hynan LS, Glanzman AM, Owens H, Nelson L, Cone SR et al. (2008) The Test of Infant Motor Performance: reliability in spinal muscular atrophy type I. *Pediatr Phys Ther* 20: 242–246.

Finkel RS, McDermott MP, Kaufmann P, Darras BT, Chung WK, Sproule DM et al. (2014) Observational study of spinal muscular atrophy type I and implications for clinical trials. *Neurol* 83: 810–817.

Glanzman AM, Mazzone E, Main M, Pelliccioni M, Wood J, Swoboda KJ et al. (2010) The Children's Hospital of Philadelphia Infant Test of *Neuromuscul Dis* (CHOP INTEND): test development and reliability. *Neuromuscul Disord* 20: 155–161.

Glanzman AM, McDermott MP, Montes J, Martens WB, Flickinger J, Riley S et al. (2011) Validation of the Children's Hospital of Philadelphia Infant Test of *Neuromuscul Dis* (CHOP INTEND). *Pediatr Phys Ther* 23: 322–326.

Glanzman AM, O'Hagen JM, McDermott MP, Martens WB, Flickinger J, Riley S et al. (2011) Validation of the Expanded Hammersmith Functional Motor Scale in spinal muscular atrophy type II and III. *J Child Neurol* 26: 1499–1507.

Goemans N, Klingels K, van den Hauwe M, Boons S, Verstraete L, Peeters C et al. (2013) Six-Minute Walk Test: Reference Values and Prediction Equation in Healthy Boys Aged 5 to12 Years. *PLoS ONE* 8(12): e84120.

Henricson E, Abresch R, Han JJ, Nicorici A, Goude Keller E, de Bie E et al. (2013) The 6-Minute Walk Test and person-reported outcomes in boys with Duchenne muscular dystrophy and typically developing controls: longitudinal comparisons and clinically-meaningful changes over one year. *PLoS Curr* 5: ecurrents.md.9e17658b007eb79fcd6f723089f79e06. doi: 10.1371/currents.md.9e17658b007eb79fcd6f723089f79e06.

Henricson EK, Abresch RT, Cnaan A, Hu F, Duong T, Arrieta A et al. (2013) The cooperative international neuromuscular research group Duchenne natural history study: glucocorticoid treatment preserves clinically meaningful functional milestones and reduces rate of disease progression as measured by manual muscle testing and other commonly used clinical trial outcome measures. *Muscle Nerve* 48: 55–67.

Hobart JC, Cano SJ, Zajicek JP, Thompson AJ (2007) Rating scales as outcome measures for clinical trials in neurology: problems, solutions, and recommendations. *Lancet Neurol* 6: 1094–1105.

Hobart J and Cano S (2009) Improving the evaluation of therapeutic interventions in multiple sclerosis: the role of new psychometric methods. *Health Technol Assess* 13(12). doi.10.3310/hta13120.

Iannaccone, ST and American Spinal Muscular Atrophy Randomized Trials Group (2002) Outcome measures for pediatric spinal muscular atrophy. *Arch Neurol* 59(9): 1445–1450.

Klingels K, Mayhew AG, Mazzone ES, Duong T, Decostre V, Werlauff U et al. (2016) Development of a patient-reported outcome measure for upper limb function in Duchenne muscular dystrophy: DMD Upper Limb PROM. *Dev Med Child Neurol* 59(2): 224–231.

Kolb SJ, Coffey CS, Yankey JW, Krosschell K, Arnold WD, Rutkove SB et al. (2016) Baseline results of the NeuroNEXT spinal muscular atrophy infant biomarker study. *Ann Clin Transl Neurol* 3: 132–145.

Krosschell KJ, Maczulski JA, Crawford TO, Scott C, Swoboda KJ (2006) A modified Hammersmith functional motor scale for use in multi-center research on spinal muscular atrophy. *Neuromuscul Disord* 16: 417–426.

Krosschell KJ, Scott CB, Maczulski JA, Lewelt AJ, Reyna SP, Swoboda KJ et al. (2011) Reliability of the Modified Hammersmith Functional Motor Scale in young children with spinal muscular atrophy. *Muscle Nerve* 44: 246–251.

Krosschell KJ, Maczulski JA, Scott C, King W, Hartman JT, Case LE et al. (2013) Reliability and validity of the TIMPSI for infants with spinal muscular atrophy type I. *Pediatr Phys Ther* 25: 140–148, discussion, p. 149.

Landfeldt E, Mayhew A, Eagle M, Lindgren P, Bell CF, Guglieri M et al. (2015) Development and psychometric analysis of the Duchenne muscular dystrophy Functional Ability Self-Assessment Tool (DMDSAT). *Neuromuscul Disord* 25: 937–944.

de Lattre C, Payan C, Vuillerot C, Rippert P, de Castro D, Bérard C et al. (2013) Motor function measure: validation of a short form for young children with neuromuscular diseases. *Arch Phys Med Rehabil* 94: 2218–2226.

Lord JP et al. (1987) Upper extremity functional rating for patients with Duchenne muscular dystrophy. *Arch Phys Med Rehabil* 68(3): 151–154.

Lyager S, Steffensen B, Juhl B (1995) Indicators of need for mechanical ventilation in Duchenne muscular dystrophy and spinal muscular atrophy. *Chest* 108: 779–785.

Maharshi V, Hasan S (2017) Nusinersen: the first option beyond supportive care for Spinal Muscular Atrophy. *Clin Drug Investig* 37: 807–817.

Main M, Kairon H, Mercuri E, Muntoni F (2003) The Hammersmith functional motor scale for children with spinal muscular atrophy: a scale to test ability and monitor progress in children with limited ambulation. *Eur J Paediatr Neurol* 7: 155–159

Mayhew A et al. (2011) Moving towards meaningful measurement: Rasch analysis of the North Star Ambulatory Assessment in Duchenne muscular dystrophy. *Dev Med Child Neurol* 53(6): 535–542.

Mayhew A, Cano S, Scott E, Eagle M, Bushby K, Muntoni F et al. (2013) Development of the Performance of the Upper Limb module for Duchenne muscular dystrophy, accessed on *Dev Med Child Neurol* 55(11): 1038–1045.

Mayhew AG, Cano SJ, Scott E, Eagle M, Bushby K, Manzur A et al. (2013) Detecting meaningful change using the North Star Ambulatory Assessment in Duchenne muscular dystrophy. *Dev Med Child Neurol* 55: 1046–1052.

Mazzone E, Bianco F, Main M, van den Hauwe M, Ash M, de Vries R et al. (2013) Six minute walk test in type III spinal muscular atrophy: a 12 month longitudinal study. *Neuromuscul Disord* 23: 624–628.

Mazzone E, De Sanctis R, Fanelli L, Bianco F, Main M, van den Hauwe M et al. (2014) Hammersmith Functional Motor Scale and Motor Function Measure-20 in non ambulant SMA patients. *Neuromuscul Disord* 24: 347–352.

Mazzone ES, Messina S, Vasco G, Main M, Eagle M, D'Amico A et al. (2009) Reliability of the North Star Ambulatory Assessment in a multicentric setting. *Neuromuscul Disord* 19: 458–461.

Mazzone ES, Vasco G, Palermo C, Bianco F, Galluccio C, Ricotti V et al. (2012) A critical review of functional assessment tools for upper limbs in Duchenne muscular dystrophy. *Dev Med Child Neurol* 54(10): 879–885.

Mazzone ES, Coratti G, Sormani MP, Messina S, Pane M, D'Amico A et al. (2016) Timed rise from floor as a predictor of disease progression in Duchenne muscular dystrophy: an observational study. *PLoS ONE* 11: e0151445.

McDonald CM, Henricson EK, Abresch RT, Florence JM, Eagle M, Gappmaier E et al. (2013) The 6-minute walk test and other endpoints in Duchenne muscular dystrophy: longitudinal natural history observations over 48 weeks from a multicenter study. *Muscle Nerve* 48: 343–356.

McDonald CM, Abresch RT, Carter GT, Fowler WM Jr, Johnson ER, Kilmer DD et al. (1995) Profiles of neuromuscular diseases. Duchenne muscular dystrophy. *Am J Phys Med Rehabil* 74(5 Suppl): S70–S94.

McDonald CM, Henricson EK, Han JJ, Abresch RT, Nicorici A, Elfring GL et al. (2010) The 6-minute walk test as a new outcome measure in Duchenne muscular dystrophy. *Muscle Nerve* 41: 500–510.

McDonald CM, Henricson EK, Abresch RT, Han JJ, Escolar DM, Florence JM et al. (2013a) The cooperative international neuromuscular research group Duchenne natural history study – a longitudinal investigation in the era of glucocorticoid therapy: design of protocol and the methods used. *Muscle Nerve* 48: 32–54.

McDonald CM, Henricson EK, Abresch RT, Florence J, Eagle M, Gappmaier E et al. (2013b) The 6-minute walk test and other clinical endpoints in duchenne muscular dystrophy: reliability, concurrent validity, and minimal clinically important differences from a multicenter study. *Muscle Nerve* 48: 357–368.

Mercuri E, Messina S, Battini R, Berardinelli A, Boffi P, Bono R et al. (2006) Reliability of the Hammersmith functional motor scale for spinal muscular atrophy in a multicentric study. *Neuromuscul Disord* 16: 93–98.

Mercuri E, McDonald C, Mayhew A, Florence J, Mazzone E, Bianco F et al. (2012) International workshop on assessment of upper limb function in Duchenne Muscular Dystrophy: Rome, 15–16 February 2012. *Neuromuscul Disord* 22(11): 1025–8. doi: 10.1016/j.nmd.2012.06.006.

Mercuri E, Coratti G, Messina S, Ricotti V, Baranello G, D'Amico A et al. (2016) Revised North Star Ambulatory Assessment for young boys with Duchenne muscular dystrophy. *PLoS ONE* 11: e0160195.

Mercuri E, Finkel R, Kirschner J, Chiriboga C, Kuntz N, Sun P et al. (2017) Efficacy and safety of nusinersen in children with later-onset spinal muscular atrophy (SMA): end of study results from the phase 3 CHERISH study. *Neuromusc Disord* 27: S210.

Montes J, Dunaway S, Montgomery MJ, Sproule D, Kaufmann P, De Vivo DC et al. (2011) Fatigue leads to gait changes in spinal muscular atrophy. *Muscle Nerve* 43: 485–488.

Montes J, Blumenschine M, Dunaway S, Alter AS, Engelstad K, Rao AK et al. (2013) Weakness and fatigue in diverse neuromuscular diseases. *J Child Neurol* 28: 1277–1283.

Morel T, Cano SJ (2017) Measuring what matters to rare disease patients – reflections on the work by the IRDiRC taskforce on patient-centered outcome measures. *Orphanet J Rare Dis* 12: 171.

Nelson L, Owens H, Hynan LS, Iannaccone ST, AmSMART Group. 2006. The gross motor function measure is a valid and sensitive outcome measure for spinal muscular atrophy. *Neuromuscul Disord* 16: 374–380.

Novick MR (1966) The axioms and principal results of classical test theory. *J Math Psychol* 3: 1–18.

O'Hagen JM, Glanzman AM, McDermott MP, Ryan PA, Flickinger J, Quigley J et al. (2007) An expanded version of the Hammersmith Functional Motor Scale for SMA II and III patients. *Neuromuscul Disord* 17: 693–697.

Palisano RJ, Hanna SE, Rosenbaum PL, Russell DJ, Walter SD, Wood EP et al. (2000) Validation of a model of gross motor function for children with cerebral palsy. *Phys Ther* 80(10): 974–985.

Pane M, Mazzone ES, Fanelli L, De Sanctis R, Bianco F, Sivo S et al. (2014) Reliability of the Performance of Upper Limb assessment in Duchenne muscular dystrophy. *Neuromuscul Disord* 24: 201–206.

Pane M, Mazzone ES, Sivo S, Fanelli L, De Sanctis R, D'Amico A et al. (2014) The 6 minute walk test and performance of upper limb in ambulant duchenne muscular dystrophy boys. *PLoS Curr* 6: ecurrents. md.a93d9904d57dcb08936f2ea89bca6fe6.

Pera MC, Coratti G, Forcina N, Mazzone ES, Scoto M, Montes J et al. (2017) Content validity and clinical meaningfulness of the HFMSE in spinal muscular atrophy. *BMC Neurol* 17: 39.

Ramsey D, Scoto M, Mayhew A, Main M, Mazzone ES, Montes J et al. (2017) Revised Hammersmith Scale for spinal muscular atrophy: A SMA specific clinical outcome assessment tool. *PLoS ONE* 12(2): e0172346. https://doi.org/10.1371/journal.pone.0172346.

Ricotti V, Ridout DA, Pane M, Main M, Mayhew A, Mercuri E et al. (2016) The NorthStar Ambulatory Assessment in Duchenne muscular dystrophy: considerations for the design of clinical trials. *J Neurol Neurosurg Psychiatry* 87: 149–155.

Russell DJ, Avery LM, Rosenbaum PL, Raina PS, Walter SD, Palisano RJ (2000) Improved scaling of the gross motor function measure for children with cerebral palsy: evidence of reliability and validity. *Phys Ther* 80(9): 873–885.

Scott E, Eagle M, Mayhew A, Freeman J, Main M, Sheehan J et al. (2012) Development of a functional assessment scale for ambulatory boys with Duchenne muscular dystrophy. *Physiother Res Int* 17(2): 101–109.

Steffensen B, Hyde S, Lyager S, Mattsson E (2001) Validity of the EK scale: A functional assessment of non-ambulatory individuals with Duchenne muscular dystrophy or spinal muscular atrophy. *Physiother Res Int* 6(3): 119–134.

Steffensen BF, Lyager S, Werge B, Rahbek J, Mattsson E (2002) Physical capacity in non-ambulatory people with Duchenne muscular dystrophy or spinal muscular atrophy: a longitudinal study. *Dev Med Child Neurol* 44: 623–632.

VanSant AF (2006) The International Classification of Functioning, Disability and Health. *Pediatr Phys Ther* 18: 237.

Vignos PJ Jr, Spencer GE Jr, Archibald KC (1963) Management of progressive muscular dystrophy in childhood. *JAMA* 184: 89–96.

Vuillerot C, Girardot F, Payan C, Fermanian J, Iwaz J, De Lattre C, Bérard C (2010) Monitoring changes and predicting loss of ambulation in Duchenne muscular dystrophy with the Motor Function Measure. *Dev Med Child Neurol* 52: 60–65.

Vuillerot C, Payan C, Girardot F, Fermanian J, Iwaz J, Bérard C et al. (2012) Responsiveness of the motor function measure in neuromuscular diseases. *Arch Phys Med Rehabil* 93(12): 2251–2256.

Vuillerot C, Payan C, Iwaz J, Ecochard R, Bérard C, MFM Spinal Muscular Atrophy Study Group (2013) Responsiveness of the motor function measure in patients with spinal muscular atrophy. *Arch Phys Med Rehabil* 94: 1555–1561.

Walton MK, Powers JH III, Hobart J, Patrick D, Marquis P, Vamvakas S et al. (2015) Clinical Outcome Assessments: Conceptual Foundation-Report of the ISPOR Clinical Outcomes Assessment – Emerging Good Practices for Outcomes Research Task Force. *Value Health* 18: 741–752.

Werlauff U, Steffensen BF, Bertelsen S, Fløytrup I, Kristensen B, Werge B (2010) Physical characteristics and applicability of standard assessment methods in a total population of spinal muscular atrophy type II patients. *Neuromuscul Disord* 20: 34–43.

WHO (2001) *The International Classification of Functioning, Disability and Health*. Geneva: World Health Organization. doi.10.1097/01.pep.0000245823.21888.71.

Wright BD, LJ (1989) Observations are always ordinal: measurements, however must be interval. *Arch Phys Med Rehabil* 70(12): 857–860.

Wright BD, Stone MH (1979) *Best Test Design: Rasch Measurement.* Chicago, IL: MESA.

# Section 3
## Overview of the Most Frequent Neuromuscular Conditions in Children and Disease Specific Medical Management

# 6
# SPINAL MUSCULAR ATROPHY AND OTHER MOTOR NEURON DISEASES

*Wendy KM Liew, Banu Sundar and Basil T Darras*

## Introduction

Spinal muscular atrophy (SMA) is a group of autosomal recessive disorders characterized by progressive muscle weakness and atrophy. SMA is associated with degeneration of motor neurons in the spinal cord and, in the most severely affected patients, of the lower brain stem motor neurons. SMA is the most common genetic cause of infant mortality and affects all populations, irrespective of ethnicity. Patients and their families benefit from a holistic and multidisciplinary approach to care that includes specialists in neurology and neuromuscular medicine, pulmonology, gastroenterology, nutrition, orthopedics, rehabilitation, and social work (Table 6.1). Understanding of the genetic basis of SMA has led to recent and ongoing advances in drug development and to the first definitive treatments for these devastating conditions.

SMA was first described by Austrian clinician Guido Werdnig at the University of Graz, Austria, and by German physician Johann Hoffmann in Heidelberg, Germany (Werdnig 1891; Hoffmann 1893). They described a neuromuscular disorder associated with the loss of anterior horn cells in the spinal cord, causing progressive neuromuscular weakness and early death, with onset in infancy. Guido Werdnig and Johann Hoffmann were the first to provide a complete description of an intermediate form of SMA; however, Werdnig–Hoffmann disease is an eponym used for the more severe subtype known as SMA type I. The types of SMA will be defined and discussed in the Clinical features section (Table 6.2).

## Epidemiology

The incidence of SMA has been estimated to be 7.8–10 per 100 000 live births, with 4.1 per 100 000 live births being SMA type I, the most severe subtype (Lefebvre et al. 1995; Mostacciuolo et al. 1992; Sugarman et al. 2012; Mailman et al. 2002). The carrier frequency for mutations in the *SMN1* gene is approximated to be between 1:38 to 1:50 in the general population, although lower frequencies have been reported as well. A 2009 North American study reported the *SMN1* mutation carrier frequency to be 1 in 37 (2.7%) in Caucasians, 1 in 46 (2.2%) in Ashkenazi Jews, 1 in 56 (1.8%) in Asians, 1 in 91 (1.1%) in African Americans, and 1 in 125 (0.8%) in Hispanic populations (Hendrickson et al. 2009). Despite the high carrier frequency, the incidence of SMA is lower than expected. This could be explained by

**TABLE 6.1**
**Specialties that contribute to care for SMA and other motor neuron disorders**

| | |
|---|---|
| Geneticists, genetic counselors | Diagnosis, social aspects |
| Neurology, neuromuscular medicine | Overall management, drug treatment |
| Pulmonology | Pulmonary function, ventilation |
| Gastroenterology | Feeding issues, gastrostomy |
| Nutrition | Failure to thrive, nutritional issues |
| Orthopedics | Scoliosis, contractures, fractures |
| Physical/Occupational therapy | Motor and functional milestones |
| Social work | Family and financial issues |

**TABLE 6.2**
**Clinical classification of spinal muscular atrophy**

| SMA subtype | Other names | Age of onset | Maximum motor milestone achieved | SMN2 copy number | Life expectancy | Incidence (%) | Prevalence (%) |
|---|---|---|---|---|---|---|---|
| 0/1A | Prenatal Congenital SMA Werdnig–Hoffmann disease | Birth to 2 weeks | Nil | 1 | <6 months, usually days–weeks | <1 | 0 |
| 1B 1C | Werdnig–Hoffmann disease Severe SMA "Non-sitters" | 1B: <3 months 1C: 3–6 months | Unable to sit unsupported | 1,2,3 | <2 years without any respiratory support | 60 | 12 |
| II | Dubowitz disease Intermediate SMA "Sitters" | 6–18 months | Able to sit unsupported but unable to walk independently | 2,3,4 | 20–40 years | 25 | 60 |
| III | Kugelberg–Welander disease Mild SMA "Walkers" | IIIA: 18 months –3 years IIIB: >3 years | Able to walk independently | 3,4,5 | Almost normal | 15 | 28 |
| IV | Adult onset | >21 years | Normal | 4,5 | Normal | <1 | 1 |

Adapted from Markowitz et al. (2012) with permission from Elsevier.

the consequences of a "0+0" *SMN1/SMN2* genotype (i.e., a patient having no SMN protein, hence resulting in fetal demise) (Prior 2010a; 2010b).

## Genetics

THE *SMN* GENE

The gene for SMA in both the acute and chronic forms was first localized in 1990 to chromosome 5q13.2, providing evidence in favor of genetic homogeneity between the two forms (Melki et al. 1990; Gilliam et al. 1990). Linkage analysis studies showed that all three forms of SMA map to chromosome 5q11.1–13.3. In 1995, Lefebvre et al. identified the *SMN* gene within this region, which was absent or interrupted in 98.6% of the patients in their group (Lefebvre et al. 1995). The structure of this chromosomal region is complex, with a large inverted duplication of a 500kb element. The *SMN1* gene, which is deleted or interrupted in patients with SMA, is located in the telomeric portion of the duplicated region. The *SMN2* gene, the result of a duplication of *SMN1* that differs from it by only ten nucleotides and a five nucleotide insertion, lies in the centromeric portion (Lefebvre et al. 1995).

The critical difference between *SMN1* and *SMN2* is a C-to-T transition in an exonic splicing enhancer located in exon 7 of the *SMN2* gene (Monani et al. 1999) (Fig. 6.1). While this C-to-T transition does not create an amino acid sequence change (translationally silent), it affects the splicing of the gene so that exon 7 is excluded from most, but not all, *SMN2* mRNA transcripts. Thus, as exon 7 is frequently spliced out of the *SMN2* mRNA, the *SMN2* gene produces about 5–10% full-length functional protein and 90–95% truncated protein (Lorson and Androphy 2000). In healthy carriers who have one *SMN1* copy and zero *SMN2* copies, having 50% functional full-length SMN protein is sufficient for normal functioning. In patients with SMA, the most common *SMN2* copy numbers are 1–2 copies in type I, 2–3 copies in type II and 3–4 copies in type III. About 50% of patients with type III have

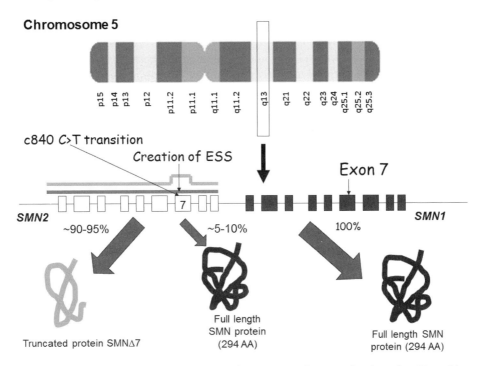

**Fig. 6.1.** Diagram of *SMN1* and *SMN2* genes on chromosome 5 demonstrating that a C-to-T transition at position 6 of *SMN2* creates an exonic splicing suppressor (ESS), which then leads to skipping of exon 7 during transcription, resulting in the production of truncated nonfunctional SMN protein. AA: amino acids. Reprinted from Darras et al. (2015) with permission from Elsevier. A colour version of this figure can be seen in the plate section at the end of the book.

3 copies of *SMN2* (Coovert et al. 1997). At a maximum range of 10% functional protein production per *SMN2* gene, these patients are predicted to have 20–30% full-length SMN protein production. Patients with milder type III, with four copies of *SMN2*, would have about 40% SMN protein, still below the 50% level seen in healthy carriers with no *SMN2* copies. Furthermore, asymptomatic individuals with 5 copies of *SMN2* and zero copies of *SMN1* have been described, and these individuals are predicted to have 50% SMN protein level (Mailman et al. 2002). The clinical severity of the disease in SMA patients depends partly on the copy number as well as on the quality of *SMN2* genes that the copies carry. Although there is a rough correlation between *SMN2* copy number, level and quality of SMN protein, and clinical severity, physicians often see a clinical overlap in the phenotypes of these patients (Lefebvre et al. 1997).

SURVIVAL MOTOR NEURON

SMN is a 38-kDa protein found in all cells, located in both the cytoplasm and the nucleus, where it localizes to structures known as Gemini of Cajal bodies, or simply "gems"; it is encoded by the *SMN* gene and its expression is ubiquitous. Fibroblasts from patients with different types of SMA showed a moderate reduction in the amount of SMN protein, particularly in patients with type I (Coovert et al. 1997). Fetal spinal cord analysis revealed a decrease in SMN protein levels in patients with types I and III SMA, with the amount of SMN protein being less in type I compared to type III (Lefebvre et al. 1997). The SMN protein in conjunction with several Gemin proteins forms an SMN complex, whose chaperone function facilitates the assembly of spliceosomal snRNP particles, essential components of the spliceosome complex, and hence plays a critical role in pre-mRNA splicing. The SMN protein may also be essential in assisting arginine methylation of some splicing-related proteins, transporting axonal mRNAs in motor neurons, and perhaps in other processes in muscle and neuromuscular junctions. The role of SMN protein in axonal mRNA trafficking and mRNA splicing may explain the selective vulnerability of spinal cord motor neurons to decreased SMN protein.

Kariya et al. demonstrated in mice structural and functional abnormalities at the level of the neuromuscular junction that precede overt symptoms, as well as structural abnormalities in the neuromuscular junctions of humans with SMA, and hence proposed that SMA may be a "synaptopathy" (Kariya et al. 2008). This concept, along with electrophysiological data suggesting dysfunction of the neuromuscular junction in patients with SMA types II and III, has led to the development of some treatment approaches directed towards enhancing neuromuscular transmission of patients with SMA (Wadman et al. 2012).

MUTATIONS

About 95% to 98% of patients with SMA harbor deletions of the telomeric *SMN1* gene (Fig. 6.2). The remainder have small intragenic mutations or have undergone gene conversions from *SMN1* to *SMN2*. In the latter case, a frameshift or point mutation of *SMN1* results in the disruption of exon 7, effectively converting *SMN1* to *SMN2* (Ogino et al. 2004). *De novo* mutations occur at a rate of about 2% (Darras 2015). The large number of repeated sequences around the *SMN1* and *SMN2* locus likely predisposes this region

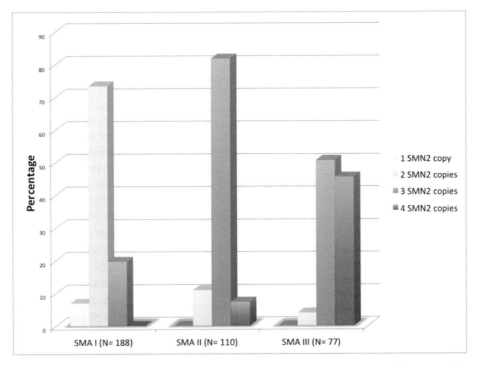

**Fig. 6.2.** Frequency of patients with SMA types I, II and III and *SMN2* copy numbers. In SMA type I, 80% of patients had 1 or 2 copies of *SMN2*; in SMA type II, 82% of patients had 3 copies of *SMN2*; and in SMA type III, 96% of patients carried 3 or 4 *SMN2* copies. Adapted from Feldkötter et al. (2002) with permission from Elsevier. A colour version of this figure can be seen in the plate section at the end of the book.

to unequal crossovers, resulting in a high rate of unequal crossover events and *de novo* mutations (especially paternally derived). This fact could explain the relatively high carrier frequency despite the mortality rate for the most severe forms of the disease (Prior 2007). More mildly affected patients seemed more likely to have undergone gene conversions of *SMN1* to *SMN2* rather than deletion of *SMN1* (DiDonato et al. 1997; Campbell et al. 1997).

The number of copies of *SMN2* per chromosome 5 varies among normal individuals, and 10–15% of the population possess no copies of *SMN2* (Ogino et al. 2004; Feldkötter et al. 2002). Among patients with SMA, an inverse correlation has been established between *SMN2* copy number and phenotypic severity. Feldkötter et al. in 2002 found in their series that 80% of patients with SMA type I had 1 or 2 copies of *SMN2*, 82% of patients with type II had 3 copies of *SMN2*, and 96% of patients with type III had 3 or 4 copies of *SMN2* (Feldkötter et al. 2002). Studies by Mailman et al. in 2002 and Arkblad et al. in 2009 found similar results: in both studies, 95–100% of patients with type I had 1 or 2 copies of *SMN2*; for patients with type III, Mailman et al. found 100% had 3 copies of *SMN2*, and Arkblad et al. found 77.8% had 3 copies and 22.8% had 4 copies of *SMN2* (Mailman et al. 2002; Arkblad et al. 2009). However, there is a degree of phenotypic overlap, and the correlation from the *SMN2* copy number alone may not absolutely predict the clinical severity. Additional evidence that *SMN2* copy number alone cannot be the sole modifying factor in disease severity is the fact that some patients with SMA type III have 5 copies of *SMN2*. Similarly, unaffected family members with homozygous *SMN1* deletions and 5 copies of *SMN2* have also been described (Mailman et al. 2002; Prior et al. 2004). In general, however, it can be said that a patient with one copy of *SMN2* is highly likely to present with severe SMA type 0 and less likely with SMA type I (Mailman et al. 2002; Feldkötter et al. 2002).

MODIFIERS OF THE *SMN2* GENE

The presence of modifiers of the *SMN2* gene may explain exceptions to the correlation between *SMN2* copy number and the clinical severity seen in the different SMA subtypes. The variant SMNG859C (c.859G>C) creates a new exonic splicing enhancer that increases exon 7 inclusion and thus the amount of full-length protein by about 20%; it has been reported in patients with types II and III SMA, and appears to be associated with a milder disease course, thus suggesting a protective effect (Vezain et al. 2010; Bernal et al. 2010). This variant has not been seen in patients with SMA type I but is seen in approximately 50% of patients with type II in the Spanish population, who often have 2 copies of *SMN2* and a milder phenotype.

Two or more siblings in a family affected with SMA often present with similar phenotypic severity and with identical *SMN2* copy numbers, suggesting that genetic modifiers often act in trans. Plastin 3 (PLS3) has also been reported as a modifier in female patients with SMA (Darras et al. 2015).

NEWBORN SCREENING

The American College of Obstetricians and Gynecologists Committee on Genetics published their opinion that routine preconception and prenatal screening for SMA should be offered to all women who are considering pregnancy or are currently pregnant and have had appropriate counseling about the possible range of severity, carrier rate, and detection rate (ACOG Committee on Genetics 2009). Newborn screening has already been approved in one state (Missouri), and pilot programs are in progress in a few other states in the United States.

## Clinical features

Patients with SMA can be divided into four broad clinical subtypes (I, II, III, IV), summarized in Table 6.2. The subtypes represent a phenotypic continuum, and within each subtype is another spectrum of clinical severity (Zerres and Davies 1999). Most clinicians and guidelines classify these patients using maximum motor function or gross motor developmental milestone achieved. Classically, patients with type I are described as "non-sitters" and present within 6 months of age; patients with type II are described as children who have achieved independent sitting ("sitters") and usually present at an age older than 6 months and younger than 18 months; patients with type III are "walkers" who typically present after 18 months of age; and patients with type IV present in adulthood (Iannaccone et al. 2000; Wang et al. 2007a).

SMA TYPE I

Patients with SMA type I, also known as Werdnig–Hoffman disease, severe SMA or "non-sitters", usually present from birth to 6 months of age with diffuse hypotonia and poor head control. Patients with SMA type I can be further subdivided into three groups: type IA/ type 0, type IB, and type IC (Dubowitz 1999).

Type IA or type 0 has been used to describe patients who lie on the most severe end of the phenotypic spectrum. These patients present in the neonatal period with severe hypotonia, weakness, severe motor impairment and respiratory failure. They may have arthrogryposis or joint contractures, suggesting a prenatal onset. Mothers sometimes report decreased fetal movements. Facial diplegia and congenital cardiac disease such as atrial septal defects have been described. Respiratory failure is usually the main cause of morbidity and mortality, with a life expectancy of days to weeks in most patients. Patients with type IB present with symptoms prior to 3 months of age, while patients with type IC present between 3 to 6 months of age.

On examination, patients with SMA type I have a characteristic alert expression, tongue fasciculations, generalized weakness affecting the lower limbs more than the upper limbs, and areflexia. They adopt a "frog-leg" posture in supine position and a "slip-through" sign on vertical suspension. They do not achieve the ability to roll independently or sit unsupported and hence are sometimes called "non-sitters". Weakness of the inspiratory respiratory muscles produces a bell-shaped chest and paradoxical breathing where the chest wall moves in during inspiration and out on expiration, the reverse of normal respiratory movements. Bulbar muscles eventually become affected and infants may present with choking during feeds, recurrent aspiration pneumonias, and poor weight gain. In the past, most children with SMA type I did not live past 2 years of age due to respiratory failure and recurrent respiratory infections; however, with the use of mechanical ventilator devices, lifespans of these children can be prolonged (Zerres and Davies 1999; O'Hagen et al. 2007; Sproule et al. 2010; Darras et al. 2015).

SMA TYPE II

Patients with SMA type II, also known as Dubowitz disease or intermediate SMA, have been described as "sitters" as they are able to sit unsupported at some stage but do not develop the ability to stand unsupported or walk independently. Onset of symptoms is classically between 6–18 months of age. Similar to patients with SMA type I, they have diffuse hypotonia, tongue fasciculations, generalized weakness affecting the lower limbs more than the upper limbs, and areflexia. Polyminimyoclonus or tremors of the hands may be present (Zerres and Davies 1999; Darras et al. 2015). Frequency of respiratory symptoms is less in this subtype of patients. However, as weakness progresses, they are faced with orthopedic issues such as scoliosis, with resulting restrictive lung disease if the scoliosis is not corrected. Joint contractures and ankylosis of the mandible are also common problems. Cognition is normal with above average verbal intelligence (von Gontard et al. 2002). Prognosis for patients with type II is better; however, depending on the degree of respiratory compromise, life expectancy can be shortened (Zerres and Davies 1999; Darras et al. 2015). Survival rates for 240 patients with SMA type II were found to be 98.5% at 5 years and 68.5% at 25 years in a natural history study.

SMA TYPE III

Patients with SMA type III, also known as Kugelberg–Welander disease, mild SMA or "walkers", are children who are able to stand unsupported and walk independently (Kugelberg and Welander 1956). These children usually present later than 18 months of age. The onset of symptoms further subdivides these patients into two groups: patients with type IIIA have onset of symptoms between 18 months and 3 years, and patients with type IIIB usually present after the age of 3 years. The distribution of weakness is similar to that seen in patients with types I and II SMA in that the lower limbs are affected more than the upper limbs, but the progression of weakness is a more gradual process; some patients may eventually become wheelchair dependent at a later stage (this is seen more frequently in patients with type IIIA). They can have polyminimyoclonus of the hands. Respiratory and orthopedic complications are less frequent in this subset of patients, with life expectancy almost similar to the normal population (Zerres and Davies 1999; Darras et al. 2015).

SMA TYPE IV

Patients with SMA type IV have onset of symptoms in adulthood, typically after the age of 21 years. Type IV is a milder clinical phenotype, with minimal respiratory or orthopedic complications and a normal lifespan (Russman 2007).

"NON-5q SMAs"

A minority of SMA patients fall under the category known as "non-5q13 spinal muscular atrophies". Non-5q SMA is a diverse group of motor neuron disorders caused by mutations in various genes. These disorders are rare compared to 5q SMA (Darras 2011; Zerres and Rudnik-Schöneborn 2003). Examples are the distal spinal muscular atrophies, distal hereditary motor neuropathies, and X-linked, autosomal dominant or autosomal recessive spinal muscular atrophies (Zerres and Davies 1999). These patients generally have distinct clinical features that help clinicians to differentiate them from the classic SMA patients (Darras 2011). These features are summarized in Table 6.3 (Darras 2015).

Besides the non-5q SMAs, other differentials of 5q SMA include the hereditary neuropathies (such as congenital hypomyelinating and axonal neuropathies) and other disorders, such as hexosaminidase A deficiency. Hexosaminidase A deficiency can present with upper motor neuron signs, progressive muscle weakness, abnormal saccades and cerebellar atrophy, and can be indistinguishable from the milder forms of SMA (Jamrozik et al. 2013).

**Biomarkers and outcome measures in spinal muscular atrophy**

Over the past decade, efforts have been dedicated to developing reliable and sensitive outcome measures for SMA. Such measures have become increasingly important as more therapeutic agents are being developed for SMA. Biomarkers can be classified into the following subtypes: (1) for prognostication of disease or clinical outcome; (2) for the monitoring of disease progression; (3) for quantifying the effect of therapeutic agents over time; and (4) as a prediction of one's clinical response to therapy. Biomarkers help the clinician to stratify therapies and to make important management decisions for the individual patient.

**TABLE 6.3**
**Non-5q spinal muscular atrophies**

| Non-5q SMAs (Distinguishing features) | Gene/Locus |
|---|---|
| ***Distal SMA/dHMN***  Autosomal recessive | |
| SMA with respiratory distress type I (SMARD1/ HMN6/ DSMA1)  • Diaphragmatic paralysis, onset within first 3 months of life  • Autonomic and sensory nerve involvement  • Ventilatory dependent | *IGHMBP2* |
| DSMA2/ HMNJ | 9p21.1–p22 |
| DSMA3/ HMN3,4 | 11q13 |
| DSMA4  • Lower motor neuron syndrome | *PLEKHG5* |
| **Autosomal dominant** | |
| HMN1  • Juvenile onset | 7q34–q36 |
| HMN2A  • Adult onset | *HSPB8* |
| HMN2B | *HSPB1* |
| HMN2C | *HSPB3* |
| HMN5A/ CMT2D  • Upper limb predominance, distal SMA | *GARS* |
| HMN5B  • Upper limb predominance  • Congenital generalized lipo-dystrophy type 2  • Silver syndrome/SPG17 | *BSCL2* |
| HMN7A  • Vocal cord paralysis | *SLCA7* |
| HMN7B  • Vocal cord paralysis | *Dynactin1* |
| ***Proximal SMA (+/- distal involvement)***  **Autosomal dominant** | |
| SMA with late-onset, Finkel type/ALS8 | *VAPB* |
| SPSMA/HMSN2C  • Congenital SMA with contractures and lower limb predominance  • Scapuloperoneal SMA  • CMT type 2C | *TRPV4* |
| SMALED  • Lower extremity predominance, ankle contractures  • Early onset, disease static or slowly progressive | *DYNC1H1, BICD2* |
| HMSNP  • proximal | *TFG* |

Continued

**TABLE 6.3**
**Continued**

| Non-5q SMAs (Distinguishing features) | Gene/Locus |
|---|---|
| **Spinal and bulbar muscular atrophies/SMA plus types** <br> **Autosomal recessive** | |
| LAAHD <br> • Lethal arthrogryposis with anterior horn cell disease | GLE1 |
| SMA-PCH1 <br> • Pontocerebellar hypoplasics, postnatal progressive microcephaly, cerebellar vermis relatively spared | VRK1, EXOCS3 |
| BVVLS <br> • Fazio-Londe disease, bulbar palsy | RFT2 (C20orf54) |
| **X-linked recessive** | |
| SBMA/SMAX1 <br> • Kennedy disease (Adult onset) | Androgen receptor gene |
| SMAX2 <br> • Infantile onset with arthrogryposis | UBA1 |
| SMAX3 | ATP7A |

Functional outcome measures have been widely used as a way to monitor motor function and changes related to disease progression. Over the years, these outcome measures have evolved from qualitative assessments of strength, such as handheld myometry, to assessments of a child's function or motor performance in everyday activities.

Examples of functional outcome measures and biomarkers include clinical scales such as the Children's Hospital of Philadelphia Infant Test of Neuromuscular Disorders (Montes et al. 2009), the Hammersmith Functional Motor Scale (Main et al. 2003), the Modified or Expanded Hammersmith Functional Motor Scale (O'Hagen et al. 2007), the Six-Minute Walk Test (Montes et al. 2010), compound muscle action potential and motor unit number estimation (Swoboda et al. 2005), quantitative muscle ultrasound (Wu et al. 2010), and SMN messenger RNA or protein levels (Singh et al. 2013b).

**Natural history of spinal muscular atrophy**
Efforts to collect data involving patients with SMA types I, II and III started as early as 1950, by Brandt et al. in Denmark and by Byers and Banker in the United States. Over the years, many more studies were published in various countries relating to the types of SMA patients and the level of supportive care that they received, as well as survival and mortality data. Historical and recent studies show a strong correlation between survival and the intensity of supportive care received by the patient, as well as the role of *SMN2* copy number as a prognostic biomarker (Darras and Finkel 2017).

SURVIVAL

In natural history studies involving patients with SMA type I, survival is related to the age of first onset of symptoms. Patients with an earlier age of symptom onset appear to have a shorter lifespan than those with later onset; however, with good supportive ventilatory and nutritional management, survival becomes more or less similar (Rudnik-Schöneborn et al. 2009; Ge et al. 2012; Ioos et al. 2004; Finkel et al. 2014). The mean age of death is approximately 6–10 months when palliative or comfort care is provided (Cobben et al. 2008); however, with proactive respiratory interventions survival increases from months to years. Although supportive care has been shown to improve survival, it does not change the natural progression of the disease; strength and motor function for these patients continue to show progressive decline after diagnosis (Mercuri et al. 2016; Finkel et al. 2018).

Compared to two decades ago, improvements in the standards of care of patients with SMA types II and III have improved the overall natural history, suggesting that early intervention and management involving nutrition and gastrostomy, scoliosis and respiratory infections can affect the progression of disease. In the first year of follow-up, decline in motor function and respiratory function is usually minimal; subsequently, different rates of clinical deterioration have been reported (Mercuri et al. 2016; Kaufmann et al. 2011). Patients with contractures, severe scoliosis or sudden weight gain appear to have a faster rate of deterioration (Finkel et al. 2018). Data on adult patients with SMA type II suggest that function and motor strength continue to decline, with an increase in orthopedic complications such as joint contractures. In particular, patients experience an increase in the limitation of mouth opening, resulting in orofacial issues affecting their speech and eating (Jeppesen et al. 2010).

Lifespan for patients with SMA type II is now commonly greater than 30 years, with one study reporting median survival beyond 40 years. Lifespan for patients with SMA type III is normal.

MOTOR FUNCTION

SMA is a progressive disease in which patients lose function over time. In children with SMA type I, motor function scales demonstrate a decline of motor skills as the disease progresses. In children with types II and III, baseline motor function abilities may vary significantly within each subtype. Longitudinal analysis shows that motor functions of these children do not change significantly when they are followed within a 12-month period (Kaufmann et al. 2011). However, motor functions start to show a decline after 12 months, suggesting that loss of motor function is a gradual process and occurs slowly (Werlauff et al. 2012).

Age-related changes are also seen in children with SMA type II: those under 5 years appear to have the potential to gain motor milestones even in the absence of any therapy; the greatest decline in function seems to fall in the 5–15 years old age group, while patients above 15 years of age are more stable (Kaufmann et al. 2011; Mercuri et al. 2016).

STRENGTH

Decline in muscle strength is very slow and can take many years to detect (Werlauff et al. 2012). Various natural history studies looking at muscle strength in patients with SMA have reached differing conclusions on muscle strength and motor function. These differences may be due to various reasons, for example: (1) the tools used to measure muscle strength may not be sufficiently sensitive, and (2) the periods during which the patients were followed may not have been long enough to detect decline in strength. More recently, new tools such as the MyoGrip handgrip and MyoPinch key pinch have been developed and are reported to be extremely sensitive in monitoring muscle strength.

PULMONARY FUNCTION

Data on pulmonary function are limited in infants with SMA type I. In patients with types II and III, pulmonary function declines over time, apparently related to the progression of the underlying disease (Souchon et al. 1996). The presence of scoliosis can contribute to a decline in pulmonary function; correction of scoliosis with surgery does not improve the pulmonary function but slows down its progressive decline (Souchon et al. 1996).

LOSS OF AMBULATION

All patients with SMA type III may lose ambulation, with the probability being higher in patients with type IIIA (Ge et al. 2012; Russman et al. 1996). Studies of patients with type III showed an ambulatory probability of 57.5–76.7% at age 10 for type IIIA compared to 85–97% for type IIIB. At age 20, the ambulatory probability for patients with type IIIA is 30–44% and 67.5–89% for type IIIB. Loss of ambulation has been associated with weight gain, onset of puberty, and infection.

*SMN2* COPY NUMBER

Studies have shown a strong correlation between *SMN2* copy number and the phenotypic severity in the different subtypes of SMA. *SMN2* copy number varies between 1 and 4, with a higher number predicting a milder form of SMA (Wirth et al. 2006; Ogino et al. 2003). Although there has been no reported correlation between *SMN2* copy number and the age of loss of ambulation, ambulatory probability is higher in patients who have a higher *SMN2* copy number (e.g., 4 copies of *SMN2* compared to 3 copies of *SMN2*).

**Care of the patient with spinal muscular atrophy**

Since SMA was first described almost a century ago, tremendous progress has been made in understanding its pathophysiology, genetics and phenotypic spectrum. The collection of natural history data and various outcome measures in this group of patients has also led to changes in their management. Good supportive management in a holistic, multidisciplinary approach can greatly affect the outcome and quality of life of these patients, resulting in improvements in survival and maximization of functional capacity.

Patients with SMA and their families benefit immensely from a multidisciplinary approach to care. Multidisciplinary care involves members from neurology/neuromuscular medicine, orthopedics, physical and occupational therapy, pulmonology, nutrition and gastroenterology. For patients with SMA type I and severe type II, early involvement of the pediatric advanced care or palliative care team can provide parents with support and assistance in making decisions that conform with their values and help to maximize the child's quality of life. In 2007, a Consensus Statement for Standard of Care in Spinal Muscular Atrophy was released by a core committee team involving neurologists, pulmonologists and patient advocacy groups regarding the current best recommendations for management of patients with SMA (Wang et al. 2007b). In 2016, these recommendations were revisited with updated data and recent literature. Issues addressed at the recent workshop included the following: (1) genetics of SMA; (2) nutrition, growth and bone healthcare; (3) pulmonary care; (4) orthopedic care; (5) physical therapy and rehabilitation; (6) involvement of other organ systems; (7) acute care in the hospital setting; (8) medications; and (9) ethical issues and palliative care (Finkel et al. 2018).

DIAGNOSIS

In a typical presentation of SMA, the first-line investigation would be genetic testing, with the criterion standard being *SMN1* deletion/mutation and *SMN2* copy number testing. The minimum standard would be *SMN1* deletion testing. Diagnosis of SMA is confirmed by the presence of homozygous absence of exons 7 and 8 ( approximately 90% of patients), or of only exon 7 of the *SMN1* gene (approximately 10% of patients). In most patients, the *SMN1* deletion is inherited from both parents; however, in 2% of patients, neither parent is a carrier, and the molecular mutation observed is *de novo* (Prior and Finanger 2016).

With the high reliability of genetic testing, the use of muscle biopsy, nerve conduction and electromyography studies is rarely indicated in a classic presentation of SMA (Finkel et al. 2018). The typical muscle biopsy findings seen in SMA patients reflect a motor neuron disorder with neurogenic grouped atrophy and type 1 fiber hypertrophy. In nerve conduction studies, the patient has normal sensory potentials, with decreased compound motor action potential amplitudes. Needle electromyography demonstrates a neurogenic picture with evidence of denervation and reinnervation. Fibrillations and positive sharp waves are present at rest; on muscle activation, high-amplitude, long-duration motor unit potentials of a reduced recruitment pattern are seen (Darras et al. 2015). Serum creatine kinase may be normal or elevated up to four fold (Darras et al. 2015).

PULMONARY

Respiratory failure is the major cause of mortality in patients with SMA types I and II. Infants with SMA type I have weak intercostal muscles with relatively preserved diaphragmatic strength. Because expiratory function depends on intercostal effort, the dominant respiratory function impairment in patients with SMA type I is the loss of expiratory power, resulting in the characteristic bell-shaped chest seen in these patients. Patients with SMA type II have weak intercostal muscles with scoliosis contributing to progressive restrictive lung disease (Iannaccone 2007; Schroth 2009). The restrictive lung disease results in insidious onset of sleep hypoventilation. In general, sleep disordered breathing is often the first sign of respiratory muscle weakness in neuromuscular disease (Mellies et al. 2004). Mellies et al. found evidence of sleep hypoventilation on overnight polysomnography in 7 out of 12 SMA patients who had vital capacities below 60%; non-invasive ventilation (BiPAP) during sleep completely eliminated disordered breathing, normalized sleep architecture and improved symptoms such as fatigue and headaches ($p < 0.05$) (Mellies et al. 2004). The dual setting of the BiPAP machine increases the tidal volume and thus targets the main respiratory functional deficit of SMA. Regarding the use of non-invasive ventilation, Oskoui et al. reviewed 143 patients with SMA type I enrolled in the International SMA Registry and found significantly increased survival for those born between 1995 and 2006 versus those born between 1980 and 1994, with a 70% reduced risk of death over mean follow-up of 49.9 months significantly affected by the increased use of ventilation (non-invasive and invasive), mechanical cough assist devices, and gastrostomy feeding (Oskoui et al. 2007). Proper use of non-invasive ventilatory support such as BiPAP, with correct pressure adjustments and mask placement, has no significant side effects on patient hemodynamics (Markström et al. 2010). Expiratory muscle weakness in patients with SMA results in reduced cough pressure and a consequent impaired airway clearance, with predisposition to hypoxemia from mucus plugging. It is recommended that patients at risk for mucus plugging be monitored with overnight oximetry during acute illnesses, and that assisted airway clearance methods be employed. These methods may include a mechanical in-/ex-sufflator device, manual assisted airway clearance, and postural drainage.

Lemoine and colleagues (2012) reported a retrospective single-site case series of 49 symptomatic patients with SMA type I, enrolled between 2002–2009 and followed for an average of 2.3 years. Those parents who elected to initiate non-invasive ventilation and cough assist within 3 months of the diagnosis of SMA type I were assigned to the "proactive" group (n = 23) and those who chose suctioning and supplemental oxygen were assigned to the "supportive" group (n = 26). In the proactive group, 6 patients died (26%) with median age at death of 7.6 months, compared with 16 deaths in the supportive group (62%) at a median age of 8.8 months. The Kaplan-Meier survival curves were congruent for the two groups for the initial 6 months of observation, and then diverged significantly, with the proactive group maintaining survival at approximately 74% while survival in the supportive group declined to approximately 38% at 4 years (Lemoine et al. 2012).

Also recommended is a low threshold for the use of antibiotics during acute illnesses in these patients due to the risk of pneumonia (Wang et al. 2007b, Iannaccone 2007; Schroth 2009). Patients should be followed regularly by a pulmonologist experienced in caring for patients with neuromuscular diseases.

GASTRO-INTESTINAL ISSUES

Patients with SMA type I fatigue easily during feedings, which can lead to failure to thrive and aspiration with recurrent respiratory infections (Iannaccone 2007). Patients with SMA may have a high incidence of silent gastro-esophageal reflux, which can contribute to aspiration (Durkin et al. 2008). In a small retrospective study, Durkin et al. (2008) found that early laparoscopic Nissen fundoplication and gastrostomy in patients with SMA type I was associated with improved nutritional status, and also perhaps with a trend towards fewer long-term aspiration events (Durkin et al. 2008). Another group also had positive outcomes in a series of patients with type I and one patient with severe SMA type II who underwent laparoscopic Nissen fundoplication and gastrostomy tube placement followed by postoperative non-invasive ventilation (Yuan et al. 2007). Lastly, patients with SMA are at risk of constipation, which can worsen reflux or even respiratory symptoms (Iannaccone 2007).

NUTRITION

Failure to thrive or growth failure is common in infants with SMA type I and in some severely affected patients with type II. However, although many patients with type II are plotted as having a "normal" BMI (often as low as third percentile for a healthy child of their age), they may actually have excessive fat mass relative to their muscle mass. Bertoli et al. reported that among 30 SMA patients (n = 15 type I and n = 15 type II), patients with type I had significantly lower total free fat mass and lean body mass compared to patients with type II (Bertoli et al. 2017). This finding may be due to the magnitude of neurofunctional impairment rather than to the nutritional status derangement in these two subtypes of patients. However, children with types I and II can have different energy requirements as a result of their specific body composition and hypermetabolism of free fat mass. Patients with SMA who are clinically high functioning (Hammersmith score ≥12) but non-ambulatory are more prone to adiposity and becoming overweight than patients who are ambulatory or who are non-ambulatory and low-functioning (Hammersmith score <12) (Sproule et al. 2009; 2010). It is now known that different individuals require different degrees of nutritional and other interventions, with a common consensus that proactive nutritional support should be practiced. However, as there is limited literature regarding nutrition in SMA patients, more research is needed in this specific area to define the best nutrition practice for these patients.

ORTHOPEDIC

Patients with SMA require close orthopedic follow-up for the development of scoliosis and contractures. Surgical intervention for scoliosis is often required, and careful coordination of peri-operative respiratory and nutritional support can help minimize complications (Wang et al. 2007b). In the 2017 ENMC International Workshop, workgroups discussed several important issues including (1) the optimal timing of surgical intervention for the correction of scoliosis, (2) the conservative management of joint contractures, and (3) the use of thoracolumbosacral orthoses in younger SMA patients for the prevention of scoliosis. These issues will be discussed in greater detail in later chapters.

A retrospective study by Wasserman et al. (2017) of 85 patients with SMA, aged 12 months to 18 years, found an incidence of 38% with femur fractures and 85% with low area bone mineral density (aBMD), Z-scores ≤ −2.0 SD. Bone health markers appeared to be progressively lower in the more severe subtypes. Fractures are also commonly seen in patients with SMA types II and III. Distal femur is the most common fracture site followed by lower leg, ankle, and upper arm. Most of the fractures can be treated conservatively (Fujak et al. 2010).

**Rehabilitation**

The main goals of physical therapy and rehabilitation in patients with SMA are to (1) maintain or improve motor function, (2) maintain joint mobility, and (3) prevent the development of orthopedic complications such as joint contractures and scoliosis (Finkel et al. 2018). Functional scales (as described in the Care of the patient with spinal muscular atrophy section) are often used in clinical evaluations. The frequency at which rehabilitation services should be provided depends on the individual patient.

## Social aspects of spinal muscular atrophy

The diagnosis of SMA impacts not only the child, but also families and caregivers. A child with a more severe subtype requires round-the-clock care at home, including respiratory care such as suctioning, gastrostomy tube feeding, and rehabilitation. These children also have numerous hospital appointments with various specialists. Financial support is also an important aspect in SMA. Frequently, a parent may have to give up a career to care for the child. Additional expenditures for items such as respiratory or other medical equipment or home modifications need to be considered. Often, the medical social worker may be able to assist the family with emotional and financial support; however, the extent of support varies between countries.

Cognition is preserved in patients with SMA. When children with SMA types II and III become older, they may find it hard to accept that they are different from their peers or unable to participate in certain physical activities with their peers. They may worry about further loss of function and independence. It is important to consider the physiological impact if a child suddenly becomes more withdrawn socially.

## Clinical trials for drug development in spinal muscular atrophy

The understanding of the genetic basis of SMA has resulted in numerous clinical trials exploring the efficacy and safety of various drug treatments. Up until December 2016, no definitive treatment for SMA was identified despite major efforts exploring pharmacological methods that could upregulate the expression of *SMN2* or produce more functional SMN protein (Markowitz et al. 2012). Now, several potential therapeutic developments are in the pipeline and showing potential, giving the SMA community around the world great hope that, one day, at least one therapeutic option may allow every SMA child to reach his or her best potential in terms of motor function. These efforts are summarized in Table 6.4 and discussed below.

Currently, histone deacetylase inhibitors and nonhistone deacetylase inhibitors are being investigated as potential therapeutic agents because they are known to increase *SMN2* gene expression, *SMN* mRNA and SMN protein. Histone deacetylase inhibitors have been shown in some studies to increase full-length *SMN2* transcript levels by inhibiting the deacetylation of histones, nonhistones, and transcription factors (Singh et al. 2013b). This class of drugs has been extensively studied; however, clinical trials with valproic acid, phenylbutyrate and hydroxyurea have been disappointing and found no significant change in the primary outcome measures.

In a pilot study of 13 patients with SMA types II and III, treatment with albuterol, a β-adrenergic agonist, was associated with increased *SMN2* full-length transcript levels and improvements in muscle strength and Hammersmith Functional Motor Scale score with no major adverse effects. Another pilot study of 23 patients with SMA type II using salbutamol, a form of albuterol, also demonstrated improved Hammersmith Functional Motor Scale Scores (Pane et al. 2008). However, these studies were not placebo-controlled and the intervention has not been subsequently evaluated in randomized, double-blinded placebo-controlled clinical trials.

**TABLE 6.4**
**Summary of experimental therapies in spinal muscular atrophy**

| Therapeutic targets | Approaches | Clinical trials |
|---|---|---|
| Increase SMN transcript and enhance *SMN2* gene expression | Histone deacetylase inhibitors | Valproic acid<br>Sodium 4-phenylbutyrate |
| | Nonhistone deacetylase inhibitors | Hydroxyurea |
| | Quinazoline | Repligen RG3039 |
| | Prolactin | |
| *SMN2* exon 7 inclusion | Antisense oligonucleotides | Nusinersen |
| | Small molecules | Roche RG7916<br>Novartis LM1070 |
| Stabilization of SMN protein | Aminoglycoside | |
| | Proteasome inhibitors | |
| | Indoprofen | |
| Neuroprotection | Neurotrophic factors | Riluzole<br>Gabapentin<br>Olesoxime (TRO19622) |
| Improving function of skeletal muscle | Skeletal muscle troponin activator | Cytokinetics CK-2127107 |
| Cell therapy | Stem cells | |
| Replacement of *SMN1* | Gene therapy | AveXis AVXS-101 |

Adapted from Swaiman et al. (2018) with permission from Elsevier.

Antisense oligonucleotides (ASOs) are synthetic RNA molecules that promote exon 7 inclusion by interfering with the physiological splicing of exons, thus increasing the production of full-length *SMN2* mRNAs (Burghes and McGovern 2010). In *in-vitro* and SMA mouse models, these effects appear to compensate for the lack of *SMN1*. ASOs can affect the splicing of *SMN2* exon 7 by blocking the binding of trans-acting protein factors by steric hindrance (Hua et al. 2008), rearranging the structure of target RNA molecules (Singh et al. 2013a, Owen et al. 2011) (Fig. 6.3). Multiple challenges arise when translating this approach into clinical practice: (1) finding an efficient and safe route of administration of ASOs into the central nervous system; and (2) timing the introduction of this therapy to affected patients. Animal models appear to suggest that intra-cerebroventricular injections of ASOs produce a higher level of *SMN2* expression in motor neurons compared to systemic administration (Singh et al. 2009; Hua et al. 2010). A preclinical study suggesting that timing of therapy is also important showed a median survival of 100 days or longer compared to 41 days in SMA mice that received the treatment immediately after birth compared to 4 days after birth.

In December 2016, the Food and Drug Administration (FDA) announced the approval of Spinraza (nusinersen) for patients with SMA, making it the first approved therapy for these patients. Nusinersen is a 2′-O-methoxyethyl phosphorothioate-modified antisense oligonucleotide therapy developed by Ionis Pharmaceuticals in conjunction with Biogen, Inc. It increases the amount of functional full-length SMN protein, deficient in SMA patients, by

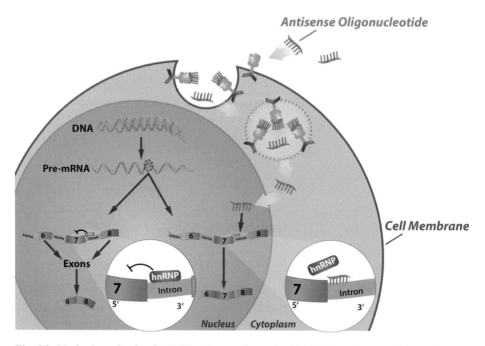

**Fig. 6.3.** Mechanism of action for SMN antisense oligonucleotide (ASO). ASOs enter the cytoplasm of the cells by endocytosis, and enter the nucleus where they bind to the *SMN2* pre-mRNA, displacing protein hnRNP which normally suppresses splicing of exon 7. This action enhances exon 7 inclusion and results in the production of full-length SMN protein. Courtesy of Frank Bennett, PhD, Ionis Pharmaceuticals, Carlsbad, CA, USA. A colour version of this figure can be seen in the plate section at the end of the book.

changing the splicing of *SMN2* pre-mRNA. In 2004, the Singh Laboratory at University of Massachusetts Medical School discovered ISS-N1 (intronic splicing silencer N1). *In vivo* studies showed that blocking ISS-N1 with an ASO enhanced *SMN2* exon 7 inclusion during splicing events, and this finding was subsequently confirmed in studies involving both SMA patient cells and mouse models. In 2010, Ionis Pharmaceuticals (previously known as ISIS Pharmaceuticals) obtained the license for exclusive use, and in 2011 Phase 1 clinical trials began with encouraging results, demonstrating the drug's safety and effectiveness in reducing the disease severity and improving the phenotype in SMA patients (Chiriboga et al. 2016). These trials were followed by Phase 2 and later Phase 3 trials.

The Phase 3 CHERISH study, a multicenter, randomized, double-blinded sham procedure-controlled study, aimed to assess the efficacy and safety of nusinersen in children with later onset SMA (types II or III) (Mercuri et al. 2018). Symptomatic children between the ages of 2 and 12 years, diagnosed with 5q SMA, and with onset of symptoms at or older than 6 months of age, were eligible to be included in this study. They were then randomized to receive four doses of 12mg of intrathecal nusinersen versus sham procedure control. The four doses of nusinersen were administered over a 15-month period. The primary endpoint of this study was the change in Hammersmith Functional Motor Scale Expanded (HFMSE) score at 15 months. Secondary endpoints included a greater or equal than 3.0 increase in baseline HFMSE score, a new World Health Organization (WHO) motor milestone, the number of new WHO motor milestones achieved, any change in the Revised Upper Limb Module (RULM) score, and the proportion of children who achieved standing alone or walking with assistance. The study found clinical and statistical differences in the change of HFMSE score between the children who received nusinersen versus those in the sham procedure comparison group. There were no significant adverse side effects from nusinersen and the therapy was generally well tolerated by the children, although there were more complaints of back pain, headache and vomiting in the nusinersen group (>5% frequency) 72 hours after the administration of the drug. These complaints were attributed to the lumbar puncture procedures rather than a direct side effect from the drug.

The ENDEAR study was a Phase 3, randomized, double-blind, sham procedure-controlled study assessing the clinical efficiency, safety and tolerability of intrathecal nusinersen in infants with SMA type I (Finkel et al. 2017). Patients between 3 weeks and 7 months of age, with genetically-confirmed 5q SMA, and with symptom onset between 3 weeks and 6 months, were eligible for inclusion. Outcome measures were event-free survival (time to death or permanent ventilation, defined as tracheostomy or greater than or equal than 16 hours of ventilatory support per day for more than 21 days in the absence of an acute reversible event), and changes in motor function and electrophysiologic assessments: the motor milestones portion of the Hammersmith Infant Neurological Exam and the Children's Hospital of Philadelphia Infant Test of Neuromuscular Disorders scores, and compound motor action potential amplitudes. Age at death or permanent ventilation was compared with natural history. The study results were encouraging. Rate of survival without ventilation assistance was higher in infants who were treated with nusinersen compared to the comparison group (hazard ratio: 0.53; p value: 0.005). Fifty-one percent of nusinersen-treated infants showed improvements in their motor function assessments versus 0% of control infants (Finkel et al. 2017). The treatments were generally well tolerated. All reported side effects were felt to be expected in infants with SMA, with some related to the lumbar puncture itself; no safety concerns were identified.

The approval of nusinersen by the United States FDA as a therapy for SMA patients is a major step for patients worldwide. Nevertheless, much work remains to be done as researchers transition to the next phase, in which the long-term efficacy of nusinersen is monitored. Follow-up trials to assess the long-term efficacy of nusinersen are in progress. Many other studies are underway, targeting other approaches or studying a less invasive route of administration for an effective delivery of drug into brain and spinal cord. In addition to studies of patients who are already symptomatic, an ongoing study (NURTURE) looks at the efficacy in preventing or delaying complications/symptoms in presymptomatic, genetically-confirmed SMA patients (Biogen 2015), and so far the results seem promising.

The following is the recommended dosage for nusinersen in SMA patients: 3 loading doses to be given 14 days apart (days 1, 15, 30) at 12mg (5ml) per dose, to be administered as an intrathecal bolus. The fourth loading dose is given 30 days after the last dose, around day 60. For maintenance, a dose every 4 months is recommended. Before each dose and as clinically indicated, recommendations include monitoring the platelet count, coagulation profile (prothrombin time and aPTT), and baseline quantitative spot urine protein testing.

Small molecule or low-molecular-weight drugs have been found to increase SMN protein in the following ways: by activation of the *SMN2* promoter and increasing its expression, or by alteration of the splicing pattern of *SMN2* resulting in the inclusion of exon 7.

Olesoxime is a molecule with cholesterol-like structure and neuroprotective properties. Preclinical studies suggest that it improves the function and survival of neurons. A Phase 2 randomized, double-blind placebo-controlled clinical trial in patients with SMA types II and III between the ages of 3 and 25 was promising at the 12-month mark, with results suggesting that olesoxime maintained motor function and prevented the deterioration of muscle function during 12 months of treatment, but results at 18 months were disappointing and development has been discontinued (Lopes 2018).

LM1070 is a small molecule (developed by Novartis) designed to alter the *SMN2* alternative splicing of exon 7, hence increasing full-length SMN. The Phase 1 trial is an open-label, first-in-human study of oral LM1070 in patients with SMA type I (Novartis Pharmaceuticals 2015). SMA patients up to 8 months of age are eligible for enrollment. This study examines the safety, tolerability, pharmacokinetics, pharmacodynamics, and efficacy after 13 weeks, as well as the maximum tolerated dose and optimal dosing regimen in this group of patients. RG7800 was another orally bioavailable small molecule which was studied in a Phase 1a/2b clinical trial, MOONFISH, involving pediatric and adult SMA patients. However, the study was terminated early after an unexpected toxicology finding in an animal study.

RG7916 is an oral *SMN2* splicing modifier (developed by Hoffman-La Roche in collaboration with PTC Therapeutics and the SMA Foundation) designed to produce more functional SMN protein. Clinical trials are being planned in Europe and the United States to involve patients with SMA type I aged 1–7 months old (FIREFISH) and patients with types II and III aged 2–25 years (SUNFISH) (Hoffmann-La Roche 2016a; 2016b). Another study, JEWELFISH, aims to enroll patients with types II and III who have already been exposed to a *SMN2* targeting therapy (such as RG7800 or nusinersen) (Hoffmann-La Roche 2017).

A novel compound (CK-2127107) designed to improve the function of skeletal muscle via a skeletal muscle troponin activator is currently in a Phase 2 clinical trial to examine its efficacy in both ambulatory and non-ambulatory SMA patients (Cytokinetics and Astellas Pharma Global Development Inc 2015). This compound is unlike others in that it is not intended to increase the levels of SMN protein. Instead, this drug slows down the rate of calcium release from the troponin complex of fast skeletal muscle fibers.

Stem cells and gene therapy have long been tested in preclinical studies and have been promising (Foust et al. 2010; Passini et al. 2010). Tremendous progress has been made in gene therapy, and various classes of viral vectors have been researched extensively to find a vector that is safe, readily made and easily administered. In the early days of gene therapy research, adenoviruses were used as gene delivery vectors; however, immunogenicity was found to be a major issue. Subsequently, recombinant adeno-associated viral vectors (rAAV) proved to be promising as a gene transfer vehicle due to their lower immunogenicity.

An open-label Phase 1 trial studying a gene therapy product (AVXS-101) given intravenously in patients with SMA type I has recently been completed; the results seem promising and similar to nusinersen in terms of event-free survival (100% of enrolled patients alive and not requiring permanent ventilation at 20 months compared with historical cohort rate of event-free survival of 8%), motor milestone acquisition (patients in the high-dose cohort achieved milestones such as sitting unassisted, rolling over, oral feeding and speaking, and two walked independently), and scores on the Children's Hospital of Philadelphia Infant Test of Neuromuscular Disorders (increase of 9.8 points and 15.4 points at 1 and 3 months respectively, compared with decline in scores in historical cohort) (Mendell et al. 2017). AVXS-101 is derived from a non-replicating adeno-associated virus serotype 9 vector that is used to deliver a functional copy of *SMN* gene via an intravenous or intrathecal injection. In preclinical studies, it demonstrated its effectiveness in targeting motor neuron cells when administered either intravenously or via an intrathecal route. Further studies for patients with types I and II will be initiated in the United States in the near future (AveXis Inc 2014) (Table 6.4).

## Conclusion

SMA is a chronic, progressive, inherited motor neuron disease. Over the years, increasing knowledge and advances in research have given families with children affected by SMA great hope and optimism. Although there is now an FDA-approved treatment for all subtypes of SMA, ongoing research is being carried out to identify new therapeutic agents through the development of novel compounds. Standards of care are also developed to guide clinicians and caregivers to optimize the holistic, multidisciplinary management of these patients. As more therapeutic agents are being developed, standards of care and treatment guidelines will continue to evolve and may encompass more proactive respiratory intervention and support in an acute hospital setting. While the availability of new drugs has given many SMA families hope, the cost of the drugs together with the vast differences in healthcare policies in countries worldwide have meant that many children still may not have access to these drugs.

Lastly, support groups such as SMA Foundation, CureSMA and Fight SMA have provided a vital role in research efforts as well as a community for families affected by SMA.

## Key points
- Spinal muscular atrophy (SMA) is a group of autosomal recessive disorders associated with degeneration of motor neurons in the spinal cord and, in the most severely affected patients, of the lower brain stem motor neurons.
- Patients with SMA experience progressive muscle weakness and atrophy along a phenotypic continuum, divided by clinical severity into four broad clinical subtypes using maximum motor function or gross motor developmental milestone achieved.
- More rare than SMA, "non-5q SMA" is a diverse group of motor neuron disorders caused by mutations in various genes; non-5q SMAs include distal spinal muscular atrophies, distal hereditary motor neuropathies, and X-linked, autosomal dominant or autosomal recessive spinal muscular atrophies.

- Patients and their families benefit from a holistic and multidisciplinary approach to care that includes specialists in neurology and neuromuscular medicine, pulmonology, gastroenterology, nutrition, orthopedics, rehabilitation, and social work.
- Understanding of the genetic basis of SMA has led to recent and ongoing advances in drug development and to the first definitive treatments for these devastating conditions.

**Clinical vignette**

An 18-month-old girl was diagnosed with SMA via DNA testing that showed a homozygous deletion of *SMN1* and 3 copies of *SMN2*. Later enrolled in a prospective multicenter national history study, she was evaluated at ages 6 years through 13 years for motor function, pulmonary function, muscle strength, electrophysiological measures, and patient-reported outcomes. Motor function improved during the first 18 months of observation, but then the patient experienced slow functional decline. Intensive rehabilitation efforts allowed the patient to walk until the age of 9 years; however, she ultimately required multiple orthopedic procedures and wheelchair dependency. Aggressive and proactive airway management was necessary to ensure adequate ventilation. This patient has SMA type IIIA, with onset before the age of 3 years. Her motor achievements, unusual for this SMA type, illustrate that rehabilitation and other management efforts can mitigate the natural course of the disease.

## REFERENCES

ACOG Committee on Genetics (2009) ACOG committee opinion No. 432: spinal muscular atrophy. *Obstet Gynecol* 113: 1194–1196.

Arkblad E, Tulinius M, Kroksmark AK, Henricsson M, Darin N (2009) A population-based study of genotypic and phenotypic variability in children with spinal muscular atrophy. *Acta Paediatr* 98: 865–872.

AveXis Inc. (2014) Gene transfer clinical trial for spinal muscular atrophy type 1. ClinicalTrials.gov Identifier: NCT02122952. https://ClinicalTrials.gov/show/NCT02122952.

Bernal S, Alías L, Barceló MJ, Also-Rallo E, Martínez-Hernández R, Gámez J et al. (2010) The c.859G>C variant in the SMN2 gene is associated with types II and III SMA and originates from a common ancestor. *J Med Genet* 47: 640–642.

Bertoli S, De Amicis R, Mastella C, Pieri G, Giaquinto E, Battezzati A et al. (2017) Spinal Muscular Atrophy, types I and II: what are the differences in body composition and resting energy expenditure? *Clin Nutr* 36: 1674–1680.

Biogen (2015) A study of multiple doses of Nusinersen (ISIS 396443) Delivered to infants with genetically diagnosed and presymptomatic spinal muscular atrophy. ClinicalTrials.gov Identifier: NCT02386553. https://ClinicalTrials.gov/show/NCT02386553.

Burghes AH, McGovern VL (2010) Antisense oligonucleotides and spinal muscular atrophy: skipping along. *Genes Dev* 24: 1574–1579.

Campbell L, Potter A, Ignatius J, Dubowitz V, Davies K (1997) Genomic variation and gene conversion in spinal muscular atrophy: implications for disease process and clinical phenotype. *Am J Hum Genet* 61: 40–50.

Chiriboga CA, Swoboda KJ, Darras BT, Iannaccone ST, Montes J, De Vivo DC et al. (2016) Results from a phase 1 study of nusinersen (ISIS-SMN(Rx)) in children with spinal muscular atrophy. *Neurology* 86: 890–897.

Cobben JM, Lemmink HH, Snoeck I, Barth PA, van der Lee JH, de Visser M (2008) Survival in SMA type I: a prospective analysis of 34 consecutive cases. *Neuromuscul Disord* 18: 541–544.

Coovert DD, Le TT, McAndrew PE, Strasswimmer J, Crawford TO, Mendell JR et al. (1997) The survival motor neuron protein in spinal muscular atrophy. *Hum Mol Genet* 6: 1205–1214.

Cytokinetics, Astellas Pharma Global Development Inc (2015) A Study of CK-2127107 in patients with spinal muscular atrophy. ClinicalTrials.gov Identifier: NCT02644668. https://ClinicalTrials.gov/show/NCT02644668.

Darras BT (2011) Non-5q spinal muscular atrophies: the alphanumeric soup thickens. *Neurology* 77: 312–314.

Darras BT (2015) Spinal muscular atrophies. *Pediatr Clin North Am* 62: 743–766.

Darras BT, Finkel RS (2017) Natural history of spinal muscular atrophy. *In* Sumner CJ, Paushkin S, Po C-P (eds), *Spinal Muscular Atrophy: Disease Mechanisms and Therapy*. San Diego: Academic Press. doi.10.1016/B978-0-12-803685-3.00025-2.

Darras BT, Markowitz JA, Monani UR, De Vivo DC (2015) Spinal muscular atrophies. In Darras BT, Jones HRJ, Ryan MM, De Vivo DC (eds), *Neuromuscular Disorders of Infancy, Childhood, and Adolescence: A Clinician's Approach*, 2nd ed. San Diego: Academic Press doi.10.1016/B978-0-12-417044-5.00008-1.

Darras BT, Monani UR, De Vivo DC (2018) Genetic disorders affecting the motor neuron: spinal muscular atrophy. In Swaiman KF, Ashwal S, Ferriero DM, Schor NF, Finkel RS, Gropman AL et al. (eds) *Swaiman's Pediatric Neurology: Principles and Practice*, 6th edn. Edinburgh: Elsevier, pp. 1057–1064.

DiDonato CJ, Ingraham SE, Mendell JR, Prior TW, Lenard S, Moxley RT III et al. (1997) Deletion and conversion in spinal muscular atrophy patients: is there a relationship to severity? *Ann Neurol* 41: 230–237.

Dubowitz V (1999) Very severe spinal muscular atrophy (SMA type 0): an expanding clinical phenotype. *Eur J Paediatr Neurol* 3: 49–51.

Durkin ET, Schroth MK, Helin M, Shaaban AF (2008) Early laparoscopic fundoplication and gastrostomy in infants with spinal muscular atrophy type I. *J Pediatr Surg* 43: 2031–2037.

Feldkötter M, Schwarzer V, Wirth R, Wienker TF, Wirth B (2002) Quantitative analyses of SMN1 and SMN2 based on real-time lightCycler PCR: fast and highly reliable carrier testing and prediction of severity of spinal muscular atrophy. *Am J Hum Genet* 70: 358–368.

Finkel RS, McDermott MP, Kaufmann P, Darras BT, Chung WK, Sproule DM et al. (2014) Observational study of spinal muscular atrophy type I and implications for clinical trials. *Neurology* 83: 810–817.

Finkel RS, Mercuri E, Darras BT, Connolly AM, Kuntz NL, Kirschner J et al. (2017) Nusinersen versus Sham Control in Infantile-Onset Spinal Muscular Atrophy. *N Engl J Med* 377: 1723–1732.

Finkel RS, Mercuri E, Meyer OH, Simonds AK, Schroth MK, Graham RJ et al. (2018) Diagnosis and management of spinal muscular atrophy: Part 2: Pulmonary and acute care; medications, supplements and immunizations; other organ systems; and ethics. *Neuromuscul Disord* 28: 197–207.

Foust KD, Wang X, McGovern VL, Braun L, Bevan AK, Haidet AM et al. (2010) Rescue of the spinal muscular atrophy phenotype in a mouse model by early postnatal delivery of SMN. *Nat Biotechnol* 28: 271–274.

Fujak A, Kopschina C, Forst R, Gras F, Mueller LA, Forst J (2010) Fractures in proximal spinal muscular atrophy. *Arch Orthop Trauma Surg* 130: 775–780.

Ge X, Bai J, Lu Y, Qu Y, Song F (2012) The natural history of infant spinal muscular atrophy in China: a study of 237 patients. *J Child Neurol* 27: 471–477.

Gilliam TC, Brzustowicz LM, Castilla LH, Lehner T, Penchaszadeh GK, Daniels RJ et al. (1990) Genetic homogeneity between acute and chronic forms of spinal muscular atrophy. *Nature* 345: 823–825.

Hendrickson BC, Donohoe C, Akmaev VR, Sugarman EA, Labrousse P, Boguslavskiy L et al. (2009) Differences in SMN1 allele frequencies among ethnic groups within North America. *J Med Genet* 46: 641–644.

Hoffmann-La Roche (2016a) A study to investigate the safety, tolerability, pharmacokinetics, pharmacodynamics and efficacy of RO7034067 in infants with type1 spinal muscular atrophy (FIREFISH). ClinicalTrials.gov Identifier: NCT02913482. https://ClinicalTrials.gov/show/NCT02913482.

Hoffmann-La Roche (2016b) A study to investigate the safety, tolerability, pharmacokinetics, pharmacodynamics and efficacy of RO7034067 in type 2 and 3 spinal muscular atrophy (SMA) participants. ClinicalTrials.gov Identifier: NCT02908685. https://ClinicalTrials.gov/show/NCT02908685.

Hoffmann-La Roche (2017) A study of RO7034067 in adult and pediatric participants with spinal muscular atrophy. ClinicalTrials.gov Identifier: NCT03032172. https://ClinicalTrials.gov/show/NCT03032172.

Hoffmann J (1893) Ueber chronische spinale muskelatrophie im kindesalter auf familiarer basis. *Dtsch Z Nervenheilkd* 3: 427–470.

Hua Y, Vickers TA, Okunola HL, Bennett CF, Krainer AR (2008) Antisense masking of an hnRNP A1/A2 intronic splicing silencer corrects SMN2 splicing in transgenic mice. Am J Hum Genet 82: 834–848.

Hua Y, Sahashi K, Hung G, Rigo F, Passini MA, Bennett CF et al. (2010) Antisense correction of SMN2 splicing in the CNS rescues necrosis in a type III SMA mouse model. *Genes Dev* 24: 1634–1644.

Iannaccone ST (2007) Modern management of spinal muscular atrophy. *J Child Neurol* 22: 974–978.

Iannaccone ST, Russman BS, Browne RH, Buncher CR, White M, Samaha FJ et al. (2000) Prospective analysis of strength in spinal muscular atrophy. *J Child Neurol* 15: 97–101.

Ioos C, Leclair-Richard D, Mrad S, Barois A, Estournet-Mathiaud B (2004) Respiratory capacity course in patients with infantile spinal muscular atrophy. *Chest* 126: 831–837.

Jamrozik Z, Lugowska A, Gołębiowski M, Królicki L, Mączewska J, Kuźma-Kozakiewicz M (2013) Late onset GM2 gangliosidosis mimicking spinal muscular atrophy. *Gene* 527: 679–682.

Jeppesen J, Madsen A, Marquardt J, Rahbek J (2010) Living and ageing with spinal muscular atrophy type 2: observations among an unexplored patient population. *Dev Neurorehabil* 13: 10–18.

Kariya S, Park GH, Maeno-Hikichi Y, Leykekhman O, Lutz C, Arkovitz MS et al. (2008) Reduced SMN protein impairs maturation of the neuromuscular junctions in mouse models of spinal muscular atrophy. *Hum Mol Genet* 17: 2552–2569.

Kaufmann P, McDermott MP, Darras BT, Finkel R, Kang P, Oskoui M et al. (2011) Observational study of spinal muscular atrophy type 2 and 3: functional outcomes over 1 year. *Arch Neurol* 68: 779–786.

Kugelberg E, Welander L (1956) Heredofamilial juvenile muscular atrophy simulating muscular dystrophy. *AMA Arch Neurol Psychiatry* 75: 500–509.

Lefebvre S, Bürglen L, Reboullet S, Clermont O, Burlet P, Viollet L et al. (1995) Identification and characterization of a spinal muscular atrophy-determining gene. *Cell* 80: 155–165.

Lefebvre S, Burlet P, Liu Q, Bertrandy S, Clermont O, Munnich A et al. (1997) Correlation between severity and SMN protein level in spinal muscular atrophy. *Nat Genet* 16: 265–269.

Lemoine TJ, Swoboda KJ, Bratton SL, Holubkov R, Mundorff M, Srivastava R (2012) Spinal muscular atrophy type 1: are proactive respiratory interventions associated with longer survival? *Pediatr Crit Care Med* 13:e161–e165.

Lopes JM (2018) Roche stops work on olesoxime after disappointing long-term results in Phase 2 trial. https://smanewstoday.com/2018/06/06/roche-stops-development-of-sma-therapy-olesoxime-after-disappointing-trial-results/

Lorson CL, Androphy EJ (2000) An exonic enhancer is required for inclusion of an essential exon in the SMA-determining gene SMN. *Hum Mol Genet* 9: 259–265.

Mailman MD, Heinz JW, Papp AC, Snyder PJ, Sedra MS, Wirth B et al. (2002) Molecular analysis of spinal muscular atrophy and modification of the phenotype by SMN2. *Genet Med* 4: 20–26.

Main M, Kairon H, Mercuri E, Muntoni F (2003) The Hammersmith functional motor scale for children with spinal muscular atrophy: a scale to test ability and monitor progress in children with limited ambulation. *Eur J Paediatr Neurol* 7: 155–159.

Markowitz JA, Singh P, Darras BT (2012) Spinal muscular atrophy: a clinical and research update. *Pediatr Neurol* 46: 1–12.

Markström A, Cohen G, Katz-Salamon M (2010) The effect of long term ventilatory support on hemodynamics in children with spinal muscle atrophy (SMA) type II. *Sleep Med* 11: 201–204.

Melki J, Abdelhak S, Sheth P, Bachelot MF, Burlet P, Marcadet A et al. (1990) Gene for chronic proximal spinal muscular atrophies maps to chromosome 5q. *Nature* 344: 767–768.

Mellies U, Dohna-Schwake C, Stehling F, Voit T (2004) Sleep disordered breathing in spinal muscular atrophy. *Neuromuscul Disord* 14: 797–803.

Mendell JR, Al-Zaidy S, Shell R, Arnold WD, Rodino-Klapac LR, Prior TW et al. (2017) Single-Dose Gene-Replacement Therapy for Spinal Muscular Atrophy. *N Engl J Med* 377: 1713–1722.

Mercuri E, Finkel R, Montes J, Mazzone ES, Sormani MP, Main M et al. (2016) Patterns of disease progression in type 2 and 3 SMA: implications for clinical trials. Neuromuscul Disord 26: 126–131.

Mercuri E, Darras BT, Chiriboga CA, Day JW, Campbell C, Connolly AM et al. (2018) Nusinersen versus Sham Control in Later-Onset Spinal Muscular Atrophy. *N Engl J Med* 378: 625–635.

Monani UR, Lorson CL, Parsons DW, Prior TW, Androphy EJ, Burghes AH et al. (1999) A single nucleotide difference that alters splicing patterns distinguishes the SMA gene SMN1 from the copy gene SMN2. *Hum Mol Genet* 8: 1177–1183.

Montes J, Gordon AM, Pandya S, De Vivo DC, Kaufmann P (2009) Clinical outcome measures in spinal muscular atrophy. *J Child Neurol* 24: 968–978.

Montes J, McDermott MP, Martens WB, Dunaway S, Glanzman AM, Riley S et al. (2010) Six-Minute Walk Test demonstrates motor fatigue in spinal muscular atrophy. *Neurology* 74: 833–838.

Mostacciuolo ML, Danieli GA, Trevisan C, Müller E, Angelini C (1992) Epidemiology of spinal muscular atrophies in a sample of the Italian population. *Neuroepidemiology* 11: 34–38.

Novartis Pharmaceuticals.(2015) An open label study of LMI070 (Branaplam) in type 1 spinal muscular atrophy (SMA). ClinicalTrials.gov Identifier: NCT02268552. https://ClinicalTrials.gov/show/NCT02268552.

O'Hagen JM, Glanzman AM, McDermott MP, Ryan PA, Flickinger J, Quigley J et al. (2007) An expanded version of the Hammersmith Functional Motor Scale for SMA II and III patients. *Neuromuscul Disord* 17: 693–697.

Ogino S, Gao S, Leonard DG, Paessler M, Wilson RB (2003) Inverse correlation between SMN1 and SMN2 copy numbers: evidence for gene conversion from SMN2 to SMN1. *Eur J Hum Genet* 11: 723.

Ogino S, Wilson RB, Gold B (2004) New insights on the evolution of the SMN1 and SMN2 region: simulation and meta-analysis for allele and haplotype frequency calculations. *Eur J Hum Genet* 12: 1015–1023.

Oskoui M, Levy G, Garland CJ, Gray JM, O'Hagen J, De Vivo DC et al. (2007) The changing natural history of spinal muscular atrophy type 1. *Neurology* 69: 1931–1936.

Owen N, Zhou H, Malygin AA, Sangha J, Smith LD, Muntoni F et al. (2011) Design principles for bifunctional targeted oligonucleotide enhancers of splicing. *Nucleic Acids Res* 39: 7194–7208.

Pane M, Staccioli S, Messina S, D'Amico A, Pelliccioni M, Mazzone ES et al. (2008) Daily salbutamol in young patients with SMA type II. *Neuromuscul Disord* 18: 536–540.

Passini MA, Bu J, Roskelley EM, Richards AM, Sardi SP, O'Riordan CR et al. (2010) CNS-targeted gene therapy improves survival and motor function in a mouse model of spinal muscular atrophy. *J Clin Invest* 120: 1253–1264.

Prior TW (2007) Spinal muscular atrophy diagnostics. *J Child Neurol* 22: 952–956.

Prior TW (2010a). Perspectives and diagnostic considerations in spinal muscular atrophy. *Genet Med* 12: 145–152.

Prior TW (2010b) Spinal muscular atrophy: newborn and carrier screening. *Obstet Gynecol Clin North Am* 37: 23–36. doi.10.1016/j.ogc.2010.03.001.

Prior TW, Swoboda KJ, Scott HD, Hejmanowski AQ (2004) Homozygous SMN1 deletions in unaffected family members and modification of the phenotype by SMN2. *Am J Med Genet A* 130A:307–310.

Prior TW, Finanger E (2016) Spinal Muscular Atrophy. 2000 Feb 24 [Updated 2016 Dec 22]. In: Adam MP, Ardinger HH, Pagon RA, et al. (eds). GeneReviews® [Internet]. Seattle (WA): University of Washington, Seattle; 1993-2019. Available from: https://www-ncbi-nlm-nih-gov.ezp-prod1.hul.harvard.edu/books/NBK1352/.

Rudnik-Schöneborn S, Berg C, Zerres K, Betzler C, Grimm T, Eggermann T et al. (2009) Genotype-phenotype studies in infantile spinal muscular atrophy (SMA) type I in Germany: implications for clinical trials and genetic counselling. *Clin Genet* 76: 168–178.

Russman BS (2007) Spinal muscular atrophy: clinical classification and disease heterogeneity. *J Child Neurol* 22: 946–951.

Russman BS, Buncher CR, White M, Samaha FJ, Iannaccone ST, The DCN/SMA Group (1996) Function changes in spinal muscular atrophy II and III. *Neurology* 47: 973–976.

Schroth MK (2009) Special considerations in the respiratory management of spinal muscular atrophy. *Pediatrics* 123(Suppl 4): S245–S249.

Singh NN, Shishimorova M, Cao LC, Gangwani L, Singh RN (2009) A short antisense oligonucleotide masking a unique intronic motif prevents skipping of a critical exon in spinal muscular atrophy. RNA Biol 6: 341–350.

Singh NN, Lawler MN, Ottesen EW, Upreti D, Kaczynski JR, Singh RN (2013a). An intronic structure enabled by a long-distance interaction serves as a novel target for splicing correction in spinal muscular atrophy. *Nucleic Acids Res* 41: 8144–8165.

Singh P, Liew WK, Darras BT (2013b). Current advances in drug development in spinal muscular atrophy. *Curr Opin Pediatr* 25: 682–688.

Souchon F, Simard LR, Lebrun S, Rochette C, Lambert J, Vanasse M (1996) Clinical and genetic study of chronic (types II and III) childhood onset spinal muscular atrophy. *Neuromuscul Disord* 6: 419–424.

Sproule DM, Montes J, Montgomery M, Battista V, Koenigsberger D, Shen W et al. (2009) Increased fat mass and high incidence of overweight despite low body mass index in patients with spinal muscular atrophy. Neuromuscul Disord 19: 391–396.

Sproule DM, Montes J, Dunaway S, Montgomery M, Battista V, Koenigsberger D et al. (2010) Adiposity is increased among high-functioning, non-ambulatory patients with spinal muscular atrophy. *Neuromuscul Disord* 20(7): 448–452. doi: 10.1016/j.nmd.2010.05.013.

Sugarman EA, Nagan N, Zhu H, Akmaev VR, Zhou Z, Rohlfs EM et al. (2012) Pan-ethnic carrier screening and prenatal diagnosis for spinal muscular atrophy: clinical laboratory analysis of >72,400 specimens. *Eur J Hum Genet* 20: 27–32.

Swoboda KJ, Prior TW, Scott CB, McNaught TP, Wride MC, Reyna SP et al. (2005) Natural history of denervation in SMA: relation to age, SMN2 copy number, and function. *Ann Neurol* 57: 704–712.

Vezain M, Saugier-Veber P, Goina E, Touraine R, Manel V, Toutain A et al. (2010) A rare SMN2 variant in a previously unrecognized composite splicing regulatory element induces exon 7 inclusion and reduces the clinical severity of spinal muscular atrophy. *Hum Mutat* 31:E1110–E1125.

von Gontard A, Zerres K, Backes M, Laufersweiler-Plass C, Wendland C, Melchers P et al. (2002) Intelligence and cognitive function in children and adolescents with spinal muscular atrophy. *Neuromuscul Disord* 12: 130–136.

Wadman RI, Vrancken AF, van den Berg LH, van der Pol WL (2012) Dysfunction of the neuromuscular junction in spinal muscular atrophy types 2 and 3. *Neurology* 79: 2050–2055.

Wang CH, Finkel RS, Bertini ES, Schroth M, Simonds A, Wong B et al. (2007a) Consensus statement for standard of care in spinal muscular atrophy. *J Child Neurol* 22(8): 1027–1049. doi.10.1177/0883073807305788.

Wang CH, Finkel RS, Bertini ES, Schroth M, Simonds A, Wong B, Aloysius A, Morrison L, Main M, Crawford TO, Trela AParticipants of the International Conference on S. M. A. Standard of Care (2007b) Consensus statement for standard of care in spinal muscular atrophy. *J Child Neurol* 22: 1027–49. doi.10.1177/0883073807305788.

Wasserman HM, Hornung LN, Stenger PJ, Rutter MM, Wong BL, Rybalsky I et al. (2017) Low bone mineral density and fractures are highly prevalent in pediatric patients with spinal muscular atrophy regardless of disease severity. *Neuromuscul Disord* 27: 331–337.

Werdnig G (1891) Zwei fruihnfantile hereditare Falle von progressive Muskelatrophie unter dem Bilde der Dystrophie, aber auf neurotischer Grundlage. *Arch Psychiatr Neurol* 22: 437–481.

Werlauff U, Vissing J, Steffensen BF (2012) Change in muscle strength over time in spinal muscular atrophy types II and III. A long-term follow-up study. *Neuromuscul Disord* 22: 1069–1074.

Wirth B, Brichta L, Schrank B, Lochmüller H, Blick S, Baasner A et al. (2006) Mildly affected patients with spinal muscular atrophy are partially protected by an increased SMN2 copy number. *Hum Genet* 119: 422–428.

Wu JS, Darras BT, Rutkove SB (2010) Assessing spinal muscular atrophy with quantitative ultrasound. *Neurology* 75: 526–531.

Yuan N, Wang CH, Trela A, Albanese CT (2007) Laparoscopic Nissen fundoplication during gastrostomy tube placement and noninvasive ventilation may improve survival in type I and severe type II spinal muscular atrophy. *J Child Neurol* 22: 727–731.

Zerres K, Davies KE (1999) 59th ENMC International Workshop: Spinal Muscular Atrophies: recent progress and revised diagnostic criteria 17–19 April 1998, Soestduinen, The Netherlands. *Neuromuscul Disord* 9: 272–278.

Zerres K, Rudnik-Schöneborn S (2003) 93rd ENMC international workshop: non-5q-spinal muscular atrophies (SMA) – clinical picture (6–8 April 2001, Naarden, The Netherlands). *Neuromuscul Disord* 13: 179–183.

# 7
# AN INTRODUCTION TO NEUROPATHIES AND INHERITED NEUROPATHIES

*Nicolas Deconinck and Lionel Paternoster*

## An Introduction to Neuropathies

Polyneuropathy is typically defined as a diffuse, generally symmetrical length-dependent disease of at least two but in most of the cases multiple nerves. A wide and heterogeneous range of etiologies can cause a polyneuropathy and determining either an acquired or an inherited origin is commonly a first way to categorize them in children.

The course of most peripheral nerve disorders is gradual and slowly progressive. One uses then the term of chronic polyneuropathy. However, toxic exposure or inflammatory conditions can cause an acute presentation of the disease (acute polyneuropathy). Bilateral, symmetric, predominantly distal involvement is shown in most peripheral neuropathies, although for example trauma could cause focal neuropathies in children. The severity of diffuse nerve injuries is related directly to axon length which means longer axons are first affected, leading to earlier and more prominent presentations in the distal lower extremities. Some neuropathies are only characterized by motor or sensory abnormalities, but most have a combined involvement.

Infantile-onset peripheral neuropathy is a rare entity compared to adults. The difference between the infantile-onset neuropathies and those presenting in adults is the inclusion of a greater number of inherited conditions (Wilmshurst and Ourvrier 2011), which is particularly true in high income countries.

Distally marked weakness is the most common motor symptom, especially in the peroneal compartment. It may present as difficulty with climbing stairs, running, impaired fine motor skills, clumsiness. Another common symptom is ataxia or balance difficulties. On the other hand sensory symptoms could include numbness or positive sensory symptoms like paresthesia, burning sensations, pain, but also abnormal response to pain. The absence of deep tendon reflexes during a neurological examination is typical (Charcot and Marie 1886).

Autonomic neuropathy could manifest solely or as a more widespread neuropathy, and in children is frequently observed in the context of acute inflammatory syndrome like Guillain–Barré syndrome (GBS). Peripheral neuropathy could be accompanied by autonomic symptoms such as cardiac arrhythmias, bowel and bladder dysfunction, abnormal sweating. In children, there could also be involvement of the central nervous system, but this is more typically associated with hereditary neurodegenerative diseases.

Suggestive symptoms of peripheral neuropathy should be investigated in a center experienced in infantile examination and the interpretation of results. The combination of needle examination (EMG) with motor/sensory examinations in infants is distressing and requires a thorough preparation of the patient (see Chapter 4).

In Chapter 7 we start with the description of inherited neuropathies in children focusing on the most frequent forms and when possible their specific management. The second part (see Chapter 8) is dedicated to acquired neuropathies with particular an emphasis on Guillain–Barré syndrome but also leprosy neuropathy still frequently encountered in lower medium income countries (LMICs).

## Inherited Neuropathies

In children, inherited polyneuropathies are particularly represented and can be separated in three groups (all including autosomal dominant, recessive or X-linked inheritance): (1) isolated neuropathies exclusively involving the peripheral nervous system; (2) multisystem neuropathies involving both central (brain and spinal cord) and peripheral nervous systems; and (3) neuropathies with multi-organ involvement affecting non-neurologic organs such as skin, heart, liver and kidney. The distinction between category 2 and 3 is not always so clear cut for a number of entities, as will be illustrated.

### Inherited neuropathies involving only the peripheral nervous system

Charcot–Marie–Tooth disease is often used as a general name that, in fact, includes a wide variety of inherited sensory and/or motor neuropathies (El-Abassi et al. 2014).

Hereditary motor sensory neuropathy (HMSN) or Charcot–Marie–Tooth (CMT) is the largest group of disorders in this category, affecting mainly lower extremity motor and primary sensory neurons. It is probably the most common neuromuscular disorder in the pediatric population. Although this is a primary group, we can distinguish five other categories of neuropathies combining different specific neurons alterations such as: (1) HSAN, affecting primary sensory and autonomic neurons, (2) HSN or hereditary sensory neuropathy without involvement of the autonomic system, (3) dHMN or distal hereditary motor neuropathy affecting distal lower motor neurons; (4) HBPN or hereditary brachial plexus neuropathy affecting the upper extremity nerves and the brachial plexus; and (5) HNPP or hereditary neuropathy with liability to pressure palsies (Brennan and Shy 2014). In the context of this book that has a specific focus on management aspects, we will only detail the description of entities that are encountered with a relative high frequency in multidisciplinary neuromuscular consultations.

*Hereditary motor sensory neuropathy or Charcot–Marie–Tooth*
Classification

Charcot–Marie–Tooth (CMT) can be categorized into different subtypes based on the pattern of inheritance and based on neurophysiological studies. Subtypes include autosomal dominant demyelinating (CMT1), autosomal dominant axonal (CMT2), autosomal recessive (CMT4), and X-linked (CMTX) (Charcot and Marie 1886) (see Table 7.1). Slow nerve conduction velocities (<38m/s upper extremities) and pathological evidence of hypertrophic demyelinating neuropathy is typical for CMT1, whereas normal nerve conduction velocities and evidence of axonal degeneration is characteristic for CMT2. Originally some patients (most often with a severe early-onset phenotype) were misclassified due to incomplete family histories, they were thought to be autosomal recessive and classified as HSMN III or Dejerine-Sottas syndrome. Advances in molecular technology led to a revision of this classification concluding that most HSMN III patients showed spontaneous mutations in dominantly inherited genes. The term HSMN III or CMT3 is no longer used, Dejerine-Sottas syndrome however is still used to describe severely affected infants with CMT with typically slow nerve conduction velocities (Dejerine and Sottas 1893).

The discovery of causal genes has led to the modification of the classification. Each type of CMT is now subdivided according to the specific genetic cause of the neuropathy (see Tables 7.1–7.3).

Prevalence

With an estimated prevalence of 1 in 2 500, CMT disease is the most common inherited neuropathy. Resulting from next generation sequencing techniques, gene discovery in CMT rapidly expanded with more than 80 genes having been identified, and many more are still to be discovered (Charcot and Marie 1886; Barreto et al. 2014; Cornett et al. 2016). A recent multicentric study including 520 children and adolescents (274 males) aged 3 to 20 showed the most prevalent types were CMT1A (*PMP22* duplication 55%), CMT2A (6.0%), CMT1B (2.9%), CMT4C (2.5%) and CMTX1 (1.9%). (Dejerine and Sottas 1893; Cornett et al. 2016; Murphy et al. 2012).

Clinical picture

The typical clinical course of CMT1 and CMT2 patients includes, despite their pheno-typic variability, normal development before sensory loss and weakness appears grad-ually within the first two decades of life; often referred to as the classic phenotype. Affected children are often slow runners and have difficulties with activities that require balance. Hands are normally less affected than feet, although fine hand movements can be impaired. On clinical examination, there is an observation of a progressive distal wasting and weakness, especially of the peroneal compartment, usually with some distal sensory impairment (touch, pain and vibration) and sometimes ataxia related to impaired joint position discrimination. Deep tendon reflexes are decreased and very often absent and some scales have recently been developed to determine severity, such as the CMT neu-ropathy score (CMTNS) or the CMT pediatric scale (CMTPedS) (Murphy et al. 2011; Burns et al. 2012). In time the patients can develop contractures (scoliosis, claw hand) and skeletal deformities (pes cavus and hammer toes). These patients often require AFOs (ankle-foot orthotics) in late childhood or adolescence. In most cases they remain ambu-lant throughout life and have a normal expectation of life. The prognosis and severity are mainly linked to function disabilities in daily life, such as limitations with walking or writing (Johnson ct al. 2014).

**TABLE 7.1**
**Demyelinating CMT 1**

| Inheritance | Denomination | Gene | Phenotype MIM number | Location | Onset | Evocative clinical features |
|---|---|---|---|---|---|---|
| AD | CMT1A | PMP22 duplication | 118220 | 17p12 | First two decades: rarely at birth | Foot deformity (pes cavus with hammertoes), scoliosis, deafness, optic neuritis |
| AD | CMT1B | MPZ/P0 | 118200 | 1q23.3 | Infantile, childhood, or adult onset | Deafness, pupillar abnormalities, steroid responsive neuropathy |
| AD | CMT1C | LITAF/SIMPLE | 601098 | 16p13.3 | Highly variable age (mean: 20 y) | Tremor |
| AD | CMT1D | EGR2 | 607678 | 10q21.1–q22.1 | 5–25 y | Pes cavus foot deformity and bilateral foot drop, Cranial nerve involvement (facial weakness, hearing loss, vocal cord involvement, ophthalmoplegia) |
| AD | CMT1E | PMP22 | 118300 | 17p12 | 5–25 y | Deafness |
| AD | CMT1F | NEFL | 607734 | 8p21.2 | 1–13 y | Tremor, deafness, sensory ataxia, pyramidal tract involvement |
| AD | – | FBLN5 | 608895 | 14q32.12 | Adulthood | Skin hyperelasticity, age-related macular degeneration |
| AD | – | GJB3/Connexin 31 | 612644 | 1p34.3 | Adulthood | Deafness, erythrokeratodermia variabilis |
| AD | – | ARHGEF10 | 608236 | 8p23.3 | Adulthood | Raynaud |
| AR | CMT4A | GDAP1 | 214400 | 8q21.11 | Infancy to early childhood | Diaphragm and vocal cord palsy, scoliosis |
| AR | CMT4B1 | MTMR2 | 601382 | 11q21 | <4 y (mean: 34 months) | Diaphragm and vocal cord palsy, deafness, scoliosis |

Continued

TABLE 7.1
Continued

| Inheritance | Denomination | Gene | Phenotype MIM number | Location | Onset | Evocative clinical features |
|---|---|---|---|---|---|---|
| AR | CMT4B2 | SBF2/ MTMR13 | 604563 | 11p15.4 | 4–13 y | Congenital glaucoma, lancinating pain, scoliosis |
| AR | CMT4B3 | SBF1/MTMR5 | 615284 | 22q13.33 | 5–11 y | Pes cavus, cognitive impairment |
| AR | CMT4C | SH3TC2/ KIAA1985 | 601591 | 5q32 | First and second decade | Severe deformations and scoliosis, deafness |
| AR | CMT4D | NDRG1 | 601455 | 8q24.3 | <10 y | Deafness, tongue atrophy, abnormal brain MRI (white matter abnormalities), scoliosis |
| AR | CMT4E | EGR2/ KROX20 | 605253 | 10q21.1– q22.1 | Birth and early infancy | Congenital hypotonia, scoliosis |
| AR | CMT4F | PRX | 614895 | 19q13.1– q13.2 | Birth and <7 y | Severe deformations and scoliosis |
| AR | CMT4G/ HMSN-Russe | HK1 | 605285 | 10q22.1 | Birth to adolescence | Scoliosis |
| AR | CMT4H | FGD4 | 609311 | 12p11.21– q13.11 | <5 y | Severe deformations and scoliosis, pes equinus |
| AR | CMT4J | FIG4/ KIAA0274/ SAC3 | 609390 | 6q21 | Early childhood to adult | Bulbar and cranial nerve involvement, scoliosis |
| AR | CCFDN | CTDP1 | 604168 | 18q23 | Birth and early infancy | Cataract, intellectual disability |
| AR | CMT4K | SURF1 | 616684 | 9q34.2 | Childhood | Ataxia, deafness, scoliosis |
| XL | CMTX1 | GJB1/ Connexin 32 | 302800 | Xq13.1 | >5 y (mean: 20 y) | Abnormal brain MRI (white matter abnormalities), deafness |

AD: autosomal dominant; AR: autosomal recessive; XL: X-linked.

**TABLE 7.2**
**Axonal CMT**

| Inheritance | Denomination | Gene | Phenotype MIM number | Location | Onset | Evocative clinical features |
|---|---|---|---|---|---|---|
| AD | CMT2A1 | *KIF1B* | 118210 | 1p36.2 | Childhood–50 y | Optic atrophy, central involvement with white matter MRI abnormalities |
| AD | CMT2A2 | *MFN2* | 609260 | 1p36.22 | Toddler to fifth decade | Proximal weakness, optic atrophy, optic neuritis, spasticity, abnormal brain MRI (white matter abnormalities), pyramidal tract involvement, diaphragm and vocal cord palsy |
| AD | CMT2B | *RAB7* | 605588 | 3q21.3 | Adolescence and young adulthood | Lancinating pain, sensory anomalies and ulcerations |
| AD | CMT2C | *TRPV4* | 606071 | 12q23–q24 | Birth to fifth decade | Diaphragm and vocal cord palsy, bone deformities, bladder dysfunction, hearing loss |
| AD | CMT2D | *GARS* | 601472 | 7p15 | Adolescence and young adulthood | Sensory involvement, predominantly upper limbs involvement, severe deformations and scoliosis, cold induced hand cramps |
| AD | CMT2E (and CMT1F) | *NEFL* | 607684 | 8p21.2 | Toddler to fifth decade | Ataxia, deafness, hypercreatinemia, hyperlipemia, diabetes, sensory involvement marked |
| AD | CMT2F | *HSPB1/HSP27* | 606595 | 7q11.23 | Childhood to sixth decade | Sensory involvement |
| AD | CMT2G | Unknown | | 12q12–q13.3 | 9–76 y (mean: 20 y) | Proximal muscle involvement, hypercreatinemia, hyperlipemia, diabetes |
| AD | CMT2I/CMT2J | *MPZ/P0* | 607677/607736 | 1q23.3 | Late onset (fourth to sixth decade)/late onset (>13 y) | Pupillar abnormalities, deafness, lancinating pain, diaphragm and vocal cord palsy, sensory involvement marked |
| AD | CMT2K | *GDAP1* | 607831 | 8q21.11 | Second to fifth decade | Ataxia, pes cavus |
| AD | CMT2L | *HSPB8/HSP22* | 608673 | 12q24.23 | Adolescence to young adulthood | Proximal muscle involvement, predominantly upper limbs involvement, severe deformations and scoliosis |

Continued

TABLE 7.2
Continued

| | | | | | | |
|---|---|---|---|---|---|---|
| AD | CMT2M | DNM2 | 606482 | 19p13.2 | Toddler to fifth decade | Congenital cataract, ophthalmoparesis and ptosis, neutropenia, muscle oedema, fatty infiltration |
| AD | CMT2N | AARS | 613287 | 16q22.1 | Early childhood to fifth decade | Neutropenia, cataract, |
| AD | CMT2O | DYNC1H1 | 60012 | 14q32.31 | Toddler to adolescence | Neuropathic pain, learning difficulties, pes cavus, pyramidal tract involvement |
| AD | CMT2P | LRSAM1 | 614436 | 9q33.3 | Second to fifth decade | Proximal muscle involvement, sensory involvement |
| AD | CMT2Q | DHTKD1 | 615025 | 10p14 | Adolescence to young adulthood | Pes cavus |
| AD | CMT2T | MME | 617017 | 3q25.2 | Third to eighth decade | Ataxia |
| AD | CMT2U | MARS | 616280 | 12q13.3 | Adulthood | – |
| AD | CMT2V | NAGLU | 616491 | 17q21.2 | Adolescence to sixth decade | Lancinating pain, ataxia |
| AD | CMT2W | HARS | 616625 | 5q31.3 | Childhood to sixth decade | Pas cavus, ataxia |
| AD | CMT2Y | VCP | 616687 | 9p13.3 | Third to fourth decade | Paget disease, dementia, cardiomyopathy |
| AD | CMT2Z | MORC2 | 616688 | 22q12.2 | Birth to second decade | Hypotonia, learning difficulties, pyramidal tract involvement |
| AD | CMT2CC | NEFH | 616924 | 22q12.2 | Infancy to fourth decade | Important sensory involvement, ALS susceptibility, ataxia |
| AD | HMSNP/CMT2P-Okinawa | TFG | 604484 | 3q12.2 | Young adulthood | Diabetes, hyperlipidemia, progressive need to walking aids |
| AD | HMN5A | BSCL2 | 600794 | 11q13 | Infancy to third decade | Spasticity, pyramidal tract involvement |
| AR | CMT2A2B | MFN2 | 617087 | 1p36.22 | Infancy to fifth decade | Optic atrophy, sensory involvement, diaphragm involvement |

Continued

TABLE 7.2
Continued

| Inheritance | Denomination | Gene | Phenotype MIM number | Location | Onset | Evocative clinical features |
|---|---|---|---|---|---|---|
| AR | CMT2B1 | LMNA | 605588 | 1q22 | Second decade | Myopathy and cardiomyopathy, proximal muscle involvement, scoliosis |
| AR | CMT2B2 | MED25/ARC92/ACID1 | 605589 | 19q13.33 | Adulthood | Sensory involvement, ataxia |
| AR | CMT2F | HSPB1/HSP27 | 606595 | 7q11.23 | Toddler to sixth decade | Sensory involvement |
| AR | CMT2H | GDAP1 | 607731 | 8q13–q23 | Childhood | Pyramidal tract involvement, diaphragm and vocal cord palsy, hyperreflexia |
| AR | CMT2K | GDAP1 | 607831 | 8q21.11 | Birth to 7 y | Diaphragm and vocal cord palsy, severe deformations and scoliosis, ataxia |
| AR | CMT2P | LRSAM1 | 614436 | 9q33.3 | Second to fifth decade | Proximal muscle involvement, sensory involvement |
| AR | CMT2R | TRIM2 | 615490 | 4q31.3 | Infancy to early childhood | Vocal cord paralysis, pes cavus |
| AR | CMT2S | IGHMBP2 | 616155 | 11q13.3 | Infancy to early adulthood | Ataxia |
| AR | CMT2T | MME | 617017 | 3q25.2 | Third to fifth decade | Ataxia |
| AR | CMT2X | SPG11 | 616668 | 15q21 | 4–35 y | Sensory involvement, pes cavus, scoliosis, bladder dysfunction, erectile dysfunction, cognitive impairment |
| XL | CMTX1 | GJB1/Connexin 32 | 302800 | Xq13.1 | >5 y (mean: 20 y) | Abnormal brain MRI (white matter abnormalities), deafness |
| XL | CMTX4 | AIFM1 | 310490 | Xq26.1 | Birth to early childhood | Intellectual disability, deafness, optic atrophy |

AD: autosomal dominant; AR: autosomal recessive; XL: X-linked; ALS: amyotrophic lateral sclerosis.

**TABLE 7.3**
**Intermediate CMT**

| Inheritance | Denomination | Gene | Phenotype MIM number | Location | Onset | Evocative clinical features |
|---|---|---|---|---|---|---|
| AD | CMTDIA | Unknown | 606483 | 10q24.1–q25.1 | First to second decade | Sensitive involvement |
| AD | CMTDIB | DNM2 | 606482 | 19p13.2 | First and second decade | Cataract, neutropenia |
| AD | CMTDIC | YARS | 608323 | 1p35.1 | 7–59 y | Sensitive involvement |
| AD | CMTDID | MPZ/P0 | 607791 | 1q23.3 | 30–50 y | Sensitive involvement, deafness, Adie's pupil |
| AD | CMTDIE | INF2 | 614455 | 14q32.33 | 5–28 y | Focal segmental glomerulosclerosis, deafness, pes cavus |
| AD | CMTDIF | GNB4 | 615195 | 3q26.33 | 5–70 y | Sensitive involvement, pes cavus, scoliosis |
| AD | CMT1C | LITAF | 601098 | 16p13.3 | Highly variable age (mean: 20 y) | Tremor |
| AD | CMT2E | NEFL | 607684 | 8p21.2 | First to fifth decade | Sensitive involvement, deafness, ataxia, postural tremor |
| AR | CMTRIA | GDAP1 | 608340 | 8q21.11 | 2–4 y | Ataxia, sensitive involvement |
| AR | CMTRIB | KARS | 613641 | 16q23.1 | 10–60 y | Dysmorphic features, vestibular schwannoma developmental delay |
| AR | CMTRIC | PLEKHG5 | 615376 | 1p36.31 | First to fifth decade | Sensitive involvement, pes cavus |
| AR | CMTRID | COX6A1 | 616039 | 12q24 | First decade | Sensitive involvement |

Continued

**TABLE 7.3**
**Continued**

| Inheritance | Denomination | Gene | Phenotype MIM number | Location | Onset | Evocative clinical features |
|---|---|---|---|---|---|---|
| XL | CMTX1 | GJB1/Connexin 32 | 302800 | Xq13.1 | >5 y (mean: 20 y) | Abnormal brain MRI (white matter abnormalities), deafness |
| XL | CMTXI | DRP2 | – | Xq22.1 | 50 y | Sensitive involvement |
| XL | CMTX2 | CMTX2 | 302801 | Xp22.2 | Infantile | Intellectual disability |
| XL | CMTX3 | CMTX3 | 302802 | Xq27.1 | 3–13 y | Sensitive involvement, pes cavus |
| XL | CMTX5 | PRPS1 | 311070 | Xq22.3 | Childhood | Deafness, optic atrophy |
| XL | CMTX6 | PDK3 | 300905 | Xp22.1 | First decade | Hand tremor, sensitivity involvement, ataxia |

AD: autosomal dominant; AR: autosomal recessive; XL: X-linked.

Early onset with severe phenotype in CMT patients is rare. Two phenotypes can be distinguished:

1. Clear prenatal/neonatal onset presenting at birth with hypotonia, arthrogryposis and respiratory insufficiency. The birth of a hypotonic child can lead to obstetric complications and birth asphyxia, masking the underlying peripheral neuropathy. To prevent early mortality ventilatory support is often required. Spinal muscular atrophy (SMA) and other early-onset motor neuron diseases form important differential diagnosis for CMT. If myelination appears to be disrupted during embryologic development, some severe cases can be classified as congenital hypomyelination (Parman et al. 2004).

2. No abnormal perinatal history but delayed motor milestones and infant-onset symptoms such as foot deformity can be observed. The most prominent clinical manifestations are delayed motor milestone (infantile onset) and areflexia, in contrast to adults where distal weakness and sensory loss are the predominant features. Facial weakness and tongue fasciculations (axonal lesions) may be present but also the presence of proximal weakness, foot deformity, scoliosis and congenital hip dysplasia is typical. The clinical features may mimic myopathy.

As already mentioned, the term Dejerine-Sottas neuropathy is currently primarily used to describe severe early-onset clinical phenotypes regardless of the inheritance pattern. Many patients have de novo autosomal dominant disorders.

### *Diagnostic strategy: importance of electrodiagnostics*

Since the first modern electrophysiologic classification schemes of hereditary motor and sensory neuropathies (HMSNs) were proposed by Dyck and Lambert in 1968, nerve conduction studies remain an important component in the classification and determination of specific genetic forms. In the context of this book, the classification of CMTs we propose in Tables 7.1–7.3 is based on the electrophysiological approach as starting point.

The impact of specific factors like age, duration of disease, severity of symptoms on electrodiagnostics is crucial in children. Indeed, "maturation" of motor and sensory conduction velocities (MCV, SCV) as well as distal latencies and F waves occur during the first 5 years of life (see Chapter 4) and interpretation of conduction speed has to be cautiously interpreted when compound motor action potential amplitude (CMAP) is flattened (for example in the context of an axonal disease).

So, in children older than 5, and if the ulnar CMAP is more than 0.5mV, a conduction velocity less than 38m/s is considered demyelinating (CMT1), and 38–45m/s is intermediate. When there is loss of CMAP and/or needle EMG denervation, a conduction velocity more than 45m/s is considered to indicate a primary axonal process (CMT2). It is more difficult to distinguish primary axonal from demyelinating forms if patients present with symptoms late in the course of their disease. With careful measurements, these conduction studies can have cut-off values similar to those in the ulnar forearm. Recently, forearm nerve conduction has been further categorized into: (1) very slow (<15m/s); (2) slow (15–35m/s); (3) intermediate

(35–45m/s); and (4) normal (>45m/s). This subdivision has proven to be helpful in selecting genetic testing for patients with inherited neuropathies (Klein et al. 2013).

The numerous forms of CMTs are presented in Tables 7.1–7.3, using the (clinical-) electrophysiological approach as starting point followed by the inheritance criteria. Table 7.1 depicts the demyelinating forms (mostly autosomal dominant CMT1 and autosomal recessive CMT4); Table 7.2 depicts the axonal forms (mostly CMT2) and Table 7.3 the intermediate forms.

*Importance of associated features*
In order to help the clinician, the combination of phenotypic features to particular CMT types can be used (Rouzier et al. 2012; Di Meglio et al. 2016; Sevilla et al. 2008). For examples, optic atrophy is often associated with a mutation in the *MFN2* gene and vocal cords palsy is associated with mutations in the *GDAP1* gene (Parman et al. 2004) with a recessive (CMT4A, AR-CMT2) or dominant inheritance (CMT2K).

Genetics
Clinical appearance alone is often not sufficient to subdivide the peripheral nerve diseases. Only in a few cases specific phenotypes are evident for the peripheral nerve disease but much more frequently there is overlap with other subtypes. This has the implication that sequential Sanger sequencing of genes according to phenotype will not be, at term, the most cost effective method. CMT specific panels with multiple genes will be a viable option in the future although will still require careful interpretation (numerous polymorphisms in certain genes, only coding regions are sequenced, poor coverage of CG-rich regions and X chromosome) (Rossor et al. 2013).

Based on prevalence, *PMP22* duplication should be the initial screen especially with motor conduction velocities of 15–35m/s and walking before the age of 15 months. If consanguinity is excluded in the family history, de novo duplications of *PMP22* are most likely to account for most sporadic demyelinating inherited neuropathies. With more than 80 genes identified a second step should be to combine next generation sequencing with detailed phenotyping (clinical course, core motor and sensory symptoms, associated symptoms and electrodiagnostics) to optimize the result (Dejerine and Sottas 1893). Among patients with axonal dominantly inherited neuropathy, genetic testing is less likely to be positive. At most, 35% of those with axonal dominantly inherited forms (defined by corrected normal or unobtainable nerve conduction velocities) had a genetic diagnosis: mutations in *MFN2*, *MPZ*, and *GJB1* were most common. Among children with axonal neuropathies with loss of ambulation, *MFN2* is the most likely mutation.

Specific forms of Charcot–Marie–Tooth and long term evolution
It is out of the scope of this chapter to detail the specific clinical description of all genes involved in CMT, and we refer readers to Brennan and Shy's chapter 'Hereditary Neuropathies in Late Childhood and Adolescence' in the book *Neuromuscular Disorders of Infancy, Childhood and Adolescence: A Clinician's Approach* (Brennan and Shy 2014). We provide

a short description of the most common forms, and this as a function of their relative prevalence in recent published studies (Cornett et al. 2016).

*CMT1A*

CMT1A, affecting 50–60% of the genetically determined CMT, is the most common form in children in most populations. Evidently, it is also the most common form of CMT type 1, accounting for 80–90% and will be the most commonly observed CMT neuropathy in late childhood and adolescence. CMT1A is usually characterized with the classic CMT phenotype including lower limb symptoms (foot deformity, walking difficulty) with onset in the first two decades of life. It is often accompanied by distal weakness, sensory loss, atrophy, hyporeflexia. Patients with the classic phenotype usually walk on time and their lifespan is not affected. They rarely require the use of a wheelchair for ambulation but often they do require ankle-foot orthotics. In extreme rare cases CMT1A patients can present an earlier onset Dejerine-Sottas phenotype. Nerve conduction velocities (NCVs) follow the rules of a demyelinating neuropathy (see the next section) and are typically in the 20s range. The sensory action potentials are either reduced or absent. Nerve biopsy is not required, but, if performed, reveals demyelination and onion bulb formation. Most patients will report a family history as this is an autosomal dominant condition, but 10% of the patients have a de novo mutation. Therefore, children and adolescents without family history but who present ulnar MNCV under 35m/s should first be screened for CMT1A before testing other genes. CMT1A is caused by a 1.4 Mb duplication on chromosome 17p11.2 in the region that carries the *PMP22* gene (Russo et al. 2011). It is the extra copy of *PMP22* that causes the neuropathy (Lupski et al. 1991).

*CMT1B*

CMT1B is clinically associated with several distinct phenotypes: (1) early infantile-onset severe phenotype presented by delayed walking and NCV less than 10m/s (Dejerine-Sottas disease); or (2) more rarely a classic CMT phenotype in about 15% of the patients, but (3) also and not so rarely an adult-onset phenotype (NCV around 40m/s). It is the third or fourth most common type of CMT. It is caused by point mutations in the myelin protein zero (*MPZ*) gene on chromosome 1q22–23. MPZ is the major component of peripheral nerve myelin, comprising at least 50% of the protein (Hayasaka et al. 1993).

*HNPP*

Hereditary neuropathy with liability to pressure palsies (HNPP) is an autosomal dominant disorder and the third most common type of CMT, typically presenting with recurrent neuropathies occurring at sites of entrapments. This particular form of neuropathy also involves *PMP22* and is commonly caused by a deletion of the 1.4Mb stretch of chromosome 17p11.2 (the same stretch which is duplicated in CMT1A). More rarely, HNPP can be caused by point mutation of the *PMP22* gene. The age at onset is similar to CMT1A although one larger study suggests an earlier age at onset presented typically by a delay in ambulation. The literature gives evidence for a wide range of onset from early childhood till adulthood. Motor NCVs are normal but slowed around sites of entrapment such as carpal tunnel, fibular head and medial epicondyle. This observation combined with prolonged distal motor latencies gives an indication for diagnosis (Li et al. 2002). Clinically, patients present with a history of recurrent focal mononeuropathies that are transient, lasting anything from hours to days or weeks and occasionally longer. Many patients develop a predominantly length-dependent large fiber sensory neuropathy as they age (Stögbauer et al. 2000).

*CMT1X*

Caused by mutations in the gap junction beta 1 (*GJB1*) gene, CMT1X is the main X-linked form of CMT. This gene encodes for the protein connexin 32 (Cx32). Males are typically more severely affected and tend to have marked atrophy of the intrinsic hand muscles and all compartments of the calf muscles. CMT1X is often characterized by a "split hand syndrome" with abductor polices brevis being weaker and more wasted than first dorsal interosseous (Siskind et al. 2011). Conduction velocities are often but not systematically in the intermediate range (Tables 7.1–7.3). First symptoms generally occur in childhood, although 20% of the patients will have a later onset. Episodes of transient stroke-like symptoms have been rarely reported, usually following a stressor. Probably these events occur because Cx32 is also expressed in oligodendrocytes in the central nervous system (CNS) (Shy et al. 2007).

*CMT2A*

Accounting for 6% of all genetic polyneuropathies in children, this is the most common form of CMT2. CMT2A often has a severe phenotype with onset in infancy or early childhood, with many patients requiring a wheelchair to ambulate by the age of 20. Genetically CMT2A is caused by mutation in the nuclear encoded mitofusin 2 or *MFN2* gene (Feely et al. 2011). This GTPase is a component of the outer mitochondrial membrane and is essential for fusion of mitochondria to each other or to the endoplasmic reticulum (Züchner et al. 2004). Commonly these patients have unrecordable CMAP amplitudes and nerve conduction speed (NCS) even in the upper extremities. These results give an indication to test for *MFN2* mutations. A high number of polymorphisms are encountered in the *MFN2* gene, so care must be taken if the mutation is indeed disease-causing. In rare cases the disease manifest later during life (childhood, adolescence, adulthood) with a milder phenotype. Some have additional clinical features such as optic atrophy or pyramidal signs as part of their disease (Züchner et al. 2006).

*CMT4C*

CMT4C is a demyelinating neuropathy with a slightly later onset than other autosomal recessive CMTs with childhood-adolescent onsets reported (Houlden et al. 2009). CMT4C is commonly characterized by scoliosis. Occasional additional clinical findings include movement disorders (ataxia and tremors), facial and bulbar weakness, sensorineural deafness, and respiratory insufficiency. It is caused by mutations in the SH3 domain and tetratricopeptide repeat domain 2 (*SH3TC2*) gene. It is the most common of the autosomal recessive CMTs in North American and Northern European populations (Senderek et al. 2003; Lassuthova et al. 2011).

Although the prevalence and genetic characterization of each type of CMT is becoming clearer, less is known about the clinical presentations of these genetic types in childhood.

CMT1A was confirmed to be more slowly progressive compared to other forms of CMT and most patients remain ambulant through their lifetime, although there is a variability in the severity and rate of progression.

Patients with CMT1B, CMT2A and CMT4C are more severely affected than patients diagnosed with CMT1A or CMT1X. Disease severity of CMT4C was similar to that of CMT2A and hand dexterity was identified as a major limitation for children and adolescents with CMT4C. CMT4C affected children commonly present with (kypho)scoliosis between the ages of 2 and 10. Slowly progressive neuropathy usually manifests in the first decade or adolescence, and occasionally earlier or later with variability and foot deformities (pes cavus, pes planus, or pes valgus are common).

MANAGEMENT

General approach

Despite the great improvement in our biologic understanding of inherited neuropathies, derived mostly from developments in molecular biology and transgenic animal models in the last 25 years, there is still no treatment available for any type of CMT.

In most inherited neuropathies treatment still remains supportive. There are different approaches with special attention to: (1) anticipating specific impairment; (2) taking care of acral appendages especially in the varieties of HSAN in which mutilating injuries and amputations are preventable; (3) arranging proper bracing and supporting devices; (4) emphasizing routine health maintenance such as weight control, early diabetes, thyroid deviations; (5) considering the increased risk for worsened neuropathy associated with certain chemotherapeutic agents, including platinum-based agents, vinca alkaloids, and probably paclitaxel, thalidomide and bortezomib products; and (6) providing reassurance that these disorders are compatible with productive lives.

A dedicated, multidisciplinary rehabilitation team can significantly contribute to the management of patients with CMT and improve functionality and quality of life. Physical therapy, occupational therapy, and a few orthopedic procedures are still the cornerstone of treatment. Next, we will focus on the management of foot and ankle deformities that are so common in CMT.

Foot and ankle manifestations

There are three common foot deformities in CMT: claw toes, forefoot (pes) cavus, and hindfoot varus (ankle inversion deformity). The most popular theory regarding the etiology explains the development of pes cavus as an imbalance between agonist and antagonist muscles although there is still much debate around the question.

The classification of pes cavus is still complex and controversial, involving several dimensions. In the context of CMT one can classify it using an antero-posterior axis, the structure of pes cavus falling into anterior, posterior and global categories. The anterior cavus (or forefoot pes cavus) is either total (indicating plantar flexion of the entire forefoot) or local (plantar flexion of the first ray only).

In CMT1A this is thought to occur due to the unopposed action of the relatively spared peroneus longus against the weakened tibialis anterior on the first ray of the foot, resulting in plantar flexion of the first metatarsal. This results in an increase in the height of the foot

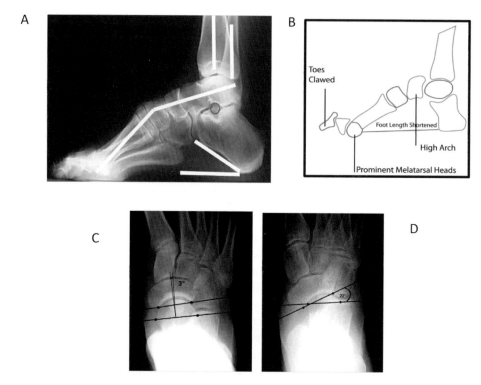

**Fig. 7.1. A** Weight-bearing X-rays of the foot and ankle of a 16-year-old CMT1A patient: evidence of a high-arch foot pattern. The heel bone has an elevated angle relative to the ground (>20°) and the 1st metatarsal bone is pointed down. **B** Skeletal structure, pes cavus foot, CMT1. **C** Normal talo-navicular coverage angle. **D** Medial peritalar subluxation with pes cavus. Usually a relatively strong posterior is unopposed by a weakened peroneus brevis tendon, producing medial subluxation of the navicular on the talus.

arch and tilting of the subtalar joint in to varus (resulting in ankle inversion). The raised arch is often accompanied by tightening of the plantar fascia. (Fig. 7.1).

The posterior (hindfoot varus) type has a high calcaneal inclination (pitch) angle but no forefoot equinus. It is often seen in idiopathic pes cavus but was historically associated with poliomyelitis due to selective plantar flexion weakness.

The global type hindfoot varus (inversion), combines both deformities and refers to the inversion of the foot at the subtalar joint (ankle) in order to compensate for the plantar flexion of the first metatarsal causing forefoot (pes) cavus. The hindfoot varus deformity predisposes the patient to recurrent inversion injuries of the ankle.

When evaluating pes cavus foot it is important to describe whether the deformity is flexible or rigid, in terms of function.

Conservative management of foot deformity in Charcot–Marie–Tooth

The nonoperative management of foot deformity in CMT includes gastrocnemius stretching exercises to prevent Achilles tendon tightening, and the prescription of ankle-foot orthoses

(AFOs). While there is no evidence that personalized AFOs prevent or slow the progression of foot deformities, they have been shown to reduce foot pain in patients with pes cavus and to improve ambulation when compared with sham AFOs (Johnson et al. 2014; Burns et al. 2006). A wide variety of AFOs exist offering different degrees of support and rigidity, and should be tailored to each individual's therapeutic needs.

Surgical Management of foot deformity in Charcot–Marie–Tooth

While many patients undergo surgery for foot deformity, there is no randomized evidence on when and how to operate. Nevertheless, the decision to plan an intervention is based on several factors, such as age of the patient, the severity of the foot deformity, and is intended to prevent further deterioration. Foot operations for patients with CMT fall into three categories (see also Chapter 23).

Soft tissue corrections

Soft tissue corrections are only likely to be effective in patients with "supple" feet without fixed deformity. The most common soft tissue procedure is lengthening of the gastrocnemius complex for Achilles tendon tightness. Complete release of the plantar fascia may also be performed to correct the secondary contracture that forms in forefoot cavus deformity.

To correct forefoot cavus deformity, transfer of the peroneus longus tendon to the peroneus brevis muscle may also be performed. This procedure on one hand allows to reduce the plantar flexing forces on the first metatarsal causing the high arch and on the second hand allows the increased additional muscle strength  generated by peroneus longus muscle on the everting peroneus brevis muscle insertion to reduce the hindfoot varus (inversion) deformity.

Osteotomies

In patients with some rigid foot deformity osteotomies may be performed to increase the flexibility of the foot and allow the correcting forces following tendon transfer to correct the forefoot cavus and hindfoot varus.

Fusions

Triple arthrodesis is the mainstay of treatment for a severely affected rigid cavovarus foot deformity. It is an option of last resort, however, and commonly results in accelerated arthritic change in the foot.

**Neuropathies including both central (brain and spinal cord) and peripheral nervous system**

Over 40 genes have now been identified as causing spinocerebellar ataxia syndromes in both dominant and recessive forms. It is important to recognize this group in the potential differential diagnosis of unexplained inherited neuropathy. These syndromes are characterized by slowly progressive cerebellar and spinal degeneration with ataxia of speech, hands, gait and eye movements. Many have areflexia and paradoxical Babinski or other upper motor neuron signs with peripheral neuropathy.

Dominantly inherited forms make up most of the hereditary ataxia varieties and are mostly seen in adults, but autosomal recessive Friedreich ataxia is the most common cause of hereditary ataxia often observed in children and adolescents.

FRIEDREICH ATAXIA

The prevalence is about 1 in 100 000 persons, this relates to the high rate of carrier expansions. Friedreich ataxia is caused by the expansion of an intronic GAA triplet repeat located within the first intron of the frataxin gene, resulting in reduced levels of frataxin in some tissues. Ataxia is the first symptom of Friedreich ataxia, with unsteadiness when walking. Over time, speech may become more slurred, handwriting may become less clear, and fine motor movements of the hands and feet may become harder to execute and patients may eventually, often in adulthood or as teenagers, become unable to stand without losing their balance and will require assistive devices such as walkers, wheelchairs or scooters to remain mobile. Patients have a sensory onset neuropathy with the clinical observation of absent reflexes, and experience stiffness and cramping in their legs. Some may be categorized as CMT2 if the ocular and other ataxic features are missed. The high incidence of diabetes in Friedreich ataxia can mistakenly lead to a diagnosis of diabetic neuropathy (Bürk 2017).

The condition also typically include an hypertrophic cardiomyopathy, heart arrhythmias and scoliosis.

GIANT AXONAL NEUROPATHY

Giant axonal neuropathy (GAN) is due to recessive mutations in the gigaxonin (*GAN*) gene, and is characterized by a severe early-onset motor and sensory axonal neuropathy with CNS involvement and characteristic kinky hair. Onset is usually within the first few years of life. Most children present with delayed development and gait difficulties. In some, CNS signs (cerebellar, oculomotor, and upper motor neuron features) are apparent early; in others these features develop later or remain absent during the course of the disease. Intellectual disability is common. In some families with confirmed *GAN* mutation kinky hair is absent. Associated features include skeletal deformities, and less commonly cranial neuropathies and seizures. The clinical course is progressive. Most affected children are wheelchair-dependent by the second decade. Nerve condition studies generally show an axonal sensorimotor neuropathy. On magnetic resonance imaging periventricular and cerebellar white matter signal abnormalities and/or cerebral, cerebellar and brainstem atrophy may be present. The pathological hallmark of GAN is giant axons (large axonal swellings in thinly myelinated/amyelinated never fibers) filled with densely packed structurally normal bundles of neurofilaments (Kuhlenbäumer et al. 2014).

AUTOSOMAL RECESSIVE SPINAL CEREBELLAR ATAXIA OF CHARLEVOIX SAGUENAY

Autosomal recessive spinal cerebellar ataxia of Charlevoix Saguenay (ARSACS) is a rare autosomal recessive disorder starting during childhood and characterized clinically initially by cerebellar ataxia, spasticity, pyramidal signs, but also quite typical retinal features with the occurrence of retinal striations on fundoscopy. A demyelinating sensorimotor neuropathy with progressive axonal degeneration is classically observed in a second time leading to skeletal foot deformities and pes cavus during childhood.

Bilateral abnormal plantar response and marked saccadic alteration of ocular pursuit are typically observed. Magnetic resonance imaging shows superior vermian cerebellar atrophy, thinning of the cervical spinal cord and pontine linear hypointensities (Bouchard et al. 1998; Duquette et al. 2013).

**Neuropathies with multi-organ involvement**

The diseases in this group, typically observed in the context of metabolic diseases, involve the peripheral nervous system but also very often the CNS (brain and spinal cord) and/or also other important organs such as the liver, heart, bones, the eye and the auditory organs.

The inherited metabolic diseases in which a peripheral neuropathy is prominent may be separated into several categories, including storage diseases, disorders of amino acid and fatty acid metabolism, and mitochondrial cytopathies. While the biochemical and molecular bases of these disorders are well established, effective treatment is quite elusive without specific therapies directed at the primary metabolic defect. In some cases, pharmacologic interventions may be helpful.

We present the most relevant forms in the pediatric population.

DISORDERS OF SPHINGOLIPID METABOLISM

A polyneuropathy occurs very often in the context of several sphingolipidoses, but with the exception of Krabbe disease and Fabry disease (trihexosylceramide lipidosis), polyneuropathy symptoms are usually not at the foreground, the disease involving mostly the CNS.

*Krabbe*

In Krabbe disease, peripheral neuropathy can be a prominent feature and the initial complaint in the infantile forms, but is mild or absent in the juvenile and adult forms. Peripheral neuropathy is associated with elevated levels of cerebrospinal fluid protein (up to 400mg/dl) and reduced nerve conduction velocities (NCV = 10m/s or lower).

*Fabry disease*

Trihexosylceramide lipidosis, Fabry disease, is an X-linked disease caused by mutations on the GLA gene, encoding the enzyme α-galactosidase A. The principal clinical manifestations involve skin, heart, kidney, and peripheral nerve. The hallmark of Fabry disease, although not specific, is its cutaneous manifestation – angiokeratoma – violaceous angiectatic lesions over the genitalia, thighs, buttocks, back, and lower abdomen. Similar lesions may be seen in the oral mucosa. Fabry disease has its onset most commonly in adolescence or early adulthood.

The most common neurological problem is a painful, involving sensory small fibers, peripheral neuropathy which generally involves typical acroparesthesias in the distal extremities that very often start during childhood (mainly in heterozygous males, later in heterozygous females). Clinical features also include both severe crises of lancinating pain and chronic, unremitting pain. The painful crises may be precipitated by exercise, fatigue, stress, or exposure to sunshine or hot weather and may last for hours or days (Luciano et al. 2002).

Decreased sweating (hypohidrosis) leads to temperature intolerance and untoward responses to sun exposure. Objective neurological signs of the neuropathy are limited, with often preservation of ankle reflexes, and classic nerve conduction studies are normal.

The degree of peripheral nerve involvement can be easily assessed by analysis of biopsy specimens. A decrease in small peripheral sensory neurons may be noted. Deficient α-galactosidase (trihexosylceramide α-galactosidase) activity in plasma and/or white cells is the basis for Fabry disease in males. In females, as the enzyme activity may overlap with normal ranges, DNA analysis is recommended.

Other common features are corneal and lenticular opacifications and retinal vasculopathies. CNS vaso-occlusive events (typically during adulthood) may be noted with a prognostic value on the overall evolution and Fabry disease should be considered in the differential diagnosis of stroke in the young individual. Corneal opacifications are the most common signs, being present in nearly three-fourths of carriers and chronic renal disease poses the major clinical problem.

As such, Fabry disease had been regarded as the best candidate among the sphingolipidoses for direct therapeutic intervention. Supportive management of painful neuropathy in Fabry disease includes the use of conventional antiepileptic and antidepressant agents. Specific treatment has been revolutionized by the availability of enzyme replacement therapy (ERT). There are two products (agalsidase alfa and agalsidase beta) both administered every 2 weeks intravenously, and which are both very expensive and subject to manufacturing shortages. To date, ERT has been shown to benefit many non-neurological manifestations of Fabry disease and some neurological features, including peripheral nerve function, although its impact on intra-epidermal nerve fiber density has been less convincing (Schiffmann et al. 2001; Eng et al. 2001). ERT is far from curative for Fabry disease, and newer specific treatments are being developed, including substrate reduction, molecular chaperones and gene therapy. Their role, either as monotherapy or in combination with ERT, is currently under investigation.

PORPHYRIAS

Porphyrias are genetic or acquired deficiencies in the activity of enzymes in the heme biosynthetic pathway. Peripheral neuropathy is a common feature of acute intermittent porphyria, although it also occurs in hereditary coproporphyria, and variegate porphyria.

Muscle weakness often begins proximally in the legs but may involve the arms or the distal extremities. Reflexes are lost. Motor neuropathy also may involve the cranial nerves or lead to bulbar paralysis, respiratory impairment, and death. Some patients develop sensory, patchy neuropathy. Autonomic dysfunction may lead to colicky abdominal pain, diarrhea or constipation, and bladder dysfunction.

Episodes of porphyria may be triggered by drugs, hormones, infections, or low carbohydrate intake, all inducing d-aminolaevulinic synthase and the accumulation of d-aminolaevulinic acid and porphobilinogen, which are neurotoxic. The urine detection of d-aminolaevulinic acid and porphobilinogen are critical for orienting the diagnosis towards genetic testing. Management requires patients to have a good carbohydrate intake, treat infections promptly and to avoid unsafe drugs (Ginsberg 2014; Anderson et al. 2001), usually with a good outcome if followed properly.

METABOLIC DISORDERS, MISCELLANEOUS

In adrenomyeloneuropathy, polyneuropathy may play a relatively minor role in contrast to the more prominent and progressive spastic paraparesia In the mucopolysaccharidosis, neuropathy may represent a complication of the underlying storage disease, such as an entrapment neuropathy.

VITAMIN E DEFICIENCY

In a rare condition called ataxia with vitamin E deficiency (AVED), vitamin E malabsorption appears to be an isolated defect, and related to mutations in the alpha-tocopherol transfer protein gene (TTP1) (Di Donato et al. 2010; Fusco et al. 2008), the last impacting vitamin E incorporation into plasma low-density lipoproteins. Although normally absorbed by the intestine, normal recycling of vitamin E is deficient and levels are low. AVED, which starts between 3 and 13 years of age is characterized by progressive ataxia, dysarthria, weakness, areflexia, and proprioceptive loss with undetectable or very low serum vitamin E levels, and this in the absence of hypolipidemia or fat malabsorption. Nerve conduction studies typically show a sensory neuropathy with normal motor conduction and absent or markedly reduced sensory nerve action potentials (SNAPs) and abnormal posterior column function is confirmed by somatosensory evoked potential studies. Dietary vitamin E supplementation can lead to clinical and electrophysiological recovery of sensory conduction and evoked potentials (Puri et al. 2005).

RIBOFLAVIN (VITAMIN B$_2$) TRANSPORT DEFICIENCY

In recent years, failure of riboflavin transport has been recognized as causing Fazio–Londe syndrome where patients were found to carry mutations in the *SLC52A2* and *SLC52A3* genes, which encode two of the three known riboflavin transporter genes (RFVT) (Bosch et al. 2012; Johnson et al. 2012; Ciccolella et al. 2013). In Fazio–Londe syndrome, children present variable degrees of a quite rapidly progressive axonal sensorimotor neuropathy manifesting with sensory ataxia, severe weakness of the upper limbs and axial muscles often with distinctly preserved strength in the lower limbs, bulbar palsy, hearing loss, optic atrophy, and often respiratory insufficiency.

Riboflavin in the dose of 10–15mg/kg/day has been used successfully and the time for response may vary up to months in some children (Ciccolella et al. 2013). Improvement in the muscle power can be seen as early as a few days and it has been documented to facilitate early recovery from respiratory paralysis even in patients on tracheostomy.

**Key points**
- Etiologies of childhood-onset peripheral neuropathies differ from those of adult-onset, with more inherited conditions.
- Charcot–Marie-Tooth (CMT) disease, is the most common neuromuscular disorder, and its genetic labels, types CMT1, CMT2, CMT4, CMTX, are the preferred sub-type terms.
- CMT, particularly in children, is caused by a wide molecular genetic heterogeneity, but its clinical presentation typically shares common clinical distal features, making the final diagnosis challenging.

- The diagnostic approach often relies on some combination of careful history taking, physical examination findings, a careful determination of family history, electrodiagnostic studies, occasionally metabolic laboratory studies and more frequently the use of gene panels based on next generation sequencing technology.
- CMT1A is, however, the most common form in children in most populations and should be looked for as one of the first steps in the diagnostic work up, especially with motor conduction velocities of 15–35m/s and in a child walking before the age of 15 months.
- For most patients worldwide, however, diagnostic studies are limited to clinical assessment, and the use of specific signs to identify specific subtypes is particularly useful such as presentation in early childhood, scoliosis, marked sensory involvement, respiratory compromise, upper limb involvement, visual or hearing impairment, pyramidal signs and intellectual disability.
- Although CMT disease is a not treatable condition, its management requires a multidisciplinary approach with some particular focus on neuro-orthopedic treatment.
- Some metabolic neuropathies (for example Fabry disease) are important to recognize as they may require early treatment including enzyme replacement therapy.

## REFERENCES

Anderson KE, Sassa S, Bishop DF, Desnick RJ (2001) Disorders of hemebiosynthesis: X-linked sideroblastic anemia and the porphyrias. In: Scriver CR, Beaudet AL, Sly WS, Valle D (eds) *The Metabolic and Molecular Bases of Inherited Disease*, 8th edn. New York, NY: Mc Graw-Hill, pp. 2991–3062.

Barreto LCL et al. (2014) Epidemiologic study of Charcot–Marie–Tooth disease: the patient's perspective. *Neuromuscul Disord* 11: 1018–1023.

Bosch AM, Stroek K, Abeling NG, Waterham HR, Ijlst L, Wanders RJ (2012) The Brown-Vialetto-Van Laere and Fazio Londe syndrome revisited: natural history, genetics, treatment and future perspectives. *Orphanet J Rare Dis* 7: 83.

Bouchard JP, Richter A, Mathieu J, Brunet D, Hudson TJ, Morgan et al. (1998) Autosomal recessive spastic ataxia of Charlevoix-Saguenay. *Neuromuscul Disord* 8: 474–479.

Brennan KM, Shy ME (2014) Hereditary Neuropathies in Late Childhood and Adolescence. In Darras BT, Royden Jones H, Ryan MM, De Vivo DC (eds) *Neuromuscular Disorders of Infancy, Childhood and Adolescence: A clinician's approach*, 2nd ed. London: Academic Press.

Bürk K (2017) Friedreich Ataxia: current status and future prospects. *Cerebellum Ataxias* 4: 4.

Burns J, Crosbie J, Ouvrier et al. (2006) Effective orthotic therapy for the painful cavus foot: an randomized controlled trial. *J Am Pod Med Assoc* 96: 205–208.

Burns J, Ouvrier R, Estilow T, Shy R, Laurá M, Pallant J et al. (2012) Validation of the Charcot–Marie–Tooth disease pediatric scale as an outcome measure of disability. *Ann Neurol* 71: 642–652.

Charcot JM, Marie P (1886) Sur une forme particulière d'atrophie musculaire progressive souvent familiale débutant par les pieds et les jambes et atteignant plus tard les mains. *Rev Med (Paris)* 6: 97–138.

Ciccolella M, Corti S, Catteruccia M, Petrini S, Tozzi G, Rizza et al. (2013) Riboflavin transporter 3 involvement in infantile Brown-Vialetto-Van Laere disease: two novel mutations. *J Med Genet* 50: 104–107.

Cornett KMD, Menezes MP, Bray P, Halaki M, Shy RR, Yum S et al. (2016) Phenotypic variability of childhood Charcot–Marie–Tooth disease. *JAMA Neurol* 73: 645–651.

Dejerine J, Sottas J (1893) Sur la nevrite interstitielle, hypertrophique et progressive de l'enfance. *C R Soc Biol* 45: 63–96.

Di Donato I, Bianchi S, Federico A (2010) Ataxia with vitamin E deficiency: update of molecular diagnosis. *Neurol Sci* 31: 511–515.

Di Meglio C, Bonello-Palot N, Boulay C, Milh M, Ovaert C, Levy et al. (2016) Clinical and allelic heterogeneity in a pediatric cohort of 11 patients carrying MFN2 mutation. *Brain Dev* 38: 498–506.

Duquette A, Brais B, Bouchard JP, Mathieu J (2013) *Clinical presentation and early evolution of spastic ataxia of Charlevoix-Saguenay. Mov Dis* 28(14) 2011–2014. doi.10.1002/mds.25604.

El-Abassi R, England JD, Carter GT (2014) Charcot–Marie–Tooth disease: an overview of genotypes, phenotypes, and clinical management strategies. *PMR* 6: 342–355.

Eng CM, Guffon N, Wilcox WR, Germain DP, Lee P, Waldek et al. (2001) Safety and efficacy of recombinant human alpha-galactosdiase A replacement therapy in Fabry's disease. *N Engl J Med* 345(1): 9–16.

Feely SM, Laurá M, Siskind CE, Sottile S, Davis M, Gibbons V et al. (2011) MFN2 mutations cause severe phenotypes in most patients with CMT2A. *Neurology* 76: 1690–1696.

Fusco C, Frattini D, Pisani F, Gellera C, Della Giustina E (2008) Isolated vitamin E deficiency mimicking distal hereditary motor neuropathy in a 13-year-old boy. *J Child Neurol* 23: 1328–1330.

Ginsberg L (2014) Inherited metabolic neuropathies. In Hilton-Jones D, Turner MR (eds) *Oxford Textbook of Neuromuscular Disorders*, Oxford: Oxford University Press, pp. 85–90.

Hayasaka K, Himoro M, Sato W, Takada G, Uyemura K, Shimizu et al. (1993) Charcot–Marie–Tooth neuropathy type 1B is associated with mutations of the myelin P0 gene. *Nat Genet* 5: 31–34.

Houlden H, Laurá M, Ginsberg L, Jungbluth H, Robb SA, Blake et al. (2009) The phenotype of Charcot–Marie–Tooth disease type 4C due to SH3TC2 mutations and possible predisposition to an inflammatory neuropathy. *Neuromuscul Disord* 19: 264–269.

Johnson JO, Gibbs JR, Megarbane A, Urtizberea JA, Hernandez DG, Foley A et al. (2012) Exome sequencing reveals riboflavin transporter mutations as a cause of motor neuron disease. *Brain* 135: 2875–2882.

Johnson NE, Heatwole CR, Dilek N, Sowden J, Kirk CA, Shereff et al. (2014) Quality-of-life in Charcot–Marie–Tooth disease: the patient's perspective. *Neuromuscul Disord* 24: 1018–1023.

Klein CJ, Duan X, Shy ME (2013) Inherited neuropathies: clinical overview and update. *Muscle Nerve* 48: 604–622.

Kuhlenbäumer G, Timmerman V, Pascale Bomont, P (2014) Giant Axonal Neuropathy Gene Reviews. Initial Posting: 9 January 2003; Last Update: October 9, 2014.

Lassuthova P, Mazanec R, Vondracek et al. (2011) High frequency of SH3TC2 mutations in Czech HMSN I patients. *Clin Genet* 80: 334–345.

Li J, Krajewski K, Shy ME, Lewis RA (2002) Hereditary neuropathy with liability to pressure palsy: the electrophysiology fits the name. *Neurology* 58: 1769–1773.

Luciano CA, Russell JW, Banerjee TK, Quirk JM, Scott LJ, Dambrosia J et al. (2002) Physiological characterization of neuropathy in Fabry's disease. *Muscle Nerve* 26: 622–629.

Lupski JR, de Oca-Luna RM, Slaugenhaupt S, Pentao L, Guzzetta V, Trask B et al. (1991) DNA duplication associated with Charcot–Marie–Tooth disease type 1A. *Cell* 66: 219–232.

Murphy SM, Herrmann DN, McDermott MP, Scherer SS, Shy ME, Reilly M et al. (2011) Reliability of the CMT neuropathy score (second version) in Charcot–Marie–Tooth disease. *J Peripher Nerv Syst* 16: 191–198.

Murphy SM, Laurá M, Fawcett K, Pandraud A, Liu YT, Davidson G et al. (2012) Charcot–Marie–Tooth disease: frequency of genetic subtypes and guidelines for genetic testing. *J Neurol Neurosurg Psychiatry* 83: 706–710.

Parman Y, Battaloglu E, Baris I, Bilir B, Poyraz M, Bissar-Tadmouri et al. (2004) Clinicopathological and genetic study of early-onset demyelinating neuropathy. *Brain* 127: 2540–2550.

Puri V, Chaudhry N, Tatke M, Prakash V (2005) Isolated vitamin E deficiency with demyelinating neuropathy. *Muscle Nerve* 32: 230–235.

Rossor AM, Polke JM, Houlden H, Reilly MM (2013) Clinical implications of genetic advances in Charcot–Marie–Tooth disease. *Nat Rev Neurol* 9: 562–571.

Rouzier C, Bannwarth S, Chaussenot A, Chevrollier A, Verschueren A, Bonello-Palot et al. (2012) The MFN2 gene is responsible for mitochondrial DNA instability and optic atrophy 'plus' phenotype. *Brain* 135: 23–34.

Russo M, Laurá M, Polke JM, Davis MB, Blake J, Brandner et al. (2011) Variable phenotypes are associated with PMP22 missense mutations. *Neuromuscul Disord* 21: 106–114.

Schiffmann R, Kopp JB, Austin HA III, Sabnis S, Moore DF, Weibel et al. (2001) Enzyme replacement therapy in Fabry disease: a randomized controlled trial. *JAMA* 285: 2743–2749.

Senderek J, Bergmann C, Stendel C, Kirfel J, Verpoorten N, De Jonghe et al. (2003) Mutations in a gene encoding a novel SH3/TPR domain protein cause autosomal recessive Charcot–Marie–Tooth type 4C neuropathy. *Am J Hum Genet* 73: 1106–1119.

Sevilla T, Jaijo T, Nauffal D, Collado D, Chumillas MJ, Vilchez J et al. (2008) Vocal cord paresis and diaphragmatic dysfunction are severe and frequent symptoms of GDAP1-associated neuropathy. *Brain* 131: 3051–3061.

Shy ME, Siskind C, Swan ER, Krajewski KM, Doherty T, Fuerst D et al. (2007) CMT1X phenotypes represent loss of GJB1 gene function. *Neurology* 68: 849–855.

Siskind CE, Murphy SM, Ovens R, Polke J, Reilly MM, Shy ME (2011) Phenotype expression in women with CMT1X. *J Peripher Nerv Syst* 16: 102–107.

Stögbauer F, Young P, Kuhlenbäumer G, De Jonghe P, Timmerman V (2000) Hereditary recurrent focal neuropathies: clinical and molecular features. *Neurology* 54: 546–551.

Wilmshurst JM, Ouvrier R (2011) Hereditary peripheral neuropathies of childhood: an overview for clinicians. *Neuromuscul Disord* 21: 763–775.

Züchner S, Mersiyanova IV, Muglia M, Bissar-Tadmouri N, Rochelle J, Dadali E et al. (2004) Mutations in the mitochondrial GTPase mitofusin 2 cause Charcot–Marie–Tooth neuropathy type 2A. *Nat Genet* 36: 449–451.

Züchner S, De Jonghe P, Jordanova A, Claeys KG, Guergueltcheva V, Cherninkova et al. (2006) Axonal neuropathy with optic atrophy is caused by mutations in mitofusin 2. *Ann Neurol* 59: 276–281.

# 8
# ACQUIRED NEUROPATHIES

*Nicolas Deconinck*

For an introduction to Neuropathies, please see Chapter 7 (page 113).

## Introduction

The major causes of acquired peripheral neuropathies, their general clinical features, and when necessary, their specific management are described in this chapter. Acquired neuropathies are usually classified following the causal agent in the following categories: inflammatory disorders, infections (such as Chagas, leprosy, HIV, Lyme disease, etc. which most of the time are not observed in Western countries with the exception of Lyme disease), in the context of organ failure such as renal or hepatic failure, or of critical illness (Verity et al. 2011). Polyneuropathy can also be observed in children with endocrine abnormalities (e.g. diabetes mellitus), in the context vitamin deficiency (Vit B1, Vit E) or excess (Vit B6), in systemic conditions such as systemic lupus erythematosus (SLE) or very rarely as a paraneoplastic complication of malignancies like lymphoma. Finally, peripheral neuropathy is a side effect of many medications, the most common associations involving antibiotics, antiretroviral agents, chemotherapeutic agents, phenytoin, and thalidomide, and can be caused by toxins including heavy metals and industrial or environmental substances such as arsenic, lead, n-hexane, organophosphorus esters, thallium, etc. As the potential causes are so numerous, a detailed description of all situations is out of the scope of this chapter. In the following paragraphs we focus and describe in greater detail some selected causes of acquired polyneuropathies because of their relative high prevalence in the pediatric population.

## Inflammatory neuropathies

Inflammatory neuropathies in children include Guillain–Barré syndrome (GBS) and chronic inflammatory demyelinating polyneuropathy (CIDP).

### GUILLAIN–BARRÉ SYNDROME

The acute immune-mediated polyneuropathies are classified under the eponym Guillain–Barré syndrome (GBS) in reference to the authors involved in the early descriptions of the disease. In the post-polio era, Guillain–Barré syndrome (GBS) is the most common cause of acute flaccid paralysis in healthy infants and children (Jones 2000). GBS occurs worldwide with an annual incidence of 0.34 to 1.34 cases per 100 000 persons aged 18 years or under (Yuki and Hartung 2012). While all age groups are affected, the incidence is lower in children than in adults. GBS occurs rarely in children younger than 2 years of age, but can occur even in infants (Buchwald et al. 1999). Males are affected approximately 1.5 times more often than females in all age groups. Historically, GBS was considered a single disorder, but it is now known to be a heterogeneous syndrome with several variant forms in both children and adults (Ryan 2005).

Most often, GBS presents as an acute monophasic paralyzing illness known as acute inflammatory demyelinating polyneuropathy (AIDP), with typical, mostly symmetric, muscle weakness and absent or depressed deep tendon reflexes. Two-thirds develop the neurologic symptoms 2 to 4 weeks after what initially appears to be a benign febrile respiratory or gastro-intestinal infection (Sladky 2004; Hicks et al. 2010). The most common symptoms at presentation in children are pain and gait difficulty, and this often before true weakness. In preschool-aged children, the most common symptoms are refusal to walk and pain in the legs (Roodbol et al. 2011).

Lower extremity symmetric or modestly asymmetric weakness may ascend over hours to days to involve the arms and the muscles of respiration in severe cases. The facial nerve is occasionally affected, resulting in bifacial weakness. Autonomic dysfunction occurs in approximately one-half of children and may include cardiac dysrhythmias (asystole, bradycardia, persistent sinus tachycardia, and atrial and ventricular tachyarrhythmias), orthostatic hypotension, transient or persistent hypertension, paralytic ileus, bladder dysfunction and abnormal sweating (Korinthenberg et al. 2007).

Most children reach their clinical nadir within 1 to 3 weeks, with subsequent return of function over the course of weeks to months, with a shorter and better long-term prognosis than in adults (Hahn 1998; Jones 1996): 85% of children with GBS have an excellent recovery. The weakness can vary from mild difficulty with walking to nearly complete paralysis of all extremity, facial, respiratory and bulbar muscles.

No single investigation can confirm or disprove the diagnosis of GBS, particularly early in its course. The use of the Brighton criteria (Roodbol et al. 2017) adapted for children in Guillian-Barré syndrome are helpful in estimating the probability of a positive diagnosis. Clinical presentation and examination are key and allow diagnosis in typical situations. However, some GBS variants present with local or regional involvement of particular muscle groups or nerves, and several have prominent cranial nerve involvement; the variable initial presentations can hinder early diagnosis.

In a child with a compatible clinical presentation, the diagnosis is generally supported by the following tests:

- The finding of cerebrospinal fluid (CSF) albumin-cytologic dissociation, characterized by an elevated CSF protein (>45mg/dl) with a normal CSF white blood cell count. The elevated protein may be due to increased permeability of the blood–nervebarrier at the level of the proximal nerve roots. Around 60% of patients with GBS present this featurein the first week after the onset of symptoms (Devos et al. 2013; Chareyre et al. 2017). Conversely around 40% of patients, when tested earlier than 1 week after symptom onset, havenormal CSF protein values, an observation that should not prompt clinicians to exclude GBS diagnosis.
- Some children with GBS may have mildly elevated CSF cell counts (Devos et al. 2013). In children with acute flaccid paralysis who have a CSF cell count >50/mm³, other

diagnoses (such as poliomyelitis, enterovirus 71 infection, West Nile virus, or Lyme disease) should be considered.

• In the demyelinating forms of GBS, electrodiagnositic studies can demonstrate a variety of abnormalities including motor conduction block (particularly frequent in children), slowing of motor and sensory nerve conduction (see the Electrodiagnostics section in Chapter 4, page 54), temporal dispersion, and prolonged distal latencies. In the axonal forms of GBS, nerve conduction studies show decreased amplitude of motor (and possibly sensory) responses, with normal conduction velocities (Nachamkin et al. 2007).

• When spine MRI with gadolinium contrast is performed, nerve root enhancement is frequently present (retrospective studies seem to show a high sensitivity), and this test modality can supplement the more traditional electrophysiological studies and cerebrospinal fluid analysis. However, spine MRI with gadolinium contrast is not very specific (Roodbol et al. 2011; Korinthenberg et al. 2007).

Additional forms of GBS have now been recognized in children. We briefly summarize two demyelinating forms that also concern children: Miller Fisher syndrome and polyneuritis cranialis. Finally, we shortly describe AMAN, the axonal form of GBS in children.

Miller Fisher syndrome (MFS) is characterized by a peculiar triad of symptoms including external ophthalmoplegia, ataxia, and areflexia (Fisher 1956). Incomplete forms include acute ophthalmoplegia without ataxia, and acute ataxic neuropathy without ophthalmoplegia (Yuki and Hartung 2012). Cerebrospinal fluid findings and electrophysiologic features are similar to those in acute inflammatory demyelinating polyneuropathy. In clinical practice, commercially available testing for serum IgG antibodies to GQ1b is useful for the diagnosis of Miller Fisher syndrome, having a sensitivity of 85–90%. Antibodies to GQ1b may also be present in GBS with ophthalmoparesis, Bickerstaff encephalitis, and the pharyngeal-cervical brachial GBS variant, but not in disorders other than GBS (Willison et al. 1993).

Brainstem auditory evoked potentials may demonstrate peripheral and central conduction defects (Wong 1997).

Patients with polyneuritis cranialis develop acute bilateral multiple cranial nerve involvement (e.g. bilateral facial weakness, dysphagia, and dysphonia) with severe peripheral sensory loss. Patients tend to be younger than those with other GBS subtypes. This variant is often associated with preceding cytomegalovirus infection (Visser et al. 1996). Cerebrospinal fluid findings and electrophysiologic features of polyneuritis cranialis are similar to those of AIDP. MRI with gadolinium shows post-contrast enhancement of the cranial nerve roots (Morosini et al. 2003). More children with this variant require ventilator support than those with the more typical presentation of GBS (Polo et al. 1992). However, most recover fully.

Axonal forms of GBS exist in children and are now well-recognized; acute motor axonal neuropathy (AMAN) is distinguished from AIDP by its involvement of predominantly motor nerves and an electrophysiologic pattern suggesting axonal damage. AMAN occurs mainly in northern China, but is also a common form of GBS in other locations, including Japan, Mexico, and South America (McKhann et al. 1993; Nachamkin et al. 2007). It is more common in developing nations, has a seasonal incidence, and is associated with a preceding *Campylobacter jejuni* infection (Sekiguchi et al. 2012; Chareyre et al. 2017).

*Pathogenenesis*

Antecedent infections are common with GBS, and are thought to trigger the immune response that leads to acute polyneuropathy (Fig. 8.1). Approximately two-thirds of patients have a history of an antecedent respiratory tract or gastro-intestinal infection. Campylobacter infection is the most commonly identified precipitant of GBS and can be demonstrated in as many as 30% of cases. Other precipitants include Cytomegalovirus, Epstein-Barr virus, Mycoplasma pneumoniae, Influenza-like illnesses, HIV etc.

Importantly for pediatricians, the available evidence suggests that there is no increased risk of GBS associated with the H1N1 influenza vaccine in children (Verity et al. 2011).

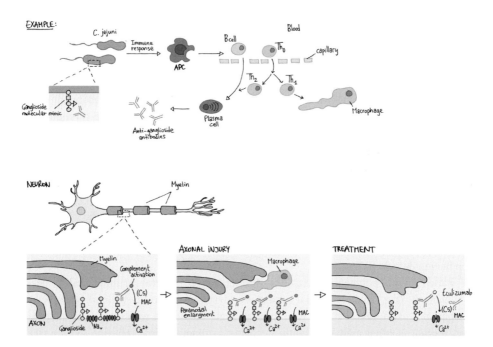

**Fig. 8.1.** The pathogenesis of Guillain–Barré syndrome (GBS). Several studies have demonstrated that anti-GM1 and anti-GQ1b autoantibodies bind to gangliosides of peripheral nerve and neuromuscular junctions, and anti-GD1a antibodies bind to the nodes of Ranvier, paranodal myelin and neuromuscular junction. This binding allows complement activation that leads to the disruption of voltage-gated sodium channel ($Na_V$) clusters, and the formation of the membrane attack complex, which in turn causes axonal intracellular calcium influx and subsequent injury. The nodal disturbed architecture and the axonal injury typically attract macrophages that find their way between the axon and myelin sheet. Complement inhibition could theoretically stop an important step of the pathogenesis at place in GBS. Eculizumab, an anti-C5 monoclonal antibody that is licensed for the treatment for paroxystic hemoglobinuria is currently being tested in two randomized, blinded, placebo-controlled trials in adults. The trigger mechanism (a molecular mimic of gangliosides) that leads to the production of anti-gangliosides in GBS is well described in the case of *Campylobacter jejuni* infection but only convincingly in the case of acute motor axonal neuropathy (AMAN). A colour version of this figure can be seen in the plate section at the end of the book.

*Management*

Important guidelines for surveillance

All patients with GBS require close surveillance of autonomic, motor (i.e. blood pressure, heart rate and sphincter function), and respiratory systems. Serial pulmonary testing (i.e. peak flow (easier), vital capacity and maximum inspiratory pressure) should be performed regularly at the bedside. As children have fewer reserves, they may deteriorate quickly, developing for example sudden apnea. In children too young to cooperate with pulmonary testing, fatigue or decreased alertness should be closely monitored.

In fact mortality in GBS is often correlated with complications that occur along the disease course such as infection, acute respiratory arrest and pneumothorax. Therefore, children with any of the following problems (which are strong predictors of likelihood of undergoing mechanical ventilation) should be admitted urgently to a pediatric intensive care unit (Agrawal et al. 2007; Lawn et al. 2001):

* flaccid quadriparesia
* rapidly progressive weakness
* reduced vital capacity ($\leq$20mL/kg)
* bulbar palsy
* significant autonomic instability.

Patients with a less severe affection can be followed in a lower intensive care setting with close monitoring of cardiac rhythm, blood pressure and vital capacity.

The following parameters warn of impending respiratory arrest and are an indication for urgent intubation (Hu et al. 2012):

* vital capacity $\leq$20mL/kg
* maximum inspiratory pressure less negative than $-30$cmH$_2$O (i.e. between $-30$ and 0cmH$_2$O)
* maximum expiratory pressure $\leq$40cmH$_2$O
* tidal volume <5mL/kg.

Pulmonary function testing is difficult in children younger than 6 years of age, and the clinician has to rely on other clinical signs such as, for example: a sustained increase of pCO$_2$ to $\geq$50mmHg, an increasing respiratory rate, increasing oxygen requirement, an overuse of accessory muscles, and sweating about the head and neck.

In the context of ventilation in the intensive care unit (ICU), one should avoid the use of particular medications such as sedatives and neuromuscular blockers in GBS. Chest physiotherapy and clearance of secretions performed by trained physiotherapists reduce the risk of pneumonia.

As autonomic dysfunction is a well-recognized feature of GBS, vasoactive or sedative drugs should be handled carefully, because dysautonomia may exaggerate the hypotensive responses to these drugs. Regarding feeding during the critical GBS phase, the use of a nasogastric tube is quite common (sometimes, gastrostomy or parental nutrition). Prevention of deep vein thrombosis is recommended.

*Immunotherapies*

Regarding immunotherapies, two types of treatment may be considered in the context of GBS in children: intravenous immuno globulins and plasma exchange.

In any case, intravenous immune globulin (IVIG) and plasma exchange for children with GBS should be reserved for those with any of the following indications:

• progressing weakness
• worsening respiratory status or need for mechanical ventilation
• significant bulbar weakness
• inability to walk unaided.

Intravenous immunoglobulin

Although no large randomized controlled trials regarding the use of immunoglobulins in children exist, data from the available small open-label randomized trials in children suggest that IVIG shortens the time to recovery compared with supportive care alone (Korinthenberg et al. 2005; Hughes et al. 2014). Similarly, most observational studies show that IVIG hastens recovery in children (Kanra et al. 1997; Singhi et al. 1999; Shahar and Leiderman 2003; Yata et al. 2003). While the effect of IVIG on long-term overall prognosis is still debated, results of existing trials are consistent with the larger randomized trials showing a beneficial effect of IVIG treatment for GBS in adults.

Plasma exchange in children can also be administrated as a first-line treatment in GBS in children. In a recent retrospective study it was shown to shorten the course of hospitalization, to reduce mortality and incidence of permanent paralysis (Maitrey Gajjar, et al. 2016). It is a safe procedure, if volume shifts, calcium supplementation, venous access and anticoagulation are carefully monitored. Minor complications such as hypotension and shivering may occur.

IVIG is still probably more widely used and preferred to plasma exchange in children because of IVIG's relative safety and ease of administration, although there are no reliable data suggesting that one or the other is superior.

IVIG and plasma exchange are not recommended for ambulatory children with GBS who have mild, non-progressive disease or for children whose symptoms have stabilized. Children who have rapid progression followed by stabilization of symptoms within the first or second week of GBS onset may still be considered candidates for treatment by some child neurologists. When a child neurologist decides to initiate an IVIG or plasma exchange treatment, this should happen during the 2 to 4 weeks after disease onset. Finally, glucocorticoids are not recommended as they have never shown any benefits in GBS (Hughes 1991; Korinthenberg and Mönting 1996).

CHRONIC INFLAMMATORY DEMYELINATING POLYNEUROPATHY

Chronic inflammatory demyelinating polyneuropathy (CIDP) is a rare acquired disorder of peripheral nerves and nerve roots. It has now been more and more recognized in children, although its exact incidence remains unclear. In terms of pathogenesis, the cause of CIDP remains unclear but both the cellular and humoral components of the immune system appear to be involved.

There is a temporal continuum between AIDP, the demyelinating form of GBS, and CIDP (McMillan et al. 2013). In its classic form, motor involvement, in general quite symmetric, is greater than sensory. Weakness is present in both proximal and distal muscles. In a series of 13 children, the most common presentation was lower extremity weakness with difficulty walking (Nevo et al. 1996). Most patients also have sensory involvement and deep tendon reflexes are quite often diminished or absent. Cranial nerve and bulbar involvement are more uncommon. The course of the disease has a relapsing-remitting character but some patients experience a prolonged stepwise monophasic course.

Increased cerebrospinal fluid protein without pleocytosis is present in over 90% of patients with CIDP. While the initial diagnosis of CIDP is clinical, electrodiagnostic testing is particularly helpful by showing signs of demyelination. One of the following demyelinating parameters are necessary:

- ≥50% prolongation of motor distal latency above the upper limit of normal (ULN) in two nerves;
- ≥30% reduction of motor conduction velocity below the lower limit of normal (LLN) in two nerves;
- ≥20% prolongation of F-wave latency above the ULN in two nerves, or >50% if the amplitude of the distal negative peak compound muscle action potential (CMAP) is <80% of the LLN;
- absence of F-waves in two nerves;
- partial motor conduction block, defined by a ≥50% amplitude reduction of the proximal negative peak CMAP relative to distal, in two nerves, or in one nerve plus at least one other demyelinating parameter (meeting any of the definite criteria) in at least one other nerve.

*Management*

As a chronic condition CIDP often requires multiple modalities of treatment over time.

Initial therapy for CIDP typically starts either with intravenous immune globulin (IVIG; typically: 2g/kg over 5 days), glucocorticoids (1mg/kg for 4 weeks, followed by slow tapering), or plasma exchange. These treatments have traditionally been regarded as being equally efficacious. A retrospective study of childhood CIDP suggested that the response to treatment was more favorable with IVIG and glucocorticoids than with plasma exchange, but very few children received plasma exchange as a first-line treatment (because of the complexity of organizing treatment provision in children). IVIG is even considered to be the preferred initial treatment by many but there are questions about cost and reimbursement issues. However, the lack of any randomized studies (due to the rarity of the disease) means that there is not a clear consensus on initial choice of treatment, nor for second-line therapies for patients in whom IVIG and corticosteroids fail, or for patients who become corticosteroid dependent. The long-term prognosis of CIDP is generally favorable, but a significant number of patients do not have complete remission of their illness, and many need intermittent, if not continuous, immunomodulatory treatment (Sekiguchi et al. 2012).

**Infections**

Peripheral neuropathies are associated with a variety of infections in children. We briefly describe the most frequent causes but their specific management is out of the scope of this book. With the exception of Lyme disease, these conditions are rare in the United States and Western Europe.

LYME DISEASE

In contrast to adults, meningoradiculitis and peripheral neuropathy in the context of Lyme disease occur rarely in children (Belman et al. 1993). Lyme disease is a multisystem inflammatory disease caused by spirochetes, known collectively as *Borrelia burgdorferi*, which are spread by the bite of infected Ixodes ticks. Adults with Lyme disease can develop a painful radiculitis manifested by neuropathic symptoms such as numbness, tingling, and burning. This radiculoneuropathy may affect the limbs (upper greater than lower extremity) or trunk. Persistent facial palsy was shown to occur in 13% of children diagnosed with Lyme neuroborreliosis (Skogman et al. 2012). With appropriate treatment, prognosis for recovery in Lyme disease is good. Neuroborreliosis is typically treated with intravenous antibiotics which cross the blood–brain barrier, such as penicillins, ceftriaxone, or cefotaxime. Small observational studies suggest ceftriaxone is also effective in children. The recommended duration of treatment is 14 to 28 days.

CHAGAS DISEASE

Chagas disease (American trypanosomiasis) is caused by infection with the protozoan parasite *Trypanosoma cruzi*. A mixed sensorimotor peripheral neuropathy with predominantly sensory symptomatology has been reported in the chronic phase of Chagas disease (Córdova et al. 2010), affecting up to 10% of patients. In addition, autonomic neuropathy (blunting of autonomic responses) is fairly common in chronic Chagas disease, with subtle changes on testing even in children (Bowman et al. 2011). Importantly, in this context, peripheral neuropathy is a known side effect of benznidazole (Miller et al. 2015), a treatment of Chagas disease.

LEPROSY

Leprosy (Hansen disease), a chronic disease caused by *Mycobacterium leprae*, is still a major public health problem in developing countries, with more than 200 000 new cases reported each year. It has a prevalence of 10–12 million cases, most of them in the countries of Asia, South America, and Africa where the affection is endemic (Wkly Epidemiol Rec. 2015), and 10% of the cases develop in children younger than 15 (mainly with the paucibacillary form). Leprosy can be observed in the US and in Europe mainly in patients immigrating from endemic regions.

Although leprosy is better known for its cutaneous manifestations, the neural involvement is responsible for the most serious complications of the disease, leading to functional and anatomical changes of the nerve that can evolve to disabilities and lifelong deformities if the disease is not treated early (Nolen et al. 2014; Lockwood and Saunderson 2012). The involvement of the nerves can be caused by local infection by the bacillus and by immunologically mediated reactions.

The hallmark clinical findings in leprosy are hypopigmented skin lesions with loss of sensation that are observed more frequently in the cooler areas of the body, such as the nose and earlobes.

Peripheral neuropathy is caused by bacterial invasion of the Schwann cells. Nerve destruction usually becomes significant only years after infection, and results from complex (not yet fully understood) mechanisms involving not only the infection but also the host immune response and an inflammatory reaction. Nerves are usually injured at two different levels in leprosy. First, as *M. leprae* has a predilection to involve initially the dermal nerves, nerve injury does not follow a specific nerve territory distribution, and affects thermal, pain, tactile, and autonomic fibers of the skin in a mosaic distribution. Secondly, later in the disease course, injury can occur in more proximal nerve trunks typically including ulnar and median nerves (claw hand), the common peroneal (foot drop), the posterior tibial (claw toes and plantar insensitivity), facial, radial cutaneous, and great auricular (coolest regions of the body). Superposition of both patterns is very suggestive of leprosy neuropathy. So an asymmetric sensory loss is typically observed as well as nerve hypertrophy although not always detected on examination. Nerve ultrasonography is effective in detecting nerve hypertrophy and should be considered in patients with idiopathic asymmetric neuropathy. Motor and sensory nerve conduction velocity is slow in both clinically involved and unaffected nerves (Wilder-Smith and Wilder-Smith 1996), but this pattern is rarely observed in children. Nerve biopsy shows loss of axons and myelin with swollen Schwann cells that contain the organism.

Early treatment is obviously recommended in order to avoid permanent nerve damage. Recent recommendations focus on regimens with shorter duration. Six months of multidrug therapy (monthly rifampicin, daily dapsone) is recommended by the World Health Organization for paucibacillary (≤5 skin lesions) patients and 12 months of multidrug therapy (monthly rifampicin (10mg/kg), daily dapsone (2mg/kg) and every other day clofazimine 1mg/kg) for multibacillary patients (>5 skin lesions) (WHO 2016). Relapses are very rare. The use of dapsone should be closely monitored, as it can cause an axonal motor neuropathy. Reconstructive surgery may be indicated in patients with soft tissue defects, particularly for plantar ulcerations in patients with leprosy.

HIV
Although the incidence of many neurologic complications has decreased in the era of highly active antiretroviral therapy (HAART), because children infected by HIV (mainly via vertical transmission) now live longer, they are at higher risk of developing neurologic complications over their lifetimes. Distal symmetric polyneuropathy (DSPN) is the most common neurologic complication of HIV infection, occurring in adults and children and can be due to HIV infection or a side effect of anti-retroviral therapy (ART) – particularly the nucleoside transcriptase inhibitors. Epidemiologic reports are scarce in children but some may indicate a prevalence rate of 15–34%, pointing however to a less severe clinical picture than the one found in adults and finally indicating a potential association with malnutrition. More attention to symptoms and signs in the follow-up of pediatric patients with HIV is needed, particularly now patients have a longer life expectancy. Management measures

that avoid more harm to the peripheral nervous system, that relieve those children from uncomfortable symptoms, and try to protect them from developing walking disabilities need to be adopted (Araújo et al. 2000; Esteban et al. 2009).

## Systemic disorders

Although rare in children, and not always present at the initial presentation of the disorder, a peripheral neuropathy can complicate several systemic diseases. The polyneuropathy may be hidden by constellations of other signs of systemic involvement, and/or may often be asymptomatic, being detected only on electro-stimulation or electromyography (EMG) studies or with a very careful clinical examination.

We review some of the clinically significant entities.

### CRITICAL ILLNESS POLYNEUROPATHY

Critical illness polyneuropathy occurs in patients with multiple organ failure who have received prolonged intensive care treatment. This condition occurs predominantly in adults, but also children although much more rarely. The disorder is associated with multiple organ dysfunction, prolonged mechanical ventilation, and sepsis. Peripheral neuropathy with myopathy may occur after prolonged neuromuscular blockade with non-depolarizing neuromuscular blocking (Watling and Dasta 1994). Affected patients have flaccid paralysis and areflexia. The diagnosis should be considered in a flaccid child who is difficult to wean from ventilator support (Wijdicks et al. 1994).

Nerve conduction studies show a generalized axonal sensory and motor neuropathy and electromyography may show varied abnormalities. Often, evidence of ongoing denervation (fibrillation potentials and positive sharp waves) is seen in conjunction with normal appearing motor units. Occasionally, electromyography shows myopathic changes, suggesting that critical illness myopathy and neuropathy form a continuum. Cerebrospinal fluid is normal. Motor function returns slowly over several months.

### SYSTEMIC LUPUS ERYTHEMATOSUS

Reports of peripheral neuropathy in children with systemic lupus erythematosus (SLE) commonly describe neuropsychiatric manifestations, which can complicate diagnosis. Three clinical presentations are described: mononeuritis multiplex, an acute sensorimotor neuropathy similar to GBS, and a distal sensory neuropathy (Omdal et al. 2001). Treatment may include standard immunomodulation and intravenous immunoglobulin. Most studies recommend regular nerve conduction studies to screen children with SLE for early evidence of subclinical neuropathy (Huynh et al. 1999).

### DIABETES MELLITUS NEUROPATHY

Peripheral neuropathy, which is a major complication of diabetes type 1 in adults, rarely has clinical impact during childhood or adolescence. However, a subclinical neuropathy is commonly seen, especially in adolescents. Nerve conduction studies (NCS) are the gold-standard method for its detection. For example, abnormalities were detected in 25% of children at their initial presentation by measurement of reduced nerve conduction velocities (Louraki et al. 2012). However, NCS is invasive, difficult to per-form and selectively detects large-fiber abnormalities. Clinical tools, such as vibration sensation thresholds (VSTs) and thermal discrimination thresholds (TDTs), are quicker and easier and, therefore, more suitable as screening tools (Donaghue et al. 1996). Poor glycemic control is the most important risk factor for the development of diabetes mel-litus neuropathy. Maintaining near-normoglycemia is the only way to prevent or reverse neural impairment. Early detection of children and adolescents with nervous system abnormalities is crucial to allow all appropriate measures to be taken to prevent the development of diabetes mellitus neuropathy.

RENAL FAILURE

The neuropathy of chronic renal failure is typically an axonal degenerative type, which in most children is asymptomatic (Makkar and Kochar 1994; Ho et al. 2012). Nerve conduction studies in long-term hemodialysis have been reported as a useful indicator of clinically asymptomatic uremic polyneuropathy, identifying this complication in almost 60% of indi-viduals in one series of children with chronic renal failure. This neuropathy usually remains stable or improves with treatment; if not, increasing the frequency and duration of dialysis may result in improvement.

VITAMIN DEFICIENCY OR EXCESS

Vitamin deficiency or excess (such as vitamin $B_6$) may result in peripheral neuropathy. Symptoms usually resolve with correction of the deficiency or elimination of the excess vitamin. We further detail two situations of specific vitamin deficiency with pediatric impact.

*Vitamin B$_1$ (thiamine) deficiency*

Thiamine, formerly known as vitamin $B_1$ deficiency is typically seen in areas where polished rice is a major portion of the diet. Breast-fed infants of thiamine-deficient moth-ers, and after the trigger of a gastroenteritis, may develop an encephalopathy (infantile encephalitic beriberi) with cardiomyopathy, dyspnea, vomiting and acute neuritis includ-ing altered sensorium, laryngeal nerve paralysis (the classic sign of voice hoarseness), and peripheral neuropathy. The latter may be obscured by the central nervous system (CNS) and systemic symptoms. If the deficiency is prolonged, a patchy, demyelinating neuropathy may develop (Cochrane et al. 1961). There is an excellent response to thia-mine supplementation.

*Vitamin E*

Progressive neurologic syndrome secondary to deficient vitamin E absorption occurs in children with longstanding obstructive liver disease, chronic intestinal malabsorption, and cystic fibrosis (Muller 2010). Children suffering from protein-energy malnutrition are also at risk of vitamin E deficiency (Kalra et al. 2001). Vitamin E deficiency is a major factor in the pathogenesis of the polyneuropathy associated with abetalipopro-teinemia and ataxia with vitamin E deficiency (AVED) (Di Donato et al. 2010; Puri et al. 2005) (see Chapter 7, page 133).

**Medications**

Peripheral neuropathy is a side effect of many medications. A detailed history, looking at patient environment and food habits is essential in order to make a correct diagnosis and the primary treatment is withdrawal of the suspected/aggressing drug. A toxic neuropathy is to be considered in the differential diagnosis of a subacute, chronic symmetrical polyneuropathy, particularly with a distal localization and with the occurrence of sensory symptoms. The most common associations are listed here, although the list of possible drugs is much longer.

ANTIBIOTICS

Antibiotic agents have been associated with peripheral nerve disorders. These agents include penicillin, chloroquine, sulfonamide, metronidazole, nitrofurantoin, isoniazid. Symptoms consist of paresthesias, motor weakness, and/or sensory abnormalities.

CHEMOTHERAPEUTIC AGENTS

Peripheral neuropathy is an important complication of chemotherapeutic agents, including vincristine, cisplatin, cytarabine, bortezomib, thalidomide, and paclitaxel (Purser et al. 2014). In some cases, this toxicity may limit the use of these drugs. However, retrospective data suggest that most children with chemotherapy-induced peripheral neuropathy have a favorable outcome, with clinical improvement during the maintenance phase or after completion of therapy.

PHENYTOIN

Peripheral neuropathy associated with the use of phenytoin has been well described (Mochizuki et al. 1981). The total dose and duration of therapy with phenytoin correlated with reduced motor conduction velocity in the posterior tibial nerve. Fortunately, phenytoin is less and less prescribed as a long-term medication in children.

THALIDOMIDE

Indications are increasing for the use of this drug to treat inflammatory and neoplastic diseases. When children receive thalidomide, it could be that, like many adults, some children will develop a motor, sensory, and autonomic polyneuropathy, which in some cases may worsen even after discontinuation of treatment (Fleming et al. 2005; Priolo et al. 2008). The diagnosis is confirmed by identification of the toxic substance in blood, urine, or body tissues (e.g. hair or nails).

N-HEXANE (GLUE SNIFFING)

N-hexane, which is contained in products such as solvents, glues, spray paints, etc., is a neurotoxin that causes giant axonal changes and potentially an axonal neuropathy. Toxicity can result from industrial exposure or addictive inhalation. A glue-sniffing neuropathy is characterized by predominant proximal as well as distal weakness; distal paresthesia has been rarely reported in children. After elimination of the exposure, recovery is slow and may be incomplete (Burns et al. 2001).

THALLIUM, ARSENIC, LEAD

Thallium is used in rodenticides and insecticides in some countries, despite recommendation against its use by the World Health Organization. Abdominal pain with nausea and vomiting occur in the acute phase and an encephalitic pattern may be prominent (tremor, ataxia, coma). A painful, rapidly progressive, and usually including ascending weakness of peripheral origin typically begins 2 to 5 days after acute exposure and dominates the clinical picture in the second or third week. Treatment consists of oral ferric hexacyanoferrate (Prussian blue), which binds thallium and prevents reabsorption but the fatality rate remains high.

Arsenic ingestion is accompanied by gastro-intestinal symptoms, and the occurrence of a rapidly progressive motor and sensory polyneuropathy

Lead neuropathy, after chronic exposure, is extremely rare in childhood, in comparison with PICA behavioral problems. Neuropathy, when it occurs, usually presents in children as distal ankle weakness with foot drop. In contrast, the arms are more likely to be affected in adults, who often develop wrist drop (Burns et al. 2001; Behse and Carlsen 1978).

## Key points

- Acquired neuropathies in children have a large number of etiologies, including neuroinfections, neuroinflammation, toxins and vitamin deficiencies some of them being quite prevalent (leprosy, HIV drug toxicity, vitamin B1, E deficiency, etc.) in lower middle income countries (LMICs).
- They are important to recognize as some of them are treatable, requiring some specific management schemes.
- Encouraging progress has been made in the management of acute inflammatory demyelinating polyneuropathy (AIDP), which is the most common acquired neuropathy of childhood.

## Clinical vignette

A 14-year-old girl had been in excellent health until 3 months ago when she noticed difficulty climbing the stairs. She also experienced hypersensitivity on the top of her right foot, but also numbness in both hands, with clumsiness. Balance when she closed her eyes was poor. No dysarthia, no bladder dysfunction were reported. Her general condition was good. On clinical examination, cranial nerves were normal. Force examination was normal in axial muscles and in the proximal muscles groups of the upper and lower limbs; measuring 3/5 in ankle and toes extensors as well as flexors. Deep tendon reflexes were present in upper limb extremities, were obtained in the knee but were absent in both ankles; sensory examination showed decreased sense of position and decreased vibratory sensation, and pinprick decreased sensation in distal parts of the limbs, and under the knees.

SUMMARY OF FINDINGS AND FIRST DIAGNOSTIC HYPOTHESIS

The clinical findings localize to the peripheral nerves. The pattern of progressive distal weakness, sensory loss, and hyporeflexia evolving for more than 2 months are suggestive of chronic polyneuropathy.

Nerve conduction studies showed a combination of slowed conduction velocities, prolonged distal latencies in peroneal median, and cubital nerves. Sural nerves sensory nerve action potentials (SNAPs) could not be recorded. Prolonged F-wave latencies were noted in the tibial and common fibular nerves, and a conduction block in ulnar nerve. The overall results are in favor of a chronic demyelinating neuropathy that may be inherited or acquired.

CSF analysis showed albumino-cytologic dissociation, with an elevated protein level measured at 70mg/dl, with <5 leukocytes/mm³. Together with the suggestive clinical and electrodiagnostic results the diagnostic of CIDP was made.

The patient was initially treated with IVIg at a dosage of 0.4g/kg/day for 5 days (total 2g/kg). The treatment was well-tolerated, other than minor adverse effects such as headache, itching and a rash.

A positive answer was observed within 10 days with drastic improvement in ankle extensors muscles and balance abilities. After 2 months a relapse was observed requiring a second cure which again resulted in an improvement but one that lasted for a longer period. After 1 year the situation was stable, although she still had a slight deficit in extension of her toes.

Another treatment option would be the prescription of oral steroids such as methyl prednisolone (typically at a dosage of 1mg/kg for 4 weeks followed by progressive tapering) or plasmapheresis. The choice of treatment modality remains however empirical, depending on the treating neurologist.

## REFERENCES

Agrawal S, Peake D, Whitehouse WP (2007) Management of children with Guillain–Barré syndrome. *Arch Dis Child Educ Pract Ed* 92: 161–168.

Araújo AP, Nascimento OJ, Garcia OS (2000) Distal sensory polyneuropathy in a cohort of HIV-infected children over five years of age. *Pediatrics* 106: E35.

Behse F, Carlsen F (1978) Histology and ultrastructure of alterations in neuropathy. *Muscle Nerve* 1: 368–374.

Belman AL, Iyer M, Coyle PK, Dattwyler R (1993) Neurologic manifestations in children with North American Lyme disease. *Neurology* 43: 2609–2614.

Bowman NM, Kawai V, Gilman RH, Bocangel C, Galdos-Cardenas G, Cabrera L et al. (2011) Autonomic dysfunction and risk factors associated with Trypanosoma cruzi infection among children in Arequipa, Peru. *Am J Trop Med Hyg* 84: 85–90.

Buchwald B, de Baets M, Luijckx GJ, Toyka KV (1999) Neonatal Guillain–Barré syndrome: blocking antibodies transmitted from mother to child. *Neurology* 53: 1246–1253.

Burns TM1, Shneker BF, Juel VC (2001) Gasoline sniffing multifocal neuropathy. *Pediatr Neurol* 25(5): 419–21.

Chareyre J, Hully M, Simonnet H, Musset L, Barnerias C, Kossorotoff M et al. (2017) Acute axonal neuropathy subtype of GuillainBarré syndrome in a French pediatric series: adequate follow-up may require repetitive electrophysiological studies. *Eur J Paediatr Neurol* 21: 891–897.

Cochrane WA, Collins-Williams C, Donohue WL (1961) Superior hemorrhagic polioencephalitis (Wernicke's disease) occurring in an infant-probably due to thiamine deficiency from use of a soya bean product. *Pediatrics* 28: 771–777.

Córdova E, Maiolo E, Corti M et al. (2010) Neurological manifestations of Chagas' disease. Neurol Res 32(3): 238–44. doi: 10.1179/016164110X12644252260637.

Devos D, Magot A, Perrier-Boeswillwald J, Fayet G, Leclair-Visonneau L, Ollivier Y et al. (2013) Guillain–Barré syndrome during childhood: particular clinical and electrophysiological features. *Muscle Nerve* 48: 247–251.

Di Donato I, Bianchi S, Federico A (2010) Ataxia with vitamin E deficiency: update of molecular diagnosis. *Neurol Sci* 31: 511–515.

Donaghue KC, Fung AT, Fairchild JM, Howard NJ, Silink M (1996) Prospective assessment of autonomic and peripheral nerve function in adolescents with diabetes. *Diabet Med* 13: 65–71.

Esteban PM, Thahn TG, Bravo JF, Roca LK, Quispe NM, Montano SM et al. (2009) Malnutrition associated with increased risk of peripheral neuropathy in Peruvian children with HIV infection. *J Acquir Immune Defic Syndr* 52(5): 656–658. doi:10.1097/QAI.0b013e3181bb268d.

Fisher M (1956) An unusual variant of acute idiopathic polyneuritis (syndrome of ophthalmoplegia, ataxia and areflexia). *N Engl J Med* 255: 57–65.

Fleming FJ, Vytopil M, Chaitow J, Jones HR Jr, Darras BT, Ryan MM (2005) Thalidomide neuropathy in childhood. *Neuromuscul Disord* 15: 172–176.

Gajjar M, Patel T, Bhatnagar N, Solanki M, Patel V, Soni S (2016) Therapeutic plasma exchange in pediatric patients of Guillain–Barré syndrome: Experience from a Tertiary Care Centre. *Asian J Transfus Sci* 10: 98–100.

Hahn AF (1998) Guillain–Barré syndrome. *Lancet* 352: 635–641.

Hicks CW, Kay B, Worley SE, Moodley M (2010) A clinical picture of Guillain–Barré syndrome in children in the United States. *J Child Neurol* 25: 1504–1510.

Ho DT, Rodig NM, Kim HB, Lidov HG, Shapiro FD, Raju GP et al. (2012) Rapid reversal of uremic neuropathy following renal transplantation in an adolescent. *Pediatr Transplant* 16: E296–E300.

Hu MH, Chen CM, Lin KL, Wang HS, Hsia SH, Chou ML et al. (2012) Risk factors of respiratory failure in children with Guillain–Barré syndrome. *Pediatr Neonatol* 53: 295–299.

Hughes RA (1991) Ineffectiveness of high-dose intravenous methylprednisolone in Guillain–Barré syndrome. *Lancet* 338: 1142.

Hughes RA, Swan AV, van Doorn PA (2014) Intravenous immunoglobulin for Guillain–Barré syndrome. *Cochrane Database Syst Rev* 19: CD002063.

Huynh C, Ho SL, Fong KY, Cheung RT, Mok CC, Lau CS (1999) Peripheral neuropathy in systemic lupus erythematosus. *J Clin Neurophysiol* 16: 164–168.

Jones HR Jr (1996) Childhood Guillain–Barré syndrome: clinical presentation, diagnosis, and therapy. *J Child Neurol* 11: 4–12.

Jones HR Jr (2000) Guillain–Barré syndrome: perspectives with infants and children. *Semin Pediatr Neurol* 7: 91–102.

Kalra V, Grover JK, Ahuja GK, Rathi S, Gulati S, Kalra N (2001) Vitamin E administration and reversal of neurological deficits in protein-energy malnutrition. *J Trop Pediatr* 47: 39–45.

Kanra G, Ozon A, Vajsar J, Castagna L, Secmeer G, Topaloglu H (1997) Intravenous immunoglobulin treatment in children with Guillain–Barré syndrome. *Eur J Paediatr Neurol* 1: 7–12.

Korinthenberg R, Mönting JS (1996) Natural history and treatment effects in Guillain–Barré syndrome: a multicentre study. *Arch Dis Child* 74: 281–287.

Korinthenberg R, Schessl J, Kirschner J, Mönting JS (2005) Intravenously administered immunoglobulin in the treatment of childhood Guillain–Barré syndrome: a randomized trial. *Pediatrics* 116: 8–14.

Korinthenberg R, Schessl J, Kirschner J (2007) Clinical presentation and course of childhood Guillain–Barré syndrome: a prospective multicentre study. *Neuropediatrics* 38: 10–17.

Lawn ND, Fletcher DD, Henderson RD, Wolter TD, Wijdicks EF (2001) Anticipating mechanical ventilation in Guillain–Barré syndrome. *Arch Neurol* 58: 893–898.

Lockwood DNJ, Saunderson PR (2012) Nerve damage in leprosy: a continuing challenge to scientists, clinicians and service providers. *Int Health* 4: 77–85.

Louraki M, Karayianni C, Kanaka-Gantenbein C, Katsalouli M, Karavanaki K (2012) Peripheral neuropathy in children with type 1 diabetes. *Diabetes Metab* 38: 281–289.

Makkar RK, Kochar DK (1994) Somatosensory evoked potentials (SSEPs); sensory nerve conduction velocity (SNCV) and motor nerve conduction velocity (MNCV) in chronic renal failure. *Electromyogr Clin Neurophysiol* 34: 295–300.

McKhann GM, Cornblath DR, Griffin JW, Ho TW, Li CY, Jiang Z et al. (1993) Acute motor axonal neuropathy: a frequent cause of acute flaccid paralysis in China. *Ann Neurol* 33: 333–342.

McMillan HJ, Kang PB, Jones HR, Darras BT (2013) Childhood chronic inflammatory demyelinating polyradiculoneuropathy: combined analysis of a large cohort and eleven published series. *Neuromuscul Disord* 23: 103–111.

Miller DA, Hernandez S, Rodriguez De Armas L, Eells SJ, Traina MM, Miller LG et al. (2015) Tolerance of benznidazole in a United States Chagas Disease clinic. *Clin Infect Dis* 60: 1237–1240.

Mochizuki Y, Suyehiro Y, Tanizawa A, Ohkubo H, Motomura T (1981) Peripheral neuropathy in children on long-term phenytoin therapy. *Brain Dev* 3: 375–383.

Morosini A, Burke C, Emechete B (2003) Polyneuritis cranialis with contrast enhancement of cranial nerves on magnetic resonance imaging. *J Paediatr Child Health* 39: 69–72.

Muller DP (2010) Vitamin E and neurological function. *Mol Nutr Food Res* 54: 710–718.

Nachamkin I, Arzarte Barbosa P, Ung H, Lobato C, Gonzalez Rivera A, Rodriguez P et al. (2007) Patterns of Guillain–Barré syndrome in children: results from a Mexican population. *Neurology* 69: 1665–1671.

151

Nevo Y, Pestronk A, Kornberg AJ, Connolly AM, Yee WC, Iqbal I et al. (1996) Childhood chronic inflammatory demyelinating neuropathies: clinical course and long-term follow-up. *Neurology* 47: 98–102.

Nolen L, Haberling D, Scollard D, Truman R, Rodriguez-Lainz A, Blum L et al. (2014) Incidence of Hansen's Disease – United States, 1994–2011. *MMWR Morb Mortal Wkly Rep* 63: 969–972.

Omdal R, Løseth S, Torbergsen T, Koldingsnes W, Husby G, Mellgren SI (2001) Peripheral neuropathy in systemic lupus erythematosus – a longitudinal study. *Acta Neurol Scand* 103: 386–391.

Petersen B, Schneider C, Strassburg HM, Schrod L (1999) Critical illness neuropathy in pediatric intensive care patients. *Pediatr Neurol* 21: 749–753.

Polo A, Manganotti P, Zanette G, De Grandis D (1992) Polyneuritis cranialis: clinical and electrophysiological findings. *J Neurol Neurosurg Psychiatry* 55: 398–400.

Priolo T, Lamba LD, Giribaldi G, De Negri E, Grosso P, De Grandis E et al. (2008) Childhood thalidomide neuropathy: a clinical and neurophysiologic study. *Pediatr Neurol* 38: 196–199.

Puri V, Chaudhry N, Tatke M, Prakash V (2005) Isolated vitamin E deficiency with demyelinating neuropathy. *Muscle Nerve* 32: 230–235.

Purser MJ, Johnston DL, McMillan HJ (2014) Chemotherapy-induced peripheral neuropathy among paediatric oncology patients.*Can J Neurol Sci* 41: 442–447.

Roodbol J, de Wit MC, Walgaard C, de Hoog M, Catsman-Berrevoets CE, Jacobs BC (2011) Recognizing Guillain–Barré syndrome in preschool children. *Neurology* 76: 807–810.

Roodbol J, de Wit MY, van den Berg B, Kahlmann V, Drenthen J, Catsman-Berrevoets CE, Jacobs BC (2017) Diagnosis of Guillain–Barré syndrome in children and validation of the Brighton criteria. *J Neurol* 264(5): 856–861.

Ryan MM (2005) Guillain–Barré syndrome in childhood. *J Paediatr Child Health* 41: 237–241.

Sekiguchi Y, Uncini A, Yuki N, Misawa S, Notturno F, Nasu S et al. (2012) Antiganglioside antibodies are associated with axonal Guillain–Barré syndrome: a Japanese-Italian collaborative study. *J Neurol Neurosurg Psychiatry* 83: 23–28.

Shahar E, Leiderman M (2003) Outcome of severe Guillain–Barré syndrome in children: comparison between untreated cases versus gamma-globulin therapy. *Clin Neuropharmacol* 26: 84–87.

Singhi SC, Jayshree M, Singhi P, Banerjee S, Prabhakar S (1999) Intravenous immunoglobulin in very severe childhood Guillain–Barré syndrome. *Ann Trop Paediatr* 19: 167–174.

Skogman BH, Glimåker K, Nordwall M, Vrethem M, Ödkvist L, Forsberg P (2012) Long-term clinical outcome after Lyme neuroborreliosis in childhood. *Pediatrics* 130: 262–269.

Sladky JT (2004) Guillain–Barré syndrome in children. *J Child Neurol* 19: 191–200.

Verity C, Stellitano L, Winstone AM, Andrews N, Stowe J, Miller E (2011) Guillain–Barré syndrome and H1N1 influenza vaccine in UK children. *Lancet* 378: 1545–1546.

Visser LH, van der Meché FG, Meulstee J, Rothbarth PP, Jacobs BC, Schmitz PI et al. (1996) Cytomegalovirus infection and Guillain–Barré syndrome: the clinical, electrophysiologic, and prognostic features. Dutch Guillain–Barré Study Group. *Neurology* 47: 668–673.

Watling SM, Dasta JF (1994) Prolonged paralysis in intensive care unit patients after the use of neuromuscular blocking agents: a review of the literature. *Crit Care Med* 22: 884–893.

WHO (2016) WHO Multidrug Therapy Regimens. Geneva: World Health Organization. http://www.who.int/lep/mdt/en/, accessed 15 April 2016.

Wijdicks EF, Litchy WJ, Harrison BA, Gracey DR (1994) The clinical spectrum of critical illness polyneuropathy. *Mayo Clin Proc* 69: 955–959.

Wilder-Smith A, Wilder-Smith E (1996) Electrophysiological evaluation of peripheral autonomic function in leprosy patients, leprosy contacts and controls. *Int J Lepr Other Mycobact Dis* 64: 433–440.

Willison HJ, Veitch J, Paterson G, Kennedy PG (1993) Miller Fisher syndrome is associated with serum antibodies to GQ1b ganglioside. *J Neurol Neurosurg Psychiatry* 56: 204–206.

Wkly Epidemiol Rec (2015) Global leprosy update, 2014: need for early case detection. *Wkly Epidemiol Rec* 90(36): 461–476.

Wong V (1997) A neurophysiological study in children with Miller Fisher syndrome and Guillain–Barré syndrome. *Brain Dev* 19: 197–204.

Yata J, Nihei K, Ohya T, Hirano Y, Momoi M, Maekawa K et al. (2003) High-dose immunoglobulin therapy for Guillain–Barré syndrome in Japanese children. *Pediatr Int* 45: 543–549.

Yuki N, Hartung HP (2012) Guillain–Barré syndrome. *N Engl J Med* 366: 2294–2304.

# 9
# DISORDERS OF THE NEUROMUSCULAR JUNCTION: INHERITED MYASTHENIC SYNDROMES AND JUVENILE MYASTHENIA GRAVIS

*Nicolas Deconinck*

## Introduction

Pediatric neuromuscular junction disorders are less common in children compared to adults, but both autoimmune and inherited subtypes of this disease category occur in the pediatric age group. Neuroanatomically, these can either be classified into presynaptic, synaptic or postsynaptic disorders. Symptoms occur when there is a disruption in the normal synthesis, storage, or release of acetylcholine, the microanatomy of the synapse, the acetylcholinesterase enzyme, or the function of the acetylcholine receptor complex. The specific clinical manifestations are dependent on the pathophysiology and severity of the disorder. The hallmarks of neuromuscular junction disorders are weakness and fatiguability, especially with extraocular muscles and bulbar muscles. However, due to the rarity of the condition and the overlap of the major symptoms with other neuromuscular or metabolic disorders, making the diagnosis can be quite challenging.

## Congenital myasthenic syndromes

Congenital myasthenic syndromes (CMS) form a heterogeneous group of inherited disorders of neuromuscular junction (NMJ) transmission. In contrast to transient neonatal myasthenia (TNM), these syndromes are caused by mutations in genes that encode proteins of the NMJ, and have no immunological basis. More than 20 genes have so far been identified as causing CMS, many of which involve private mutations. Their function at the level of the neuromuscular junction have been extensively studied, involving proteins localized either at the pre-, post- or synaptic level. Prevalence of CMS is estimated at 1 in 500 000 in Europe (Engel et al. 2015), although accurate prevalence is difficult to ascertain.

Fatigable muscle weakness, especially affecting the ocular and other cranial muscles, a positive family history, and a decremental electromyographic response presenting early in life (at birth to early childhood) is the hallmark of this group of disorders as a whole. However, each genetic subtype of CMS has its own specific phenotypical characteristics

**TABLE 9.1**
**Proposed treatment for specific forms of Congenital myasthenic syndromes**

| | *Treatment options* |
|---|---|
| ChAT | AChE inhibitors, 3,4-DAP (see text) |
| AChR deficiency | AChE inhibitors, 3,4-DAP |
| Rapsyn | AChE inhibitors, 3,4-DAP |
| Fast channel syndrome | AChE inhibitors, 3,4-DAP |
| Slow channel syndrome | Fluoxetine, quinidine[a] |
| Acetylcholinesterase deficiency (COLQ) | Ephedrine, salbutamol |
| DOK7 | Ephedrine, salbutamol (can be very striking), 3,4-DAP[b] |

[a]However, quinidine requires therapeutic drug monitoring and carries the risk of QT interval prolongation.
[b]May also worsen symptoms.
ChAT: choline acetyltransferase; AchE: acetylcholinesterase; 3,4-DAP: 3,4-diaminopyridine; AChR: acetylcholine receptors; DOK: downstream of kinase 7.

although overlap exists making gene panel analysis often necessary to obtain the final diagnosis. Eye signs can often be of considerable help in directing genetic testing.

CMS has a variable impact on patients' lives, with a spectrum of patients, harboring pathogenic mutations, ranging from asymptomatic to having severe physical disabilities.

We provide a short description of the most frequent congenital myasthenic syndromes, stressing their key differentiating clinical presentation (differential oculomotor semiology may be interesting regarding this), natural history and their specific pharmacologic and management aspects (Table 9.1).

ACETYLCHOLINE RECEPTOR DEFICIENCY

This postsynaptic form of CMS is the most frequent one with genetic screening most often revealing two different mutations in the ε subunit of the acetylcholine receptor (i.e. compound heterozygotes). A common mutation, 1267 delG, has been reported to be present on at least one allele in 20% of a large cohort of patients (Palace and Beeson 2008).

Symptom onset is usually at birth or in infancy. Feeding difficulties in early life and ptosis are common presenting features and motor milestones are typically delayed.

Ophthalmoplegia is a striking and very common feature in this type of CMS. Generalized weakness is typically present and mild bulbar weakness and respiratory weakness may be observed. The severity of this condition is highly variable but most patients have a stable lifetime course (Fig. 9.1).

RAPSYN

Rapsyn (receptor associated protein of the synapse) is a key protein in the initiation and maintenance of synaptic structures and specifically in clustering of acetylcholine receptors (AChR) at the muscle endplate. The N88K missense mutation is a common cause of rapsyn CMS in Europeans (Müller et al. 2003). The phenotypes of this recessive CMS (Burke et al. 2004) are different to AChR deficiency syndromes due to AChR subunit mutations. Typically, onset is at birth or early infancy with respiratory failure, feeding difficulties, or generalized hypotonia. Fetal akinesia in utero gives rise to characteristic dysmorphic

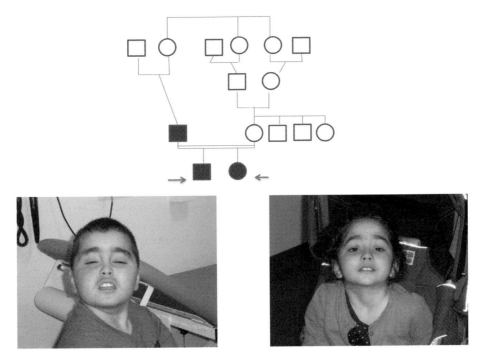

**Fig. 9.1.** Male patient presenting with swallowing difficulties at the age of 2 months. At the age of 12 months he had bilateral ptosis and moderate generalized muscle weakness and had a delay in milestones acquisition (sitting, standing up, etc.). He had no ophthalmoparesia. His sister presented the same symptoms 2 years later. A homozygous mutation was found in the Ɛ subunit of the acetylcholine receptor (Ɛ 1276delG). The father presented similar symptoms during infancy. Inheritance was recessive although mimicking a dominant pattern (compare with consanguinity).

facies and usually mild arthrogryposis which tends to resolve with physiotherapy. Quite specific to this form of CMS, patients commonly have a high arched palate. Weakness is typically generalized, also including facial muscles. Ophthalmoplegia is not a feature, but ptosis may be present. Strabismus, usually divergent, is very common in rapsyn CMS and is a useful distinguishing feature. However, the main caveat to this is the high frequency of strabismus, convergent more than divergent, in the general population. Exacerbations are frequent in the first few years of life and usually, but not always, occur in the context of intercurrent infection. Similar to ChAT CMS, these episodic exacerbations can be associated with respiratory failure and apnea and little weakness in between attacks.

Rapsyn CMS has a good long-term prognosis, often improving during childhood and many adults are able to substantially reduce or even stop treatment.

## DOK7

DOK7 (downstream of kinase 7) is a cytoplasmic protein that is essential for normal synaptogenesis. It interacts with MuSK (muscle-specific tyrosine kinase) signaling pathways responsible for postsynaptic differentiation including AChR clustering.

Infants are often asymptomatic with normal early motor milestones. Affected children present with difficulties in walking during early childhood. However, more severe cases may present with neonatal stridor or feeding difficulties from birth (Jephson et al. 2010). Weakness in DOK7 CMS is usually generalized and most often proximal giving rise to a limb-girdle phenotype. Ptosis is often moderate to severe and extraocular muscles are spared. Bulbar and respiratory weakness is common and can present later in the course of the disease. DOK7 patients can report variation in their symptoms over longer time periods, i.e. weeks to months but are very rarely dramatic.

ACETYLCHOLINESTERASE DEFICIENCY

Mutations in the acetylcholinesterase (AChE) collagen-like tail subunit gene (*COLQ*) account for approximately 6% of genetically diagnosed CMS, known as COLQ CMS. It is considered as a synaptic form of CMS. *COLQ* mutations cause loss of AChE enzyme activity, resulting in prolonged acetylcholine lifetime in the synapse with consequent desensitization of the AChR, prolonged end plate potentials (EPPs) and depolarization blockade.

Typically, the condition causes severe and progressive weakness from birth or early infancy. However, later onset and milder phenotypes are also recognized. Weakness often affects the respiratory muscles, with both respiratory crises and chronic hypoventilation occurring. A slow pupillary response to light is pathognomonic, but is observed in 25% of patients. Neurophysiological tests may show a repetitive compound muscle action potential (CMAP) response to single stimuli.

SLOW CHANNEL SYNDROME

This is the only dominantly inherited CMS. Here, the mutations in the genes encoding AChR subunits result in abnormally prolonged AChR channel opening with consequent prolonged end plate potentials (EPPs). Like AChE deficiency it is associated with a depolarization blockade associated with CMAP decrement. Mutations may occur in any of the adult receptor subunits.

The age at onset of symptoms is widely variable but tends to happen later and the severity tends to be milder than the other CMS subtypes. Asymptomatic relatives are occasionally identified. Most patients present in childhood with neck flexion weakness or difficulty running. A pattern of selective weakness of cervical and upper limb muscles, particularly affecting the distal arm and hand, has been identified (Engel et al. 1982; Oosterhuis et al. 1987). While ophthalmoplegia is common it does not tend to be as severe as in AChR deficiency or fast channel syndrome.

FAST CHANNEL SYNDROME

This syndrome is caused by a recessive mutation in one allele of an acetylcholine receptor subunit, and in the vast majority of cases accompanied by a null or low-expressor mutation. Mutations cause channel opening that is abnormally brief (opposite to slow channel syndrome), owing to a decreased probability that the acetylcholine receptor channel is opened by physiological concentrations of acetylcholine.

Patients with fast channel syndrome tend to be symptomatic from birth or early infancy, with the majority of patients presenting at birth with bulbar symptoms, ptosis, hypotonia, and weak cry (Palace et al. 2012). Respiratory symptoms may require respiratory support at birth. Stridor paralysis was specifically documented following bronchoscopy. Sudden life-threatening apneas often leading to repeated admissions to intensive care is a major concern.

CHOLINE ACETYLTRANSFERASE DEFICIENCY

The enzyme choline acetyltransferase (ChAT) is active in the presynaptic nerve terminal where it functions in the resynthesis of acetylcholine molecules, making ChAT deficiency a presynaptic form of CMS. This very rare condition is typically associated with sudden episodes of respiratory distress with apnea and bulbar weakness, and patients may be relatively strong in between such crises. These episodes of dyspnea may appear early during the first weeks after birth and continue episodically following initial improvement or may appear later in childhood. Some patients experienced prolonged respiratory weakness, requiring days to weeks of artificial ventilation (Beeson et al. 2005), and infection can trigger crises, which tend to reduce with age. Ptosis may be a feature but extraocular muscles are spared (Kraner et al. 2003).

To demonstrate abnormal NMJ transmission it has been recommended that the tested muscle should be fatigued, either with exercise or with 10Hz stimulation for up to 5 min (Kaminski 2008), which is challenging in young patients.

## Diagnosing congenital myasthenia

Besides a suggestive clinical description, electrodiagnostic testing has a crucial role in the diagnostic work up of a CMS. Typically, sensory nerves action potentials (SNAPs), CMAP amplitudes, and conduction velocities are normal. The clue is found in the observation of a decremental response defined as a greater than 10% decrease of the amplitude or area of the fourth, compared to the first, evoked compound motor action potential, or an abnormal single-fiber electromyographic response. However, in the context of CMS a decremental electromyographic response might be detected only after prolonged subtetanic stimulation and the absence of a positive decrement does not exclude CMS diagnosis.

Tests for anti-acetylcholine receptor and anti-muscle-specific tyrosine kinase (anti-MuSK) antibodies should be done in sporadic patients after the age of 1 year and in arthrogrypotic infants, even if the mother has no myasthenic symptoms to exclude autoimmune myasthenia.

The genetic diagnosis of a specific CMS is greatly helped when clinical and electromyographic studies point to a candidate gene. Tests for CMS-causing mutations in previously identified CMS genes are now commercially available, but these are best used in a targeted manner based on specific phenotypes. Whole-exome sequencing has been used to identify novel CMS-causing mutations.

## Treatment options for congenital myasthenic syndromes

Current therapies for CMS include:

• *cholinergic agonists*: pyridostigmine and amifampridine (3,4-DAP);

- *long-lived open-channel blockers of the acetylcholine receptor ion channel*: fluoxetine and quinidine;
- *adrenergic agonists*: salbutamol and ephedrine.

As illustrated in Table 9.1, the selection of a particular medication has to be made on the basis of a particular CMS subtype and its linked pathophysiology. One has to bear in mind that some drugs may benefit one type of CMS but can be ineffective or harmful in another type. For example, patients harboring low-expressor or fast channel mutations in acetylcholine receptors show improvement with cholinergic agonists, whereas patients with slow channel mutations in acetylcholine receptors deteriorate on these drugs and those with COLQ CMS can experience significant clinical deterioration with AChE inhibitors or 3,4-DAP medication.

### Juvenile myasthenia gravis

Myasthenia gravis (MG) is an autoimmune disease in which antibodies are directed at the postsynaptic membrane of the neuromuscular junction, leading to varying degrees of muscle weakness and fatigability. When myasthenia gravis presents before 19 years of age, it is termed juvenile myasthenia gravis (JMG). Although JMG shares many features with the more common adult MG, there are many important differences.

PATHOGENESIS

The exact pathogenesis is not known but myasthenia gravis is related to circulating antibodies to various muscle receptors, including, in most patients, to the nicotinic acetylcholine receptor (AChR) and, rarely, muscle-specific receptor tyrosine kinase (MuSK). The thymus is thought to trigger antibody production in the form with anti-AChR antibodies. AChR antibodies are however probably less frequent in prepubertal patients than in adolescent and adult patients (30–50%) (Andrews et al. 1994; Evoli et al. 1998). It is currently unknown whether anti-low-density lipoprotein receptor-related protein 4 (LRP4) antibodies have been reported in some seronegative patients. The disorder can also be drug-induced.

EPIDEMIOLOGY AND CLINICAL FEATURES

JMG is a rare disorder of childhood, but its incidence and prevalence vary geographically. Pediatric presentation of myasthenia gravis is more common in Oriental than in Caucasian populations (Chiu et al. 1987). Up to 50% of all cases of myasthenia gravis in Chinese populations present in childhood, mostly with ocular features, with a peak age at presentation of 5–10 years (Zhang et al. 2007). The most frequent clinical presentation of JMG is ptosis, which is often associated with other ocular symptoms, namely unilateral or asymmetric ophthalmoplegia, strabismus, and lid twitch, which may only be elicited after sustained upgaze (Parr and Jayawant 2007). These symptoms cause particular problems in children as, if severe, they may cause persistent amblyopia (Ellenhorn et al. 1986). Most children also develop generalized muscle weakness, which presents as painless fatigability of the bulbar and limb musculature, with resultant dysphonia, dysphagia, and proximal limb weakness. Weakness is often fluctuating and usually becomes more pronounced through the day and improves with rest. Children are at risk of choking or aspiration and are at increased risk of chest infection. Occasionally, impairment of the respiratory muscles necessitates ventilatory support. This is known as myasthenic crisis. Prepubertal children presenting with JMG have some interesting and distinct clinical features compared with those who present around or after puberty (Evoli et al. 1998; Chiu et al. 1987). Prepubertal JMG is more likely to manifest as ocular myasthenia (Chiang et al. 2009). There is an equal male:female ratio (Haliloglu et al. 2002), in contrast to the female predominance that is seen in peri-/postpubertal children, and a better prognosis, with a higher rate of spontaneous remission in prepubertal presenters (Evoli et al. 1998; Haliloglu et al. 2002). Peri- or postpubertal patients presenting with JMG share more similarities with adult-onset myasthenia gravis. Ocular myasthenia gravis (OMG) (by definition, myasthenia gravis restricted to the oculomotor muscles for 2 years without becoming generalized) in children tends to remain limited contrary to adults in whom up to 80% patients with OMG at presentation will progress to generalized disease (Luchanok and Kaminski 2008; Oosterhuis 1997; Bever et al. 1983; Pineles et al. 2010). Progression may be even less frequent in prepubertal children (Kim et al. 2003).

DIAGNOSIS OF JUVENILE MYASTHENIA GRAVIS
JMG is primarily a clinical diagnosis with classic patterns of fluctuating weakness and fatigability as described above (Della Marina et al. 2014; Castro et al. 2013). A number of diagnostic tools are available to aid with diagnosis. In very young children it is particularly important to distinguish between autoimmune myasthenia and CMS as the treatment options, prognosis, and genetic implications are very different. CMS usually presents in the first years of childhood with variable disability. There is often a positive family history, and diagnosis is aided, primarily by electrophysiology and DNA analysis and occasionally by muscle biopsy (Beeson et al. 1997).

Detection of antibodies to the AChR supports the diagnosis of JMG. In young children where AChR antibodies are negative this can lead to difficulty in differentiating from CMS.

A variable percentage of myasthenia gravis patients without AChR antibodies are found to have antibodies against another neuromuscular junction protein, the muscle-specific tyrosine kinase (MuSK) (Vincent and Leite 2005). MuSK-positive myasthenia gravis is rare in children, and these children represent a distinct subgroup of JMG, with a marked female predominance. MuSK antibodies appear to be associated with more severe disease with prominent facial and bulbar weakness and frequent respiratory crises (Pasnoor et al. 2010). Patients without antibodies to AChR or MuSK are described as having seronegative myasthenia gravis (SNMG). Low affinity antibodies to clustered AChRs can be found in 60% of previously defined SNMG patients. These antibodies are found in all age groups (Leite et al. 2008).

*Using pharmacological investigation for diagnosis*
The Tensilon test involves intravenous infusion of edrophonium, a fast-acting, short duration cholinesterase inhibitor, looking for a transient improvement in previously documented weakness, for example, ptosis, dysphonia. This test is not without risk and should only be performed by staff experienced in pediatric resuscitation, due to the cholinergic effects of edrophonium, which can result in bradycardia, nausea, and excess salivation. Alternatively,

159

in subacute clinical presentation, evaluation of mestinon per os could be considered in the first-line as a diagnostic test.

*Electrophysiology*

Repetitive nerve stimulation in JMG will show a decrement in the compound motor action potential of more than 10% by the fourth or fifth stimulation. Single-fiber EMG (SFEMG) is especially useful in diagnosis of seronegative myasthenia gravis and congenital myasthenic syndromes. It can be technically more difficult in children due to discomfort of the procedure and the level of cooperation required.

*Imaging*

Although thymoma in children is rare, the thymus must be imaged (usually by computed tomography) once JMG has been diagnosed. AChR seropositive myasthenia gravis is frequently associated with changes in the thymus, thymus hyperplasia being the most commonly observed (Hayashi et al. 2007).

MANAGEMENT

Treatment of JMG has largely been extrapolated from adult studies and experience with adult patients. There are few studies looking specifically at interventions in children, particularly prepubertal children.

*Acetylcholinesterase inhibitors*

Acetylcholinesterase inhibitors are first-line treatment in JMG and provide symptomatic relief and may be sufficient in mild cases and in some cases of ocular myasthenia gravis. Pyridostigmine is a long-acting cholinesterase inhibitor that is commonly used. Dosing is usually 4–6 times per day and is tailored to effects. Cautious use in MuSK-positive children is advised due to risk of acetylcholine hypersensitivity.

*Thymectomy*

Because of the presumed role of the thymus in the pathogenesis of myasthenia gravis, thymectomy is a recognized aspect of management (Punga et al. seropositive for MuSK antibody, 2006). A systematic review of the literature, but mainly based on adult publications, concluded that thymectomy increases the probability of remission or improvement of symptoms in AChR seropositive, non thymomatous, autoimmune myasthenia gravis (Gronseth and Barohn 2000; Rodriguez et al. 1983). More recent reviews of children, including prepubertal patients, also suggested increased remission rates after thymectomy (Hennessey et al. 2011; Tracy et al. 2009). Caution needs to be taken in early childhood due to subsequent immunosuppression and the high rates of spontaneous remission in prepubertal presenters. Current evidence suggests that thymectomy should not be recommended in MuSK-positive disease as it is unclear whether it confers any benefit (Skeie et al. 2010; Sanders et al. 2003; Evoli et al. 2003).

*Immunosuppressive therapies*

Frequently, some form of immunosuppression or immunomodulation is required to improve symptoms of JMG. Corticosteroids are often effective and are the mainstay of therapy but can worsen symptoms in the first few weeks of use, particularly if started at high doses (Schneider-Gold et al. 2005). Because of the numerous adverse effects associated with long-term high-dose steroids in children, steroids are often used in combination with a steroid-sparing immunosuppressant, for example, azathioprine.

Azathioprine is a purine analogue that suppresses B and T cell proliferation. It has been found to be effective when used alone (Mertens et al. 1981), but is most commonly used in combination with prednisolone as a steroid-sparing agent. Beneficial effects may take months to appear (Gold et al. 2008) but eventually result in tapering off or eventually stopping of the steroid doses (Palace et al. 1998). Some studies have suggested that azathioprine or corticosteroids may reduce the likelihood of progression of ocular myasthenia gravis to the generalized form of disease (Kupersmith 2004; Sommer et al. 1997). Although these studies included some children in their case series, these were not specifically pediatric studies, and given the lower rates of progression in prepubertal children anyway, these findings are of uncertain relevance in pediatric practice.

Patients unresponsive or intolerant to azathioprine should be considered for other immunosuppressive agents, which could include cyclosporin A and cyclophosphamide, although experience in JMG is limited and one has to take into consideration the safety profile of these drugs before initiating them in children. Mycophenolate mofetil (MMF), a purine synthesis blocking agent that selectively inhibits proliferation of activated T and B lymphocytes (Allison and Eugui 1996), showed some benefit when used either as a monotherapy or in conjunction with prednisolone, but again experience is limited in children. Maximum effects may not be seen until after 1 year of treatment (Hehir et al. 2010). Isolated reports describe a benefit of the use of rituximab or tacrolimus in refractory JMG (Wylam et al. 2003; Mori et al. 2013).

*Plasma exchange/intravenous immunoglobulin*

Improvement in symptoms after plasma exchange or administration of intravenous immunoglobulin (IVIG) is usually temporary (from 4 to 10 weeks). Their use is therefore largely reserved to optimize condition for surgery before thymectomy and in management of myasthenic crisis (Selcen et al. 2000; Gajdos et al. 2002; 2008) (see Clinical vignette). A single randomized controlled trial showed; however, no evidence for superior benefit of plasma exchange over IVIG in treatment of myasthenic crisis (Gajdos et al. 1997).

*Outcome*

Outcomes in JMG have improved significantly over the last decade, with better recognition, diagnosis, and more effective therapies, and long-term prognosis is good (Grob et al. 2008). Children with JMG exhibit higher rates of remission than adults. This includes spontaneous remission and remission following a period of drug therapy. Prepubertal children have the highest rates of spontaneous remission. Remission rates also appear to be influenced by ethnic origin (Evoli et al. 1998).

**Key points**
- Congenital myasthenic syndromes (CMS) form a heterogeneous group of inherited disorders of neuromuscular junction (NMJ) transmission that are caused by mutations in genes that encode proteins of the NMJ.

- Symptoms in CMS generally include fatigable muscle weakness especially affecting the ocular and other cranial muscles, a positive family history, and a decremental electromyographic response presenting early in life (at birth to early childhood, the absence of it, nevertheless, does not exclude the diagnosis).
- Although each genetic subtype of CMS has its own specific phenotypical characteristics, overlap exists making gene panel analysis often necessary.
- Depending on the physiopathology, current therapies for CMS include cholinergic agonists such as pyridostigmine and amifampridine (3,4-DAP), long-lived open-channel blockers of the acetylcholine receptor ion channel, such as fluoxetine and quinidine, and adrenergic agonists, salbutamol and ephedrine.
- Juvenile myasthenia gravis (JMG) is a rare condition of childhood and has particularities that are distinct from adult myasthenia gravis.
- Prepubertal children in particular have a higher prevalence of isolated ocular symptoms, lower frequency of acetylcholine receptor antibodies, and a higher probability of achieving remission.
- Diagnosis in young children can be complicated by the need to differentiate from congenital myasthenic syndromes, which do not have an autoimmune basis.
- Treatment commonly includes anticholinesterases, a cautious use of corticosteroids with or without steroid-sparing agents, and newer immune modulating agents. Plasma exchange and intravenous immunoglobulin (IVIG) are effective in preparation for surgery and in treatment of myasthenic crisis.

**Clinical vignette**

A 10-year-old female was admitted at the pediatric emergency because of respiratory distress. Parents reported that their daughter had been complaining of fatigue while running that started 4 months ago. She also presented fluctuating abnormal gait, and decreased strength. Moreover, parents observed fluctuating strabismus and face amimia.

On physical examination, the girl had dyspnea. Her saturation $SpO_2$ was recorded fluctuating between 85 and 93%. On neurological examination there were clear signs of bilateral palsy, but outward gaze limitations with bilateral ptosis. She also mentioned occasional swallowing difficulties. On muscle testing, she had proximal weakness (3+/5) in both upper and lower limbs. Deep tendon reflexes were present although reduced in amplitude.

Supplemental oxygenotherapy (8l/min) was provided and she was admitted to the intensive care unit, in order to initiate non invasive ventilation. A repetitive nerve stimulation recorded a pathological decrement of 25% and 35%, respectively in the facial and ulnar nerves. AChR antibodies returned negative; however, MuSK antibody titers returned positive (titer levels of 1:2600), signing the diagnosis of MuSK seropositive myasthenia. A chest computed tomography scan did not show any sign of thymoma.

IVIG infusion was started at the dosage of 0.4g/Kg/day for 5 days but without clear improvement. Nephrologists and neurologists together recommended initiation of plasmapheresis of which she completed four rounds. After the third round she her respiratory function improved and she was stable on room air.

She was discharged from the intensive care unit, after 2 weeks. As she presented ongoing facial and proximal weakness, she received increasing doses of pyridostigmine (anticholinesterase therapy) until 40mg 4 times a day but without any improvement. As she had no contraindication for the use of steroids, prednisolone was started at a dose of 1.5–2mg/Kg/day for 3 months with an excellent clinical response on proximal muscle weakness. In order to avoid long-term use of steroids (important in a child), azathioprine (1mg/Kg/day) was added, followed by progressive prednisone taper off. After one year she only complained about occasional weakness in proximal upper limbs, she was attending school regularly without specific adaptations. Her treatment comprised a combination of prednisone (0.2mg/Kg/day) and azathioprine (1mg/Kg).

Myasthenic crisis can be life-threatening and often involves critical care monitoring. It is defined as an acute neuromuscular respiratory failure due to a relative decrease in the amount of acetylcholine at the NMJ. Triggers include stress, infection, and surgery, though sometimes the etiology is idiopathic. It is vital to assess respiratory function and be prepared to provide support whether it is in the form of noninvasive ventilation or intubation and mechanical ventilation until the patient receives appropriate immunomodulatory therapy (plasmapheresis or IVIG). As it has been recognized by several authors, plasmapheresis is more effective than IVIG in anti-MuSK MG.

Pyridostigmine therapy should not be used in myasthenic crisis. Neurology and the critical care team should be contacted promptly for care management.

## REFERENCES

Allison AC, Eugui EM (1996) Purine metabolism and immunosuppressive effects of mycophenolate mofetil (MMF). *Clin Transplant* 10: 77–84.

Andrews PI, Massey JM, Howard JF Jr, Sanders DB (1994) Race, sex, and puberty influence onset, severity, and outcome in juvenile myasthenia gravis. *Neurology* 44: 1208–1214.

Beeson D, Palace J, Vincent A (1997) Congenital myasthenic syndromes. *Curr Opin Neurol* 10: 402–407.

Beeson D, Hantaï D, Lochmüller H Engel A (2005) 126th International workshop: Congenital Myasthenic Syndromes, 24–26 September 2004, Naarden, The Netherlands. *Neuromuscul Disord* 15(7): 498–512. doi: 10.1016/j.nmd.2005.05.001.

Bever CT Jr, Aquino AV, Penn AS, Lovelace RE, Rowland LP (1983) Prognosis of ocular myasthenia. *Ann Neurol* 14: 516–519.

Burke G, Cossins J, Maxwell S, Robb S, Nicolle M, Vincent A et al. (2004) Distinct phenotypes of congenital acetylcholine receptor deficiency. *Neuromuscul Disord* 14: 356–364.

Castro D, Derisavifard S, Anderson M, Greene M, Iannaccone S (2013) Juvenile myasthenia gravis: a twenty-year experience. *J Clin Neuromuscul Dis* 14: 95–102.

Chiang LM, Darras BT, Kang PB (2009) Juvenile myasthenia gravis. *Muscle Nerve* 39: 423–431.

Chiu HC, Vincent A, Newsom-Davis J, Hsieh KH, Hung T (1987) Myasthenia gravis: population differences in disease expression and acetylcholine receptor antibody titers between Chinese and Caucasians. *Neurology* 37: 1854–1857.

Della Marina A, Trippe H, Lutz S, Schara U (2014) Juvenile myasthenia gravis: recommendations for diagnostic approaches and treatment. *Neuropediatrics* 45: 75–83.

Ellenhorn N, Lucchese N, Greenwald M (1986) Juvenile myasthenia gravis and amblyopia. *Am J Ophthalmol* 101: 214–217.

Engel AG, Lambert EH, Mulder DM, Torres CF, Sahashi K, Bertorini TE et al. (1982) A newly recognized congenital myasthenic syndrome attributed to a prolonged open time of the acetylcholine-induced ion channel. *Ann Neurol* 11: 553–569.

Engel AG, Shen XM, Selcen D, Sine SM (2015) Congenital myasthenic syndromes: pathogenesis, diagnosis, and treatment. *Lancet Neurol* 14: 420–434.

Evoli A, Batocchi AP, Bartoccioni E, Lino MM, Minisci C, Tonali P (1998) Juvenile myasthenia gravis with prepubertal onset. *Neuromuscul Disord* 8: 561–567.

Evoli A, Tonali PA, Padua L, Monaco ML, Scuderi F, Batocchi AP et al. (2003) Clinical correlates with anti-MuSK antibodies in generalized seronegative myasthenia gravis. *Brain* 126: 2304–2311.

Gajdos P, Chevret S, Clair B, Tranchant C, Chastang C, Myasthenia Gravis Clinical Study Group. (1997) Clinical trial of plasma exchange and high-dose intravenous immunoglobulin in myasthenia gravis. *Ann Neurol* 41: 789–796.

Gajdos P, Chevret S, Toyka K (2002) Plasma exchange for myasthenia gravis. *Cochrane Database Syst Rev* 4:CD002275.

Gajdos P, Chevret S, Toyka K (2008) Intravenous immunoglobulin for myasthenia gravis. *Cochrane Database Syst Rev* 23:CD002277.

Gold R, Hohlfeld R, Toyka KV (2008) Progress in the treatment of myasthenia gravis. *Ther Adv Neurol Disorder* 1: 36–51.

Grob D, Brunner N, Namba T, Pagala M (2008) Lifetime course of myasthenia gravis. *Muscle Nerve* 37: 141–149.

Gronseth GS, Barohn RJ (2000) Practice parameter: thymectomy for autoimmune myasthenia gravis (an evidence-based review): report of the Quality Standards Subcommittee of the American Academy of Neurology. *Neurology* 55: 7–15.

Haliloglu G, Anlar B, Aysun S, Topcu M, Topaloglu H, Turanli G et al. (2002) Gender prevalence in childhood multiple sclerosis and myasthenia gravis. *J Child Neurol* 17: 390–392.

Hayashi A, Shiono H, Ohta M, Ohta K, Okumura M, Sawa Y (2007) Heterogeneity of immunopathological features of AChR/MuSK autoantibody-negative myasthenia gravis. *J Neuroimmunol* 189: 163–168.

Hehir MK, Burns TM, Alpers J, Conaway MR, Sawa M, Sanders DB (2010) Mycophenolate mofetil in AChR-antibody-positive myasthenia gravis: outcomes in 102 patients. *Muscle Nerve* 41: 593–598.

Hennessey IA, Long AM, Hughes I, Humphrey G (2011) Thymectomy for inducing remission in juvenile myasthenia gravis. *Pediatr Surg Int* 27: 591–594.

Jephson CG, Mills NA, Pitt MC, Beeson D, Aloysius A, Muntoni F et al. (2010) Congenital stridor with feeding difficulty as a presenting symptom of Dok7 congenital myasthenic syndrome. *Int J Pediatr Otorhinolaryngol* 74: 991–994.

Kaminski HJ (2008) *Myasthenia Gravis and Related Disorders*. Berlin: Springer.

Kim JH, Hwang JM, Hwang YS, Kim KJ, Chae J (2003) Childhood ocular myasthenia gravis. *Ophthalmology* 110: 1458–1462.

Kraner S, Laufenberg I, Strassburg HM, Sieb JP, Steinlein OK (2003) Congenital myasthenic syndrome with episodic apnea in patients homozygous for a CHAT missense mutation. *Arch Neurol* 60: 761–763.

Kupersmith MJ (2004) Does early treatment of ocular myasthenia gravis with prednisone reduce progression to generalized disease? *J Neurol Sci* 217: 123–124.

Leite MI, Jacob S, Viegas S, Cossins J, Clover L, Morgan BP et al. (2008) IgG1 antibodies to acetylcholine receptors in 'seronegative' myasthenia gravis. *Brain* 131: 1940–1952.

Luchanok U, Kaminski HJ (2008) Ocular myasthenia: diagnostic and treatment recommendations and the evidence base. *Curr Opin Neurol* 21: 8–15.

Mertens HG, Hertel G, Reuther P, Ricker K (1981) Effect of immunosuppressive drugs (azathioprine). *Ann N Y Acad Sci* 377(1 Myasthenia Gr): 691–699.

Mori T, Mori K, Suzue M, Ito H, Kagami S (2013) Effective treatment of a 13-year-old boy with steroid-dependent ocular myasthenia gravis using tacrolimus. *Brain Dev* 35: 445–448.

Müller JS, Mildner G, Müller-Felber W et al. (2003) Rapsyn N88K is a frequent cause of congenital myasthenic syndromes in European patients. *Neurology* 60(11): 1805–10.

Oosterhuis HJ (1997) *Myasthenia Gravis*. Groningen: Groningen Neurological Press.

Oosterhuis HJ, Newsom-Davis J, Wokke JHJ, Molenaar PC, Weerden TV, Oen BS et al. (1987) The slow channel syndrome. Two new cases. *Brain* 110: 1061–1079.

Palace J, Beeson D (2008) The congenital myasthenic syndromes. *J Neuroimmunol* 201–202: 2–5.

Palace J, Newsom-Davis J, Lecky B, Myasthenia Gravis Study Group. (1998) A randomized double-blind trial of prednisolone alone or with azathioprine in myasthenia gravis. *Neurology* 50: 1778–1783.

Palace J, Lashley D, Bailey S, Jayawant S, Carr A, McConville J et al. (2012) Clinical features in a series of fast channel congenital myasthenia syndrome. *Neuromuscul Disord* 22: 112–117.

Parr JR, Jayawant S (2007) Childhood myasthenia: clinical subtypes and practical management. *Dev Med Child Neurol* 49: 629–635.

Pasnoor M, Wolfe GI, Nations S, Trivedi J, Barohn RJ, Herbelin L et al. (2010) Clinical findings in MuSK-antibody positive myasthenia gravis: a S experience. *Muscle Nerve* 41: 370–374.

Pineles SL, Avery RA, Moss HE, Finkel R, Blinman T, Kaiser L et al. (2010) Visual and systemic outcomes in pediatric ocular myasthenia gravis. *Am J Ophthalmol* 150: 453–459.e3.

Punga AR, Flink R, Askmark H, Stålberg EV (2006) Cholinergic neuromuscular hyperactivity in patients with myasthenia gravis seropositive for MuSK antibody. *Muscle Nerve* 34: 111–115.

Rodriguez M, Gomez MR, Howard FM Jr, Taylor WF (1983) Myasthenia gravis in children: long-term follow-up. *Ann Neurol* 13: 504–510.

Sanders DB, El-Salem K, Massey JM et al. (2003) Clinical aspects of MuSK antibody positive seronegative MG. *Neurology* 60(12): 1978–1980.

Schneider-Gold C, Gajdos P, Toyka KV, Hohlfeld RR (2005) Corticosteroids for myasthenia gravis. *Cochrane Database Syst Rev* 18:CD002828.

Selcen D, Dabrowski ER, Michon AM, Nigro MA (2000) High-dose intravenous immunoglobulin therapy in juvenile myasthenia gravis. *Pediatr Neurol* 22: 40–43.

Skeie GO, Apostolski S, Evoli A, Gilhus NE, Illa I, Harms L et al. (2010) Guidelines for treatment of auto-immune neuromuscular transmission disorders. *Eur J Neurol* 17: 893–902.

Sommer N, Sigg B, Melms A, Weller M, Schepelmann K, Herzau V et al. (1997) Ocular myasthenia gravis: response to long-term immunosuppressive treatment. *J Neurol Neurosurg Psychiatry* 62: 156–162.

Tracy MM, McRae W, Millichap JG (2009) Graded response to thymectomy in children with myasthenia gravis. *J Child Neurol* 24: 454–459.

Vincent A, Leite MI (2005) Neuromuscular junction autoimmune disease: muscle specific kinase antibodies and treatments for myasthenia gravis. *Curr Opin Neurol* 18: 519–525.

Wylam ME, Anderson PM, Kuntz NL, Rodriguez V (2003) Successful treatment of refractory myasthenia gravis using rituximab: a pediatric case report. J Pediatr 143: 674–677.

Zhang X, Yang M, Xu J, Zhang M, Lang B, Wang W et al. (2007) Clinical and serological study of myasthenia gravis in HuBei Province, China. *J Neurol Neurosurg Psychiatry* 78: 386–390.

# 10
# AN INTRODUCTION TO MUSCULAR DYSTROPHIES AND DUCHENNE AND BECKER MUSCULAR DYSTROPHIES

*Nathalie Goemans*

## An Introduction to Muscular Dystrophies

The muscular dystrophies are inherited degenerative muscle diseases characterized by a muscle breakdown due to mutations in genes involved in muscle membrane and muscle structure. These diseases have been historically classified based on clinical presentation, onset of symptoms, distribution of weakness, disease progression and mode of inheritance such as Duchenne–Becker muscular dystrophy (DMD/BMD), Limb-girdle muscular dystrophy (LGMD), facio scapulo humeral muscular dystrophy (FSHD), congenital muscular dystrophy (CMD) and Emery Dreifuss muscular dystrophy (EDMD) (Emery, 2002). Improved insights in the underlying molecular defects of these diseases have highlighted the wide phenotypical expression of these genetic diseases and challenged the original classification of muscular dystrophies and inherited myopathies. Mutations in a single gene may result in symptoms across the whole spectrum of the disease from mild to severe , blurring the borders between the severe "congenital" dystrophies and the milder "limb-girdle" dystrophies. On the other hand mutations in a variety of distinct genes may result in a similar phenotype as observed in the large group of LGMD. Further unraveling of the underlying genetic defects in inherited muscle disorders demonstrated that mutation in a single gene could be responsible for either a "dystrophy" or a "myopathy", the latter being characterized by structural abnormalities of the muscle on histopathological examination and by a more stable disease course, hence questioning the original classification between these two entities.

Ongoing reclassification of these diseases, based on the underlying molecular deficit is important in the context of targeted therapy development for these diseases, however the original classification is still useful in a clinical context.

## Duchenne muscular dystrophy

Duchenne muscular dystrophy (DMD), an X-linked inherited disorder, is the most common and severe form of muscular dystrophy, with an incidence worldwide of 1 in 3 500 to 1 in 6 000 male live births (Emery 1991). A prevalence of 19.5 cases per 100 000 live male births was reported based on newborn screening in Wales (Moat et al. 2013). A pooled prevalence of DMD among males worldwide of 4.78 per 100.00 (95% confidence intervals 1.94–11.81) has been reported based on a meta-analysis of the published epidemiological data (Mah et al. 2014). Originally described by Edward Meyron in 1851, who detailed the clinical and histopathological aspects of this progressive muscular disorder affecting boys, this disease has been eponymously associated with Duchenne de Boulogne who provided later further clinical and pathological description of the disease (Emery 2002).

DMD is caused by a mutation in the *DMD* gene (locus Xp21) which encodes for the dystrophin protein (Hoffman et al. 1987). Other clinical presentations of dystrophinopathies include the milder Becker muscular dystrophy (BMD), the intermediate type (IMD) and X-linked cardiomyopathy (XLCM) (Emery 1991). The prevalence of BMD, is 1–17 500 to 1 in 50 000 (Emery 1991).

## Molecular genetics and pathophysiological aspects

THE DYSTROPHIN GENE

The dystrophin gene is a 2.4Mb gene located on the short arm of chromosome X; it is one of the largest human genes. Its coding sequence, however, is limited to 0.6% of the gene (11kb), dispersed over 79 exons, separated by large introns. Gene transcription is driven by different promotors, resulting in dystrophin isoforms named after their predominant site of expression. Three isoforms, Brain (Dp427c), Muscular (Dp427m) and Purkinje (Dp457p), are full-length dystrophin, while four internal promotors generate shorter tissue specific isoforms (Retinal Dp260,Brain specific Dp140, Schwann cell Dp116 and General Dp71) (Muntoni et al. 2003).

The muscle isoform is the best-known protein product of this locus. Muscle dystrophin protein is a subsarcolemmal protein anchoring the cytoskeleton to the plasma membrane and basal lamina. Dystrophin is considered to contribute to membrane stability as part of the large transmembraneous dystrophin-associated protein complex, which forms a structural bridge between the extracellular matrix and the cytoskeleton (Hoffman et al. 1987; Koenig and Kunkel 1990). The rod-shape structure of the dystrophin protein hints at a protecting role of dystrophin against the repeated contraction-induced mechanical damage to muscle fibers by stabilizing the sarcolemma. Multiple linking domains, anchoring with structural and signaling proteins, suggest that the role of the dystrophin protein is not limited to a mechanical linking and protecting function but that this protein plays a key role in cell signaling as well (Le Rumeur et al. 2010) (Fig. 10.1).

Absence of the dystrophin protein will lead to membrane leakage and increased permeability inducing a pathophysiological cascade of events resulting in muscle necrosis and fibrosis. An increased influx of calcium through the dystrophin-deficient membrane will result in disrupted calcium homeostasis and activation of calcium dependent proteases, ultimately inducing cell death. Impaired hemodynamic responses to exercise, due to mislocalization of neuronal nitric oxide synthase (nNOS,) will cause additional cell damage. Ultimately, chronic inflammatory responses and extracellular matrix gene upregulation will result in an end-stage necrosis and fibrosis of the muscle (Deconinck and Dan 2007).

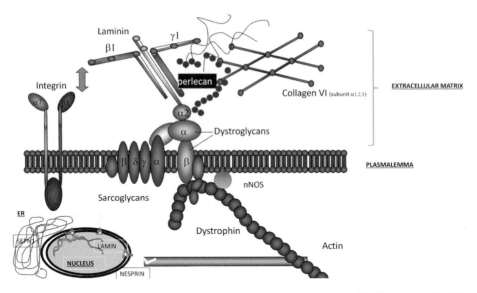

**Fig. 10.1.** Representation of the cellular localisation of the proteins involved in CMDs, DMD/BMD and LGMD. Most genetic defects causing CMD and the milder LGMD affect proteins of plasma membrane–extracellular matrix interface. The three $\alpha$-chains of Collagen VI, a major component of the extracellular matrix, associate with the basal lamina. Laminin $\alpha$2 interacts with the $\alpha$-dystroglycan complex, which is also located in the extracellular matrix, linking the extracellular matrix with the dystrophin-associated glycoprotein (DAG) complex, the sarcoglycans and dystrophin, the latter being involved in Duchenne/Becker dystrophinopathies. A smaller proportion of muscular dystrophies *s* is caused by mutations in genes encoding intracellular proteins, such as Lamin A/C and Nesprin located at the inner nuclear membrane or encoding proteins of the endoplasmatic reticulum such as Selenoprotein1. A colour version of this figure can be seen in the plate section at the end of the book.

Intragenic deletions and duplications of one or more exons account for 72% and 7% of the reported mutations, respectively; the remaining approximately 20% being microdeletions, point mutations and translocations. Most mutations cluster around the hot spot regions of exons 45–55 and exons 2–19 (Aartsma-Rus et al. 2006).

The phenotype resulting from a mutation is not related to the size of the deletion but will depend on the ensuing effect of the mutation on the translation according to the reading frame hypothesis. Mutations in the *DMD* gene disrupting the transcriptional open reading frame will lead to prematurely aborted dystrophin translation, resulting in the absence of the dystrophin protein at the sarcolemmal membrane. However, mutations that maintain the translational reading frame usually lead to internally deleted but partially functional dystrophin proteins, with preserved N-terminal, cysteine rich and C-terminal domains, and are associated with the typically much milder BMD phenotype (Monaco and Kunkel 1988).

The majority of patients with BMD show slowly progressive symptoms of proximal weakness in adolescence or early adulthood but do preserve ambulation and do not evolve towards full-time wheelchair dependency. Respiratory function is preserved as well; however, cardiac involvement is common, with dilated cardiomyopathy as the most common cause of death. Large in-frame deletions involving almost 50% of the gene have been described in the milder BMD phenotype, indicating that some parts of the central rod domain may be truncated with minimal impact on protein function (Muntoni et al. 2003). This reading frame rule has shown a 88–91% predictive accuracy in different cohorts (Aartsma-Rus et al. 2006). Other clinical phenotypes of dystrophinopathies include intermediate muscular dystrophy (IMD) and pure cardiac X-linked dilated cardiomyopathy (XLCM). Being an X-linked recessive inherited disorder, female carriers are generally asymptomatic; however, mild to more severe presentations are well described, due to non-random X inactivation of the normal X chromosome, with a spectrum of symptoms ranging from mild myalgia and cramps to overt muscle weakness, which can present in a limb girdle pattern and follow a full blown pattern of DMD as well as in an asymmetrical, focal involvement of a limb. An increased incidence of dilated cardiomyopathy (5%) has been reported and regular cardiac surveillance is advised in female carriers (Bushby et al. 2003).

Genetic modifiers

The advances in whole genome sequencing techniques have improved our insights in polymorphisms among large populations. Recent studies have highlighted the role of genetic modifiers on the DMD disease course and/or response to glucocorticosteroid treatment such as osteopontin (OPN), the protein product of *SPP1* that interacts with the inflammatory pathway and muscle regeneration in DMD. A modified response to glucocorticoid treatment has been shown in patients carrying a polymorphism in the secreted phosphoprotein 1 (SPP1) promoter (rs28357094) (Vianello et al. 2017). Additionally, a disease-modifying role has been ascribed to CD40 and ACTN3 (Bello et al. 2016; Hogarth et al. 2017). Further unraveling of these genetic modifiers may open new perspectives for targeted treatment strategies and will have to be taken into consideration in the design of clinical trials.

**Clinical aspects and natural course**

DMD is a progressive myopathy with onset in early childhood. It is characterized by a predictable clinical course, affecting primordially striated and cardiac muscles. Affected boys may present with delayed motor development at an early age followed by a progressive weakness of the skeletal muscles during childhood. This muscle weakness may be overlooked at an early age, as the motor delay may be considered as part of a more global developmental delay, which can be the presenting symptom and reason for referral. Indeed, the presence of a cognitive impairment is well described in a proportion of patients with DMD, with a wide spectrum of general deficits in multiple areas of cognition and adaptive functioning, ranging from subtle learning and verbal memory disorders to attention-deficit–hyperactivity disorder (ADHD), autism spectrum disorder and severe intellectual disability. Overall mean IQ (82) is approximately one standard deviation (SD) below the normal population (Banihani et al. 2015; Pane et al. 2013). Children missing all brain isoforms, due to mutations in the distal part of the gene, and especially children missing the Dp140 brain isoform, have a higher risk of showing neurodevelopmental disorders (Chamova et al. 2013).

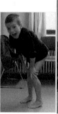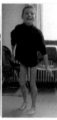

**Fig. 10.2.** Gowers' maneuver reflecting limb girdle weakness in a boy with Duchenne muscular dystrophy.

Young children with DMD may come to clinical attention by the incidental finding of high creatine kinase (CK) leaking in the blood circulation due to the damaged striated muscle membrane, or by the finding of an associated rise in aspartate aminotransferase (AST) and alanine aminotransferase (ALT) of muscular origin. Raised transaminases are often mistaken for an underlying hepatic disease by uninformed clinicians and may lead to unnecessary ancillary hepatic investigations. Creatine kinase levels are typically increased to more than 10 times the upper limit of normal, with a maximum value around the ages of 1 to 6 years old, followed by a progressive decline due to loss of muscle mass (Zatz et al. 1991).

The first clinical manifestations of muscle weakness include gait abnormalities and difficulties in climbing stairs and rising from the floor, with the typical Gowers' sign (broad-based stance and climbing upright by using of the support of the hands on the thighs) by the age of 3–4 years (Fig. 10.2). Affected boys will develop a typical waddling gait pattern with a tendency to tiptoeing due to progressive pelvic girdle weakness and muscle contractures. Muscle pseudohypertrophy may be striking, especially at the level of the calves; however, spectacular pseudohypertophic muscle mass may also develop at the level of the shoulder girdle and paraspinal musculature. If untreated, ambulation will be lost by age 13 years, with subsequent progressive loss of upper limb function (Emery 2002). Full-time wheelchair dependency and axial weakness lead to the development of scoliosis and joint contractures in upper and lower limbs. Progressive weakness of respiratory muscles results in difficulties in coughing and breathing, with the need for assistance in airway clearance and ventilatory support from the late second or third decade on. With increasing age, DMD patients typically develop a progressive dilated cardiomyopathy, eventually leading to symptomatic congestive heart failure and an increased risk of cardiac arrhythmia and sudden death (Muntoni et al. 2003). Progressive cardiac and respiratory involvement will result in a reduced life expectancy and early death in the second or third decade of life, if untreated.

**Diagnosing Duchenne muscular dystrophy**
A diagnosis of DMD should be suspected in any young boy with a motor or more general developmental delay and/or with clinical signs and symptoms of a proximal muscle weakness. Delay in walking, difficulties with running, hopping, jumping or climbing stairs, a

positive Gowers' sign or gait abnormalities should alert the clinician and trigger an assessment of creatine kinase levels in serum. Raised creatine kinase levels of more than 10 times the upper limit of normal will confirm this suspicion and trigger further investigations. The incidental finding of raised creatine kinase and/or transaminases in an apparently asymptomatic young boy should raise suspicions as well, which should be further investigated by genetic analysis. Quantitative assays of all exons using multiplex ligation-dependent probe amplification (MLPA) will detect whole exon deletions and duplications (approximately 75% of mutations). This technique characterizes the borders of most rearrangements and can be used for carrier testing of females. If this assay is negative, and in the presence of a strong clinical suspicion, further sequencing of the DMD gene is indicated to detect point mutations or small rearrangements (Birnkrant et al. 2018b). Although an additional muscle biopsy is not strictly required, in cases where clinical suspicion has been confirmed by genetic diagnosis, it may provide useful additional information by giving an indication of the amount of dystrophin and dystrophin-positive revertant fibers especially in less common mutations where the genotype–phenotype correlations are not always clear or when the open reading frame rule does not seem to fit the clinical picture.

The recent advances in pharmacological therapies for DMD have boosted the interest in newborn screening programs, which is feasible by measuring creatine kinase in a dried blood spot. A raised creatine kinase would then prompt genetic testing to further characterize the dystrophy (Moat et al. 2013). The idea behind is to provide timely genetic counselling to the affected families and an earlier access to disease-modifying therapies. So far, however, newborn screening of creatine kinase is not included in any national screening program.

## Treatment and management

Major efforts have been made in the past decade to develop therapies for DMD by targeting the molecular defect or the subsequent pathophysiological cascade of events, resulting in the approval by the European Medical Agency (EMA) and the Food and Drug Administration (FDA) of some disease-modifying compounds; however, there is still no cure for this disease.

Nevertheless, a multidisciplinary approach to symptoms has been shown to be effective in altering the natural course of the disease and life expectancy. With good care and coordinated medical, surgical and rehabilitative interventions, patients with DMD may now expect to live into adulthood (Eagle et al. 2007; Moxley et al. 2010; Saito et al. 2017). Guidelines on coordinated multidisciplinary care were published in 2010, based on the recommendations of the DMD Care Considerations Working Group, and have been recently updated (Birnkrant et al. 2018b).

MEDICAL TREATMENT

*Treatment with corticosteroids*

Chronic glucocorticosteroid (GCS) treatment, initiated in the ambulant stage of the disease, has been established as a standard of care (Birnkrant et al. 2018b). Corticosteroid use has been proven to increase muscle strength and function (Henricson et al. 2013), to delay the loss of ambulation and the progression of cardiac and respiratory function (McDonald et al.

2017b) as well as to prevent the development of severe scoliosis (Moxley et al. 2010). The mechanism of action relates to a combination of anti-inflammatory and immunosuppressive properties and interaction with expression of genes involved in protein synthesis and calcium metabolism (Fisher et al. 2005).

Both prednisone/prednisolone and deflazacort, an oxazoline derivative of prednisolone, have been shown effective in increasing muscle strength and delaying disease progression (Bello et al. 2015; Manzur et al. 2008). Uncontrolled studies suggest slightly different (side-) effect profiles for those compounds, such as higher efficacy and less weight gain but an increased incidence of cataract for deflazacort (Lamb 2016; McDonald 2017b). Deflazacort (Emflaza*)* has received FDA approval as treatment for DMD (FDA 2017) but deflazacort is not registered and/or commercialized in all countries.

GCS treatment is most often initiated between 3 to 6 years, optimally, before the child shows signs of decline. The standard dosage is 0.75mg/kg/day prednisone or the equivalent of 0.9mg/kg/day deflazacort. Classic contraindications for GCS, including active tuberculosis and other active bacterial, viral, parasitic or mycotic infections, should be excluded.

A wide range of regimens are currently used across the world among which daily, alternated day or intermittent schedules (10d on 10d off or weekend dosing) are the most commonly used (Griggs et al. 2013). Daily steroids have been proven more effective to improve strength and function compared to alternate day administration; however, alternate day or intermittent schedules have been associated with a milder side-effect profile (Griggs et al. 2013; Ricotti et al. 2012; Straathof et al. 2009). High-dose weekend prednisone was shown to be as effective as daily prednisone with a milder side-effect profile (Escolar et al. 2011).

A international multicentric study (FOR-DMD; Clinical Trials identifier: NCT01603407) is currently comparing the side-effect profile and efficacy of prednisone 0.75mg/kg/day, prednisone 0.75mg/kg/day 10 days on and 10 days off treatment, and deflazacort 0.9mg/kg/day as disease-modifying treatments for DMD (Guglieri et al. 2017).

The prevention and management of the known side-effects such as cushingoid features, weight gain and growth inhibition, impaired fat and glucose metabolism, fluid retention and hypertension, osteoporosis with increased risk of vertebral fractures, and cataract, should be integrated in the care of patients with DMD. Patients and families and their care givers should be alerted about the risks and symptoms of adrenal suppression, and stress dose protocols should be discussed in case of emergencies or planned surgical interventions. Guidelines are available online (https://www.parentprojectmd.org/wp-content/uploads/2018/03/PJ-Nicholoff-Steroid-Protocol.pdf) (Kinnett and Noritz 2017).

Corticosteroid treatment is currently continued into the non-ambulant stage of the disease. The dosage and regimen of the steroid treatment is then most often tailored to the individual side-effects profile. Data on the very long-term effects and risk-versus-benefit of chronic use of corticosteroids in the adult DMD population should be further collected. A recent publication of the data from a large prospective, international cohort study with up to 10 years of follow-up provides additional evidence of the long-term positive effects of glucocorticosteroids in DMD on motor function as well as on survival; however, data on the multisystemic side-effects for the very long term are lacking (McDonald et al. 2017b).

*Recently approved pharmacological therapies*

Molecular genetic advances and new insights into the underlying disease mechanisms have generated new concepts for therapeutic approaches for DMD, some of which are currently approved by the EMA or FDA.

Antisense-mediated exon skipping strategy

The antisense-mediated exon skipping strategy for DMD is based on the open reading frame rule and uses sequence-specific single stranded antisense oligonucleotides (AON) to interfere with transcription and translation, hiding selected exons from the splicing machinery, in order to restore an open reading frame. This would theoretically allow the production of truncated but partially functional dystrophin proteins, associated with typically much milder phenotypes as seen in Becker muscular dystrophy (Aartsma-Rus et al. 2002). Exon skipping is a mutation specific therapeutic approach; however, the skipping of one exon may correct different mutations. As an example, exon skipping 51 would theoretically be applicable to 13% of all DMD mutations.

Currently, one AON, a phosphorodiamidate morpholino oligomers (PMO), targeting the restoration of exon 51 skippable mutations (Eteplirsen, EXONDYS 51), has received accelerated approved by the FDA based on data from a placebo-controlled study and its long-term open label extension in 12 participants (Clinical trial identifiers: NCT01396239/ NCT01540409), showing a positive risk/benefit profile for this compound and a statistically significant mean increase in dystrophin levels in muscle biopsies, including additional muscle biopsy data from 13 participants included in a Phase 3 study (Clinical trial identifiers: NCT02255552) after 48 weeks of 30mg/kg/week-treatment (Mendell et al. 2016).

This accelerated FDA approval has raised heated controversies questioning the efficacy of the compound and the probability of the dystrophin findings translating into clinical benefit (Kesselheim and Avorn 2016).

Suppression of stop codon mutations

Ataluren (Translarna) is a small molecule known to specifically induce ribosomal read-through of premature stop codons caused by nonsense mutations. This approach aims at restoring dystrophin by interfering with mRNA translation and could theoretically be applicable in approximately 13% of all DMD patients. This compound has received a conditional approval from the EMA for the treatment of ambulant boys above age 5 with DMD caused by nonsense mutations. This conditional approval has recently been expanded for younger boys as well (age 2 to 5). A large Phase 3 study (ACT DMD; Clinical trial identifier: NCT01826487) did not meet its primary outcome; however, a clinical and statistical significant positive effect on ambulatory capacity was observed in a pre-specified subgroup of patients with a baseline Six Minute Walking Distance test result of 30m or more to less than 400m, compared to natural history studies and data from placebo arms (McDonald et al. 2017a).

MULTIDISCIPLINARY CARE

*Respiratory care*

Progressive involvement of the respiratory muscles will result into respiratory insufficiency and inadequate clearance of secretions leading to an early death. Improved respiratory care with the provision of ventilatory support, together with coughing and clearing assisting techniques and devices, has changed life expectancy considerably since the 1980s (Kieny et al. 2013; Passamano et al. 2012). More recently, a Japanese cohort of 118 long-term survivors was reported, highlighting the effects of multidisciplinary care on survival (Saito et al. 2017).

Guidelines for respiratory care in DMD have been published (Birnkrant et al. 2018a, Finder et al. 2004) and include the use of assisted coughing and clearing techniques and the timely instauration of ventilatory support in the presence of hypoventilation, which may start insidiously and first be limited to deep sleep stages, reflecting dystrophic involvement of the diaphragm. The use of non-invasive ventilation through a nose or a mouth piece is advocated; however, invasive ventilation through tracheostomy may be indicated in individuals where non-invasive techniques fail.

Assessment of respiratory function should be done yearly as long as the child is ambulant. Once ambulation is lost, respiratory function, in/expiratory mouth pressure and coughing abilities should be monitored twice a year. Symptoms of sleep-disordered breathing such as morning headaches and fatigue, anorexia, frequent nocturnal awakenings, hypersomnolence and difficulties in concentration should trigger sleep studies with capnography to detect and treat nocturnal hypoventilation (Birnkrant et al. 2018a).


*Cardiac management*

Cardiac involvement in DMD is characterized by the development of a progressive dilated cardiomyopathy, resulting in congestive heart failure, conduction abnormalities (prolonged QTc) ventricular/supraventricular arrhythmia and risk of sudden early death (Kieny et al. 2013; Passamano et al. 2012). Improvement in respiratory care with the provision of ventilator support has resulted in a shift in causes of death. Acute cardiac events and cardiac insufficiency are nowadays the leading cause of death in DMD.

Cardiac management includes early detection and follow-up of cardiac abnormalities and the standard treatment of cardiac symptoms of insufficiency and arrhythmias. Clinical symptoms of cardiomyopathy may emerge only in adolescence or young adulthood; however, early regional myocardial damage and myocardiac changes can be detected in young people with DMD using imaging techniques such as magnetic resonance imaging (MRI), tissue Doppler measurements, and myocardial velocity gradients (Mertens et al. 2008).

The early initiation of angiotensin-converting-enzyme inhibitors (ACE-I) as a cardioprotective treatment is recommended for patients approaching the age of 10 years by the 2014 National Heart Lung and Blood Institute Working Group (McNally et al. 2015) based on the results of a randomized trial on the development of cardiomyopathy and overall survival (Duboc et al. 2007; Kamdar and Garry 2016). Corticosteroid treatment has been shown to be beneficial in delaying cardiac symptomatology in DMD, refuting earlier concerns that improving skeletal muscle strength and exercise capacity with corticosteroids could, in the long term, be detrimental to the cardiac muscle by increasing the load to the dystrophic cardiac muscle (Barber et al. 2013; Schram et al. 2013).

*Orthopedic management and rehabilitation*

The natural course of DMD is characterized by the development of limb muscle contractures and scoliosis. Orthopedic management requires specific expertise for the care of patients with DMD, embedded in a multidisciplinary approach. The indication for orthopedic interventions and surgical procedures should be assessed and planned with the members of a team, involving physiotherapists, occupational therapists and orthotists. The overall aim of the orthopedic management is to optimize or preserve the weakened muscle function or to prevent severe deformities such as collapsing scoliosis.

Muscle contractures

With age, retractions of Achilles tendons, knee and hip flexors and iliotibial bands will negatively affect the stability and the gait pattern in ambulant DMD patients. Mobilization, stretching and standing programs and the use of ankle-foot orthoses (AFOs) at night are advocated as preventive measures to optimize joint positioning (Birnkrant et al. 2018a, McDonald 1998). Prolongation of ambulation and/or standing ability can be obtained by providing knee-ankle-foot orthoses. This often requires surgical release of the Achilles tendon to achieve an optimal positioning, and an intensive postoperative rehabilitation (Bakker et al. 2000). In the non-ambulant stage, further attention should be paid to adequate sitting posture and to the prevention of contractures in the upper limbs, and hands, which could otherwise impair fine motor activities in a later stage (see Orthopedic management and rehabilitation section).

Scoliosis

Corticosteroid treatment has reduced the occurrence of severe scoliosis requiring surgery in adolescent DMD, which is present in up to 90% in the natural course of the disease (Alman et al. 2004; Yilmaz et al. 2004). However, careful clinical and radiological monitoring of the spine is still indicated, as a spine curve can develop at a later age, especially when corticosteroids are stopped (Birnkrant et al. 2018a). Posterior spinal fusion is recommended to prevent further evolution in participants with progressive spinal curve. The operative risks should be limited by involving a multidisciplinary team, including a (pediatric) neurologist, anesthesiologist, cardiologist, pulmonologist and physiotherapist with experience in neuromuscular disorders. An anticipatory coordinated approach should optimize the postoperative care and rehabilitation. Data are lacking on the development of scoliosis in the emerging adult generation on very long-term corticosteroids. Bone demineralization and collapsing vertebral fractures due to the chronic use of corticosteroids are additional risks to be monitored in the spinal management of this population (see Orthopedic management and rehabilitation section).

*Endocrinological management*

The beneficial effects of corticosteroids on the disease course and survival in DMD are associated with treatment related multisystemic side-effects, raising new issues in the care and management of patients with DMD. Growth and puberty, bone health, glucose and fat metabolism, which are compromised in DMD, will be further affected by GCS. Guidelines for the management of endocrine aspects are currently based on expert opinion-papers, limited non-controlled studies, and the clinical experience with corticosteroids in other diseases underscoring the need for additional research in these areas (Bianchi et al. 2011; Birnkrant et al. 2018b, Leung et al. 2011).

Bone health

Impaired bone metabolism with reduced bone mineralization is a well-known feature of DMD, which is further negatively affected by corticosteroid therapy. Osteoporosis and an increased incidence of long bone and vertebral fractures cause significant morbidity in DMD (Bianchi et al. 2003; Bothwell et al. 2003). Leg fractures require prompt and adequate treatment aiming at limiting immobilization to a minimum, as this can precipitate definite loss of ambulation in weak ambulant DMD children. Bone health management includes periodic bone density assessment and the prescription of adequate calcium and vitamin D intake. Fall prevention, regular physical therapy and safe weight-bearing exercises, within the limits of the underlying disease, are recommended as part of bone health management. Vertebral compression fractures should be excluded at a regular base using lateral spine X-ray and treated with intravenous bisphosphonates (Birnkrant et al. 2018a).

Growth and puberty

Boys with DMD have, in general, a short stature below the mid-parental height, falling within the $5^{th}$ percentile for height as an adult, irrespective of any corticosteroid treatment (Nagel et al. 1999). Chronic corticosteroid treatment has an additional detrimental effect and will result in severely stunted growth with adolescent height falling below the $3^{rd}$ percentile.

Published data from the MD-STAR surveillance network in the UK demonstrated that an earlier initiation, daily dosing, longer duration, and greater dosages predicted shorter stature with prednisone. Treatment with deflazacort predicted a shorter stature, but a lighter weight, compared to prednisone (Lamb et al. 2016).

Treatment with recombinant human growth hormone has been reported in small studies in DMD patients (Rutter et al. 2012); however, the short duration and small sample size of these studies and the lack of data on long-term safety preclude recommendations about the use of this treatment, which should be reserved for individuals with proven growth hormone deficiency (Birnkrant et al. 2018b).

Hypogonadism and delayed puberty are additional potential complications associated with the long term use of corticosteroids. Induction of puberty with testosterone in DMD patients is commonly used in clinical practice following the standards of care in the treatment of pathological pubertal delay in the general pediatric population. However, data on the outcome of treating delayed puberty with androgens in this population are lacking. A retrospective study reported the positive effect of testosterone in young man with DMD (Wood et al. 2015).

Weight gain, glucose and fat metabolism

Treatment with glucocorticoids is often associated with an increase in appetite, resulting in an excessive weight gain and insulin resistance. This a major concern as even without steroids boys with DMD are at risk of developing overweight from the age of 7 years onwards. Excessive weight gain has a negative impact on motor function and can obscure the benefit gained by corticosteroid treatment. Overweight increases the risk of comorbidities such as arterial hypertension, glucose intolerance and hyperlipidemia. Adequate dietary advice should be embedded in the multidisciplinary care plan and provided from the time of diagnosis. Particular emphasis should be made on appetite control at the time of corticosteroids initiation. Dietary advices on caloric intake should be adjusted to the decline in the physical activity in DMD patients.

*Gastro-intestinal management and nutrition*

Dystrophin expression has been identified in the visceral smooth muscles and there is evidence of functional smooth-muscle impairment in Duchenne dystrophy (Jaffe et al. 1990). With age, DMD patients will typically develop gastro-intestinal symptoms such as delayed gastric emptying and intestinal paresis, requiring preventive measures and pharmacological interventions targeting gastro-esophageal reflux and constipation (Goemans and Buyse 2014). Weakness of the masticory muscles, swallowing difficulties and dysphagia, due to oropharangeal weakness and oesophageal dysmotility, may jeopardize safe and adequate intake and result in undernutrition. The placement of a percutaneous endoscopic gastrostomy tube should be considered to optimize nutritional status and prevent aspiration when adjustment of food consistency and nutritional advice are insufficient to palliate malnutrition. Gastric protection with proton pump inhibitors should be associated with the treatment of corticosteroids.

*Renal and urinary tract management*

Despite clear evidence of signs and symptoms of bladder dysfunction, such as urgency or hesitancy of stream, in the older DMD population, this area has been poorly investigated. Small capacity, hyperreflexic bladder, and detrusor sphincter dyssynergia have been demonstrated on video urodynamics in a small cohort (MacLeod et al. 2003). These lower urinary tract symptoms may have an important impact on quality of life and deserve further attention, with appropriate urological management and treatment (Bertrand et al. 2016).

Several dystrophin isoforms are expressed in the kidney (Dp71, Dp40, Dp140), raising the hypothesis of renal dysfunction being an integral part of the multisystemic nature of DMD. The most common dystrophin isoform that is found in the kidney (Dp 71) seems to be localized in the mesangial and endothelial cells, interstitial capillaries and the macula densa. The exact function of the renal dystrophin-associated complex is not clarified yet, although its molecular structure suggests multiple functional roles related to ion transport mechanisms and to the mechanical protection of renal epithelial cells for the high osmotic pressure of the hypertonic interstitial fluid (Haenggi et al. 2005). Renal dysfunction has been reported as a frequent complication in patients with advanced stage DMD, aggravated by inadequate fluid intake and the use of diuretics (Matsumura et al. 2012). An additional issue in monitoring renal function in DMD is the low serum and urinary level of creatinine as a consequence of the low muscle mass. This hampers the use of serum creatinine as a marker of renal function and its use in equations assessing glomerular filtration rate (Braat et al. 2015).

*Ophthalmological management*

Regular ophthalmological monitoring is part of the standard care of DMD as patients treated with chronic corticosteroids are at risk of developing cataract, particularly with the use of deflazacort. The role of the retinal dystrophin isoforms Dp260 and Dp71 is not fully elucidated; however, impairments in photopic and scotopic electroretinogram (ERG) responses have been reported in DMD as well as mild red–green color vision impairment (Costa et al. 2007; Pascual Pascual et al. 1998; Pillers et al. 1999). Research on ophthalmologic manifestations in DMD deserves further attention as the development of DMD specific clinical symptoms of retinal abnormalities could be anticipated with increased longevity.

*Dental and maxillofacial issues*

The typical distribution of facial and masticatory muscle weakness and hypertrophy together with the occurrence of tongue hypertrophy results in a typical dental conformation and maxillofacial appearance, with a risk of dental malocclusion deserving specialized orthodontic management by dental and maxillofacial specialists with experience in neuromuscular disorders (van den Engel-Hoek et al. 2016).

*Neurodevelopmental aspects*

A wide variety of neurodevelopmental and neuropsychological disorders have been described in DMD with 30% of boys with DMD showing a cognitive impairment with an IQ below 70 (Cotton et al. 2001). A higher incidence of attention-deficit–hyperactivity disorder, anxiety, autism spectrum and obsessive compulsive disorder has been reported compared to the general population (Banihani et al. 2015).

Several brain dystrophin isoforms are expressed in many brain regions responsible for higher order functions such as learning and memory, including the cerebral cortex, hippocampus, and cerebellum: Dp427c (cortex–hippocampus), Dp427p (Purkinje cells), Dp140 and Dp71 (cortex and cerebellum) (Doorenweerd et al. 2017). The risk of neurodevelopmental problems seems to be related to the location of the mutation, with patients missing all brain isoforms, due to a mutation in the distal part of the gene, being the most at risk. The absence of the Dp140 isoform is particularly associated with the lowest scores on all neuropsychological tests (general cognition, verbal memory, attention and executive function). This has been confirmed by the neuropathological finding of reduced grey matter volume and alteration in the white matter microstructure in patients missing the Dp140 isoform (Doorenweerd et al. 2014). The different isoforms show large changes in expression through pre- and postnatal life. Moreover, the expression of these isoforms are significantly associated with genes implicated in neurodevelopmental disorders such as autism spectrum or attention-deficit–hyperactivity disorder (Doorenweerd et al. 2017). Further research to improve our insights and to provide guidelines on management and treatment of the neurodevelopmental aspects in DMD is crucial considering the major impact of these deficits on the functioning and quality of life of these patients and their families.

THERAPIES IN DEVELOPMENT

The discovery of the DMD gene and the unraveling of the pathophysiological processes have fueled the research for therapy in DMD resulting in a number of therapeutic strategies that moved into clinical development during the past decade. Updated information about ongoing clinical trials is available on the http://www.clinicaltrials.gov website. A brief summary of the current therapeutic strategies is given below, including their Clinical Trials identifier (NCT).

*Genetic therapies to restore dystrophin production*

Exon skipping therapy and the use of read-through molecules, targeting the dystrophin production at a RNA level, have been described in the Molecular genetics and pathophysiological aspects section. These therapies target specific genetic subgroups of DMD (exon skip amenable mutations, nonsense point mutations). Exondys51 and Translarna are the first compounds that have received approval (conditional for Translarna) from the FDA and the EMA, respectively, as treatments for DMD (McDonald et al. 2017a; Mendell et al. 2016). Antisense oligonucleotides targeting exons 45 and 53 and antisense molecules with improved backbone are in development (PPMO: SRP-5051-NCT03375255; Morpholino: NS-065/NCNP-01; Stereopure antisense oligonucleotide (WVE-210201): NCT02740972).

Gene transfer therapy

The discovery of the defective gene in DMD has triggered a tremendous effort in the development of a gene therapy for DMD. Enormous hurdles such as the huge size of the gene, the difficulties of delivery of the corrected gene into the muscles throughout the body, and the issues of immuno-rejection have delayed the development of gene therapy as a therapeutic strategy for DMD. Despite these obstacles, progress have been made and gene therapy has currently moved into human clinical trials (Chamberlain and Chamberlain 2017).

Delivery of a synthetic dystrophin gene (micro dystrophin) encoding for a functional dystrophin protein surrogate, using a adeno associated viral ( AVV) vector, is being investigated by different research groups: two using a recombinant AAV9 viral vector carrying a truncated human dystrophin gene (Solid Bioscience NCT03368742; Pfizer NCT03362502); the other using rAAVrh74.MHCK7 to incorporate a microdystrophin (Nationwide Children's Hospital: NCT03375164).

GALGT2 gene therapy uses an AAV vector delivering a *GALGT2* gene. In animal models, overexpression of *GALGT2* has been shown to stimulate the expression of dystrophin and laminin α2 surrogates and has led to normal muscle function, even in the absence of dystrophin (Chicoine et al. 2014). Delivery of rAAVrh74.MCK.GALGT2 by limb infusion is currently in clinical research (Nationwide Children's Hospitals NCT03333590).

*Targeting muscle growth and regeneration*

Non-dystrophin specific therapeutic approaches interfering with mechanisms involved in growth and regeneration of skeletal muscle mass are currently under investigation in neuromuscular disorders. The rationale, to interfere with the myostatin pathway, a major negative regulator of skeletal muscle mass, or with its activin II receptors, is based on the observation of a remarkable increase in muscle mass in naturally occurring myostatin null animals and the functional improvement of the dystrophic muscle by myostatin blockade (Bogdanovich et al. 2002). Two compounds are currently in clinical research BMS-986089 (Hoffmann-La Roche-NCT03039686) and PF-06252616 Domagrozumab (Pfizer-NCT02907619.

*Utrophin upregulation*

Utophin is a subsarcolemmal protein expressed during fetal development and muscle cell regeneration. The strong homology of utrophin to dystrophin has fueled the research of utrophin upregulation as a potential disease-modifying approach for DMD. Utrophin is persistently expressed at the neuromuscular junction in normal mature muscle. The utrophin muscle specific promotor can be manipulated to increase utrophin RNA and expression of full length utrophin has been shown to be effective to prevent muscular dystrophy in mdx mice (Tinsley 1998; Chakravarty 2017). The utrophin modulator SMT C1100 – Ezutromid (SummitTherapeutics, Oxford) has successfully increased utrophin expression both in human cells and in the mdx mice. Early stage clinical development (NCT02858362) showed promising results (Tinsley et al. 2011). Unfortunately, this drug development program was stopped following disappointing results from the PhaseOut DMD trial, a Phase 2 proof of concept trial.

*Targeting the pathophysiological cascade*

Numerous indirect approaches targeting the pathophysiological cascade of events downstream of the dystrophin deficiency, and aiming at reducing the dystrophic process, are under investigation in preclinical and clinical phases. These include strategies aiming at reducing oxidative stress or at preventing necrosis and fibrosis.

Reduction of oxidative stress and improvement of respiratory chain function

Idebenone [2-(10-hydroxy-decyl)-5,6-dimethoxy-3-methyl-1,4-benzoquinone] is a potent antioxidant of the quinone family. It interacts also as an electron carrier in the mitochondrial chain transport and supports adenosine triphosphate (ATP) production. Idebenone may, hence, interfere with the pathophysiological cascade of events in DMD by improving mitochondrial function and stimulating cell energy production. In DMD patients, a statistically significant effect was observed in respiratory function decline over 48 weeks compared to placebo in non-steroid treated DMD patients, as assessed by peak expiratory flow measurement in a double-blind placebo-controlled study (DELOS; NCT01027884) (Buyse et al. 2017). A study on the effects of idebenone in steroid-treated boys with DMD is currently ongoing (SIDEROS; NCT02814019).

Anti-inflammatory and anti-fibrotic agents

Pamrevlumab (FG-3019) is a monoclonal antibody to connective tissue growth factor (CTGF). The rationale for the use of FG-3019 in DMD is to reduce muscle fibrosis and improve muscle function based on encouraging data from a preclinical study in mdx mice

(Morales et al. 2013). FG-3019 is currently in Phase 2 trial in non-ambulatory participants with DMD (NCT02606136).

Givinostat is a histone deacetylase (HDAC) inhibitor currently in Phase 3 clinical development (NCT02851797). The rationale for exploring HDAC inhibitors as a potential therapy in DMD is based on their positive effects on myogenesis and reduction of muscle breakdown in vitro in mdx mice by promoting the transcription of a number of factors that are key in muscle regeneration. In addition, Givinostat has potent anti-inflammatory effects and is expected to reduce fibrosis and fatty infiltration (Bettica et al. 2016).

CAT-1004 inhibits nuclear factor kappa B (NF-κB) and could be beneficial in DMD by reducing chronic inflammation. NF-κB is activated early in the disease and induces muscle inflammation, fibrosis and degeneration. Reduction of NF-κB has shown protective properties in mdx mice, CAT-1004 was found safe and was well-tolerated in a Phase 1 study and is currently being explored in a Phase 2 trial in DMD (NCT02439216) (Donovan et al. 2017).

Hematopoeitic prostaglandin D synthase (HPDS) plays an important role in the pathophysiological cascade in DMD. TAS–205 is a highly selective inhibitor of hematopoeitic HPDS that has shown beneficial effects on muscle necrosis in mdx mice and is currently in Phase 2 study for children with DMD (NCT02752048) (Mohri et al. 2009).

Vamorolone (VBP15 compound) is a steroid-like compound, inhibitor of NF-kB in myoblasts, with potentially a better side-effects profile compared with prednisone, as it does not bind to glucocorticoid receptors (Hoffman et al. 2018). The safety and tolerability of vamorolone in boys with DMD between the ages of 4–6.9 years is currently being assessed in a Phase 2b study comparing the efficacy and safety of vamorolone to prednisone and placebo (NCT03439670).

MNK-1411 (Cosyntropin) is a synthetic melanocortin receptor agonist (synthetic equivalent of adrenocorticotrope hormone ACTH) and could be beneficial in delaying disease progression through its potent anti-inflammatory properties. Its safety and efficacy is currently being assessed in a Phase 2 study in DMD (NCT03400852).

Tamoxifen is an example of the repositioning of a drug that has been approved for other indications being used as treatment in DMD based on its antifibrotic properties and its positive effects on muscle repair (Dorchies et al. 2013). Its safety and efficacy in DMD is currently being explored in a randomized double-blind placebo-controlled study (NCT03354039).

Others

Rimeporide is an inhibitor of the Na/H-exchanger-1, initially developed for heart failure that could have a beneficial effect in DMD. Rimeporide regulates sodium, pH, calcium overload, reduces inflammation in a number of muscles, decreases skeletal, diaphragm, and cardiac fibrosis as well as muscle cell degeneration in the animal model. Rimeporide is currently in the clinical stage of development, assessing safety and tolerability in a Phase 1b study (NCT02710591).

CAP-1002 is a cell therapy using cardiosphere derived cells (CDC), known to secrete numerous bioactive elements (growth factors, exosomes) with immunomodulatory, antifibrotic and regenerative properties (Chakravarty et al. 2017). A Phase 1 study (NCT02485938) demonstrated that a single dose of CAP-1002 cells could effectively impact on cardiac muscle hypertrophy. In addition, CAP-1002 cells were also found to improve skeletal muscle function as measured by upper limb function in non-ambulant DMD.

**Key points**

- Duchenne muscular dystrophy (DMD), the most common and severe type of dystrophinopathy, is a complex disorder requiring a coordinated multidisciplinary approach to address its multisystemic manifestations and secondary problems.
- Care guidelines have been published, based on the available literature and expert consensus.
- DMD has evolved from a pediatric disease to an adult condition. Transition to adult care should be anticipated and well prepared to provide optimal surveillance and management to the young men with DMD that have outgrown the pediatric care and who may develop new disease manifestations with improved life expectancy.
- Improved insights into the pathophysiology of DMD have boosted clinical research and therapy development. Today, even if there is no cure, several disease-modifying compounds are available and new compounds are in clinical development.
- However, even if disease-modifying therapeutic strategies may prove successful, a multidisciplinary approach and research aiming at improving guidelines for the care of this progressive multisystem disorder, will remain mandatory to further optimize the health and the quality of life of individuals with DMD/BMD.

**Clinical vignette**

A 12-year-old boy with Duchenne muscular dystrophy was referred to our center. He had lost ambulation a few months earlier, following a fracture of the tibia. He had been diagnosed at the age of 5, presenting with a global developmental delay and high creatine kinase. Diagnosis was genetically confirmed by the finding of a exon 44–50 deletion in the DMD gene. He was treated with prednisone 0.75mg/kg/d. At clinical examination he was wheelchair bound, unable to bear weight, with contractures of his Achilles tendon. Management was discussed within the multidisciplinary team. Knee-ankle-foot orthoses (KAFO) were proposed after assessing the patient's motor abilities and his wishes and abilities to cope with an intense rehabilitation program. After surgical release of the Achilles tendon, this young boy was casted and trained to bear weight in his casts. Customized KAFO with ischial bearing were provided and a rehabilitation program was started. He achieved independent standing and walking with KAFOs in the following weeks (see Fig. 10.3). He maintained ambulation in KAFOs for another 2 years. At the age of 20, the KAFOs are still used to stand and provide him a better balance when sitting in his wheelchair. This case illustrates the risk of loss of ambulation following a trauma of the lower limbs and the importance of a multidisciplinary management.

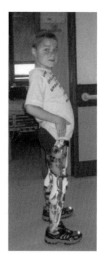

**Fig. 10.3.** Rehabilitation in Knee-Ankle-Foot ortheses in DMD.

This kind of rehabilitation program could not be successful without the dialogue and close collaboration between the patient, the patient's family, the psychologist, physiotherapist, orthopedic surgeon and orthotist.

## REFERENCES

Aartsma-Rus A, Bremmer-Bout M, Janson AA, den Dunnen JT, van Ommen GJ, van Deutekom JC (2002) Targeted exon skipping as a potential gene correction therapy for Duchenne muscular dystrophy. *Neuromuscul Disord* 12 (Suppl 1): S71–S77.

Aartsma-Rus A, Janson AA, Heemskerk JA, De Winter CL, Van Ommen GJ, Van Deutekom JC (2006) Therapeutic modulation of DMD splicing by blocking exonic splicing enhancer sites with antisense oligonucleotides. *Ann N Y Acad Sci* 1082: 74–76.

Alman BA, Raza SN, Biggar WD (2004) Steroid treatment and the development of scoliosis in males with Duchenne muscular dystrophy. *J Bone Joint Surg Am* 86-A: 519–524.

Bakker JP, de Groot IJ, Beckerman H, de Jong BA, Lankhorst GJ (2000) The effects of knee-ankle-foot orthoses in the treatment of Duchenne muscular dystrophy: review of the literature. *Clin Rehabil* 14: 343–359.

Banihani R, Smile S, Yoon G, Dupuis A, Mosleh M, Snider A et al. (2015) Cognitive and Neurobehavioral Profile in Boys With Duchenne muscular dystrophy. *J Child Neurol* 30: 1472–1482.

Barber BJ, Andrews JG, Lu Z, Meaney FJ, Price ET, Gray A et al. (2013) Oral corticosteroids and onset of cardiomyopathy in Duchenne muscular dystrophy. *J Pediatr* 163: 1080–4e1. L, Flanigan KM, Weiss RB United Dystrophinopathy Project, Spitali P, Aartsma-Rus A et al.(2016) Association study of exon variants in the NF-κB and TGFβ pathways identifies CD40 as a modifier of Duchenne muscular dystrophy. *Am J Hum Genet* 99: 1163–1171.

Bertrand LA, Askeland EJ, Mathews KD, Erickson BA, Cooper CS (2016) Prevalence and bother of patient-reported lower urinary tract symptoms in the muscular dystrophies. *J Pediatr Urol* 12: 398 e1–398 e4.

Bettica P, Petrini S, D'Oria V, D'Amico A, Catteruccia M, Pane M et al. (2016) Histological effects of givinostat in boys with Duchenne muscular dystrophy. *Neuromuscul Disord* 26: 643–649.

Bianchi ML, Mazzanti A, Galbiati E, Saraifoger S, Dubini A, Cornelio F et al. (2003) Bone mineral density and bone metabolism in Duchenne muscular dystrophy. Osteoporos Int 14: 761–767.

Bianchi ML, Biggar D, Bushby K, Rogol AD, Rutter MM, Tseng B (2011) Endocrine aspects of Duchenne muscular dystrophy. *Neuromuscul Disord* 21: 298–303.

Birnkrant DJ, Bushby K, Bann CM, Alman BA, Apkon SD, Blackwell A et al. (2018a). Diagnosis and management of Duchenne muscular dystrophy, part 2: respiratory, cardiac, bone health, and orthopaedic management. *Lancet Neurol* 17: 347–361.

Birnkrant DJ, Bushby K, Bann CM, Apkon SD, Blackwell A, Brumbaugh D et al. (2018b). Diagnosis and management of Duchenne muscular dystrophy, part 1: diagnosis, and neuromuscular, rehabilitation, endocrine, and gastrointestinal and nutritional management. *Lancet Neurol* 17: 251–267.

Bogdanovich S, Krag TO, Barton ER, Morris LD, Whittemore LA, Ahima RS et al. (2002) Functional improvement of dystrophic muscle by myostatin blockade. *Nature* 420: 418–421.

Bothwell JE, Gordon KE, Dooley JM, MacSween J, Cummings EA, Salisbury S (2003) Vertebral fractures in boys with Duchenne muscular dystrophy. *Clin Pediatr (Phila)* 42: 353–356.

Braat E, Hoste L, De Waele L, Gheysens O, Vermeersch P, Goffin K et al. (2015) Renal function in children and adolescents with Duchenne muscular dystrophy. *Neuromuscul Disord* 25: 381–387.

Bushby K, Muntoni F, Bourke JP (2003) 107th ENMC international workshop: the management of cardiac involvement in muscular dystrophy and myotonic dystrophy. 7th–9th June 2002, Naarden, The Netherlands. *Neuromuscul Disord* 13: 166–172.

Buyse GM, Voit T, Schara U, Straathof CS, D'Angelo MG, Bernert G et al. (2017) Treatment effect of idebenone on inspiratory function in patients with Duchenne muscular dystrophy. *Pediatr Pulmonol* 52: 508–515.

Chakravarty T, Makkar RR, Ascheim DD, Traverse JH, Schatz R, DeMaria A et al. (2017) ALLogeneic Heart STem Cells to Achieve Myocardial Regeneration (ALLSTAR) Trial: rationale and design. *Cell Transplant* 26: 205–214.

Chamberlain JR, Chamberlain JS (2017) Progress toward gene therapy for Duchenne muscular dystrophy. *Mol Ther* 25: 1125–1131.

Chamova T, Guergueltcheva V, Raycheva M, Todorov T, Genova J, Bichev S et al. (2013) Association between loss of dp140 and cognitive impairment in Duchenne and Becker dystrophies. *Balkan J Med Genet* 16: 21–30.

Chicoine LG, Rodino-Klapac LR, Shao G, Xu R, Bremer WG, Camboni M et al. (2014) Vascular delivery of rAAVrh74.MCKGALGT2 to the gastrocnemius muscle of the rhesus macaque stimulates the expression of dystrophin and laminin α2 surrogates. *Mol Ther* 22: 713–724.

Costa MF, Oliveira AG, Feitosa-Santana C, Zatz M, Ventura DF (2007) Red–green color vision impairment in Duchenne muscular dystrophy. *Am J Hum Genet* 80: 1064–1075.

Cotton S, Voudouris NJ, Greenwood KM (2001) Intelligence and Duchenne muscular dystrophy: full-scale, verbal, and performance intelligence quotients. *Dev Med Child Neurol* 43: 497–501.

Deconinck N, Dan B (2007) Pathophysiology of Duchenne muscular dystrophy: current hypotheses. *Pediatr Neurol* 36: 1–7.

Donovan JM, Zimmer M, Offman E, Grant T, Jirousek M (2017) A novel nf-κb inhibitor, Edasalonexent (CAT-1004), in development as a disease-modifying treatment for patients with Duchenne muscular dystrophy: phase 1 safety, pharmacokinetics, and pharmacodynamics in adult subjects. *J Clin Pharmacol* 57: 627–639.

Doorenweerd N, Straathof CS, Dumas EM, Spitali P, Ginjaar IB, Wokke BH et al. (2014) Reduced cerebral gray matter and altered white matter in boys with Duchenne muscular dystrophy. Ann Neurol 76: 403–411.

Doorenweerd N, Mahfouz A, van Putten M, Kaliyaperumal R, T′ Hoen PAC, Hendriksen JGM et al. (2017) Timing and localization of human dystrophin isoform expression provide insights into the cognitive phenotype of Duchenne muscular dystrophy. *Sci Rep* 7: 12575.

Dorchies OM, Reutenauer-Patte J, Dahmane E, Ismail HM, Petermann O, Patthey-Vuadens O et al. (2013) The anticancer drug tamoxifen counteracts the pathology in a mouse model of Duchenne muscular dystrophy. *Am J Pathol* 182: 485–504.

Duboc D, Meune C, Pierre B, Wahbi K, Eymard B, Toutain A et al. (2007) Perindopril preventive treatment on mortality in Duchenne muscular dystrophy: 10 years' follow-up. *Am Heart J* 154: 596–602.

Eagle M, Bourke J, Bullock R, Gibson M, Mehta J, Giddings D et al. (2007) Managing Duchenne muscular dystrophy – the additive effect of spinal surgery and home nocturnal ventilation in improving survival. *Neuromuscul Disord* 17: 470–475.

Emery AE (1991) Population frequencies of inherited neuromuscular diseases – a world survey. *Neuromuscul Disord* 1: 19–29.

Emery AE (2002) The muscular dystrophies. *Lancet* 359: 687–695.

Escolar DM, Hache LP, Clemens PR, Cnaan A, McDonald CM, Viswanathan V et al. (2011) Randomized, blinded trial of weekend vs daily prednisone in Duchenne muscular dystrophy. *Neurology* 77: 444–452.

FDA (2017) FDA approves drug to treat Duchenne muscular dystrophy, 9 February. https://wayback.archive-it.org/7993/20180424212953/https://www.fda.gov/NewsEvents/Newsroom/PressAnnouncements/ucm540945.htm.

Finder JD, Birnkrant D, Carl J, Farber HJ, Gozal D, Iannaccone ST et al. (2004) Respiratory care of the patient with Duchenne muscular dystrophy: ATS consensus statement. *Am J Respir Crit Care Med* 170: 456–465.

Fisher I, Abraham D, Bouri K, Hoffman EP, Muntoni F, Morgan J (2005) Prednisolone-induced changes in dystrophic skeletal muscle. *FASEB J* 19: 834–836.

Goemans N, Buyse G (2014) Current treatment and management of dystrophinopathies. *Curr Treat Options Neurol* 16: 287.

Griggs RC, Herr BE, Reha A, Elfring G, Atkinson L, Cwik V et al. (2013) Corticosteroids in Duchenne muscular dystrophy: major variations in practice. *Muscle Nerve* 48: 27–31.

Guglieri M, Bushby K, McDermott MP, Hart KA, Tawil R, Martens WB et al. (2017) Developing standardized corticosteroid treatment for Duchenne muscular dystrophy. *Contemp Clin Trials* 58: 34–39.

Haenggi T, Schaub MC, Fritschy JM (2005) Molecular heterogeneity of the dystrophin-associated protein complex in the mouse kidney nephron: differential alterations in the absence of utrophin and dystrophin. *Cell Tissue Res* 319: 299–313.

Henricson EK, Abresch RT, Cnaan A, Hu F, Duong T, Arrieta A et al. (2013) The cooperative international neuromuscular research group Duchenne natural history study: glucocorticoid treatment preserves clinically meaningful functional milestones and reduces rate of disease progression as measured by manual muscle testing and other commonly used clinical trial outcome measures. *Muscle Nerve* 48: 55–67.

Hoffman EP, Brown RH Jr, Kunkel LM (1987) Dystrophin: the protein product of the Duchenne muscular dystrophy locus. *Cell* 51: 919–928.

Hoffman EP, Riddle V, Siegler MA, Dickerson D, Backonja M, Kramer WG et al. (2018) Phase 1 trial of vamorolone, a first-in-class steroid, shows improvements in side effects via biomarkers bridged to clinical outcomes. *Steroids* 134: 43–52.

Hogarth MW, Houweling PJ, Thomas KC, Gordish-Dressman H, Bello L, Pegoraro E et al. (2017) Evidence for ACTN3 as a genetic modifier of Duchenne muscular dystrophy. *Nat Commun* 8: 14143.

Jaffe KM, McDonald CM, Ingman E, Haas J (1990) Symptoms of upper gastrointestinal dysfunction in Duchenne muscular dystrophy: case-control study. *Arch Phys Med Rehabil* 71: 742–744.

Kamdar F, Garry DJ (2016) Dystrophin–deficient cardiomyopathy. *J Am Coll Cardiol* 67: 2533–2546.

Kesselheim AS, Avorn J (2016) Approving a problematic muscular dystrophy drug: implications for FDA Policy. *JAMA* 316: 2357–2358.

Kieny P, Chollet S, Delalande P, Le Fort M, Magot A, Pereon Y et al. (2013) Evolution of life expectancy of patients with Duchenne muscular dystrophy at AFM Yolaine de Kepper centre between 1981 and 2011. *Ann Phys Rehabil Med* 56: 443–454.

Kinnett K, Noritz G (2017) The PJ Nicholoff Steroid Protocol for Duchenne and Becker Muscular Dystrophy and Adrenal Suppression. *PLoS Curr* 9: 9.

Koenig M, Kunkel LM (1990) Detailed analysis of the repeat domain of dystrophin reveals four potential hinge segments that may confer flexibility. *J Biol Chem* 265: 4560–4566.

Lamb MM, West NA, Ouyang L, Yang M, Weitzenkamp D, James K et al. (2016) Corticosteroid treatment and growth patterns in ambulatory males with Duchenne muscular dystrophy. *J Pediatr* 173: 207–213 e3.

Le Rumeur E, Winder SJ, Hubert JF (2010) Dystrophin: more than just the sum of its parts. *Biochim Biophys Acta* 1804: 1713–1722.

Leung DG, Germain-Lee EL, Denger BE, Wagner KR (2011) Report on the Second Endocrine Aspects Of Duchenne Muscular Dystrophy Conference December 1–2, 2010, Baltimore, Maryland, USA *Neuromuscul Disord* 21: 594–601.

MacLeod M, Kelly R, Robb SA, Borzyskowski M (2003) Bladder dysfunction in Duchenne muscular dystrophy. *Arch Dis Child* 88: 347–349.

Mah JK, Korngut L, Dykeman J, Day L, Pringsheim T, Jette N (2014) A systematic review and meta-analysis on the epidemiology of Duchenne and Becker muscular dystrophy. *Neuromuscul Disord* 24: 482–491.

Manzur AY, Kuntzer T, Pike M, Swan A (2008) Glucocorticoid corticosteroids for Duchenne muscular dystrophy. *Cochrane Database Syst Rev* (1): CD003725.

Matsumura T, Saito T, Fujimura H, Sakoda S (2012) [Renal dysfunction is a frequent complication in patients with advanced stage of Duchenne muscular dystrophy]. Renal dysfunction is a frequent complication in patients with advanced stage of Duchenne muscular dystrophy. *Rinsho Shinkeigaku* 52: 211–217.

McDonald CM (1998) Limb contractures in progressive neuromuscular disease and the role of stretching, orthotics, and surgery. *Phys Med Rehabil Clin N Am* 9: 187–211.

McDonald CM, Campbell C, Torricelli RE, Finkel RS, Flanigan KM, Goemans N et al. Clinical Evaluator Training Group, ACT DMD Study Group. (2017a). Ataluren in patients with nonsense mutation Duchenne muscular dystrophy (ACT DMD): a multicentre, randomised, double-blind, placebo-controlled, phase 3 trial. *Lancet* 390: 1489–1498.

McDonald CM, Henricson EK, Abresch RT, Duong T, Joyce NC, Hu F et al. (2017b). Long-term effects of glucocorticoids on function, quality of life, and survival in patients with Duchenne muscular dystrophy: a prospective cohort study. *Lancet* 391 (10119):451–461.

McNally EM, Kaltman JR, Benson DW, Canter CE, Cripe LH, Duan D et al. (2015) Contemporary cardiac issues in Duchenne muscular dystrophy. Working Group of the National Heart, Lung, and Blood Institute in collaboration with Parent Project Muscular Dystrophy. *Circulation* 131: 1590–1598.

Mendell JR, Goemans N, Lowes LP, Alfano LN, Berry K, Shao J et al. (2016) Longitudinal effect of eteplirsen versus historical control on ambulation in Duchenne muscular dystrophy. *Ann Neurol* 79: 257–271.

Mertens L, Ganame J, Claus P, Goemans N, Thijs D, Eyskens B et al. (2008) Early regional myocardial dysfunction in young patients with Duchenne muscular dystrophy. *J Am Soc Echocardiogr* 21: 1049–1054.

Moat SJ, Bradley DM, Salmon R, Clarke A, Hartley L (2013) Newborn bloodspot screening for Duchenne muscular dystrophy: 21 years experience in Wales (UK). *Eur J Hum Genet* 21: 1049–1053.

Mohri I, Aritake K, Taniguchi H, Sato Y, Kamauchi S, Nagata N et al. (2009) Inhibition of prostaglandin D synthase suppresses muscular necrosis. *Am J Pathol* 174: 1735–1744.

Monaco AP, Kunkel LM (1988) Cloning of the Duchenne/Becker muscular dystrophy locus. *Adv Hum Genet* 17: 61–98.

Morales MG, Gutierrez J, Cabello-Verrugio C, Cabrera D, Lipson KE, Goldschmeding R et al. (2013) Reducing CTGF/CCN2 slows down mdx muscle dystrophy and improves cell therapy. *Hum Mol Genet* 22: 4938–4951.

Moxley RT III, Pandya S, Ciafaloni E, Fox DJ, Campbell K (2010) Change in natural history of Duchenne muscular dystrophy with long-term corticosteroid treatment: implications for management. *J Child Neurol* 25: 1116–1129.

Muntoni F, Torelli S, Ferlini A (2003) Dystrophin and mutations: one gene, several proteins, multiple phenotypes. *Lancet Neurol* 2: 731–740.

Nagel BH, Mortier W, Elmlinger M, Wollmann HA, Schmitt K, Ranke MB (1999) Short stature in Duchenne muscular dystrophy: a study of 34 patients. *Acta Paediatr* 88: 62–65.

Pane M, Scalise R, Berardinelli A, D'Angelo G, Ricotti V, Alfieri P et al. (2013) Early neurodevelopmental assessment in Duchenne muscular dystrophy. *Neuromuscul Disord* 23: 451–455.

Pascual Pascual SI, Molano J, Pascual-Castroviejo I (1998) Electroretinogram in Duchenne/Becker muscular dystrophy. *Pediatr Neurol* 18: 315–320.

Passamano L, Taglia A, Palladino A, Viggiano E, D'Ambrosio P, Scutifero M et al. (2012) Improvement of survival in Duchenne muscular dystrophy: retrospective analysis of 835 patients. *Acta Myol* 31: 121–125.

Pillers DA, Fitzgerald KM, Duncan NM, Rash SM, White RA, Dwinnell SJ et al. (1999) Duchenne/Becker muscular dystrophy: correlation of phenotype by electroretinography with sites of dystrophin mutations. *Hum Genet* 105: 2–9.

Ricotti V, Ridout DA, Scott E, Quinlivan R, Robb SA, Manzur AY et al. (2012) Long-term benefits and adverse effects of intermittent versus daily glucocorticoids in boys with Duchenne muscular dystrophy. *J Neurol Neurosurg Psychiatry* 84(6): 698–705.

Rutter MM, Collins J, Rose SR, Woo JG, Sucharew H, Sawnani H et al. (2012) Growth hormone treatment in boys with Duchenne muscular dystrophy and glucocorticoid-induced growth failure. *Neuromuscul Disord* 22: 1046–1056.

Saito T, Kawai M, Kimura E, Ogata K, Takahashi T, Kobayashi M et al. (2017) Study of Duchenne muscular dystrophy long-term survivors aged 40 years and older living in specialized institutions in Japan. *Neuromuscul Disord* 27: 107–114.

Schram G, Fournier A, Leduc H, Dahdah N, Therien J, Vanasse M et al. (2013) All-cause mortality and cardiovascular outcomes with prophylactic steroid therapy in Duchenne muscular dystrophy. *J Am Coll Cardiol* 61: 948–954.

Straathof CS, Overweg-Plandsoen WC, van den Burg GJ, van der Kooi AJ, Verschuuren JJ, de Groot IJ (2009) Prednisone 10 days on/10 days off in patients with Duchenne muscular dystrophy. *J Neurol* 256: 768–773.

Tinsley JM, Fairclough RJ, Storer R, Wilkes FJ, Potter AC, Squire SE et al. (2011) Daily treatment with SMTC1100, a novel small molecule utrophin upregulator, dramatically reduces the dystrophic symptoms in the mdx mouse. *PLoS One* 6:e19189.

van den Engel-Hoek L, de Groot IJ, Sie LT, van Bruggen HW, de Groot SA, Erasmus CE et al. (2016) Dystrophic changes in masticatory muscles related chewing problems and malocclusions in Duchenne muscular dystrophy. *Neuromuscul Disord* 26: 354–360.

Vianello S, Pantic B, Fusto A, Bello L, Galletta E, Borgia D et al. (2017) SPP1 genotype and glucocorticoid treatment modify osteopontin expression in Duchenne muscular dystrophy cells. *Hum Mol Genet* 26: 3342–3351.

Wood CL, Cheetham TD, Guglieri M, Bushby K, Owen C, Johnstone H et al. (2015) Testosterone Treatment of Pubertal Delay in Duchenne muscular dystrophy. *Neuropediatrics* 46: 371–376.

Yilmaz O, Karaduman A, Topaloğlu H (2004) Prednisolone therapy in Duchenne muscular dystrophy prolongs ambulation and prevents scoliosis. *Eur J Neurol* 11: 541–544.

Zatz M, Rapaport D, Vainzof M, Passos-Bueno MR, Bortolini ER, Pavanello RC et al. (1991) Serum creatine-kinase (CK) and pyruvate-kinase (PK) activities in Duchenne (DMD) as compared with Becker (BMD) muscular dystrophy. *J Neurol Sci* 102: 190–196.

# 11
# LIMB-GIRDLE MUSCULAR DYSTROPHIES

*Nathalie Goemans*

For an introduction to Muscular Dystrophies, please see Chapter 10 (page 166).

**Introduction and classification**

The term limb-girdle muscular dystrophies (LGMD) was first introduced by John Walton in 1954 to distinguish a heterogeneous group of autosomal muscular dystrophies from the clinically and/or genetically well-defined muscular dystrophies such as X-linked Duchenne–Becker muscular dystrophies (DMD/BMD), facioscapulohumeral dystrophy (FSHD), congenital muscular dystrophies (CMD), myotonic dystrophy (MD) and Emery–Dreifuss muscular dystrophy (EMD) (Walton and Nattrass 1954).

LGMD currently covers a very heterogeneous group of rare autosomal (dominant or recessive) inherited muscle diseases, characterized by a progressive muscular dystrophy with degenerative muscle changes on muscle biopsy or muscle imaging, associated with elevated creatine kinase (CK) activity in blood, affecting predominantly the pelvic and shoulder girdle, with a wide clinical spectrum and etiology. Today, seven autosomal dominant inherited LGMD and 31 autosomal recessive LGMD have been identified (Table 11.1), and this list is increasing because of the availability of next generation sequencing technologies (NGS). Currently, the classification of the subtypes of LFMD is based on a consensus nomenclature, dividing LGMD by pattern of inheritance: "1" being assigned to the dominant types and "2" for the recessively inherited subtypes. Further, subclassification is based on the order of discovery, with the assignment of a letter of the alphabet (Bushby 1995).

These pre-set rules of classification are, however, challenged by the discovery of an increasing number of causative genes and the unraveling of a wide variety of pathophysiological mechanisms resulting in LGMD. Genes defects causing LGMD are found in genes which encode a wide spectrum of proteins involved in muscle fiber structure and function, including structural proteins of the nucleus, the sarcolemma, the sarcoplasma and the extracellular matrix, as well as enzymes such as Calpain-3 (Straub and Bushby 2006; Nigro and Savarese 2014; Domingos et al. 2017). The improved insights in the underlying gene defects and pathophysiological mechanisms as well as the wide heterogeneity in the resulting phenotypes prompted an initiative to revisit LGMD nomenclature in a ENMC workshop (ENMC 2017). Consensus was reached on a classification system that incorporates the name of the protein affected in the muscle cell and includes the mode of inheritance (Straub et al. 2018).

**TABLE 11.1**

**The genetic and clinical characteristics of autosomal dominant LGMD1**

| Disease | Gene | | Age at onset | Creatine kinase | Clinical features | | |
| --- | --- | --- | --- | --- | --- | --- | --- |
| | Name | Protein product | | | Specific features | Cardiac involvement | Respiratory involvement |
| LGMD1A | MYOT | Myotilin | Adulthood | 1–15x | Distal weakness Striking involvement of semimembranosus Dysarthria | + | + |
| LGMD1B | LMNA | Lamin A/C | 0–60 | 1–20x | Rigid spine Limb contractures Fatal arrhythmias | Frequent | + |
| LGMD1C | CAV3 | Caveolin 3 | 5–25 | 2–30x | Myalgia Rippling muscle Rhabdomyolysis | Frequent | |
| LGMD1D | DNAJB6 | DNJa.J/Hsp40 homolog | Adult and childhood onset | 1–5x | Rimmed vacuoles Proximal and distal muscle involvement | Not observed | + |
| LGMD1E | DES | Desmin | 15–50 | 1–4x | Myofibrillar myopathy Cardiomyopathy Distal weakness: Semitendinosus, gracilis, sartorius | Frequent | |
| LGMD1F | TPNO3 | Transportin 3 | 10–40 | 1–15x | Distal weakness, joint contractures | Not observed | + |
| LGMD1G | HNRPDL | Heterogeneous-nuclear ribonucleoprotein D-like | 30–47 | 1 | South American population, Progressive finger and toe contractures Rimmed vacuoles | Not observed | – |
| LGMD1H | ? | ? | 16–50 | 1–10x | Calf hypertrophy, HyperCK, slow progression | Not observed | – |

Adapted from Nigro and Savarese (2014), Murphy and Straub (2015), Domingos et al. (2017), Neuromuscular Disorders gene table, http://www.musclegenetable.fr/

**Prevalence**

The prevalence worldwide is estimated to be 1 in 14 500–45 000 (Mah et al. 2016). The incidence of the different subtypes is widely variable and is sometimes limited to specific ethnic populations based on founder mutations. Some subtypes have only been described in a few families. Dominant LGMD1 is relatively rare representing less than 10% of all LGMD. LGMD2A is the most common subtype (26.5–30%), followed by LGMD2I (19%); however, there is a wide variance among different ethnicities (Straub and Bertoli 2016). Calpainopathies (8%) and dysferlinopathies (5%) are the most common causes of LGMD in Australia (Lo et al. 2008; Sveen et al. 2006). In contrast to European populations, cases of LGMD2I are rare in Australasia (van der Kooi et al. 1996; Lo et al. 2008; Norwood et al. 2009; Stensland et al. 2011; Fanin et al. 2005; Magri et al. 2017).

**Clinical features**

From a clinical standpoint it is hard to define a homogeneous phenotype. LGMD, as a group, are characterized clinically by a large variability among subgroups in age at onset and severity of symptoms and disease course. The common symptom is muscle weakness affecting predominantly the shoulder and pelvic girdle, but with the achievement of independent walking at some point. Axial and distal muscles are often also affected within the disease course and may even be the presenting symptom in some subtypes. The age at onset, degree of severity, association with cardiomyopathy, respiratory involvement and joint contractures is widely variable among subtypes (Domingos et al. 2017). Some LGMD, such as the sarcoglycanopathies LGMD2C, LGMD2E and LGMD2F, may have a severe, early-onset, Duchenne-like course, associated with cardiac and respiratory involvement while others, such as LGMD2L and LGMD2B, are characterized by a late onset and a slow disease progression. Even within a subtype, clinical features may reach both extremes of the spectrum from a mild adult form of muscular dystrophy to severe childhood or even congenital-onset muscular dystrophy, blurring the barriers between LGMD and CMD (LGMD2I, K, M, N, O) (Fig. 11.1). Creatine kinase (CK) levels are also variable, with some of the LGMD reaching creatine kinase levels in the range of DMD and others with only a limited rise.

Some LGMD may have specific features such as striking tightness of the Achilles tendon or a rigid spine (LGMD1B and LGMD2) or the occurrence of rhabdomyolysis symptoms (LGMD2L), myasthenia (LGMD2T) or "rippling muscle" (LGMD1C) (Domingos et al. 2017; Murphy and Straub 2015).

The natural history of LGMD patients as a group is hard to define, considering the broad range of underlying etiologies, and the variability in phenotypical expression; however, natural history data are emerging for the most common types, such as LGMD2I and LGMD2B (Willis et al. 2013; JAIN 2015; ClinicalTrials.gov NCT01676077).

**Diagnosis**

A thorough history taking, including family history, and clinical examination, complemented by targeted genetic analysis, will exclude well-defined dystrophies such as DMD/BMD, FSHD and Emery–Dreifuss muscular dystrophy (EDMD) that may present with a

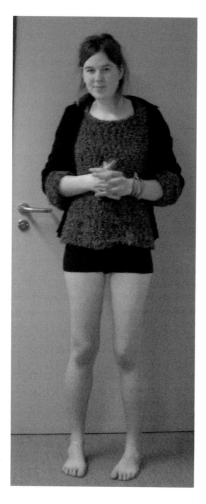

**Fig. 11.1.** LGMD 2I: Homozygous deletion c.826C>A in the fukutin related protein gene (FKRP). First clinical signs at age 5. Highly elevated CK. Progressive weakness with LGMD pattern of involvement. Loss of ambulation at age 26. Non-invasive night time ventilatory support from age 30.

pelvic girdle weakness. Pompe disease, spinal muscular atrophy type 3, congenital myopathies such as Bethlem myopathy and congenital myasthenia may share clinical features with LGMD and should be included in the differential diagnosis.

The clinical features, disease onset, pattern of involvement, association with cardiac and/or respiratory involvement, and creatine kinase (CK) level may give a clue to a specific LGMD type, to be confirmed by targeted genetic testing. The use of muscle MRI in the diagnostic journey has proven successful in identifying patterns of involvement that may help to distinguish certain subgroups of LGMD from others (Tasca et al. 2018).

Muscle biopsy with immunohistochemical staining and western blot analysis may confirm a dystrophic picture and the absence of a specific protein marker, providing further information for additional genetic testing; however, the introduction of new genome sequencing technologies has considerably lowered the threshold to go straight to genetic testing. Today, the use of targeted gene sequencing panels has considerably improved the diagnostic yield of genetic testing in LGMD and has become the favored approach for LGMD diagnosis. However, this approach may miss deletions, duplications and repeat sequences and may result in reporting a considerable amount of variants of unknown significance.

## Treatment

There is no causative treatment available for LGMD so far; management should aim at a comprehensive multidisciplinary approach of the muscular and extra muscular symptoms of the disease and their consequences (Narayanaswami et al. 2014). Some subtypes are characterized by severe cardiomyopathy or cardiac conduction disturbances requiring a specific approach, such as the implantation of defibrillators in LGMD1B (van Rijsingen et al. 2012).

The use of glucocorticosteroids is not generally recommended in LGMD, although some good responses have been observed in cases of sarcoglycanopathies, LGMD2I and LGMD2M (Godfrey et al. 2006).

The improved understanding of the pathophysiological mechanisms of these diseases have fueled therapeutic research targeting the underlying gene defects, such as gene therapy using adeno-associated vectors, gene transfer of mini-dysferlin and exon-skipping (Potter et al. 2018; Sondergaard et al. 2015; Mendell et al. 2009; Azakir et al. 2012; Barthélémy et al. 2011; Xu et al. 2013). Encouraging results in animal models raise the hope for translation of these techniques to clinical application. However, these approaches face the same hurdles and barriers experienced in the therapy development for other neuromuscular disease. The limited number of patients, the heterogeneity of the disease course and the lack of natural history data and meaningful, validated clinical outcome measures for most LGMD are additional challenges in the translation to clinical research (Straub and Bertoli 2016).

The genetic and clinical characteristics of autosomal dominant LGMD1 and autosomal recessive LGMD2 are summarized in Tables 11.1 and 11.2. Allelic presentations with CMD phenotypes (see Chapter 12) are highlighted as well. Note: The LGMD nomenclature is currently being revisited, with a proposal for a new nomenclature (Straub et al. 2018).

## Key points

- The term limb-girdle muscular dystrophies (LGMD) covers a very heterogenous group of rare (dominant or recessive) inherited muscle diseases characterized by progressive degenerative muscle changes, affecting predominantly the pelvic and shoulder girdle.
- Gene defects causing LGMD encode for a wide spectrum of proteins involved in muscle fiber structure and function.
- The classification of the LGMD subtypes has been based on a consensus nomenclature dividing LGMD by pattern of inheritance: "1" being assigned to the dominant types and "2" for the recessively inherited subtypes.
- With the discovery of an increasing number of causative genes resulting in a LGMD, a revised classification system that incorporates the name of the protein affected in the muscle cell and includes the mode of inheritance has been proposed.
- The age at onset, degree of severity, association with cardiomyopathy, respiratory involvement and joint contractures is widely variable among subtypes of LGMD.

## TABLE 11.2
### The genetic and clinical characteristics of autosomal recessive LGMD2

| Gene | | | sCK | Clinical features | | Allelic disorders |
|---|---|---|---|---|---|---|
| Disease | Name | Protein product | | Specific features | Cardiomyopathy | |
| LGMD2A | CAPN3 | Calpain 3 | 3–20x | Most frequent worldwide<br>Highly variable course<br>Childhood/teens onset<br>Loss of ambulation from 5–39 years<br>Respiratory involvement<br>Calf hypertrophy<br>Scapular winging<br>Relative sparing of sartorius, gracilis and vastus lateralis | Rarely observed | |
| LGMD2B | DYSF | Dysferlin | 5–40x | Common form (5–35%)<br>Highly variable clinical presentation<br>Late teens/early adulthood onset<br>Distal involvement (Miyoshi myopathy)<br>Rigid spine<br>Asymptomatic hyper CK | Possible | Miyoshi Muscular Dystrophy 1 (254130)<br>Myopathy, distal, with anterior tibial onset (606768) |
| LGMD2C | SGCG | γ-Sarcoglycan | 10–70x | 10–20% | Often severe | |
| LGMD2D | SGCA | α-Sarcoglycan | 10–70x | Childhood onset<br>Duchenne like progression | Often severe | |
| LGMD2E | SGCB | β-Sarcoglycan | 10–70x | Limb extensors spared compared to flexors | Often severe | |
| LGMD2F | SGCD | δ-Sarcoglycan | 10–70x | Calf hypertrophy<br>Scapular winging<br>Macroglossia<br>MRI: thigh adductors, glutei and posterior thigh groups most affected, lower leg muscles relatively spared | Rarely observed | Cardiomyopathy, dilated, CMD 1L (606685) |
| LGMD2G | TCAP | Telethonin | 10x | Adolescent onset<br>Slow progression | Possible | Hypertrophic cardiomyopathy CMH25 related to TCAP (607487) |

Continued

TABLE 11.2
Continued

| Disease | Gene | | | Clinical features | | |
|---|---|---|---|---|---|---|
| | Name | Protein product | sCK | Specific features | Cardiomyopathy | Allelic disorders |
| LGMD2H | TRIM32 | Tripartite motif-containing 32 | 10x | Adulthood onset<br>Proximal weakness and atrophy<br>Slow progression | Not observed | Bardet-Biedl syndrome (209900) |
| LGMD2I | FKRP | Fukutin related protein | 10–20x | Highly variable onset (congenital to late adulthood)<br>Most common in North Europe<br>Respiratory and cardiac involvement<br>Calf hypertrophy<br>Scapular winging<br>Macroglossia<br>MRI: iliopsoas and thigh muscle adductors most affected | yes | |
| LGMD2J | TTN | Titin | 10–40x | Childhood onset<br>Distal weakness<br>Cardiac and respiratory involvement | yes | Cardiomyopathy, dilated, 1G (604145)<br>Cardiomyopathy, familial hypertrophic, 9 CMH9 (613765)<br>Myopathy, early-onset, with fatal cardiomyopathy (611705)<br>Myopathy, proximal, with early respiratory muscle involvement (603689)<br>Tibial muscular dystrophy, tardive (600334) |

Continued

**TABLE 11.2**
Continued

| Gene | | | Clinical features | | |
|------|------|-----------------|------|------|------|
| Disease | Name | Protein product | sCK | Specific features | Cardiomyopathy | Allelic disorders |
| LGMD2K | *POMT1* | Protein-O-mannosyl Transferase 1 | 10–40x | CMD phenotype with brain abnormalities more frequent<br>Occasional childhood onset with milder progression. | Not observed | Muscular dystrophy-dystroglycanopathy (congenital with intellectual disability), type B, 1 (613155)<br>Muscular dystrophy-dystroglycanopathy (congenital with brain and eye anomalies), type A, 1 (236670)<br>Muscular dystrophy-dystroglycanopathy (limb girdle), type C, 1 (609308) |
| LGMD2L | *NO5* | Anoctamin 5 | 1–15x | Common in North Europe (15–40%)<br>LGMD phenotype or distal myopathy<br>Variable onset (Teens to Adulthood)<br>Wide phenotype from asymptomatic hyper CKemia to loss of ambulation<br>Cardiorespiratory involvement not reported | Not observed | Gnathodiaphyseal dysplasia (166260)<br>Miyoshi muscular dystrophy 3 (613319) |

Continued

**TABLE 11.2**
Continued

|  | Gene | |  | Clinical features | | |
|---|---|---|---|---|---|---|
| Disease | Name | Protein product | sCK | Specific features | Cardiomyopathy | Allelic disorders |
| LGMD2M | *FKTN* | Fukutin | 10–70x | CMD phenotype with or without brain abnormalities more frequent<br>Occasional childhood onset with milder progression<br>Muscle hypertrophy | Possible | Cardiomyopathy, dilated, 1X (611615)<br>Muscular dystrophy-dystroglycanopathy (congenital with brain and eye anomalies), type A, 4 (253800)<br>Muscular dystrophy-dystroglycanopathy (congenital with intellectual disability), type B, 1 (613155) |
| LGMD2N | *POMT2* | Protein-O-mannosyl transferase 2 | 5–15x |  | Rarely observed | Muscular dystrophy-dystroglycanopathy (congenital with brain and eye anomalies), type A, 2 (613150)<br>Muscular dystrophy-dystroglycanopathy (congenital with intellectual disability), type B, 2 (613156) |

Continued

TABLE 11.2
Continued

| | Gene | | | Clinical features | | |
|---|---|---|---|---|---|---|
| Disease | Name | Protein product | sCK | Specific features | Cardiomyopathy | Allelic disorders |
| LGMD2O | POMGnT1 | Protein-O-linked mannose beta 1, 2-N-acetyl-glucosaminyl transferase | 2–10x | | Not observed | Muscular dystrophy-dystroglycanopathy (congenital with brain and eye anomalies), type A, 3 (253280) Muscular dystrophy-dystroglycanopathy (congenital with intellectual disability), type B, 3 (613151) Muscular dystrophy-dystroglycanopathy (limb girdle), type C, 3 (613157) |
| LGMD2P | DAG1 | Dystroglycan | 20x | | Not observed | |
| LGMD2Q | PLEC1 | Plectin | 10–50x | Rare Early childhood onset Slow progression | Not observed | Epidermolysis bullosa simplex with pyloric atresia (612138) Epidermolysis bullosa simplex Ogna type (131950) Muscular dystrophy with epidermolysis bullosa simplex (226670) |
| LGMD2R | DES | Desmin (structural; intermediate filament) | 1x | Onset in teens Facial weakness Arrhythmias | A-V conduction block | Muscular dystrophy, limb girdle, type 2R, (615325) Cardiomyopathy, dilated, 1I (604765) Myopathy, myofibrillar 1 (601419) Scapuloperoneal syndrome, neurogenic, Kaeser type (181400) |

Continued

TABLE 11.2
Continued

| Gene | | | Clinical features | | |
|---|---|---|---|---|---|
| Disease | Name | Protein product | sCK | Specific features | Cardiomyopathy | Allelic disorders |
| LGMD2S | TRAPPC11 | Transport protein particle complex 11 | 9–16x | Occasional<br>Childhood to young adulthood<br>Slow progression<br>Alacrima, achalasia, movement disorders, cataract, hepatic steatosis | Not observed | |
| LGMD2T | GMPPB | GDP-mannose pyrophosphor-ylase B | | CMD phenotype with or without brain abnormalities more frequent<br>Occasional childhood onset<br>Cataract | Possible | Muscular dystrophy-dystroglycanopathy (congenital with brain and eye anomalies), type A, 14 (615150)<br>Muscular dystrophy-dystroglycanopathy (congenital with intellectual disability), type B, 14 (615151) |
| LGMD2U | ISPD | Isopenoid syn-thase domain containing | 6–50x | Occasional<br>Rapid to moderate progression<br>Childhood onset<br>Calf hypertrophy<br>Scapular winging | Possible | Muscular dystrophy-dystroglycanopathy (congenital with brain and eye anomalies), type A, 7 (614643) |
| LGMD2V | GAA | Alpha-1, 4-glucosidase | 1–20x | Later onset Pompe disease<br>Occasional<br>Variable progression (rapid to slow)<br>Axial and respiratory muscle involvement | Possible | Glycogen storage disease II5232300° |
| LGMD2W | LIMS2 | LIM and senescent cell antigen-like domains 2 | | Rare<br>Childhood onset<br>Macroglossia, triangular tongue<br>Calf hypertrophy<br>Left ventricular dysfunction | Possible | |

Continued

**TABLE 11.2**
**Continued**

| Disease | Gene | | | Clinical features | | |
| | Name | Protein product | sCK | Specific features | Cardiomyopathy | Allelic disorders |
|---|---|---|---|---|---|---|
| LGMD2X | BVES | Blood vessel epicardial substance | | Rare<br>Adulthood onset<br>Cardiac arrhythmia | Yes | |
| LGMD2Y | TOR1AIP1 | Lamina-associated polypeptide 1B (LAP1B) | | Rare<br>Childhood onset<br>Proximal and distal weakness<br>Rigid spine, respiratory involvement<br>Interphalangeal joint contractures | Yes | |
| LGMD-LAMA2 | LAMA2 | Laminin α2 | Mild elevation | Childhood onset<br>Demyelinating polyneuropathy<br>CNS involvement<br>cardiomyopthathy | Yes | Congenital muscular dystrophy with white matter abnormalities (607855) |

sCK: serum creatine kinase.
Adapted from Nigro and Savarese (2014), Murphy and Straub (2015), Domingos et al. (2017), Neuromuscular Disorders gene table, http://www.musclegenetable.fr/

## REFERENCES

Azakir BA, Di Fulvio S, Kinter J, Sinnreich M (2012) Proteasomal inhibition restores biological function of mis-sense mutated dysferlin in patient-derived muscle cells. *J Biol Chem* 287: 10344–10354.

Barthélémy F, Wein N, Krahn M, Lévy N, Bartoli M (2011) Translational research and therapeutic perspectives in dysferlinopathies. *Mol Med* 17: 875–882.

Bushby KM (1995) Diagnostic criteria for the limb-girdle muscular dystrophies: report of the ENMC Consortium on Limb-Girdle Dystrophies. *Neuromuscul Disord* 5: 71–74.

Domingos J, Sarkozy A, Scoto M, Muntoni F (2017) Dystrophinopathies and limb-girdle muscular dystrophies. *Neuropediatrics* 48: 262–272.

ENMC (2017) Limb girdle muscular dystrophies, nomenclature and reformed classification, 229th ENMC workshop, March 2017; Naarden, The Netherlands. http://www.enmc.org/publications/workshop-reports.

Fanin M, Nascimbeni AC, Fulizio L, Angelini C (2005) The frequency of limb girdle muscular dystrophy 2A in northeastern Italy. *Neuromuscul Disord* 15: 218–224.

Godfrey C, Escolar D, Brockington M, Clement EM, Mein R, Jimenez-Mallebrera C et al. (2006) Fukutin gene mutations in steroid-responsive limb girdle muscular dystrophy. *Ann Neurol* 60: 603–610.

JAIN (2015) International clinical outcome study for dysferlinopathy. JAIN Foundation. http://www.jain-foundation.

Lo HP, Cooper ST, Evesson FJ, Seto JT, Chiotis M, Tay V et al. (2008) Limb-girdle muscular dystrophy: diagnostic evaluation, frequency and clues to pathogenesis. *Neuromuscul Disord* 18: 34–44.

Magri F, Nigro V, Angelini C, Mongini T, Mora M, Moroni I et al. (2017) The Italian limb girdle muscular dystrophy registry: relative frequency, clinical features, and differential diagnosis. *Muscle Nerve* 55: 55–68.

Mah JK, Korngut L, Fiest KM, Dykeman J, Day LJ, Pringsheim T et al. (2016) a systematic review and meta-analysis on the epidemiology of the muscular dystrophies. *Can J Neurol Sci* 43: 163–177.

Mendell JR, Rodino-Klapac LR, Rosales-Quintero X, Kota J, Coley BD, Galloway G et al. (2009) Limb-girdle muscular dystrophy type 2D gene therapy restores alpha-sarcoglycan and associated proteins. *Ann Neurol* 66: 290–297.

Murphy AP, Straub V (2015) The classification, natural history and treatment of the limb girdle muscular dystrophies. *J Neuromuscul Dis* 2(s2):S7–S19.

Narayanaswami P, Weiss M, Selcen D, David W, Raynor E, Carter G et al. (2014) Evidence-based guideline summary: diagnosis and treatment of limb-girdle and distal dystrophies: report of the guideline development subcommittee of the American Academy of Neurology and the practice issues review panel of the American Association of Neuromuscular & Electrodiagnostic Medicine. *Neurology* 83: 1453–1463.

Nigro V, Savarese M (2014) Genetic basis of limb-girdle muscular dystrophies: the 2014 update. *Acta Myol* 33: 1–12.

Norwood FL, Harling C, Chinnery PF, Eagle M, Bushby K, Straub V (2009) Prevalence of genetic muscle disease in Northern England: in-depth analysis of a muscle clinic population. *Brain* 132: 3175–3186.

Potter RA, Griffin DA, Sondergaard PC, Johnson RW, Pozsgai ER, Heller KN et al. (2018) Systemic delivery of dysferlin overlap vectors provides long-term gene expression and functional improvement for dysferlinopathy. *Hum Gene Ther* 29(7):749–762.

Sondergaard PC, Griffin DA, Pozsgai ER, Johnson RW, Grose WE, Heller KN et al. (2015) AAV.dysferlin overlap vectors restore function in dysferlinopathy animal models. *Ann Clin Transl Neurol* 2: 256–270.

Stensland E, Lindal S, Jonsrud C, Torbergsen T, Bindoff LA, Rasmussen M et al. (2011) Prevalence, mutation spectrum and phenotypic variability in Norwegian patients with Limb Girdle Muscular Dystrophy 2I. *Neuromuscul Disord* 21: 41–46.

Straub V, Bertoli M (2016) Where do we stand in trial readiness for autosomal recessive limb girdle muscular dystrophies? *Neuromuscul Disord* 26: 111–125.

Straub V, Bushby K (2006) The childhood limb-girdle muscular dystrophies. *Semin Pediatr Neurol* 13: 104–114.

Straub V, Murphy A, Udd B, Group LWS (2018) 229th ENMC international workshop: Limb girdle muscular dystrophies – Nomenclature and reformed classification Naarden, the Netherlands, 17–19 March 2017. *Neuromuscul Disord* 28(8):702–710.

Sveen ML, Schwartz M, Vissing J (2006) High prevalence and phenotype-genotype correlations of limb girdle muscular dystrophy type 2I in Denmark. *Ann Neurol* 59: 808–815.

Tasca G, Monforte M, Díaz-Manera J, Brisca G, Semplicini C, D'Amico A et al. (2018) MRI in sarcogly-canopathies: a large international cohort study. *J Neurol Neurosurg Psychiatry* 89: 72–77.

van der Kooi AJ, Barth PG, Busch HF, de Haan R, Ginjaar HB, van Essen AJ et al. (1996) The clinical spectrum of limb girdle muscular dystrophy. A survey in The Netherlands. *Brain* 119: 1471–1480.

van Rijsingen IA, Arbustini E, Elliott PM, Mogensen J, Hermans-van Ast JF, van der Kooi AJ et al. (2012) Risk factors for malignant ventricular arrhythmias in lamin a/c mutation carriers a European cohort study. *J Am Coll Cardiol* 59: 493–500.

Walton JN, Nattrass FJ (1954) On the classification, natural history and treatment of the myopathies. *Brain* 77: 169–231.

Willis TA, Hollingsworth KG, Coombs A, Sveen ML, Andersen S, Stojkovic T et al. (2013) Quantitative muscle MRI as an assessment tool for monitoring disease progression in LGMD2I: a multicentre longitudinal study. *PLoS One* 8:e70993.

Xu L, Lu PJ, Wang CH, Keramaris E, Qiao C, Xiao B et al. (2013) Adeno-associated virus 9 mediated FKRP gene therapy restores functional glycosylation of α-dystroglycan and improves muscle functions. *Mol Ther* 21: 1832–1840.

# 12
# CONGENITAL MUSCULAR DYSTROPHIES

*Nathalie Goemans*

For an introduction to Muscular Dystrophies, please see Chapter 10 (page 166).

**Introduction**

The congenital muscular dystrophies are a heterogeneous group of muscular disorders characterized by an early-onset muscle disease, present from birth or early infancy, together with histopathological evidence of a dystrophic process. The use of this definition has proven useful to identify specific clinical entities that are different from well-defined dystrophies such as Duchenne muscular dystrophy/Becker muscular dystrophy, Emery–Dreifuss muscular dystrophy (EDMD), myotonic dystrophy (MD) and to separate them from congenital myopathies with distinct histopathological features (Bonnemann et al. 2014). Historically, this term was associated with a severe form of congenital myopathy described by Batten in the early twentieth century (Batten 1903). Subsequently, other distinct phenotypes such as Ullrich atonic sclerotic muscular dystrophy, characterized by a severe course and the combination of joint contractures and joint laxity (Ullrich 1930), and Fukuyama CMD, a severe CMD associated with cerebral involvement prevalent in Japanese population, were reported (Fukuyama et al. 1981). Muscle Eye Brain (MEB) disease, described by Santavuori in the Finnish populations and Walker–Warburg syndrome (WWS) expanded the spectrum of severe CMD with central nervous system changes (Santavuori et al. 1989; Warburg 1978).

In 1994 Tomé found that the severe form of occidental CMD with diffuse white matter abnormality was caused by lack of laminin $\alpha 2$ (laminin M, merosin chain in the extra cellular matrix) (Tomé et al. 1994; Helbling-Leclerc et al. 1995). This was the first molecular defect reported in CMD. Subsequent improvements in molecular diagnosis and better insights in the underlying pathophysiological mechanisms have further unraveled the causes of the CMD phenotypes, challenging the clinico-histopathological classification. Causative gene defects associated with CMD result in a wide variety of clinico-pathological expression, blurring the barriers between limb-girdle muscular dystrophy (LGMD) and CMD (see Table 11.2 in Chapter 11) as well as between CMD and congenital myopathies with overlaps at the clinical, morphological and genetic levela. For example, mutations in *FKRP* result in the most frequent form of CMD in the Japanese population (Fukuyama CMD); however, mutations in the same gene have been reported in much milder autosomal recessive LGMD2I phenotype (Driss et al. 2000). Similarly, mutations in the COL 6A subunits, alpha 1, 2, 3, have been associated with a wide clinical spectrum of expression, from the severe Ullrich CMD to the milder Bethlem myopathy (Bushby et al. 2014; Baker et al. 2005; Bonnemann 2011).

## Clinical presentation

Children with CMD may present at birth or soon after with hypotonia and weakness with or without joint contractures. Facial involvement is common and respiratory muscle weakness may be associated. Some forms of CMD are associated with typical features such as a striking distal joint laxity (COL6A) and rigid spine (SEPN1-CMD) or a dropped head (LMNA-CMD). Spinal muscular atrophy (SMA), metabolic myopathies, congenital myotonic dystrophy, congenital myasthenia as well as congenital myopathies should be considered in the differential diagnosis. In milder cases, diagnosis may be delayed into childhood or even adulthood. Affected children may present with delay in motor development and muscle weakness. Exercise intolerance and progressive joint contractures may be present as well. In contrast with other form of muscular dystrophies, CMD may have a relatively stable course of disease although some subgroups such as LAMA2-related CMD and Ullrich-type CMD may develop progressive and severe joint contractures and a progressive restrictive respiratory insufficiency, requiring the use of ventilatory support.

## Diagnosis

Some clinical features will point to a specific form of congenital dystrophy such as the distribution of weakness or pattern of involvement as assessed by muscle magnetic resonance imaging (MRI) (Mercuri et al. 2010). Specific clinical features such as a rigid spine, dropped head syndrome or the association with the central nervous system (CNS) and ophthalmological involvement may guide the diagnostic pathway. Muscle (and brain) MRI, neurophysiological assessment (electromyography (EMG) and nerve conduction velocity (NCV), muscle biopsy and targeted biochemical and genetic testing are important tools that may contribute to exclude other conditions and to reach a final diagnosis.

## Incidence

The overall prevalence of CMD is estimated to be 0.99 per 100 000 (Mah et al. 2016); however, some types may be characteristic for some regions and rare in other part of the world, such as the Fukuyama type CMD, which is the most frequent muscular dystrophy in Japan.

## Classification

Today, CMD can be classified based on the primary genetic and biochemical defect (Bonnemann et al. 2014; Schorling et al. 2017). Most of the genes associated with CMD are coding for proteins involved in the plasma membrane-extracellular interface (Schorling et al. 2017) (Fig. 12.1). Table 12.1 gives an overview of the most common congenital muscular dystrophies.

## Abnormalities in extra cellular matrix proteins

Merosin-deficient congenital muscular dystrophy
(Laminin α2-related congenital muscular dystrophy)

*LAMA2* encodes for the α2 chain of merosin (laminin α2) that interacts with the alpha-dystroglycan complex. Mutations in *LAMA2* result in a reduction or absence of laminin α2,

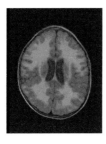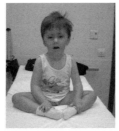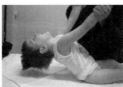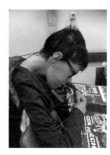

**Fig. 12.1.** Merosin-deficient congenital muscular dystrophy (LAMA2) with early-onset of proximal and facial weakness. This young man never achieved ambulation, developed a severe scoliosis and has lost head control with time. Extensive white matter changes on brain MRI. Mild cognitive impairment.

which can be demonstrated in muscle and skin biopsies by immunohistochemical staining with antibodies against the two fragments (80 and 300kDa) of the laminin α2 chain. The phenotypical expression correlates with the residual amount of laminin α2: absence of this protein will result in a classic, severe type of CMD characterized by an early-onset hypotonia and muscle weakness, joint contractures, facial and respiratory involvement, together with a severe dystrophic picture on muscle biopsy. Ambulation is rarely achieved, and orthopedic deformities are frequent (Helbling-Leclerc et al. 1995). Respiratory function is reduced and night-time hypoventilation is often observed, as well as failure to thrive (Geranmayeh et al. 2010). This CMD is associated with striking and extensive white matter abnormalities in T2-weighted MRI; CNS structural abnormalities are, however, rarely reported (Philpot et al. 2000). Intelligence is typically within the normal range (Mercuri et al. 1999) (Fig. 12.1). A higher incidence of epilepsy (30%) is reported (Philpot et al. 2000). A demyelinating neuropathy may be noted after the age of 6 months, reflecting the involvement of the Schwann cells in the disease process (Shorer et al. 1995). Incomplete absence of merosin results in a milder LGMD phenotype, with a later onset of symptoms and milder course of disease (Jones et al. 2001).

COL6A3 RELATED DYSTROPHIES (ULLRICH CONGENITAL MUSCULAR
DYSTROPHY – BETHLEM MYOPATHY)
COL6A1, COL6A2, and COL6A3 encode the three alpha chains of collagen 6, which is a major component of the extra cellular matrix. Collagen 6 forms a reticular extracellular network, linking extracellular proteins with the basal lamina. Mutations in one of these alpha chains may result in muscle diseases with a wide variety in disease severity, with the severe Ullrich CMD at one end and a mild adult-onset myopathy (Bethlem) at the other end of the spectrum (Ullrich 1930; Bethlem et al. 1966).

Ullrich CMD is most commonly autosomal recessively inherited, although dominant mutations have been reported as well (Baker et al. 2005). Ullrich CMD has an early onset and is characterized by delay in motor development, the development of severe joint contractures, scoliosis, rigidity of spine and thorax, resulting in a deterioration of respiratory function with age. Hyperkeratosis pilaris, striking distal hyperlaxity, a round face, high

**TABLE 12.1**

**Overview of the most common congenital muscular dystrophies**

| Disease | Gene/OMIM number | Protein product | Clinical features | CNS involvement | Inheritance |
|---|---|---|---|---|---|
| | | | *Disorders of the extracellular matrix components* | | |
| | | | **Laminin α2-related dystrophy** | | |
| Merosin-deficient CMD | *LAMA2* 156225 | Laminin α2 | Early onset of weakness with proximal and facial pattern<br>Delayed motor development<br>Ambulation rarely achieved<br>Respiratory involvement<br>Epilepsy in 30%<br>Normal cognitive development | White matter changes | AR |
| | | | **Collagen VI-related dystrophies** | | |
| Ullrich CMD | *COL 6A1* 120220<br>*COL 6A2* 120240<br>*COL 6A3* 1200250 | Collagen VI subunit α1<br>Collagen VI subunit α2<br>Collagen VI subunit α3 | Characteristic phenotype with proximal contractures and distal joint hyperextensibility<br>Severe progressive sclerosis and joint contractures<br>No ambulation or loss of ambulation in severe cases<br>Respiratory involvement | No | AR<br>AR<br>AR |
| Bethlem myopathy | *COL 6A1* 120220<br>*COL 6A2* 120240<br>*COL 6A3* 1200250 | Collagen VI subunit α1<br>Collagen VI subunit α2<br>Collagen VI subunit α3 | Allelic disorder to Ullrich CMD<br>Characteristic phenotype with hyperlaxity and joint contractures<br>Milder phenotype<br>Broad range of severity | No | AD |
| | | | **Integrin-related dystrophies** | | |
| CMD related to Integrin α7 | *ITGA7* 600536 | Integrin alpha 7 | Rare<br>Delayed motor milestones<br>Cognitive impairment possible<br>Probably mostly cardiac phenotype | No structural abnormalities | AR |

Continued

**TABLE 12.1**
Continued

| Disease | Gene/OMIM number | Protein product | Clinical features | CNS involvement | Inheritance |
|---|---|---|---|---|---|
| | | | **Dystroglycanopathies** | | |
| Fukuyama CMD | *FKTN* 607440 | Fukutin | Most prevalent severe and progressive CMD in Japan<br>No ambulation or loss of ambulation<br>Severe cognitive impairment<br>Epilepsy<br>Cardiac involvement | Lissencephaly<br>Micropolygyria<br>White matter abnormalities | AR |
| CMD related to defective glycosylation | *POMT1* 607423 | Protein O-mannosyltransferase | Very severe congenital weakness, often without motor development<br>Severe cognitive impairment<br>With or without epilepsy<br>With or without ocular involvement (microphthalmia, cataract etc.)<br>Wide variety of phenotypes:<br>• Walker–Warburg syndrome<br>• Muscle–eye–brain disease<br>• Fukuyama-like CMD<br>• CMD with cerebellar involvement<br>• CMD with intellectual disability and a structurally normal brain<br>• CMD with no intellectual disability; no evidence of abnormal cognitive development | Lissencephaly type II,<br>Pachygyria<br>Brainstem hypoplasia<br>Occipital encepha-locele<br>Cerebellar atrophy<br>Cerebellar cysts<br>Cerebellar Dysplasia<br>Microcephalia<br>White matter changes | AR |
| | *POMT2* 607439 | Protein O-mannosyltransferase 2 | | | |
| | *POMGnT1* 606822 | O-linked mannose β-1, 2-N-acetylglucosamin-yltransferase | | | |

**TABLE 12.1**
**Continued**

| Disease | Gene/OMIM number | Protein product | Clinical features | CNS involvement | Inheritance |
|---|---|---|---|---|---|
| | LARGE 603590 | Acetylglucosaminyl-transferase-like-protein | | | |
| | FKTN 607440 | Fukutin | | | |
| | FKRP 606596 | Fukutin-related protein | | | |
| | ISPD 614631 | Isoprenoid synthase domain containing protein | | | |
| | B3GNT1 605517 | B-Gal-b1,3N acetyl-glucosaminyltrans-ferase1 | | | |
| | B3GALNT2 610194 | B-1,3-acetylgalac-tosaminyltransferase 2 | | | |
| | GMPPB 615320 | GDP-mannose pyro-phosphorylase B | | | |
| | DPM1 603503 | Dolichophosphate mannosyltransferase 1 | | | |
| | DPM2 603564 | Dolichophosphate mannosyltransferase polypeptide 2 | | | |
| | GTDC2 614828 | Glycosyltransfer-ase-like domain containing 2 | | | |

Continued

TABLE 12.1
Continued

| Disease | Gene/OMIM number | Protein product | Clinical features | CNS involvement | Inheritance |
|---|---|---|---|---|---|
| **Abnormalities of nuclear envelope proteins** | | | | | |
| **LMNA-related dystrophy** | | | | | |
| LMNA-CMD | *LMNA* 150330 | Laminin A/C | Early onset, striking and severe weakness of axial and neck muscles, Dropped-head syndrome Contractures Cardiac involvement with life threatening conduction defects Normal cognitive development Nesprin-related dystrophies | No | AD |
| NESP-CMD | *NESP* | Nesprin 1 | CMD with adducted thumbs Variable phenotype and cardiac involvement | No | AD |
| **Abnormalities at the level of the endoplasmatic reticulum** | | | | | |
| **SELENON-related myopathy** | | | | | |
| CMD with rigid spine Multiminicore myopathy | *SELENON (SEPN1)* 606210 | Selenoprotein N1 | Delayed motor development Ambulation achieved in most patients Early axial muscular weakness, scoliosis, rigidity of spine Early respiratory insufficiency No cardiac involvement Normal cognitive development | No | AR |

Adapted from Bonnemann et al. (2014), Schorling et al. (2017), and the Neuromuscular Disorders gene table: http://www.musclegenetable.fr December 2017.
CMD: congenital mucular dystrophy; AR: autosomal recessive; AD: autosomal dominant.

forehead, round eyes may be associated and provide a clinical clue to the diagnosis (Bushby et al. 2014; Bonnemann 2011).

Ambulation may be achieved, however, is lost with progression of the disease in the Ullrich-type CMD. There is no associated cardiac or CNS involvement. Bethlem myopathy, most often autosomal dominantly inherited, has a later onset with milder course; however, motor function and respiratory capacity may slowly deteriorate with age. A characteristic feature of Bethlem myopathy is the progressive contractures of interphalangeal joints, elbows and ankles.

A whole spectrum of severity in between the typical Ullrich CMD and Bethlem myopathy has been described with variable hypotonia, delay in motor development, girdle weakness and/or contractures as clinical features (Bonnemann 2011).

INTEGRIN-RELATED DYSTROPHIES

Integrin alpha 7 is a transmembrane laminin receptor. Deficiency in integrin alpha 7 have been associated with a rare CMD phenotype characterized by delayed motor milestones, progressive weakness, scoliosis and respiratory insufficiency. No additional cases have been reported since the initial publication (Hayashi et al. 1998).

An Ullrich-like CMD has been associated with a mutation in integrin alpha 9 in French–Canadian families (Eagle et al. 2007).

DYSTROGLYCANOPATHIES

Alpha-dystroglycan is a heavily glycosylated peripheral membrane component of the dystrophin-associated glycoprotein complex (DAGP) that play a pivotal role in linking the actin-associated cytoskeleton to components of extra cellular matrix (laminin, perlecan, agrin etc.). Mutations in *FKTN, POMGnT1, POMT1, POMT2, FKRP, LARGE, GMPPB* and *ISPD* affect the O-mannosyl linked glycosylation of alpha-dystroglycan (α-DG) and result in different types of CMD most often associated with CNS involvement, including neuronal migration defects such as lissencephaly, pachygyria and abnormalities of the cerebellum and brainstem. A variety of associated congenital ocular anomalies has been reported as well (glaucoma, cataract, myopia etc.) (Schorling et al. 2017; Bonnemann et al. 2014).

Fukuyama CMD, the most prevalent muscular dystrophy in Japan, is due to a mutation in the fukutin gene (*FKTN*) and is characterized by an early-onset CMD with delay in motor development and severe cognitive involvement. Microcephaly and epilepsy may be associated features. MRI of the brain may reveal cortical migration defects (cobble stone lissencephaly type II, polymicrogyria, hydrocephalus and midbrain and/or pontocerebellar hypoplasia). Abnormalities in cerebellar foliation, and cerebellar cysts have been reported as well.

Ambulation is seldom achieved, and the disease course is severe (Osawa et al. 1991; Fukuyama et al. 1981). Ophthalmological involvement is less striking compared to the MEB- and WWS-type CMD (Warburg 1978; Dobyns et al. 1989; Santavuori et al. 1989). These CMD subtypes, characterized by a striking association of CNS involvement and ophthalmological malformations, were initially reported to be due to respectively *POMGnT1* and *POMT1* mutations (Beltran-Valero et al. 2002).

Improvements in molecular diagnoses have currently broaden the spectrum of causative genes for these historical phenotypes and highlighted the overlap between the different clinical entities as mutations in *POMT2*, *FKRP*, *LARGE*, *GMPPB* and *ISPD* may result in a variety of muscular dystrophies with a wide range of severity and CNS involvement. The phenotypic severity depends upon how severely the mutation affects the glycosylation of alpha-dystroglycan more than upon which gene is primarily mutated. A dilated cardiomyopathy has been reported with mutations in FKRP and FKTN (Murakami et al. 2006).

LGMD2 I (*FKRP*), K (*POMT1*), M (*FKTN*), N (*POMT2*), O (*POMGnT1*) and T (*GMPPB*) are allelic LGMD disorders of these alpha-dystroglycan related CMDs (Driss et al. 2000; Kang et al. 2015; Narayanaswami et al. 2014; Murakami et al. 2006; Carss et al. 2013).

## Abnormalities of nuclear envelop proteins

LMNA: CONGENITAL MUSCULAR DYSTROPHY WITH DROPPED HEAD — ALLELIC TO EMERY–DREIFUSS MUSCULAR DYSTROPHY

Mutations in LMNA, coding for lamin A/C, a major protein of the nuclear envelope result in a broad range of disorders (laminopathies) with marked phenotypical heterogeneity including non-muscular disorders such as Hutchinson–Gilford progeria and type 2 familial lipo-dystrophia (Quijano-Roy et al. 2008). Neuromuscular phenotypes are widely heterogenous (Mercuri et al. 2005a) and include EDMD type 3, LGMD 1B, CMT 2B1 and a form of CMD characterized by a striking weakness of the cervical muscles (CMD with dropped head) in combination with congenital contractures, a rigid hyperlordotic posture of the spine and respiratory muscle involvement ( Chemla et al. 2010). There is a high risk of sudden death due to cardiac involvement with typical conduction abnormalities and eventually dilated cardiomyopathy (Meune et al. 2006). There is no CNS involvement; cognitive development is unaffected.

NESPRIN: CONGENITAL MUSCULAR DYSTROPHY WITH ADDUCTED THUMBS

Nesprin-2 is a multi-isomeric protein that binds lamin and emerin at the nuclear envelope and forms a subcellular network in skeletal muscle. Mutations in nesprin have been described in a CMD with adducted thumbs (Zhou et al. 2017).

## Abnormalities at the level of the endoplasmatic reticulum

*SELENON* (previously named *SEPN1*) encodes a selenocysteine containing protein which is expressed in skeletal muscle and localized within the endoplasmic reticulum (Marino et al. 2015). There is a high expression of selenocysteine in cultured myoblasts, which is down-regulated in differentiating myotubes, suggesting a role for SELENON in early development and in cell proliferation or regeneration. Mutations result in a milder type of congenital muscular dystrophy with rigid spine (CMD-RSMD1) (Moghadaszadeh et al. 2001). Ambulation is most often preserved but early rigidity of the spine together with respiratory insufficiency and nocturnal hypoventilation is characteristic for this disease. This entity is, again, an example of the floating boundaries between CMD and congenital myopathies as SELENON-related CMD with rigid spine is allelic with multiminicore disease, a congenital myopathy with structural abnormalities and typical "cores" on muscle biopsy (Ferreiro et al. 2002).

The same applies for mutations in the ryanodine receptor gene *RYR1* causing a wide range of muscular phenotypes with variable severity. The congenital and severe forms (mostly autosomal recessive) present with generalized muscle weakness, congenital hip luxation, scoliosis, respiratory involvement and nocturnal hypoventilation together with the presence of core on muscle biopsy. Mutations in *RYR1* result in a dysfunction of calcium release in muscle and are associated with a high risk for malignant hyperthermia (Rooney et al. 2015).

Improvement in molecular diagnosis and further deciphering of the genome is resulting in an expanding list of genes involved in monogenic neuromuscular diseases, challenging the historical clinico-pathological classification of muscular dystrophies and myopathies. An exhaustive gene table is accessible at http://www.musclegenetable.fr/.

## Treatment

Currently, there is no curative treatment for CMD; however, a multidisciplinary approach for all aspects of the disease, including prevention of contractures, treatment of scoliosis, optimalization of nutritional aspects, cardio-respiratory care with provision of ventilatory support and cardiac surveillance, have improved survival and quality of life of these patients (Kang et al. 2015). Better insight in the underlying genetic causes and pathophysiological pathway will help to identify therapeutic targets for these diseases (Collins and Bonnemann 2010). New animal models have been developed and potential therapeutic strategies are in preclinical development, such as the upregulation of LARGE, Galgt2 or other α-DG glycosylation enzymatic activities for the alpha-dystroglycanopathies. Suppression of apoptosis is being explored as a potential therapeutic strategy in laminin-α2 deficiency and COL6A-related CMD. Restoration of the link between muscle and basement membrane by developing a mini-agrin binding to laminin in the basement membrane and to α-DG on the muscle is another example of the targeted therapeutic approach for CMD ( Collins and Bonnemann 2010).

## Key points
- The congenital muscular dystrophies are a heterogeneous group of muscular disorders characterized by an early-onset muscle disease, present from birth or early infancy, together with histopathological evidence of a dystrophic process.
- Causative gene defects associated with CMD result in a wide variety of clinico-pathological expression, blurring the barriers between LGMD and CMD as well as between CMD and congenital myopathies.
- Most of the genes associated with CMD code for proteins involved in the plasma membrane-extracellular interface.
- Currently, there is no curative treatment for CMD; however, a multidisciplinary approach to all aspects of the disease have improved survival and quality of life of these patients.

• Better insight in the underlying genetic causes and pathophysiological pathway will help to identify therapeutic targets for these diseases.

**Clinical vignette**

A 4-month-old boy was referred to our clinic with failure to thrive. Clinical examination revealed a hypotonic little boy with joint laxity, atrophic muscle mass, small chest with pectus deformity, high arched palate and poor mimic with alert eyes and adequate social contact. A congenital myopathy was suspected. Muscle biopsy showed a severe increase of fibrosis, variation in fiber size and small clusters of atrophic fibers. Creatine kinase was normal, and there was no heart involvement. Brain MRI was normal. Mutational analysis of collagen VI demonstrated a heterozygous COL6A2: 1332bp deletion (del exon 6–7). Mother appeared to be a mosaic carrier of this COL6A2: 1332 deletion. The motor milestones were delayed: with the acquisition of independent walking at age 3 year. Gait pattern deteriorated subsequently with loss of ambulation at age 4.

Despite physiotherapy and orthoses, contractures of the Achilles tendon, hips and knees, elbows and torticollis increased dramatically, associated with a progressive and severe general muscle wasting. Respiratory function deteriorated as well; nocturnal non-invasive ventilation was started from age 7 years. Despite adequate feeding through gastrostomy the young man became extremely dystrophic, with a weight of 18kg at the age of 21 years and evolving to a stage of extremely severe, generalized contractures of all joints, in contrast with a striking hyperlaxity of the fingers.

All his muscle mass seemed to have vanished and was replaced by fibrotic tissue. He developed a very small chest, with rigid wall and minimal excursion when breathing, with a forced vital capacity (FVC) that dropped to 0.27l (9%). He was ventilated non-invasively, first only at night but extending to daytime with progression of the disease. Despite the severe muscle wasting and retractions he kept the ability to develop some muscle power in the range of 4 – in biceps and quadriceps on the Medical Research Council (MRC) scale within his very limited range of movement. He developed a mid-facial hypoplasia. Eye movements were preserved. He died at home at the age of 25 years.

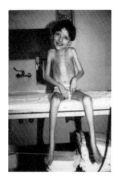 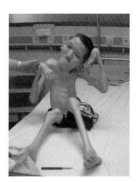 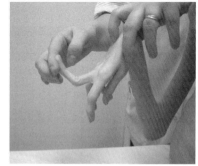

**Fig. 12.2.** Severe disease progression in Ullrich CMD. Striking association of severe progressive joint contractures and distal hyperlaxity.

COMMENT

Ullrich CMD is a severe form of CMD cause by mutations in one of the three COL 6A chains. The disease course is characterized by severe muscle wasting, fibrosis, the development of contractures and a severe restrictive respiratory disorder requiring ventilator support.

While Ullrich CMD is most often caused by recessive mutations, cases of dominant inheritance have been reported.

REFERENCES

Baker NL, Morgelin M, Peat R, Goemans N, North KN, Bateman JF et al. (2005) Dominant collagen VI mutations are a common cause of Ullrich congenital muscular dystrophy. *Hum Mol Genet* 14: 279–293.

Batten F (1903) Three cases of myopathy, infantile type. *Brain* 26: 147–148.

Beltran-Valero De Bernabe D, Currier S, Steinbrecher A, Celli J, Van Beusekom E, Van Der Zwaag B et al. (2002) Mutations in the O-mannosyltransferase gene POMT1 give rise to the severe neuronal migration disorder Walker–Warburg syndrome. *Am J Hum Genet* 71: 1033–1043.

Bethlem J, van Gool J, Hulsmann WC, Meijer A E (1966) Familial non-progressive myopathy with muscle cramps after exercise. A new disease associated with cores in the muscle fibres. *Brain* 89: 569–588.

Bonnemann CG (2011) The collagen VI-related myopathies Ullrich congenital muscular dystrophy and Bethlem myopathy. *Handb Clin Neurol* 101: 81–96.

Bonnemann CG, Wang CH, Quijano-Roy S, Deconinck N, Bertini E, Ferreiro A et al. (2014) Diagnostic approach to the congenital muscular dystrophies. *Neuromuscul Disord* 24: 289–311.

Bushby KM, Collins J, Hicks D (2014) Collagen type VI myopathies. *Adv Exp Med Biol* 802: 185–199.

Carss KJ, Stevens E, Foley AR, Cirak S, Riemersma M, Torelli S et al. (2013) Mutations in GDP-mannose pyrophosphorylase B cause congenital and limb-girdle muscular dystrophies associated with hypoglycosylation of alpha-dystroglycan. *Am J Hum Genet* 93: 29–41.

Chemla JC, Kanter RJ, Carboni MP, Smith E C (2010) Two children with "dropped head" syndrome due to lamin A/C mutations. *Muscle Nerve* 42: 839–841.

Collins J, Bonnemann C G (2010) Congenital muscular dystrophies: toward molecular therapeutic interventions. *Curr Neurol Neurosci Rep* 10: 83–91.

Dobyns WB, Pagon RA, Armstrong D, Curry CJ, Greenberg F, Grix A et al. (1989) Diagnostic criteria for Walker–Warburg syndrome. *Am J Med Genet* 32: 195–210.

Driss A, Amouri R, BEN Hamida C, Souilem S, Gouider-Khouja N, BEN Hamida M et al. (2000) A new locus for autosomal recessive limb-girdle muscular dystrophy in a large consanguineous Tunisian family maps to chromosome 19q13.3. *Neuromuscul Disord* 10: 240–246.

Eagle M, Bourke J, Bullock R, Gibson M, Mehta J, Giddings D et al. (2007) Managing Duchenne muscular dystrophy – the additive effect of spinal surgery and home nocturnal ventilation in improving survival. *Neuromuscul Disord* 17: 470–475.

Ferreiro A, Quijano-Roy S, Pichereau C, Moghadaszadeh B, Goemans N, Bonnemann C et al. (2002) Mutations of the selenoprotein N gene, which is implicated in rigid spine muscular dystrophy, cause the classical phenotype of multiminicore disease: reassessing the nosology of early-onset myopathies. *Am J Hum Genet* 71: 739–749.

Fukuyama Y, Osawa M, Suzuki H (1981) Congenital progressive muscular dystrophy of the Fukuyama type – clinical, genetic and pathological considerations. *Brain Dev* 3: 1–29.

Geranmayeh F, Clement E, Feng LH, Sewry C, Pagan J, Mein R et al. (2010) Genotype-phenotype correlation in a large population of muscular dystrophy patients with LAMA2 mutations. *Neuromuscul Disord* 20: 241–250.

Hayashi YK, Chou FL, Engvall E, Ogawa M, Matsuda C, Hirabayashi S et al. (1998) Mutations in the integrin alpha7 gene cause congenital myopathy. *Nat Genet* 19: 94–97.

Helbling-Leclerc A, Zhang X, Topaloglu H, Cruaud C, Tesson F, Weissenbach J et al. (1995) Mutations in the laminin alpha 2-chain gene (LAMA2) cause merosin-deficient congenital muscular dystrophy. *Nat Genet* 11: 216–218.

Jones KJ, Morgan G, Johnston H, Tobias V, Ouvrier RA, Wilkinson I et al. (2001) The expanding phenotype of laminin alpha2 chain (merosin) abnormalities: case series and review. *J Med Genet* 38: 649–657.

Kang PB, Morrison L, Iannaccone ST, Graham RJ, Bonnemann CG, Rutkowski A et al. (2015) Evidence-based guideline summary: evaluation, diagnosis, and management of congenital muscular dystrophy: Report of the Guideline Development Subcommittee of the American Academy of Neurology and the Practice Issues Review Panel of the American Association of Neuromuscular & Electrodiagnostic Medicine. *Neurology* 84: 1369–1378.

Mah JK, Korngut L, Fiest KM, Dykeman J, Day LJ, Pringsheim T et al. (2016) A systematic review and meta-analysis on the epidemiology of the muscular dystrophies. *Can J Neurol Sci* 43: 163–177.

Marino M, Stoilova T, Giorgi C, Bachi A, Cattaneo A, Auricchio A et al. (2015) SEPN1, an endoplasmic reticulum-localized selenoprotein linked to skeletal muscle pathology, counteracts hyperoxidation by means of redox-regulating SERCA2 pump activity. *Hum Mol Genet* 24: 1843–1855.

Mercuri E, Gruter-Andrew J, Philpot J, Sewry C, Counsell S, Henderson S et al. (1999) Cognitive abilities in children with congenital muscular dystrophy: correlation with brain MRI and merosin status. Neuromuscul Disord 9: 383–387.

Mercuri E, Brown SC, Nihoyannopoulos P, Poulton J, Kinali M, Richard P et al. (2005) Extreme variability of skeletal and cardiac muscle involvement in patients with mutations in exon 11 of the lamin A/C gene. *Muscle Nerve* 31: 602–609.

Mercuri E, Clements E, Offiah A, Pichiecchio A, Vasco G, Bianco F et al. (2010) Muscle magnetic resonance imaging involvement in muscular dystrophies with rigidity of the spine. *Ann Neurol* 67: 201–208.

Meune C, Van Berlo JH, Anselme F, Bonne G, Pinto YM, Duboc et al. (2006) Primary prevention of sudden death in patients with lamin A/C gene mutations. *N Engl J Med* 354: 209–210.

Moghadaszadeh B, Petit N, Jaillard C, Brockington M, Quijano-Roy S, Merlini L et al. (2001) Mutations in SEPN1 cause congenital muscular dystrophy with spinal rigidity and restrictive respiratory syndrome. *Nat Genet* 29: 17–18.

Murakami T, Hayashi YK, Noguchi S, Ogawa M, Nonaka I, Tanabe Y et al. (2006) Fukutin gene mutations cause dilated cardiomyopathy with minimal muscle weakness. *Ann Neurol* 60: 597–602.

Narayanaswami P, Weiss M, Selcen D, David W, Raynor E, Carter G et al. (2014) Evidence-based guideline summary: diagnosis and treatment of limb-girdle and distal dystrophies: report of the Guideline Development Subcommittee of the American Academy of Neurology and the Practice Issues Review Panel of the American Association of Neuromuscular & Electrodiagnostic Medicine. *Neurology* 83: 1453–1463.

Osawa M, Arai Y, Ikenaka H, Murasugi H, Sugahara N, Sumida S et al. (1991) Fukuyama type congenital progressive muscular dystrophy. *Acta Paediatr Jpn* 33: 261–269.

Philpot J, Pennock J, Cowan F, Sewry CA, Dubowitz V, Bydder G et al. (2000) Brain magnetic resonance imaging abnormalities in merosin-positive congenital muscular dystrophy. *Eur J Paediatr Neurol* 4: 109–114.

Quijano-Roy S, Mbieleu B, Bonnemann CG, Jeannet PY, Colomer J, Clarke NF et al. (2008) De novo LMNA mutations cause a new form of congenital muscular dystrophy. *Ann Neurol* 64: 177–186.

Rooney J, Byrne S, Heverin M, Tobin K, Dick A, Donaghy C et al. (2015) A multidisciplinary clinic approach improves survival in ALS: a comparative study of ALS in Ireland and Northern Ireland. *J Neurol Neurosurg Psychiatry* 86: 496–501.

Santavuori P, Somer H, Sainio K, Rapola J, Kruus S, Nikitin T et al. (1989) Muscle-eye-brain disease (MEB). *Brain Dev* 11: 147–153.

Schorling DC, Kirschner J, Bonnemann C G (2017) Congenital muscular dystrophies and myopathies: an overview and update. *Neuropediatrics* 48: 247–261.

Shorer Z, Philpot J, Muntoni F, Sewry C, Dubowitz V (1995) Demyelinating peripheral neuropathy in merosin-deficient congenital muscular dystrophy. *J Child Neurol* 10: 472–475.

Tomé FM, Evangelista T, Leclerc A, Sunada Y, Manole E, Estournet B et al. (1994) Congenital muscular dystrophy with merosin deficiency. *C R Acad Sci III,* 317: 351–357.

Ullrich O (1930) Kongenitale atonisch-sklerotische Muskeldystrophie, ein weiterer Typus der heredodegenerativen Erkrankungen des neuromuskulären Systems. *Z Gesamte Neurol Psychiatr* 126: 171–201.

Warburg M (1978) Hydrocephaly, congenital retinal nonattachment, and congenital falciform fold. *Am J Ophthalmol* 85: 88–94.

Zhou C, Li C, Zhou B, Sun H, Koullourou V, Holt I et al. (2017) Novel nesprin-1 mutations associated with dilated cardiomyopathy cause nuclear envelope disruption and defects in myogenesis. *Hum Mol Genet* 26: 2258–2276.

# 13
# FACIOSCAPULOHUMERAL MUSCULAR DYSTROPHY

*Nicolas Deconinck*

For an introduction to Muscular Dystrophies, please see Chapter 10 (page 166).

## Introduction

Facioscapulohumeral dystrophy (FSHD) is a muscular dystrophy characterized by progressive weakness and atrophy of the facial (facio-), shoulder–upper arm (scapulohumeral-), axial-, and leg muscles (Padberg 1982; Tawil and Van Der Maarel 2006; Mul et al. 2016). FSHD is one of the most prevalent muscular dystrophies with an estimated prevalence of 12 in 100 000 (Deenen et al. 2014). One of the hallmarks of FSHD is its clinical heterogeneity; the spectrum varies from severely affected, wheelchair-bound children to asymptomatic carriers in late adulthood, even within families with the same repeat contraction of the polymorphic D4Z4 macrosatellite repeat array (Padberg 1982; Gaillard et al. 2014; Tonini et al. 2004) (see the Genetics, epigenetics and pathology section). Typically, FSHD has an onset in adolescence and life expectancy is not impaired (Richard et al. 2014). However, a subgroup of patients with a childhood-onset, also called infantile FSHD (IFSHD), is associated with more severe disease progression. FSHD is increasingly recognized as an epigenetic disease which could be an explanation for its clinical heterogeneity.

## Classification and prevalence

Traditionally, children with IFSHD (Brooke, 1977) have been classified as a distinct disease identity based on the following criteria (Brouwer et al. 1994):

- signs or symptoms of facial weakness before the age of 5, and
- signs or symptoms of scapular weakness before the age of 10.

Accordingly, recent articles mostly classify the disease severity according to the repeat length of the genetic defect in FSHD type 1 (Trevisan et al. 2008; Chen et al. 2013; Nikolic et al. 2016). However, the correlation between disease severity and repeat length is inconsistent and is influenced by other genetic and environmental modifiers (Sacconi et al. 2013; Lemmers et al. 2015; Himeda et al. 2014). A generally accepted definition of severely affected FSHD, or early-onset classic patients, is currently lacking.

Studies investigating the prevalence of IFSHD are scarce and have used different selection criteria. Estimations of early-onset FSHD vary between 3–21% of the total FSHD population (Padberg 1982; Dorobek et al. 2015) and 58% of the pediatric FSHD population (onset at any age <18 years) (Klinge et al. 2006).

**Typical muscle symptoms**

One of the main characteristics of FSHD is the early and often asymmetrical involvement of the facial muscles. Facial weakness is not necessarily present, and it often goes unrecognized. The most obviously affected facial muscles are the orbicularis oculi and oris. Weakness of the orbicularis oculi may lead to incomplete eye closure, which may cause Bell phenomenon, exposure keratitis, and corneal scarring.

Over 80% of patients notice shoulder-girdle weakness as the first symptom of the disease (Fig. 13.1). Limited anteflexion and abduction, and abduction due to weakness of the scapulofixators, causes difficulties in handling objects above shoulder height; for example, when combing hair. When attempting anteflexion of the arms one can see a characteristic high rise of the winged scapula due to relative preservation of the deltoid muscle. Weakness typically spreads to the upper arm affecting the triceps, followed by the biceps and brachioradialis although progression beyond the shoulder is never observed in about 30% of patients (Tyler and Stephens 1950; Flanigan et al. 2001). At the same stage most patients develop foot extensor weakness. Very occasionally, foot drop may be the presenting symptom.

In about one-fifth of cases with progression beyond shoulder-girdle involvement, weakness of the pelvic girdle and upper legs precedes that of the lower legs. Pelvic-girdle weakness gives a waddling gait and difficulties in rising from a chair or climbing stairs.

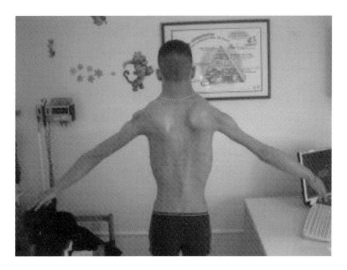

**Fig. 13.1.** A 15-year-old patient with a facioscapulohumeral dystrophy diagnosis. Notice the severe shoulder-girdle weakness with limited abduction of the arms due to the weakness of the scapulofixator muscles. This causes difficulties in handling objects above shoulder height. Notice the rise of the winged scapula and the relative preservation of deltoid muscles.

**Extramuscular symptoms**

Various extramuscular symptoms such as epilepsy, hearing difficulties, retinal abnormalities (Coats syndrome), intellectual disability and cardiac arrhythmias are associated with FSHD and they are most frequently described in the early-onset subgroup (Brouwer et al. 1994; Trevisan et al. 2008; Chen et al. 2013; Nikolic et al. 2016; Klinge et al. 2006; Funakoshi et al. 1998; Lutz et al. 2013) but with little knowledge regarding their prevalence and etiology.

**Genetics, epigenetics and pathology**

FSHD is increasingly recognized as an epigenetic disease. The most frequent cause of FSHD is contraction of the polymorphic D4Z4 macrosatellite repeat array in the subtelomere of chromosome 4 at 4q35 resulting in FSHD type 1 (FSHD1) (Wijmenga et al. 1990). This mutation explains more than 95% of the adult cases and all known infantile cases. Healthy individuals have between 11 and 100 D4Z4 repeat units on each 4q35 copy, whereas patients with FSHD1 have 1–10 repeats on one copy of the 4q35 chromosome region and a disease-permissive allele 4A on the chromosome 4q subtelomere.

Each D4Z4 repeat contains an open reading frame that encodes for the *DUX4* retrogene. Although the exact role of DUX4 is still being investigated, DUX4 protein expression causes cell death in several tissues, particularly in muscle tissue. In healthy patients with the absence of a polyadenylation (poly A) signal, transcripts from the *DUX4* retrogene are generally not stable (4B non-permissive allele). In contrast the 4A permissive allele contains an additional *DUX4* exon which provides the transcript with a poly A signal that enables the stabilization of the *DUX4* transcript emanating from the distal D4Z4 unit; hence, explaining its muscle toxicity (Lemmers et al. 2002).

However, the inverse correlation between residual repeat length and disease severity (short repeat lengths are associated with an earlier onset, wheelchair-dependency and extramuscular involvement) (Lunt et al. 1995; Tawil et al. 1996) is imperfect; for example, it does not explain the intra-familial differences in phenotype. Other mechanisms, such as aberrant epigenetic regulation of the D4Z4 chromatin structure, are thought to play an important role in explaining this clinical heterogeneity. Epigenetic disruptions in FSHD include chromatin relaxation through the *SMCHD1* or *DNMT3B* gene defects causing FSHD type 2 (FSHD2) (Sacconi et al. 2013; Lemmers et al. 2012), hypomethylation (Lemmers et al. 2015), alternative RNA splicing and nucleosome remodeling (Himeda et al. 2014). Investigating novel (epi)genetic characteristics in children with FSHD and linking this genetic profile to disease severity and age at onset will contribute to better predictors of prognosis and understanding of the pathogenesis.

Recently, several studies showing magnetic resonance imaging (MRI) changes (in particular with the use of the short tau inversion recovery [STIR] signal, which is sensitive to the presence of free water in tissues) in FSHD muscle suggest that MRI might be a measure of disease progression and a method to identify muscles with active disease based on histopathology and/or DUX4 expression (Hamel and Tawil, 2018).

**Management**

Specific etiology-related effective treatments are still lacking in FSHD. None of the following drugs showed any significant improvement in the context of clinical placebo-controlled trials: steroids, salbutamol, creatine, calcium antagonists (diltiazem), myostatin neutralizing antibodies (MYO-029) (Van der Kooi et al. 2014).

However, targeted therapies for FSHD focusing on disrupting *DUX4* expression or blocking one or more of several downstream effects of DUX4 are being developed by several pharmaceutical companies. A better understanding of the relationship between DUX4 activity, muscle pathology and muscle MRI changes will be crucial both to understand disease mechanisms and for the design of well designed future clinical trials (Hamel and Tawil 2018).

The absence of current therapeutic treatment makes interventions aimed at the preservation of muscle function and the patient's functional capabilities of major importance and this is achieved in the context of a multidisciplinary team involving close interactions between physiotherapists, orthopedics and pediatric sub-specialties. Surgical and non-surgical approaches for scapular winging and foot drop are possible and regular physiotherapy training is recommended (Orrell et al. 2010). These approaches are detailed in Chapter 23.

Clinically significant hearing loss (high-frequency bilateral sensorineural) appears to be a prominent feature of infantile-onset FSHD. Audiological evaluation is advised in these patients as hearing aids may be necessary.

The European Neuromuscular Centre recommends that patients with FSHD, particularly children with early-onset disease, should be referred to an ophthalmologist for dilated ophthalmoscopy to exclude the eventuality of a symptomatic exsudative retinopathy (Coat syndrome) that would require timely photocoagulation to preserve sight.

Sometimes, incomplete lid closure may lead to exposure keratitis and corneal scarring that requires eye drops, cream or eye patches (Van der Kooi et al. 2014).

Although very rare, tongue atrophy and dysphagia have been reported in early-onset FSHD, typically associated with more pronounced general and facial weakness. Patients with swallowing difficulties should be referred to a speech therapist. Speech therapy is also recommended for young patients with articulation problems due to orofacial weakness. Aspiration pneumonia has been reported, albeit rarely, in FSHD. Seizures have been described, although the exact incidence is not known. Their management is standard.

**Key points**
- Infantile FSHD (IFSHD) with onset in infancy or early childhood is a rare condition and has a more severe course than in adult-onset FSHD1. What makes the disease more severe has not been thoroughly elucidated, but patients tend to have larger deletions in *D4Z4*.
- Both genetic mechanisms of FSHD1 and FSHD2 converge at the level of chromatin relaxation, transcription of *DUX4* mRNA, and inappropriate expression of DUX4 protein in myonuclei. There is consensus that *DUX4* expression is toxic to skeletal muscle and causes FSHD.
- The absence of therapeutic treatment makes interventions aimed at the preservation of muscle function and the patient's functional capabilities of major importance and this is achieved in the context of a multidisciplinary team involving close interactions between physiotherapists, orthopedics and pediatric sub-specialties.

• Patients suffering from IFSHD should be screened for hearing loss and vision problems (Coats disease and retinal telangiectasia).

## REFERENCES

Brooke MH (1977) Clinical examination of patients with neuromuscular disease. *Adv Neurol* 17: 25–39.

Brouwer OF, Padberg GW, Wijmenga C, Frants RR (1994) Facioscapulohumeral muscular dystrophy in early childhood. *Arch Neurol* 51: 387–394.

Chen TH, Lai YH, Lee PL, Hsu JH, Goto K, Hayashi YK et al. (2013) Infantile facioscapulohumeral muscular dystrophy revisited: expansion of clinical phenotypes in patients with a very short EcoRI fragment. *Neuromuscul Disord* 23: 298–305.

Deenen JC, Arnts H, van der Maarel SM, Padberg GW, Verschuuren JJ, Bakker E et al. (2014) Population-based incidence and prevalence of facioscapulohumeral dystrophy. *Neurology* 83: 1056–1059.

Dorobek M, van der Maarel SM, Lemmers RJ, Ryniewicz B, Kabzińska D, Frants RR et al. (2015) Early-onset facioscapulohumeral muscular dystrophy type 1 with some atypical features. *J Child Neurol* 30: 580–587.

Flanigan KM, Coffeen CM, Sexton L, Stauffer D, Brunner S, Leppert MF (2001) Genetic characterization of a large, historically significant Utah kindred with facioscapulohumeral dystrophy. *Neuromuscul Disord* 11: 525–529.

Funakoshi M, Goto K, Arahata K (1998) Epilepsy and mental retardation in a subset of early onset 4q35-facioscapulohumeral muscular dystrophy. *Neurology* 50: 1791–1794.

Gaillard MC, Roche S, Dion C, Tasmadjian A, Bouget G, Salort-Campana E et al. (2014) Differential DNA methylation of the D4Z4 repeat in patients with FSHD and asymptomatic carriers. *Neurology* 83: 733–742.

Hamel J, Tawil R (2018) Facioscapulohumeral muscular dystrophy: update on pathogenesis and future treatments. *Neurotherapeutics* 15(4):863–871. doi: 10.1007/s13311-018-00675-3.

Himeda CL, Debarnot C, Homma S, Beermann ML, Miller JB, Jones PL et al. (2014) Myogenic enhancers regulate expression of the facioscapulohumeral muscular dystrophy-associated DUX4 gene. *Mol Cell Biol* 34: 1942–1955.

Klinge L, Eagle M, Haggerty ID, Roberts CE, Straub V, Bushby KM (2006) Severe phenotype in infantile facioscapulohumeral muscular dystrophy. *Neuromuscul Disord* 16: 553–558.

Lemmers RJ, de Kievit P, Sandkuijl L, Padberg GW, van Ommen GJ, Frants RR et al. (2002) Facioscapulo-humeral muscular dystrophy is uniquely associated with one of the two variants of the 4q subtelomere. *Nat Genet* 32: 235–236.

Lemmers RJ, van der Vliet PJ, Klooster R, Sacconi S, Camaño P, Dauwerse JG et al. (2010) A unifying genetic model for facioscapulohumeral muscular dystrophy. Science 329: 1650–1653.

Lemmers RJ, Tawil R, Petek LM, Balog J, Block GJ, Santen GW et al. (2012) Digenic inheritance of an SMCHD1 mutation and an FSHD-permissive D4Z4 allele causes facioscapulohumeral muscular dystrophy type 2. Nat Genet 44: 1370–1374.

Lemmers RJ, Goeman JJ, van der Vliet PJ, van Nieuwenhuizen MP, Balog J, Vos-Versteeg M et al. (2015) Inter-individual differences in CpG methylation at D4Z4 correlate with clinical variability in FSHD1 and FSHD2. *Hum Mol Genet* 24: 659–669.

Lunt PW, Jardine PE, Koch MC, Maynard J, Osborn M, Williams M et al. (1995) Correlation between fragment size at D4F104S1 and age at onset or at wheelchair use, with a possible generational effect, accounts for much phenotypic variation in 4q35-facioscapulohumeral muscular dystrophy (FSHD). *Hum Mol Genet* 4: 951–958.

Lutz KL, Holte L, Kliethermes SA, Stephan C, Mathews KD (2013) Clinical and genetic features of hearing loss in facioscapulohumeral muscular dystrophy. *Neurology* 81: 1374–1377.

Mul K, Lassche S, Voermans NC, Padberg GW, Horlings CG, van Engelen BG (2016) What's in a name? The clinical features of facioscapulohumeral muscular dystrophy. *Pract Neurol* 16: 201–207.

Nikolic A, Ricci G, Sera F, Bucci E, Govi M, Mele F et al. (2016) Clinical expression of facioscapulohumeral muscular dystrophy in carriers of 1–3 D4Z4 reduced alleles: experience of the FSHD Italian National Registry. *BMJ Open* 6:e007798.

Orrell RW, Copeland S, Rose MR (2010) Scapular fixation in muscular dystrophy. *Cochrane Database Syst Rev* 1:CD003278.

Padberg GW (1982) Facioscapulohumeral Disease (thesis). Leiden: Leiden University.

Richard JLF, Lemmers P, Daniel G, van der Maare SM (2014) Facioscapulohumeral Muscular Dystrophy. 1999 Mar 8 [Updated 2014 Mar 20]. In: Adam MP, Ardinger HH, Pagon RA et al. (eds). GeneReviews® [Internet]. Seattle (WA): University of Washington, Seattle. https://www.ncbi.nlm.nih.gov/books/NBK1443/.

Sacconi S, Lemmers RJ, Balog J, van der Vliet PJ, Lahaut P, van Nieuwenhuizen MP et al. (2013) The FSHD2 gene SMCHD1 is a modifier of disease severity in families affected by FSHD1. *Am J Hum Genet* 93: 744–751.

Tawil R, Forrester J, Griggs RC, Mendell J, Kissel J, McDermott M et al. (1996) Evidence for anticipation and association of deletion size with severity in facioscapulohumeral muscular dystrophy. *Ann Neurol* 39: 744–748.

Tawil R, Van Der Maarel SM (2006) Facioscapulohumeral muscular dystrophy. *Muscle Nerve* 34: 1–15.

Tonini MM, Pavanello RC, Gurgel-Giannetti J, Lemmers RJ, van der Maarel SM, Frants RR et al. (2004) Homozygosity for autosomal dominant facioscapulohumeral muscular dystrophy (FSHD) does not result in a more severe phenotype. *J Med Genet* 41:e17.

Trevisan CP, Pastorello E, Tomelleri G, Vercelli L, Bruno C, Scapolan S et al. (2008) Facioscapulohumeral muscular dystrophy: hearing loss and other atypical features of patients with large 4q35 deletions. *Eur J Neurol* 15: 1353–1358.

Tyler FH, Stephens FE (1950) Studies in disorders of muscle. II Clinical manifestations and inheritance of facioscapulohumeral dystrophy in a large family. *Ann Intern Med* 32: 640–660.

Van der Kooi E, Van der Maarel S, Van Engelen B (2014) Facioscapulohumeral muscular dystrophy. In: Hilton-Jones D, Turner MR (eds) *Oxford Textbook of Neuromuscular Disorders*, Oxford: Oxford University Press, 254–263.

Wijmenga C, Frants RR, Brouwer OF, Moerer P, Weber JL, Padberg GW (1990) Location of facioscapulohumeral muscular dystrophy gene on chromosome 4. *Lancet* 336: 651–653.

# 14
# CONGENITAL MYOPATHIES

*Sandra Coppens*

## Introduction

The congenital myopathies (CM) are a broad group of genetic muscle disorders characterized by hypotonia and muscle weakness with a neonatal or early onset and a stable or slowly progressive course. The prevalence of congenital myopathies was estimated at 1 in 26 000 in the United States (Amburgey et al. 2011) and at 1 in 20 000 in Sweden (Darin and Tulinius 2000).

## Classification

Classically, congenital myopathies are classified into four main subtypes based on the main histological findings from muscle biopsies (Fig. 14.1):

- nemaline myopathies (NM);
- core myopathies (central core disease [CCD] or multiminicore disease [MmD]);
- congenital fibre type disproportion (CFTD);
- centronuclear myopathies (CNM).

It is important to note that many patients with congenital myopathies cannot be classified into one of these four main histological subtypes due to the presence of non-specific changes in the muscle biopsy or to the presence of features overlapping several histological subtypes. Muscle biopsy alone is often not sufficient for an efficient aetiologic diagnosis of the congenital myopathies (North et al. 2014). Combining clinical assessment, muscle histology, muscle magnetic resonance imaging (MRI) and modern genetic tools now allows a rapid and efficient aetiologic diagnosis in more than 50% of patients with a congenital myopathy.

## Clinical features

The first signs of the congenital myopathies can be present during the prenatal period with decreased fetal movements, polyhydramnios and joint contractures (club feet, arthrogryposis). Prematurity is more frequent in patients with congenital myopathies (especially with *MTM1*-related myopathy). At birth, patients are usually hypotonic (floppy infant) and weak, in contrast to babies with central nervous system lesions that are hypotonic but have a normal limb strength. Some congenital myopathies patients have a myopathic facies (long and narrow facies with open mouth), ophthalmoplegia and signs of bulbar weakness (difficulty with sucking and swallowing, weak cry, high-arched palate). At examination, patients

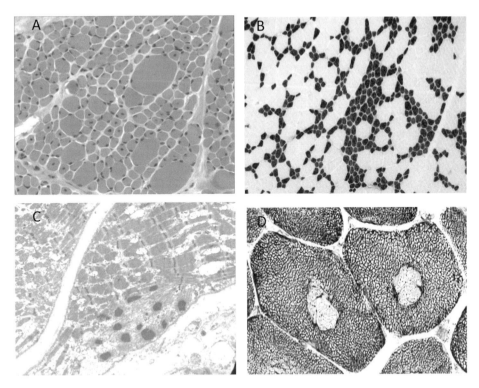

**Fig. 14.1.** Definitions and illustrations of histological subtypes. **A** Haematoxylin-eosin staining showing an increase in the number of fibres with centralized nuclei, characteristic of centronuclear myopathy (magnification ×160). **B** ATPase (pH 4.6) staining showing type 1 fibre predominance and selective type 1 fibre hypotrophy compared to type 2 fibres, characteristic of congenital fibre type disproportion myopathy (magnification ×200). **C** Electron microscopy showing nemaline rods and disruption of the sarcomere, characteristic of nemaline myopathy (magnification ×4 400). **D** NADH staining with core-like image in two fibres (magnification ×800). Courtesy of Prof. Hazim Kadhim, Department of Anatomic Pathology and Reference Center for Neuromuscular Pathology, Brugmann University Hospital, Université Libre de Bruxelles (ULB).

display an abnormal traction response with head lag. On vertical suspension, they slip through the examiner's hands because of the weakness of the shoulder girdle. Lower limbs are extended and externally rotated (frog-legged lower limb posture) with few or absent spontaneous movements. Reflexes are depressed or absent. Contractures are usually milder than in congenital muscular dystrophies or COL6-related myopathies but Achilles tendon contractures are frequent. Intellect is usually normal (North et al. 2014).

The presence or absence of extraocular muscle weakness can help to guide the genetic diagnosis. Ophthalmoplegia is common in centronuclear myopathies (associated with *MTM1*, *BIN1*, *DNM2* mutations); in multi-minicore myopathies associated with *RYR1* mutations and in myopathies associated with *MYH2* mutations. The presence of ophthalmoplegia should also make the consultant consider alternative diagnoses, such as neuromuscular junction diseases, mitochondrial myopathies and Moebius syndrome. Some mutations in the *TPM2* and

*TPM3* genes are associated with a hypercontractile phenotype with congenital muscle stiffness and frequent contractures (Marttila et al. 2014). For some genes (*SEPN1, ACTA1*), there is a clinical overlap between congenital myopathies phenotypes and congenital muscular dystrophy with rigid spine phenotypes (Moghadaszadeh et al. 2001; O'Grady et al. 2015).

If weakness is mild, patients may not present until infancy or early childhood. Children can present with a delay in the development of motor milestones (sitting, walking) or even later with difficulties for walking long distances, running or climbing stairs. The clinical course of congenital myopathies is usually stable or only slowly progressive. However, in a natural history study of congenital myopathies, 9% of ambulant patients lose their ability to walk and become wheelchair-dependant. Those patients were always late walkers and it is suggested that weight gain could be implicated (Colombo et al. 2015).

Involvement of the respiratory muscles is common in many forms of congenital myopathy and may necessitate mechanical ventilation. Untreated hypoventilation with chronic hypoxemia and hypercapnia can lead to right-heart failure or sudden death, but non-invasive nocturnal ventilation is almost always effective if patients can tolerate it. Respiratory impairment can increase with age. For this reason, careful monitoring of respiratory function with lung function tests and/or sleep studies is very important in congenital myopathies (Rutkowski et al. 2015).

Primary cardiac involvement is very rare in congenital myopathies but has been infrequently described in association with *ACTA1, DNM2, TPM2* mutations (Wang et al. 2012), and with some newly described congenital myopathy genes (see Table 14.1).

**Investigations**

Creatine kinase (CK) levels are usually normal or only mildly elevated (<3 × normal) in congenital myopathies. Elevated creatine kinase (>3 × normal) should suggest a diagnosis of congenital muscular dystrophy. Nerve conduction tests are usually normal and electromyography (EMG) may be normal or show myopathic changes in congenital myopathies. EMG can be useful to exclude a differential diagnosis with congenital myasthenic syndromes or motor neuron diseases.

Muscle MRI can be of significant help for the diagnosis of congenital myopathies, as many congenital myopathies present with a distinguishable pattern of muscle involvement on MRI (Quijano-Roy et al. 2011). For example, in *RYR1*-related myopathy, the gluteus maximus (GM) is the most severely affected muscle. In the thigh, the anterior compartment is more severely affected than the posterior compartment. Sparing of the rectus femoris (RF), adductor longus (AL) and gracilis (GRA) is common. In the lower leg, the soleus is more affected than the gastrocnemius (Klein et al. 2011, see Fig. 14.2). In *SEPN1*-related myopathy, the gastrocnemius is more affected than the soleus. Whole-body MRI might also help to differentiate *SEPN1*-related myopathy as there is a severe involvement of the sternocleidomastoid muscle (SCM) (Hankiewicz et al. 2015).

**Genetic diagnosis**

Mutations in 25 different genes have already been implicated in the congenital myopathies. Many mutations involved in the congenital myopathies reside in genes encoding for proteins

**TABLE 14.1**
**Genes implicated in early-onset congenital myopathies**

| Nemaline myopathy (NEM) | Core myopathy |
|---|---|
| *NEM1*; α-tropomyosin 3 (*TPM3*): AR/AD | *RYR1*: AD/AR (CCD or MmD) |
| *NEM2*; Nebulin (*NEB*): AR | *SEPN1*: AR (MmD) |
| *NEM3*; α-Actin (*ACTA1*): AR/AD | *MEGF10*: AR (MmD); also implicated in |
| *NEM4*; β-tropomyosin (*TPM2*): AR/AD | Early-onset myopathy, areflexia, respiratory distress |
| *NEM5*; Troponin T1 (*TNNT1*): AR | and dysphagia – EMARDD |
| *NEM6*; *KBTBD13*: AD | *CCDC78*: AD (+ central nuclei) |
| *NEM7*; Cofilin-2 (*CFN2*): AR | *MYH7*: AD (+ cardiopathy) |
| *NEM8*; *KLHL40*: AR | |
| *NEM9*; *KLHL41*: AR | |
| *NEM10*; *LMOD3*: AR | |
| *NEM11*; MYPN: AR | |
| *MYO18B* (+ cardiopathy) | |
| *TNNT3*: AR | |

| Congenital fibre type disproportion (CFTD) | Centronuclear myopathy (CNM) |
|---|---|
| *CFTD1*; *ACTA1*: AD | *CNMX*; *MTM1* |
| *CFTD2*; *Xq13*: Recessive | *CNM1*; *DNM2*: AD |
| *CFTD3*; *SEPN1*: AR | *CNM2*; *BIN1*: AR/AD |
| *CFTD4*; *TPM3*: AD | *CNM3*; *MYF6*: AD |
| *CFTD5*; *TPM2*: AD | *CNM4*; *CCDC78*: AD (+ atypical cores) |
| *MYL2*: AR | *CNM5* (+ *DCM*): SPEG: AR |
| *PTPLA*: AR | *CNM6*; *ZAK*: AR |
| *MYH7*: AD | *RYR1*: AR |
| | *TTN*: AR |

| Other congenital myopathies | |
|---|---|
| *MYMK*: AR; Carey-Fineman-Ziter Syndrome (CM with Möbius and Robin sequences) | *CACNA1S*: AR; CM with ophthalmoplegia |
| *MYBPC3*: AR; Congenital skeletal myopathy and fatal cardiomyopathy | *SPTBN4*: AR; CM with neuropathy and deafness |
| *CNTN1*: AR; Congenital lethal myopathy | *MAP3K20*: AR; CM with neuropathy and deafness |
| *SCN4A*: AR; CM linked to AR *SCN4A* mutations | *HRAS*: AR/AD; CM with excess of muscle spindles |
| | *PYROXD1*: AR; Early-onset myopathy with internal nuclei and myofibrillar disorganization |
| | *SECISBP2*: AR; multisystem selenoprotein deficiency (photosensitivity, azoospermia) |

AR: autosomal recessive inheritance; AD: autosomal dominant inheritance; CM: congenital myopathy.
Adapted from the Neuromuscular Disorders gene table, http://www.musclegenetable.fr/, WUSTL Neuromuscular, https://neuromuscular.wustl.edu/ and Pubmed searches, www.ncbi.nlm.nih.gov/pubmed/.

involved in the sarcomere structure (skeletal muscle alpha-actin, myosins, tropomyosins etc.) or in calcium release from the sarcoplasmic reticulum, a process also called excitation-contraction coupling (ryanodine receptor 1, myotubularin, dynamin 2 etc.) (Ravenscroft et al. 2015). With the widespread use of next generation sequencing (NGS), the phenotypic spectrum of mutations in several genes has been significantly expanded, blurring the boundaries between the classic histological subtypes of the congenital myopathies.

In a large natural history study of congenital myopathies, *RYR1* was the most frequently implicated gene (44% of patients) followed by *ACTA1* (17%), *SEPN1* (16%),

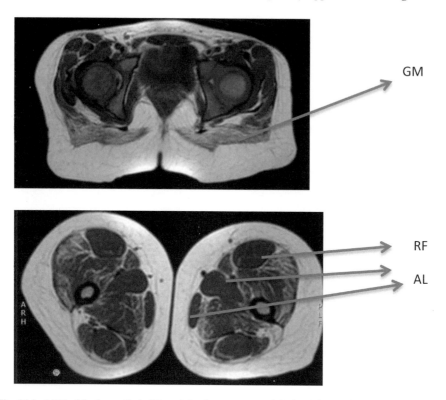

**Fig. 14.2.** MRI of the lower limb (T1-weighted sequences, axial plane) in a patient with *RYR1*-related myopathy showing a major involvement of the gluteus maximus (GM) and sparing of rectus femoris (RF), adductor longus (AL) and gracilis (GRA).

*MTM1* (8%) and *NEB* (8%) (Colombo et al. 2015). It is important to note that genetic diagnosis in this study was mostly performed with Sanger sequencing of dozens of genes. For the huge *NEB* and *RYR1* genes, only hotspot mutations were investigated. NGS allows a broader sequencing of *NEB* and *RYR1* but also of the biggest gene of the human genome, *TTN*, also responsible for some congenital myopathy phenotypes (Böhm et al. 2013). Many new genes responsible for the congenital myopathies have been discovered in recent years. In the future, the frequency of the different genes implicated should be reassessed in this context.

In the next section, some specific phenotypic and natural history features associated with the more frequent congenital myopathy genes of will be described.

### Phenotypic features of the most common congenital myopathy genes

RYR1-RELATED MYOPATHY

The *RYR1* gene encodes ryanodine receptor 1, the principal calcium release channel from the sarcoplasmic reticulum, and is thus implicated in excitation-contraction coupling. *RYR1* mutations are the most common cause of the congenital myopathies and can be transmitted in a dominant or in a recessive manner. Classically, *RYR1*-related myopathy is known to be associated with central core myopathy but 50% of the patients have another prominent histological pattern (for example, MmD, CNM, CFTD) (Amburgey et al. 2013). Onset of symptoms is usually at birth or in early childhood but can be delayed to late adulthood for some dominant mutations. Classically, patients present with congenital hypotonia and weakness, sometimes associated with hip dislocation. Patients have delayed motor milestones but finally acquire independent ambulation. Respiratory impairment is often mild. Rarely, *RYR1* mutations can be associated with fetal akinesia syndrome or severe neonatal presentations with respiratory insufficiency and severe early-onset scoliosis with some motor improvement, but generally no acquisition of independent ambulation. External ophthalmoparesis and facial weakness can be present but are more often associated with non-central core histological patterns (CNM, MmD, CFTD). Some *RYR1* mutations can also be associated with malignant hyperthermia susceptibility (MHS), a predisposition to adverse reactions with halogenated anaesthetics or succinylcholine, or with exertional rhabdomyolysis (ERM) (Jungbluth et al. 2016). Some *RYR1* mutations leading to MHS can also give rise to haemorrhagic disorders, the most common being severe menorrhagia and postpartum haemorrhage (Lopez et al. 2016).

## ACTA1-RELATED MYOPATHY

The *ACTA1* gene encodes the skeletal alpha-actin protein, the predominant actin isoform of the adult sarcomere. Mutations in *ACTA1* can lead to nemaline myopathy, intranuclear rod myopathy, actin myopathy and CFTD; 90% of *ACTA1*-related myopathies are caused by de novo dominant mutations and 10% by recessive truncating mutations (Nowak et al. 2013). The phenotype is often very severe with prenatal or neonatal onset. Patients present with severe weakness, hypotonia and severe respiratory insufficiency necessitating mechanical ventilation. Patients have a myopathic facies and difficulties for sucking and swallowing with an high-arched palate. Ophthalmoplegia is never present due to the expression of the cardiac alpha-actin in extraocular muscles. Death in the neonatal period is not infrequent. Some patients have a milder phenotype with predominant facial, bulbar, axial and respiratory weakness contrasting with a more preserved limb strength that can allow the acquisition of independent walking. Respiratory function should be monitored closely in those patients who often need nocturnal non-invasive ventilation (Wallgren-Pettersson et al. 2004).

## SEPN1-RELATED MYOPATHY

*SEPN1* encodes the selenoprotein N, an enzyme located at the membrane of the endoplasmic reticulum, where it is involved in redox and calcium homeostasis (Marino et al. 2015). *SEPN1*-related myopathy can be associated with several different histological patterns that often have in common the presence of multiminicores (Ferreiro et al. 2002). The natural history of *SEPN1*-related myopathy has been thoroughly described in a large cohort of 41 patients: 36% had a congenital onset with the most frequent symptom being neonatal hypotonia; 46% had an onset during the first few years of life with delayed motor milestones. All patients acquired independent ambulation and almost all maintained it throughout life.

The involvement of the neck, axial and respiratory muscles was particularly frequent and severe. Respiratory involvement required the use of nocturnal non-invasive ventilation in 50% and 75% of the patients at the age of 15 and 20 years, respectively. Abnormal nocturnal oxygen saturation can be present very early (2 years) suggesting that sleep studies should be started soon after diagnosis. Scoliosis affected 70% of patients with a mean age of 10 years and required spinal fusion in 34% at a mean age of 14 years. Spinal rigidity was frequently associated. Underweight was a frequent complication without obvious swallowing of chewing difficulties (Scoto et al. 2011).

MTM1-RELATED MYOPATHY

Mutations in the *MTM1* gene, encoding myotubularin, cause the very severe X-linked centronuclear myopathy (XLCNM) also called myotubular myopathy. Onset of the symptoms is often prenatal with poor fetal movements, polyhydramnios and frequent preterm births. Male patients present in the neonatal period with severe hypotonia, generalized weakness including face and eyes, respiratory insufficiency usually necessitating invasive ventilation and bulbar weakness requiring tube or gastrostomy feeding. The natural history of 50 patients with *MTM1* mutations surviving the neonatal period has been described (Amburgey et al. 2017): 96% of the patients need ventilator support, of which 76% have a tracheostomy and 66% need ventilation more than 16 hours a day. Only 11% are ambulant and 52% can sit when placed; 72% have scoliosis; 82% are fed by gastrostomy and most are seriously dependant for the activities of daily living. Mortality is lower than previously reported with only 76% of patients being alive at 10 years. Evolution of the disease is broadly stable. It is important to note that this study was carried out in North America where there is a higher level of medical intervention (invasive ventilation, gastrostomy) for *MTM1* patients compared to European countries. Patients harbouring non-truncating mutations tend to have a milder phenotype than patients with truncating mutations (McEntagart et al. 2002). Female carriers are usually asymptomatic or can present mild symptoms such as asymmetric weakness or growth or facial/ocular weakness. Nevertheless, some female carriers can have a more severe condition with mild to moderate limb weakness with or without respiratory impairment (Biancalana et al. 2017).

**Complications and their management**

Patients with congenital myopathies should be followed in a multidisciplinary neuromuscular clinic. Reaching a specific genetic diagnosis is very helpful for informing the family about prognosis and the recurrence risk for future pregnancies. A specific diagnosis can also help with closely monitoring the occurrence of complications that occur frequently with that specific diagnosis, and proposing participation in targeted therapy protocols.

Feeding and swallowing impairments are frequent in congenital myopathies especially during the first year of life. Growth and nutritional assessments are an essential part of the follow-up. Good positioning during meals and adaptation of the texture of food can be helpful in congenital myopathy patients with mild difficulties. Nasogastric tubes or gastrostomy tube insertion can be required especially if growth is delayed due to insufficient nutritional intake or if recurrent respiratory infections occur due to food aspiration.

ORTHOPAEDIC COMPLICATIONS

Regular exercise and stretching are essential to maintaining muscle strength and joint range of motion. Assistive mobility devices with adapted seating and/or environmental adaptations (ramps, shower chair etc.) should be provided when necessary to promote independent mobility and activities of daily living.

Some specific orthopaedic complications of the congenital myopathies will be discussed. Congenital hip dislocation is particularly common in *RYR1*-related myopathy and is mainly treated by abduction splinting. Splinting should not be extended beyond 3 months to avoid the occurrence of contractures. Contractures in knees and ankles are usually less severe than in the muscular dystrophies but are nevertheless frequent and should be managed carefully. Stretching and night splints can be useful. Occasionally, surgery is needed if the progression of contractures results in functional decline. Scoliosis is a common complication in congenital myopathies affecting 40% of patients, whether or not they are ambulant. A very regular clinical evaluation and if required a radiological evaluation is thus critical in the follow-up of congenital myopathies. Early scoliosis can be treated with spinal bracing. If it is required, surgical management is ideally delayed until adolescence when spinal growth is nearly achieved and allows treatment by definitive spinal fusion. If the progression of scoliosis is severe and surgery cannot be delayed, growing rods can correct and stabilize the spinal deformity while permitting further growth of the spine. Scoliosis is very often associated with respiratory impairment complicating the bracing and/or surgical management. Surgery is more often needed in patients with early and severe axial hypotonia and weakness such as patients with mutations in *SEPN1*, *MTM1*, *NEB*, or *TTN* (Wang et al. 2012).

RESPIRATORY COMPLICATIONS

Spirometry and respiratory muscle strength assessments are an essential part of the monitoring of most congenital myopathy patients. Abnormalities of breathing during sleep usually precede abnormalities during wakefulness. Thus, polysomnography with oxymetry and capnography should be performed periodically in patients with altered spirometry or in patients were spirometry is impossible (especially young patients under 5 years) to screen for nocturnal hypoventilation and obstructive apnoea. Respiratory impairment is mostly present in patients with poor axial tonus, no acquisition of walking or the presence of severe scoliosis with spinal rigidity (Rutkowski et al. 2015). Patients with *MTM1*, *SEPN1*, *ACTA1*, *TPM3*, *DNM2* and *NEB* mutations are considered as having a higher risk of severe respiratory impairent that can be out of proportion with the limb weakness. Those patients should thus be screened more often. Patients with respiratory impairment should benefit from influenza and pneumococcal vaccinations. If necessary secretion mobilization and assisted cough techniques should be used as well as nocturnal non-invasive ventilation. For more information about diagnosis and care of respiratory impairment, see Chapter 25.

MALIGNANT HYPERTHERMIA SUSCEPTIBILITY

Malignant hyperthermia susceptibility (MHS) should be considered in every patient with congenital myopathy who is undergoing anaesthesia, even if it is much more frequently associated with *RYR1* mutations. When possible, succinylcholine and halogenated anaesthetics should be avoided in congenital myopathy patients (Wang et al. 2012).

Carrier testing and appropriate genetic counselling should be proposed to the family members of patients with *RYR1*-related myopathy as the carrier status of some recessive *RYR1* mutations can be associated with MHS.

**Specific therapies**

Many animal/cellular models have been developed to dissect the physiopathological mechanisms of the congenital myopathies, paving the way for the development of targeted therapies (Ravenscroft et al. 2015). Besides treatment development, animal models could also be helpful in finding biomarkers which reflect the physiopathology of the different congenital myopathies.

The small numbers of patients and the involvement of many different genes in the congenital myopathies are major obstacles in the development of targeted therapies. International patient registries with detailed clinical and genetic information would greatly facilitate the recruitment of patients for clinical studies. Prospective multicentric natural history studies are also lacking for most of the congenital myopathies. These could help with the development of clinically relevant outcome measures, bearing in mind that the congenital myopathies are relatively stable in their evolution in contrast to the muscular dystrophies. Standardization of care for congenital myopathies between different neuromuscular centres would also facilitate the setting up of clinical trials (Wang et al. 2012).

Gene transfer therapy with adeno-associated virus 8 (AAV8) represents a promising approach for myotubular myopathy. The efficacy of systemic AAV8-mediated myotubularin delivery has been demonstrated in mice and dog models (Childers et al. 2014; Mack et al. 2017) and the first clinical trial in myotubular patients was started in September 2017 in the USA.

However, gene therapy with AAV8 is not well suited for the transfer of huge genes due to the limited cargo capacity of the adeno-associated virus, nor is it a suitable therapy for disease caused by dominant mutations with gain-of-function effects. In the future, genome engineering therapies using CRISPR-Cas9 could be a powerful approach for the correction of disease-causing mutations or for the repression of dominant disease-causing alleles in many neuromuscular disorders (Nelson et al. 2017).

Dynamin 2 modulation therapies have demonstrated their efficacy in a mouse model of myotubular myopathy and could also represent a promising approach for other types of congenital myopathy (Cowling et al. 2014; Cowling et al. 2017). N-acetylcysteine (NAC) has shown a decrease in oxidative stress and an improvement in muscle function in several animal models for *RYR1*- and *SEPN1*-related myopathy and are currently under investigation in clinical trials. Malignant hyperthermia and haemorrhagic disorders associated with *RYR1* mutations can be efficiently treated with dantrolene (Lopez et al. 2016).

**Key points**
• Congenital myopathies are characterized by early-onset hypotonia and muscle weakness with a stable or slowly progressive course.

- More than 25 genes have already been implicated in the congenital myopathies and new genes continue to be discovered each year.
- Clinical assessment, muscle biopsy and muscle MRI, together with modern genetic techniques, allow a precise aetiologic diagnosis in more than 50% of patients with a congenital myopathy.
- Scoliosis and respiratory insufficiency are major complications of congenital myopathies and should be monitored closely.
- *RYR1* mutations are the most common cause of congenital myopathies and can cause malignant hyperthermia susceptibility (MHS). Each child with congenital myopathies should be considered as being at risk for MHS and succinylcholine/halogenated anaesthetics should be avoided.

**Clinical vignette**

The patient was born preterm (31 weeks gestational age) from healthy non-consanguine-ous parents, after a pregnancy complicated by polyhydramnios. Immediately after birth, he required cardio-respiratory resuscitation and mechanical ventilation via a nasotracheal tube.

Physical examination showed hydrops fetalis, severe generalized hypotonia, lack of spontaneous movements, generalized areflexia, clinodactyly of the 2nd and 5th left fingers, high-arched palate and bilateral cryptorchidism. Sucking or swallowing movements were completely absent. No improvement in respiratory function was observed and the patient died at 2 months of age. Creatine kinase levels were normal. EMG showed no spontaneous activity and an absence of motor response upon electrostimulation. A muscle biopsy carried out at 20 days disclosed fibre atrophy and size variability at optic microscopy and severe myofibrillar disorganization (Fig. 14.3 A) with large zones of thin myofilament accumula-tion (Fig. 14.3 B) on electron microscopy. This picture was suggestive of actin myopathy and the sequencing of the *ACTA1* gene disclosed a de novo dominant c.442G>A (p.Gly-148Ser) mutation. This clinical vignette illustrates the severe prenatal onset phenotype frequently associated with *ACTA1* dominant mutations.

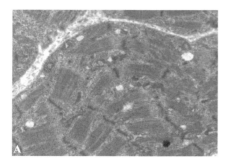 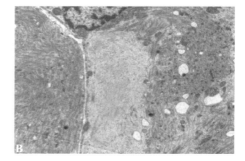

**Fig. 14.3.** Muscle biopsy showing fibre atrophy and size variability and focal myofibrillar disorga-nization. **A** Electron microscopy (magnification ×7 000) showing focal myofibrillar disorganization. **B** Electron microscopy (magnification ×4 400) showing large zones of accumulation of thin myofil-aments. Courtesy of Prof. Hazim Kadhim, Department of Anatomic Pathology and Reference Center for Neuromuscular Pathology, Brugmann University Hospital, Université Libre de Bruxelles (ULB).

## REFERENCES

Amburgey K, McNamara N, Bennett LR, McCormick ME, Acsadi G, Dowling JJ (2011) Prevalence of congenital myopathies in a representative pediatric united states population. *Ann Neurol* 70: 662–665.

Amburgey K, Bailey A, Hwang JH, Tarnopolsky MA, Bönnemann CG, Medne L et al. (2013) Genotype-phenotype correlations in recessive RYR1-related myopathies. *Orphanet J Rare Dis* 8: 117.

Amburgey K, Tsuchiya E, de Chastonay S, Glueck M, Alverez R, Nguyen CT et al. (2017) A natural history study of X-linked myotubular myopathy. *Neurology* 89: 1355–1364.

Biancalana V, Scheidecker S, Miguet M, Laquerrière A, Romero NB, Stojkovic T et al. (2017) Affected female carriers of MTM1 mutations display a wide spectrum of clinical and pathological involvement: delineating diagnostic clues. *Acta Neuropathol* 134: 889–904.

Böhm J, Vasli N, Malfatti E, Le Gras S, Feger C, Jost B et al. (2013) An integrated diagnosis strategy for congenital myopathies. *PLoS ONE* 8(6): p.e67527. doi: 10.1371/journal.pone.0067527.

Childers M, Joubert R, Poulard K, Moal C, Grange R, Doering J et al. (2014) Gene therapy prolongs survival and restores function in murine and canine models of myotubular myopathy. *Science Translational Medicine* 6(220): 220ra10. doi: 10.1126/scitranslmed.3007523.

Colombo I, Scoto M, Manzur AY, Robb SA, Maggi L, Gowda V et al. (2015) Congenital myopathies: natural history of a large pediatric cohort. *Neurology* 84: 28–35.

Cowling BS, Chevremont T, Prokic I, Kretz C, Ferry A, Coirault C et al. (2014) Reducing dynamin 2 expression rescues X-linked centronuclear myopathy. *J Clin Invest* 124: 1350–1363.

Cowling BS, Prokic I, Tasfaout H, Rabai A, Humbert F, Rinaldi B et al. (2017) Amphiphysin (BIN1) negatively regulates dynamin 2 for normal muscle maturation. *J Clin Invest* 127: 4477–4487.

Darin N, Tulinius M (2000) Neuromuscular disorders in childhood: a descriptive epidemiological study from western Sweden. *Neuromuscul Disord* 10: 1–9.

Ferreiro A, Quijano-Roy S, Pichereau C, Moghadaszadeh B, Goemans N, Bönnemann C et al. (2002) Mutations of the selenoprotein N gene, which is implicated in rigid spine muscular dystrophy, cause the classical phenotype of multiminicore disease: reassessing the nosology of early-onset myopathies. *Am J Hum Genet* 71: 739–749.

Hankiewicz K, Carlier RY, Lazaro L, Linzoain J, Barnerias C, Gómez-Andrés D et al. (2015) Whole-body muscle magnetic resonance imaging in SEPN1-related myopathy shows a homogeneous and recognizable pattern. *Muscle Nerve* 52: 728–735.

Jungbluth H, Dowling J, Ferreiro A, Muntoni F, Bönnemann C et al. (2016) 217th ENMC International Workshop: RYR1-related myopathies, Naarden, The Netherlands, 29–31 January 2016. *Neuromusc Dis* 26(9): 624–633. doi: 10.1016/j.nmd.2016.06.001.

Klein A, Jungbluth H, Clement E, Lillis S, Abbs S, Munot P et al. (2011) Muscle magnetic resonance imaging in congenital myopathies due to ryanodine receptor type 1 gene mutations. *Arch Neurol* 68: 1171–1179.

Lopez RJ, Byrne S, Vukcevic M, Sekulic-Jablanovic M, Xu L, Brink M et al. (2016) An RYR1 mutation associated with malignant hyperthermia is also associated with bleeding abnormalities. *Sci Signal* 9: ra68–ra68.

Mack DL, Poulard K, Goddard MA, Latournerie V, Snyder JM, Grange RW et al. (2017) Systemic AAV8-mediated gene therapy drives whole-body correction of myotubular myopathy in dogs. *Mol Ther* 25: 839–854.

Marino M, Stoilova T, Giorgi C, Bachi A, Cattaneo A, Auricchio A et al. (2015) SEPN1, an endoplasmic reticulum-localized selenoprotein linked to skeletal muscle pathology, counteracts hyperoxidation by means of redox-regulating SERCA2 pump activity. *Hum Mol Genet* 24: 1843–1855.

Marttila M, Lehtokari VL, Marston S, Nyman TA, Barnerias C, Beggs AH et al. (2014) Mutation update and genotype-phenotype correlations of novel and previously described mutations in TPM2 and TPM3 causing congenital myopathies. *Hum Mutat* 35: 779–790.

McEntagart M, Parsons G, Buj-Bello A, Biancalana V, Fenton I, Little M et al. (2002) Genotype-phenotype correlations in X-linked myotubular myopathy. *Neuromuscul Disord* 12: 939–946.

Moghadaszadeh B, Petit N, Jaillard C, Brockington M, Quijano-Roy S, Merlini L et al. (2001) Mutations in SEPN1 cause congenital muscular dystrophy with spinal rigidity and restrictive respiratory syndrome. *Nat Genet* 29: 17–18.

Nelson CE, Robinson-Hamm JN, Gersbach CA (2017) Genome engineering: a new approach to gene therapy for neuromuscular disorders. *Nat Rev Neurol* 13: 647–661.

North KN, Wang CH, Clarke N, Jungbluth H, Vainzof M, Dowling JJ (2014) Approach to the diagnosis of congenital myopathies. *Neuromuscul Disord* 24: 97–116.

Nowak KJ, Ravenscroft G, Laing NG (2013) Skeletal muscle α-actin diseases (actinopathies): pathology and mechanisms. *Acta Neuropathol* 125: 19–32.

O'Grady GL, Best HA, Oates EC, Kaur S, Charlton A, Brammah S et al. (2015) Recessive ACTA1 variant causes congenital muscular dystrophy with rigid spine. *Eur J Hum Genet* 23: 883–886.

Quijano-Roy S, Carlier RY, Fischer D (2011) Muscle imaging in congenital myopathies. *Semin Pediatr Neurol* 18: 221–229.

Ravenscroft G, Laing NG, Bönnemann CG (2015) Pathophysiological concepts in the congenital myopathies: blurring the boundaries, sharpening the focus. *Brain* 138: 246–268.

Rutkowski A, Chatwin M, Koumbourlis A, Fauroux B, Simonds A, CMD Respiratory Physiology Consortium (2015) 203rd ENMC international workshop: respiratory pathophysiology in congenital muscle disorders: implications for pro-active care and clinical research 13–15 December, 2013, Naarden, The Netherlands. *Neuromuscul Disord* 25: 353–358.

Scoto M, Cirak S, Mein R, Feng L, Manzur AY, Robb S et al. (2011) SEPN1-related myopathies: clinical course in a large cohort of patients. *Neurology* 76: 2073–2078.

Wallgren-Pettersson C, Pelin K, Nowak KJ, Muntoni F, Romero NB, Goebel HH et al. (2004) Genotype-phenotype correlations in nemaline myopathy caused by mutations in the genes for nebulin and skeletal muscle alpha-actin. *Neuromuscul Disord* 14: 461–470.

Wang CH, Dowling JJ, North K, Schroth MK, Sejersen T, Shapiro F et al. (2012) Consensus statement on standard of care for congenital myopathies. *J Child Neurol* 27: 363–382.

# 15
# MYOTONIC DYSTROPHIES

*Liesbeth De Waele*

## Introduction

Myotonic dystrophies (Dystrophia Myotonica, DM) are autosomal dominant, multisystemic diseases characterized by myotonia (the inability of muscles to relax after contraction), muscular dystrophy, cardiac conduction defects, cataracts, gastro-intestinal and endocrine disorders (Meola and Cardani 2015). Steinert et al. first described the classic type of myotonic dystrophy in 1909, but the underlying genetic cause was only determined in 1992. Type 1 myotonic dystrophy (myotonic dystrophy type 1, Steinert disease, OMIM 160900) is caused by an expansion of an unstable $(CTG)_n$ trinucleotide repeat in the myotonic dystrophy protein kinase (*DMPK*) gene, encoding for a myosin kinase expressed in skeletal muscle (Mahadevan et al. 1992). Individuals with more than 50 repeats are almost invariably symptomatic, and longer repeats (up to 3 000) are usually associated with earlier onset (possible from birth) and more severe disease (Turner and Hilton-Jones 2010) (Table 15.1). Type 2 myotonic dystrophy (myotonic dystrophy type 2, proximal myotonic myopathy [PROMM], OMIM 602668) is caused by an unstable $(CCTG)_n$ tetranucleotide repeat expansion in the cellular nucleic acid-binding protein (*CNBP*) gene (previously known as zinc finger 9 gene, *ZFN9*), ranging from 75 to a mean of about 5 000 repeats (Day et al. 2003). Unlike in myotonic dystrophy type 1, the size of the repeated DNA expansion in myotonic dystrophy type 2 does not appear to make a difference in the age at onset (8 to 60 years) or severity of the disease (Turner and Hilton-Jones 2010).

When transcribed into CUG/CCUG-containing RNA, mutant transcripts aggregate in muscle fibers, smooth muscle cells, cardiomyocytes and neurons, as nuclear foci that sequester RNA-binding proteins, resulting in spliceopathy of downstream effector genes (Meola and Cardani 2015). For example, mis-splicing of the *ClC-1* chloride channel leads to reduced chloride conductance in muscle fibers, resulting in myotonia (Lueck et al. 2007). However, it is now clear that additional pathogenic mechanisms, such as changes in gene expression, protein translation and micro-RNA metabolism, may also contribute to RNA toxicity and disease pathology (Bachinski et al. 2014; Mahadevan 2012).

## Epidemiology

Myotonic dystrophy affects about 1 in 8 000 Caucasians to 1 in 20 000 in Asian, Japanese and African populations; males and females are affected approximately equally. Founder effects may occur in specific regions such as Quebec, which has a prevalence as high as 1

**TABLE 15.1**
**Clinically defined forms of myotonic dystrophy type 1**
**based on the age at onset and CTG repeat size**

| Size of CUG repeat | Phenotype |
| --- | --- |
| n ≥ 1 000 | Congenital onset |
| n ≥ 800 | Childhood onset |
| n = 50–2 000 | Adult onset |
| n = 50–150 | Late onset |
| n = 38–49 | "Premutation" |
| n = 5–37 | Normal |

in 550 (Suominen et al. 2011; Udd et al. 2006). Myotonic dystrophy type 1 patients can be found worldwide, while myotonic dystrophy type 2 incidence is more limited to Europe.

## Clinical features

MYOTONIC DYSTROPHY TYPE 1

Myotonic dystrophy type 1 has a severe congenital form being apparent at birth, Congenital myotonic dystrophy (CMD), and milder childhood-onset and adult-onset forms. In CMD (15% of myotonic dystrophy type 1-affected individuals) prenatal manifestations may include reduced fetal movements, polyhydramnios, talipes equinovarus or borderline ventriculomegaly (Zaki et al. 2007). At birth patients present with neonatal hypotonia, poor feeding and respiratory problems, with an overall neonatal mortality of 18% (Campbell et al. 2013). Later in childhood, delayed motor milestones, oropharyngeal weakness and facial diplegia (Fig. 15.1) with dysarthria, learning disabilities, impairment of expressive more than receptive communication, and autism spectrum disorder can be observed (Ekström et al. 2009).

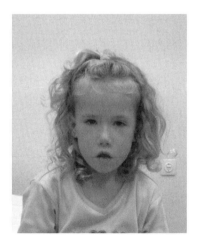

**Fig. 15.1.** Typical "facial diplegia" in young girl with congenital myotonic dystrophy type 1 (3.8 kb expansion).

Children with onset of myotonic dystrophy between 1 and 10 years of age often present with predominant cognitive, behavioural and psychiatric features without muscle problems (Ekström et al. 2009; Douniol et al. 2012). About half of these children have intellectual impairment (IQ in the range of 50–70). Attention deficit hyperactivity disorder, anxiety and mood disorders may occur, but autism is uncommon (Douniol et al. 2012).

Around 75% of patients with myotonic dystrophy type 1 develop symptoms in the second, third or fourth decade, known as classic myotonic dystrophy type 1. A useful clinical clue for diagnosis of myotonic dystrophy is the failure of spontaneous release of the hands following a strong handshake due to myotonia (delayed relaxation of muscles after contraction), being more pronounced after rest and improving with muscle activity (warm-up phenomenon) (Logigian et al. 2005). Physical examination shows action and percussion myotonia, and muscle weakness and wasting mainly of the muscles of the face (ptosis, dysarthria, tongue weakness, mild limitation of ocular motility, atrophy of the m. temporalis and m. masseter), the neck, the trunk and the distal limbs (preferentially the long finger flexors and ankle dorsiflexors). Diaphragmatic weakness may occur early in the disease. Proximal weakness of the shoulder- and hip-girdle generally develops later in the disease course. The phenotype generally worsens and occurs earlier from generation to generation (anticipation) due to increase of the CTG expansion by more than 200 repeats when transmitted from one generation to the next (De Temmerman et al. 2004).

MYOTONIC DYSTROPHY TYPE 2

Myotonic dystrophy type 2, also known as proximal myotonic myopathy (PROMM), generally has a milder phenotype (with a normal life expectancy) presenting at an older age (median age 48 years), and anticipation occurs less (Day et al. 2003). Grip myotonia often is the first symptom, but some patients present with a slowly progressive form of limb-girdle weakness without apparent myotonia (Day et al. 2003). Limb-girdle, neck flexor and elbow extensor muscles are selectively affected, and, to a lesser extent than in myotonic dystrophy type 1, also the long finger flexors. Myotonic dystrophy type 2 patients much more commonly have prominent muscle pain, stiffness and fatigue. There is no congenital disease in myotonic dystrophy type 2, muscle weakness is less pronounced and there is less facial and respiratory muscle weakness.

**Systemic features**

In both myotonic dystrophy type 1 and myotonic dystrophy type 2 cardiac disease may occur, including cardiac dysrhythmia, or prolongation of the PR interval or QRS duration. These conduction defects are progressive and may lead to severe complications such as bradycardia or asystole due to atrioventricular block. Atrial tachycardias (flutter, fibrillation, sinus tachycardia), ventricular tachycardias and heart failure may also occur (Bhakta et al. 2010). Cardiac dysrhythmia is the second leading cause of death in myotonic dystrophy, after respiratory failure (de Die-Smulders et al. 1998).

Premature cataracts, before the age of 55 years, are common in myotonic dystrophy type 1 and less frequent in myotonic dystrophy type 2. They appear as nonspecific punctate opacities by direct ophthalmoscopy, but by slit lamp examination they have a very typical multi-coloured iridescent appearance and are located in the posterior lens capsule.

Central nervous system manifestations vary in myotonic dystrophy type 1, but behavioural effects and changes of cognition are common, including anxiety, avoidant behaviour, apathy, memory impairment, executive dysfunction, and problems with visuospatial processing (Bugiardini and Meola 2014). In both types of myotonic dystrophy brain magnetic resonance imaging (MRI) may show extensive white matter alterations, especially in the frontal and temporal lobes, and loss of specific regions of grey matter (Minnerop et al. 2011; Wozniak et al. 2013).

Sleep disturbance with excessive daytime sleepiness (EDS) and respiratory failure (due to respiratory muscle weakness with poor cough and reduced vital capacity) are very common in myotonic dystrophy type 1 and often significantly reduce quality of life (Bogaard et al. 1992). Respiratory failure is the most frequent cause of death (40% of all cases) (Mathieu et al. 1999). EDS, primarily from primary central nervous system dysfunction, occurs in at least 39% of myotonic dystrophy type 1 patients (van der Werf et al. 2003). This may be coupled with a general disorganization of sleep habits and diurnal rhythm (Yu et al. 2011).

Myotonic dystrophy type 1 patients often show symptoms of gastro-intestinal dysfunction with abdominal pain (55%), dysphagia (45%), emesis (35%), chronic or episodic diarrhoea often alternating with constipation (33%), swallowing difficulties with aspiration (33%), and anal incontinence (30%) (Rönnblom et al. 2002; Heatwole et al. 2012).

Other less common features of myotonic dystrophy are insulin resistance with hyperinsulinemia, increased cholesterol, hypertriglyceridemia, disturbed liver function tests, disturbances in thyroid, parathyroid and hypothalamus function, early balding, testicular atrophy with reduced fertility and erectile dysfunction in men, and habitual abortion and menstrual irregularities in women (Turner and Hilton-Jones 2010).

Although myotonic dystrophy type 1 and myotonic dystrophy type 2 have similar symptoms, they clearly have a number of different features making them separate diseases.

**Diagnosis**

The basis for the diagnosis of myotonic dystrophy is usually the clinical picture and family history. The diagnosis is confirmed by genetic testing, which is definite and cost-effective. Electromyography (EMG) and muscle biopsy have become unnecessary, but can be informative. Nerve conduction studies are usually normal but can show mild length-dependent axonal polyneuropathy. EMG shows myotonic discharges in all patients with myotonic dystrophy type 1 and in 90–100% of patients with myotonic dystrophy type 2 (Day et al. 2003). In myotonic dystrophy type 1, muscle biopsy shows atrophy of type I fibers, increased internalized nuclei, ring fibers, sarcoplasmic masses, small angulated fibers, and atrophic fibers with pyknotic clumps. Myotonic dystrophy type 2 may show similar features but milder and with atrophy of type II fibers, in contrast. Creatine kinase levels can be normal or slightly elevated (Day et al. 2003).

**Management and treatment**

There is currently no cure for myotonic dystrophy, but an accurate diagnosis is important to assist with appropriate medical monitoring and management of symptoms. Moreover, patients with myotonic dystrophy have a higher risk for malignant hyperthermia, a potentially life-threatening complication of the use of inhaled anaesthetics. Because of the high risk of transmission, genetic counselling is very important. Prenatal testing (via chorionic villus sampling) and preimplantation genetic diagnosis are available for both forms (De Rademaeker et al. 2009).

The management of myotonic dystrophy is based on genetic counselling, preserving function and independence, preventing cardiopulmonary complications, and providing symptomatic treatment of myotonia, EDS, gastro-intestinal symptoms and pain. A main objective of the medical care is improving the quality of life.

Preventive and symptomatic orthopaedic and physiotherapeutic management consists of ankle-foot-orthotics (AFOs) to overcome the weakness of ankle dorsiflexors. Upper and lower limb weakness may lead to the need of mobility aids (wheelchairs), and visual impairment and myotonia may be compensated by functional adaptive equipment. An occupational therapist can help with home adaptations if needed.

Lung function measurements (forced vital capacity and forced expiratory volume in 1 second) should be monitored annually and the threshold to perform a polysomnographic investigation should be low (Poussel et al. 2014). In cases of obstructive sleep apnoea syndrome, noninvasive ventilation (NIV) should be offered.

All patients should undergo and electrocardiogram (ECG) annually, and Holter monitoring every 2 years. Pacemaker implantation should be considered in patients with second and third degree heart block, or prolonged pauses. Patients with ventricular arrhythmia or significant left ventricle dysfunction should be referred for implantable cardiac defibrillator (ICD) implantation (Lau et al. 2015).

EDS may be successfully treated with psychostimulant medications such as methylphenidate. The use of modafinil showed mixed results (Wintzen et al. 2007; Hilton-Jones et al. 2012). Mexiletine, and various anticonvulsant and antiarrhythmic drugs, showed reduction of grip myotonia by membrane stabilization (Logigian et al. 2010). Pain can be treated with tricyclic antidepressants and nonsteroidal anti-inflammatory drugs (NSAIDs).

When swallowing difficulties with suspicion of aspiration occur a speech therapy assessment and videofluoroscopy should be performed. Cholestyramine may improve diarrhoea, incontinence and abdominal pain. Norfloxacin, other quinolones and doxycycline may be effective by treating bacterial overgrowth, and erythromycin or domperidone may help to improve gastric emptying (Rönnblom et al. 2002).

Physical activity, specifically aerobic exercise via stationary bicycle training, was found to be safe and effective in improving fitness in myotonic dystrophy type 1 patients by promoting muscle and cardiorespiratory function, while preventing further disuse atrophy (Orngreen et al. 2005; Voet et al. 2010).

**Future therapies**

Recent advances in our understanding of the underlying molecular mechanisms involved in myotonic dystrophy have generated new approaches for more specific and effective treatments for myotonic dystrophy type 1 and myotonic dystrophy type 2. Genetic treatments (antisense oligonucleotide therapy, AON) have been used successfully in in vitro and animal models to reverse the physiological, histopathological and transcriptomic features of myotonic dystrophy (Wheeler et al. 2012). Molecular therapeutics will probably bridge the gap between bench and bedside in the near future.

**Key points**
- Myotonic Dystrophy (Dystrophia Myotonica, DM) is the most common muscular dystrophy in adults, inherited in an autosomal dominant way.
- Myotonic dystrophy type 1 is caused by expansion of a CTG triplet repeat in the gene *DMPK*; myotonic dystrophy type 2 results from repeat expansion in the gene *ZNF9/ CNBP.*
- Both disorders show progressive multisystemic features, including myotonic myopathy, cataract and cardiac conduction problems.
- The wide clinical phenotype of myotonic dystrophy type 1 ranges from an asymptomatic to a severe, life-threatening congenital form; myotonic dystrophy type 2 is less common and less severe.
- There is currently no cure for myotonic dystrophy, but proactive management is important in reducing morbidity and mortality.

**Clinical vignette**

A little girl was transferred to our hospital at day 1 of life. She was born at 34.5 weeks post-menstrual age by urgent caesarean section for fetal distress. Her weight was 1 810 g for a length of 45cm and a head circumference of 32cm. Because of respiratory insufficiency with bradycardia and apnoea she received respiratory support by nasal continuous positive airway pressure (CPAP) ventilation for 15 days. Neonatal hypotonia, mild dysmorphia (high forehead, micro- and retro-gnathia), feeding problems (with need for tube feeding) and a weak cry suggested the diagnosis of a neuromuscular disorder. A cranial ultrasound at day 2 showed a mildly increased reflectivity of the periventricular white matter in the left parieto-occipital region. Brain MRI at day 10 demonstrated multiple punctiform haemorrhagic white matter lesions in the frontoparietal region bilaterally. Metabolic screening was negative. At day 27 the genetic confirmation of CMD, was obtained by detection of expansion of 1 700 CTG repeats in the *DMPK* gene. Both parents were tested and the mother was diagnosed with myotonic dystrophy type 1. At that moment she did not experience any symptoms but her facial expression was rather weak and she had mild grip myotonia when shaking hands.

Physiotherapy was started to stimulate the psychomotor development as much as possible. The little girl showed a positive evolution with increase in muscle tone and spontaneous movements, and improvement of drinking skills. She was discharged at the age of 2 months with intensive physiotherapy and psychological support for the family.

**Comment**

Diagnosis of myotonic dystrophy type 1 is often made in young parents following the diagnosis of the congenital form in a neonate. This phenomenon of the worsening of the phenotype and earlier onset when the disease is transmitted to the next generation is known as anticipation.

## REFERENCES

Bachinski LL, Baggerly KA, Neubauer VL, Nixon TJ, Raheem O, Sirito M et al. (2014) Most expression and splicing changes in myotonic dystrophy type 1 and type 2 skeletal muscle are shared with other muscular dystrophies. *Neuromuscul Disord* 24: 227–240.

Bhakta D, Groh MR, Shen C, Pascuzzi RM, Groh WJ (2010) Increased mortality with left ventricular systolic dysfunction and heart failure in adults with myotonic dystrophy type 1. *Am Heart J* 160: 1137–41, 1141.e1.

Bogaard JM, van der Meché FG, Hendriks I, Ververs C (1992) Pulmonary function and resting breathing pattern in myotonic dystrophy. *Lung* 170: 143–153.

Bugiardini E, Meola G (2014) Consensus on cerebral involvement in myotonic dystrophy. *Neuromuscul Disord* 24: 445–452.

Campbell C, Levin S, Siu VM, Venance S, Jacob P (2013) Congenital myotonic dystrophy: Canadian population-based surveillance study. *J Pediatr* 163: 120–5.e1–3.

Day JW, Ricker K, Jacobsen JF, Rasmussen LJ, Dick KA, Kress W et al. (2003) Myotonic dystrophy type 2: molecular, diagnostic and clinical spectrum. *Neurology* 60: 657–664.

de Die-Smulders CE, Höweler CJ, Thijs C, Mirandolle JF, Anten HB, Smeets HJ et al. (1998) Age and causes of death in adult-onset myotonic dystrophy. *Brain* 121: 1557–1563.

De Rademaeker M, Verpoest W, De Rycke M, Seneca S, Sermon K, Desmyttere S et al. (2009) Preimplantation genetic diagnosis for myotonic dystrophy type 1: upon request to child. *Eur J Hum Genet* 17: 1403–1410.

De Temmerman N, Sermon K, Seneca S, De Rycke M, Hilven P, Lissens W et al. (2004) Intergenerational instability of the expanded CTG repeat in the DMPK gene: studies in human gametes and preimplantation embryos. *Am J Hum Genet* 75: 325–329.

Douniol M, Jacquette A, Cohen D, Bodeau N, Rachidi L, Angeard N et al. (2012) Psychiatric and cognitive phenotype of childhood myotonic dystrophy type 1. *Dev Med Child Neurol* 54: 905–911.

Ekström AB, Hakenäs-Plate L, Tulinius M, Wentz E (2009) Cognition and adaptive skills in myotonic dystrophy type 1: a study of 55 individuals with congenital and childhood forms. *Dev Med Child Neurol* 51: 982–990.

Heatwole C, Bode R, Johnson N, Quinn C, Martens W, McDermott MP et al. (2012) Patient-reported impact of symptoms in myotonic dystrophy type 1 (PRISM-1). *Neurology* 79: 348–357.

Hilton-Jones D, Bowler M, Lochmueller H, Longman C, Petty R, Roberts M et al. (2012) Modafinil for excessive daytime sleepiness in myotonic dystrophy type 1 – the patients' perspective. *Neuromuscul Disord* 22: 597–603.

Lau JK, Sy RW, Corbett A, Kritharides L (2015) Myotonic dystrophy and the heart: A systematic review of evaluation and management. *Int J Cardiol* 184: 600–608.

Logigian EL, Blood CL, Dilek N, Martens WB, Moxley RT IV, Wiegner AW et al. (2005) Quantitative analysis of the "warm-up" phenomenon in myotonic dystrophy type 1. *Muscle Nerve* 32: 35–42.

Logigian EL, Twydell P, Dilek N, Martens WB, Quinn C, Wiegner AW et al. (2010) Evoked myotonia can be "dialed-up" by increasing stimulus train length in myotonic dystrophy type 1. *Muscle Nerve* 41: 191–196.

Lueck JD, Mankodi A, Swanson MS, Thornton CA, Dirksen RT (2007) Muscle chloride channel dysfunction in two mouse models of myotonic dystrophy. *J Gen Physiol* 129: 79–94.

Mahadevan M (2012) Myotonic dystrophy: is a narrow focus obscuring the rest of the field? *Curr Opin Neurol* 25: 609–613.

Mahadevan M, Tsilfidis C, Sabourin L, Shutler G, Amemiya C, Jansen G et al. (1992) Myotonic dystrophy mutation: an unstable CTG repeat in the 3′ untranslated region of the gene. *Science* 255: 1253–1255.

Mathieu J, Allard P, Potvin L, Prévost C, Bégin P (1999) A 10-year study of mortality in a cohort of patients with myotonic dystrophy. *Neurology* 52: 1658–1662.

Meola G, Cardani R (2015) Myotonic dystrophy type 2: an update on clinical aspects, genetic and pathomolecular mechanism. *J Neuromuscul Dis* 2(s2): S59–S71.

Minnerop M, Weber B, Schoene-Bake JC, Roeske S, Mirbach S, Anspach C et al. (2011) The brain in myotonic dystrophy 1 and 2: evidence for a predominant white matter disease. *Brain* 134: 3530–3546.

Orngreen MC, Olsen DB, Vissing J (2005) Aerobic training in patients with myotonic dystrophy type 1. *Ann Neurol* 57: 754–757.

Poussel M, Kaminsky P, Renaud P, Laroppe J, Pruna L, Chenuel B (2014) Supine changes in lung function correlate with chronic respiratory failure in myotonic dystrophy patients. *Respir Physiol Neurobiol* 193: 43–51.

Rönnblom A, Andersson S, Hellström PM, Danielsson A (2002) Gastric emptying in myotonic dystrophy. *Eur J Clin Invest* 32: 570–574.

Suominen T, Bachinski LL, Auvinen S, Hackman P, Baggerly KA, Angelini C et al. (2011) Population frequency of myotonic dystrophy: higher than expected frequency of myotonic dystrophy type 2 (DM2) mutation in Finland. *Eur J Hum Genet* 19: 776–782.

Turner C, Hilton-Jones D (2010) The myotonic dystrophies: diagnosis and management. *J Neurol Neurosurg Psychiatry* 81: 358–367.

Udd B, Meola G, Krahe R, Thornton C, Ranum LP, Bassez G et al. (2006) 40th ENMC International Workshop: myotonic Dystrophy DM2/PROMM and other myotonic dystrophies with guidelines on management. *Neuromuscul Disord* 16: 403–413.

van der Werf S, Kalkman J, Bleijenberg G, van Engelen B, Schillings M, Zwarts M et al. (2003) The relation between daytime sleepiness, fatigue, and reduced motivation in patients with adult onset myotonic dystrophy. *J Neurol Neurosurg Psychiatry* 74: 138–139.

Voet NB, Van Der Kooi EL, Riphagen II, Lindeman E, van Engelen BG, Geurts AC (2010) Strength training and aerobic exercise training for muscle disease. *Cochrane Database Syst Rev* CD003907.

Wheeler TM, Leger AJ, Pandey SK, MacLeod AR, Nakamori M, Cheng SH et al. (2012) Targeting nuclear RNA for in vivo correction of myotonic dystrophy. *Nature* 488: 111–115.

Wintzen AR, Lammers GJ, van Dijk JG (2007) Does modafinil enhance activity of patients with myotonic dystrophy?: a double-blind placebo-controlled crossover study. *J Neurol* 254: 26–28.

Wozniak JR, Mueller BA, Bell CJ, Muetzel RL, Lim KO, Day JW (2013) Diffusion tensor imaging reveals widespread white matter abnormalities in children and adolescents with myotonic dystrophy type 1. *J Neurol* 260: 1122–1131.

Yu H, Laberge L, Jaussent I, Bayard S, Scholtz S, Raoul M et al. (2011) Daytime sleepiness and REM sleep characteristics in myotonic dystrophy: a case-control study. *Sleep (Basel)* 34: 165–170.

Zaki M, Boyd PA, Impey L, Roberts A, Chamberlain P (2007) Congenital myotonic dystrophy: prenatal ultrasound findings and pregnancy outcome. *Ultrasound Obstet Gynecol* 29: 284–288.

# 16
# AN INTRODUCTION TO METABOLIC MYOPATHIES AND POMPE DISEASE

*Boglárka Bánsági and Peter Witters*

**An Introduction to Metabolic Myopathies**

Metabolic myopathies comprise a large number of inborn errors of metabolism. Nearly all are related to energy metabolism within the muscle. Largely, they can be subdivided in glycogen storage disorders (GSD), mitochondrial diseases and fatty acid oxidation (FAO) defects.

Glycogen storage disorders are clinically characterised by exercise intolerance with a typical second wind phenomenon (i.e. after an initial period of physical activity, muscle complaints improve as muscle metabolism becomes more dependent on FAO during sustained exercise). Glycogen storage disorders can be associated with a hepatic phenotype (hepatomegaly, elevated transaminases and development of liver cirrhosis) with episodes of ketotic hypoglycaemia. Failure to thrive and hypotonia are notable features. Treatment is largely nutritional aimed at pre-exercise and avoiding hypoglycaemia (Darras and Friedman 2000a; 2000b). Pompe disease is a special type of GSD (GSD II), presenting more as a lysosomal disorder. This will be discussed in detail in the Pompe disease section.

Mitochondrial disorders often have a (severe) multisystem involvement with for instance central and peripheral nervous system involvement, deafness, reinopathy, external ophthalmoplegia, ataxia and lactic acidosis (see Chapter 17). No known therapies exist.

Fatty acid oxidation disorders can present with muscle disease and hypoketotic hypoglycaemia. Chronic weakness, post-exercise cramps and rhabdomyolysis are typical. Metabolic decompensation with metabolic acidosis can be triggered by excessive fasting, high-fat diet or intercurrent illness. Associated features can include cardiomyopathy or eye disease (Darras and Friedman 2000a; 2000b).

While a detailed description of all possible diseases is beyond the scope of this chapter, an initial biochemical work-up is shown in Table 16.1. In Table 16.2 there is a non-exhaustive list of underlying entities.

**Pompe Disease**

Pompe disease is an autosomal recessive lysosomal disorder characterised by progressive and generalised glycogenosis due to deficiency of lysosomal acid alpha-1,4-glucosidase enzyme (GAA) encoded by the glucosidase acid alpha gene (*GAA*).

**TABLE 16.1**
**Investigations in metabolic myopathies**

| First-line | Creatine kinase, lactate dehydrogenase (including isoforms), AST (SGOT), ALT (SGPT), total and free carnitine, plasma or blood spot acylcarnitine profile, plasma lactate and pyruvate, phosphate, calcium, thyroid hormone, plasma and urine amino acids, urinary organic acids, acid glucosidase alpha (GAA) |
|---|---|
| Second-line functional tests | Non-ischemic forearm test, exercise test, fasting test (after excluding fatty acid oxidation defects) |
| Third-line | Electromyogram, chest X-ray, electrocardiogram, echocardiogram, muscle biopsy |
| Fourth-line | Directed enzymatic testing on fibroblasts or lymphocytes, molecular diagnosis |

AST: aspartate aminotransferase; SGOT: serum glutamic-oxaloacetic transaminase; ALT: alanine aminotransferase; SGPT: serum glutamic-pyruvic transaminase.
Reprinted from Hoffmann et al. (2016) with persmission from Springer.

**TABLE 16.2**
**Metabolic myopathies**

**Glycogen storage disorders:**
GSD II (Pompe disease)
GSD III (Debrancher deficiency)
GSD IV (Branching enzyme deficiency)
GSD V (McArdle)
GSD VII (Phosphofructokinase deficiency)
GSD IX (Phosphoglycerate kinase deficiency)
GSD XII (Aldolase A deficiency)

**Fatty acid metabolism:**
Carnitine transporter deficiency (primary carnitine deficiency)
Translocase deficiency
CPTII deficiency (Carnitine palmitoyltransferase II)
VLCAD (Very-long-chain acyl-CoA dehydrogenase deficiency)
LCHAD (Long-chain acyl-CoA dehydrogenase)/trifunctional enzyme

**Mitochondrial diseases:**
Many disorders with mutations in either mtDNA or nuclear DNA
CoQ deficiency

**Glycolysis defects:**
Muscle phosphofructokinase deficiency
Phosphoglycerate kinase deficiency
Phosphoglycerate mutase deficiency
Lactate dehydrogenase deficiency (GSD XI)
β–enolase deficiency

**Lipid storage myopathies**
Neutral lipid storage disease with ichtyosis
Neutral lipid storage disease with myopathy
Multiple acyl-coa dehydrogenase deficiency (MADD)
Primary carnitine deficiency

A Dutch pathologist, called Pompe, described in 1932 the first infant, who died of cardiac hypertrophy and muscle weakness and showed generalised excessive accumulation of "vacuolar" glycogen. The disease has been classified as glycogen storage disease type II (OMIM#232300) highlighting the abnormal glycogen metabolism (Cori and Schulman 1954). In 1963 a Belgian biochemist, Hers, discovered that Pompe patients have acid maltase deficiency, a lysosomal enzyme required for glycogen hydrolysis (van der Ploeg and Reuser 2008; Lim, Li and Raben 2014; Remiche et al. 2014; van Capelle et al. 2016; Pascarella et al. 2018).

Pompe disease presents with a broad clinical spectrum that varies in age at onset, rate of progression, presence or absence of concomitant cardiomyopathy, degree of muscle and other organ involvement. The wide phenotypic heterogeneity can be attributed to numerous (>500) and diverse pathogenic variants in the *GAA* gene and associated residual enzyme activity (Johnson et al. 2017).

The classic infantile Pompe disease (IOPD) is the most severe of the clinical spectrum with a rather homogenous manifestation due to completely deficient GAA. Early onset and rapidly progressive symptoms of hypertrophic cardiomyopathy and generalised muscle weakness cause cardiorespiratory failure and death within the first year of life in untreated patients. Milder phenotypes are characterised by later disease onset (>1 year) and lack of cardiomyopathy. Late-onset Pompe disease (LOPD) encompasses childhood, juvenile and adult-onset forms without distinctive clinical subtypes. In general, they show slowly progressive skeletal and respiratory muscle dysfunction leading to mobility problems and respiratory mortality. A non-classic or atypical infantile form (Atypical IOPD) has been differentiated in LOPD with early symptom presentation (<1 year) but no cardiomyopathy and a less severe disease course (van der Ploeg and Reuser 2008; van Capelle et al. 2016; Chan et al. 2017; Mori et al. 2017; Rairikar et al. 2017).

**Epidemiology**

The estimated combined prevalence of Pompe disease is about 1 in 40 000 to 1 in 60 000 in the general population. There is a variability in the incidence among ethnicities and geographic regions attributed to founder effects (e.g. 1 in 40 000 Dutch and 1 in 146 000 Australians) (van den Hout et al. 2003; van der Ploeg and Reuser 2008; Kroos et al. 2012; Remiche et al. 2014; Mori et al. 2017).

**Clinical features**

Classic Infantile Pompe disease

The combination of hypertrophic cardiomyopathy, generalised muscle weakness and hypotonia in a young infant suggests the diagnosis of classic Infantile Pompe disease (IOPD). Prominent truncal and proximal limb weakness is accompanied by reduced or absent tendon reflexes and motor milestones can be never achieved. Oropharyngeal weakness and macroglossia cause feeding difficulties and subsequent failure to thrive. Accumulation of glycogen in multiple organs results in hepatomegaly, sensorineural hearing loss, central hypotonia, scoliosis and osteopenia. The progressive respiratory weakness complicated by recurrent infections requires early ventilation support. Cardiac manifestations encompass progressive cardiomegaly with outflow tract obstruction and repolarisation disturbances inducing arrhythmias. If left untreated, the rapidly progressive nature of the disease leads to death within the first 12 months of life (van den Hout et al. 2003; van der Ploeg and Reuser 2008; Tarnopolsky et al. 2016).

There is a wide phenotype heterogeneity in Late-onset Pompe disease (LOPD). The age at onset ranges from infancy to late adulthood and the progression of symptoms is variable. Childhood-onset forms (<15 years) tend to deteriorate more rapidly. There is a male predominance among young patients and male sex is associated with a more severe clinical course regardless of the genotype background (Tarnopolsky et al. 2016; van Capelle et al. 2016).

Skeletal muscle dysfunction and motor delay are the first symptoms in childhood. The limb girdle predominant weakness presents with positive Gowers' sign, difficulties in climbing stairs and frequent falls. A disproportional weakness of the neck flexors is characteristic and causes difficulties in standing up from supine. Scapular winging, scoliosis and joint contractures are frequent findings. Deep tendon reflexes are low or absent. The progressive muscle weakness results in mobility problems and wheelchair dependence. The respiratory weakness seems not to precede the limb girdle weakness in childhood, but major peripheral muscle involvement is likely to associate with restricted pulmonary functions. Glycogen accumulation in the cervical ganglions and phrenic nerves impairs the diaphragm and intercostal muscle function (Boentert et al. 2016). The respiratory muscle weakness complicated by decreased airway clearance, recurrent infections and nocturnal hypoventilation raises the risk of respiratory failure and mortality. Sporadic cardiovascular complications involve cardiac hypertrophy, arrhythmias and dilative arteriopathy. Hepatomegaly can be present and a large proportion of the children are underweight. Less typical symptoms, such as unexplained fatigue, subtle muscle weakness or persistent diarrhoea, might also suggest the diagnosis (van der Ploeg and Reuser 2008; Remiche et al. 2014; van Capelle et al. 2016; Almeida et al. 2017).

Presentation in adulthood shows a somewhat different distribution of skeletal muscle weakness. The involvement of axial muscles is more severe than in other neuromuscular diseases, although the neck flexors are less affected than in childhood (van Capelle et al. 2016).

**Aetiology and pathophysiology**

The *GAA* gene located on chromosome 17q25.2 q.25.3 is expressed in all cell types and encodes the GAA enzyme. GAA undergoes posttranslational modifications, including proteolytic cleavage and addition of mannose-6-phosphate (M6P) for the trafficking of the enzyme to the lysosomes. The function of GAA is to degrade the glycogen in the lysosomes. Biallelic, mostly compound heterozygous *GAA* mutations, cause complete or partial GAA deficiency. The many various mutations affect gene splicing, transcription, mRNA stability and GAA biosynthesis (van der Ploeg and Reuser 2008; Kroos et al. 2012; Lim et al.

2014; Johnson et al. 2017; Mori et al. 2017). The residual GAA activity is determined by the nature of the *GAA* mutation, determining the severity of the phenotype, although the correlation is not strict (van der Ploeg and Reuser 2008; Kroos et al. 2012; Lim et al. 2014).

Some recurrent *GAA* variants have a founder effect. The c.-32-13T>G mutation is the most frequent pathogenic variant in ethnic white patients with LOPD. Recurrent non-intronic 1 splice variant (IVS1) pathogenic variants cause complete loss of GAA activity and severe IOPD. Other founder mutations include large deletions of exon18 in the ethnic white population, frameshift c.525delT in the Netherlands (van der Ploeg and Reuser 2008; Mori et al. 2017).

**Diagnosis**

Establishing early diagnosis in Pompe patients has become important regarding available therapy. The clinical variability and the rare nature of the disease cause diagnostic difficulties. The natural history of IOPD helps in the differentiation of other infantile-onset conditions, such as spinal muscular atrophy, Danon disease, carnitine uptake disorder, glycogen storage disease types IIIa and IV, mitochondrial disorders and hypertrophic cardiomyopathy (Tarnopolsky et al. 2016). The diagnosis of LOPD is more challenging as the non-specific presentation might delay and mislead the diagnosis. There is a clinical overlap with other neuromuscular conditions, including limb-girdle muscular atrophy, Becker muscular dystrophy, glycogen storage diseases and polymyositis (Chan et al. 2017).

Creatine kinase and transaminase levels are elevated in most but not all patients (van den Hout et al. 2003; Ünver et al. 2016). Electromyography is normal in the limb muscles but paraspinal recordings might show myotonic discharges (Tarnopolsky et al. 2016; Almeida et al. 2017). A muscle ultrasound serves as screening tool for Pompe patients by detecting atrophic muscle changes (Hwang et al. 2017). Muscle MRI scans identify early fatty muscle degeneration on T1-weighted sequences and the truncal pattern of fatty infiltration characterises Pompe disease (Figueroa-Bonaparte et al. 2016; Lollert et al. 2018). Adult muscle biopsy specimens show periodic acid Schiff (PAS) positive glycogen vacuoles along with abnormal lysosomal abundance. However, skeletal muscle findings are often normal while imposing unnecessary risk in childhood (Vissing, Lukacs and Straub 2013; Tarnopolsky et al. 2016).

Patients manifesting skeletal muscle weakness should be tested for GAA activity using dried blood spots (DBS) as the first tier diagnostic step, which is a quick, non-invasive and cost-effective method. Positive DBS results should be followed by confirmatory diagnostic tests either with genetic analysis or with GAA tissue assay. The identification of biallelic pathogenic variants in the *GAA* gene confirms the diagnosis. In genetically undefined cases GAA activity should be measured in tissues, such as fibroblasts, skeletal muscle or leukocytes for further analysis. The criterion standard method is the use of skin biopsy derived fibroblast cell culture for the enzyme assay. GAA tissue assay definitely confirms the diagnosis but it requires specific laboratory techniques and it is time consuming. The diagnostic process should take as little time as possible, as delays in treatment in IOPD correlate clearly with a worse prognosis (Winchester et al. 2008; Vissing, Lukacs and Straub 2013; Ünver et al. 2016; Johnson et al. 2017).

**Management and treatment**

The ability of cells to secrete and uptake the GAA precursor by cation-independent M6P receptors makes enzyme replacement therapy (ERT) possible. The recombinant human GAA enzyme (rhGAA; alglucosidase alpha, Myozyme, Genzyme) is the only European Medical Agency (EMA) and Food and Drug Administration (FDA) approved disease-specific treatment for Pompe disease. The rhGAA is taken up from the circulation mostly by the liver cells and undergoes proteolytic cleavage to achieve mature form. A therapeutic dose of 20mg/kg is necessary to reach a threshold level in the skeletal muscle, which is low in M6P receptors. The half-life of rhGAA is short, hence life-long twice weekly infusions are needed. Long-term ERT has beneficial cardiac effects, which have dramatically improved the disease survival. On the other hand, skeletal muscle effects are limited and non-reversal leading to better prognosis with early initiated therapy. The high immunogenicity of rhGAA induces antibody production that can attenuate the therapeutic response. Furthermore, the inability of the enzyme to cross the blood–brain barrier fails to influence the concomitant neuronal pathology (van der Ploeg and Reuser 2008; Lim, Li and Raben 2014; Bond, Kishnani and Koeberl 2017; Puzzo et al. 2017; Rairikar et al. 2017).

CLASSIC INFANTILE POMPE DISEASE

ERT drastically improves the cardiac and respiratory survival and changes the natural history of IOPD. The therapy should be initiated shortly after birth at a dose of 20mg/kg every other week. Cross-reacting immune material (CRIM) negative infants produce high rhGAA antibody levels due to the complete lack of native enzyme. Determination of the CRIM status is required before ERT to consider immune modulation for a better response. In CRIM negative IOPD patients an honest discussion has to take place acknowledging the possibility of refraining from any treatment, as outcome is likely to be very poor (e.g. ventilator dependence in a few years) (Case et al. 2012; Tarnopolsky et al. 2016; Rairikar et al. 2017).

The distribution of the residual muscle weakness defines a distinct neuromuscular phenotype in treated patients. Selective weakness in the neck flexors, ankle dorsiflexors and hip extensors causes compensatory deformities and characteristic gait pattern. Scoliosis cannot be found in treated ambulant children. Decreased exercise tolerance and fatigue are common (Case et al. 2012). Disease biomarkers are entitled to monitor the therapy outcome and progression. Progressive muscle involvement is accompanied by elevated creatine kinase and transaminase levels. Decrease in urinary glucose tetrasaccharide is related to the therapy induced glycogen clearance (Tarnopolsky et al. 2016). Skeletal muscle histopathology correlates with the clinical outcome (Schänzer et al. 2017). Muscle ultrasound and MRI are non-invasive tools to identify atrophic muscle groups that correspond with functional muscle scales (Figueroa-Bonaparte et al. 2016; Hwang et al. 2017; Lollert et al. 2018). Hypertrophic cardiomyopathy is monitored by echocardiography measurement of the diastolic ventricular thickness. Left ventricular outflow obstruction should be treated with beta-blockers and cautious fluid control. Cardiac arrhythmia remains a long-term complication in infantile patients regardless of ERT. Adequate nutritional intake should be maintained via enteral feeding and immunisations are required for prevention (Tarnopolsky et al. 2016).

LATE-ONSET POMPE DISEASE

Long-term ERT has the capacity to improve or stabilise skeletal muscle strength in LOPD. Early therapy initiation, less advanced muscle disease and female sex correspond with a better outcome. ERT has limited respiratory muscle effects and many treated patients require ventilation support. Younger age and less severe disease manifestation are correlated with better respiratory response. ERT should be initiated at a dose of 20mg/kg in patients with measurable disease-specific symptoms. Pre-symptomatic treatment is not recommended due to lack of clinical evidence, impact of life-long therapy and high costs (Tarnopolsky et al. 2016; Ünver et al. 2016; van der Ploeg et al. 2017).

Patients are evaluated using a minimal dataset to monitor outcome and therapy response. Skeletal muscle evaluation consists of Medical Research Council (MRC) grading of muscle strength and functional muscle scales (Six Minute Walk Test). Respiratory function is best monitored by forced vital capacity while maximal inspiratory pressure measures respiratory muscle weakness. Postural drop in the forced vital capacity sensitively indicates diaphragm involvement and sleep disordered breathing. The expanded version of the Paediatric Evaluation of Disability Inventory (PEDI), a physical functioning scale serves to assess quality of life outcomes. Measuring the level of rhGAA antibodies is indicated when therapy response is insufficient. Disease progression, non-compliance, allergic reactions and comorbid conditions may lead to therapy cessation. Potentially treatable patients can be followed by muscle scans, while cerebrovascular malformations can be screened by neuroimaging. The timely recognition and correction of nocturnal hypoventilation may prevent major respiratory deterioration. Adequate nutrition, sufficient protein intake, vitamin D supplementation and immunisations are required. Targeted muscle training and balanced aerobic exercise improves endurance, muscle strength and prevents scoliosis (Schoser et al. 2015; Boentert et al. 2016; Montagnese et al. 2016; Tarnopolsky et al. 2016).

**Future therapies**

The limited effects of ERT has prompted research toward novel therapy approaches. Currently ongoing clinical trials aim to improve the efficacy of ERT by enhancing enzyme uptake in the muscles via M6P receptors (albuterol, carbohydrate remodelling) or via lysosomal targeting (fusion with IGF-2) and by stabilising the enzyme and increasing its activity using a pharmacological chaperone (duvoglustat hydrochloride; AT2220, 1-deoxynojirimycin hydrochloride) (Lim et al. 2014; Llerena Junior et al. 2016).

Other approaches target the disordered lysosomal autophagy as the key pathology of the disease. Genetic suppression of autophagy combined with ERT prevented autophagic build-up and reduced glycogen storage in the skeletal muscle of animal models (Lim et al. 2014; Pascarella et al. 2018). Impaired mechanistic target of rapamycin complex 1 (mTORC1) activity and the disturbed signalling cascade might be reversed by arginine (Lim et al. 2017). Activated transcription factor EB (TFEB) stimulates autophagy and promotes lysosomal functions in different cell types through nuclear regulation of lysosomal genes. Intramuscular injection of an adeno-associated virus (AAV)-TFEB vector in mice improved the muscle structure and enhanced glycogen clearance in targeted muscles. Systemic delivery and subsequent TFEB overexpression delayed the disease progression and improved motor and cardiac function in a murine model (Lim et al. 2014; Gatto et al. 2017).

Gene therapy is an alternative approach promising full correction and reversibility by targeting all diseased organs. The clinical trial using intradiaphragmatic delivery of AAV1-mediated *GAA* gene therapy was safe and revealed modest respiratory improvement. Intramuscular delivery of the AAV9-GAA transgene results in localised muscular effects and the related high immunogenicity requires immunosuppression (Lim et al. 2014; Puzzo et al. 2017). Intrathecal administered AAV-mediated gene transfer has corrected the neuronal pathology, improved cardiac symptoms and partially restored motor functions (Hordeaux et al. 2017). Immunomodulatory gene therapy using liver-directed AAV vectors has the potential to systematically correct Pompe disease while ensuring continuous enzyme production and antigen-specific immune tolerance (Bond, Kishnani and Koeberl 2017; Puzzo et al. 2017). Antisense oligonucleotides may provide a potential therapy for Pompe patients with the intronic 1 splice variant (IVS1) variant by blocking a cryptic splice site to restore canonical exon 2 splicing (van der Wal et al. 2017).

**Key points**
- Metabolic myopathies are diverse conditions that can be classified in the major groups of glycogen storage disorders, glycolysis defects, fatty acid oxidation defects, lipid storage and mitochondrial myopathies.
- Pompe disease is an autosomal recessive lysosomal glycogen storage disorder caused by the deficient function of the alpha-glucosidase enzyme.
- The wide phenotype-genotype heterogeneity enables to differentiate clinical subgroups within Pompe disease – infantile onset, late onset and atypical forms.
- In case of relevant symptoms, the activity of the alpha-glucosidase enzyme should be screened using dried blood spots and confirmed by tissue enzyme assay or genetic testing.
- Early diagnosis is of utmost importance regarding available enzyme replacement therapy, which proved to have beneficial long term effects and outcome.

**Clinical vignette**
A 10-month-old boy from a Turkish consanguineous family was referred for further cardiology evaluation due to an incidental finding of cardiac muscle thickness during an episode of pneumonia. His previous medical history was unremarkable other than that his gross motor milestones were delayed. Clinically, he had a myopathic face with protruding large tongue, prominent axial hypotonia with poor head control and proximal limb muscle weakness. Deep tendon reflexes were preserved. There were no signs of tongue fasciculation and neuromuscular scoliosis. His creatine kinase was mildly increased (481U/l). His liver was moderately enlarged accompanied by elevation of the transaminase levels (AST 194U/l, ALT 147U/l). No cardiomegaly was seen on a thoracic X-ray. Electrocardiogram (ECG) showed QRS changes indicating ventricular hypertrophy and repolarisation disturbances. Echocardiography described hypertrophic cardiomyopathy with normal left ventricular contraction and outflow.

Regarding the characteristic symptom constellation, the activity of the alpha-glucosidase (GAA) was measured in dried blood spots. The enzyme activity was below its respective reference ranges with repeated testing. An enzyme assay on skin biopsy derived fibroblast cell culture confirmed the low GAA activity. Simultaneously, the histological analysis of his muscle biopsy described numerous muscle fibres containing PAS positive sarcoplasmic vacuolisation. The diagnosis was confirmed by molecular analysis by the detection of the known pathogenic homozygous c.2015G>A, (p.Arg672Gln) mutation in the *GAA* gene.

By the age of 1 year, the diagnosis of Infantile Pompe disease was established and the recombinant GAA enzyme therapy (Myozyme) at a dose of 20mg/kg could be started. He was proven to have a CRIM positive status – detectable residual GAA protein by Western blot analysis – indicating a favourable treatment outcome. No antibody production has been noted during the twice weekly administered Myozyme therapy. His follow-up echocardiography visualised the normalisation of the septal and left ventricular hypertrophy with normal contractile function after 1 year of enzyme replacement therapy. He started to walk independently and remained ambulant at the age of 3 with some residual limb weakness. No respiratory complications have been noted.

COMMENT

The timely recognition of the combination of muscle weakness, cardiac hypertrophy and respiratory complications and a subsequent appropriate diagnostic approach can lead to an early diagnosis in Infantile Pompe disease. An early initiated enzyme replacement therapy results in a better outcome and survival.

## REFERENCES

Almeida V, Conceição I, Fineza I, Coelho T, Silveira F, Santos M et al. (2017) Screening for Pompe disease in a Portuguese high risk population. *Neuromuscul Disord* 27: 777–781.

Boentert M, Prigent H, Várdi K, Jones HN, Mellies U, Simonds AK et al. (2016) Practical recommendations for diagnosis and management of respiratory muscle weakness in late-onset pompe disease. *Int J Mol Sci* 17: 1735.

Bond JE, Kishnani PS, Koeberl DD (2017) Immunomodulatory, liver depot gene therapy for Pompe disease. *Cell Immunol* S0008-8749(17)30238-1.

Case LE, Beckemeyer AA, Kishnani PS (2012) Infantile Pompe disease on ERT: update on clinical presentation, musculoskeletal management, and exercise considerations. *Am J Med Genet C Semin Med Genet* 160C:69–79.

Chan J, Desai AK, Kazi ZB, Corey K, Austin S, Hobson-Webb LD et al. (2017) The emerging phenotype of late-onset Pompe disease: A systematic literature review. *Mol Genet Metab* 120: 163–172.

Cori GT, Schulman JL (1954) Glycogen storage disease of the liver. II. Enzymic studies. *Pediatrics* 14: 646–650.

Darras BT, Friedman NR (2000a). Metabolic myopathies: a clinical approach; part I. *Pediatr Neurol* 22: 87–97.

Darras BT, Friedman NR (2000b). Metabolic myopathies: a clinical approach; part II. *Pediatr Neurol* 22: 171–181.

Figueroa-Bonaparte S, Segovia S, Llauger J, Belmonte I, Pedrosa I, Alejaldre A et al. (2016) Muscle MRI findings in childhood/adult onset pompe disease correlate with muscle function. *PLoS One* 11:e0163493.

Gatto F, Rossi B, Tarallo A, Polishchuk E, Polishchuk R, Carrella A et al. (2017) AAV-mediated transcription factor EB (TFEB) gene delivery ameliorates muscle pathology and function in the murine model of Pompe Disease. *Sci Rep* 7: 15089.

Hoffmann GF, Zschocke J, Nyhan WL (2016) *Inherited Metabolic Diseases: A Clinical Approach.* Berlin: Springer, pp. 293–312.

Hordeaux J, Dubreil L, Robveille C, Deniaud J, Pascal Q, Dequéant B et al. (2017) Long-term neurologic and cardiac correction by intrathecal gene therapy in Pompe disease. *Acta Neuropathol Commun* 5: 66.

Hwang H-E, Hsu T-R, Lee Y-H, Wang H-K, Chiou H-J, Niu D-M (2017) Muscle ultrasound: A useful tool in newborn screening for infantile onset pompe disease. *Medicine (Baltimore)* 96:e8415.

Johnson K, Töpf A, Bertoli M, Phillips L, Claeys KG, Stojanovic VR et al. (2017) Identification of GAA variants through whole exome sequencing targeted to a cohort of 606 patients with unexplained limb-girdle muscle weakness. *Orphanet J Rare Dis* 12: 173.

Kroos M, Hoogeveen-Westerveld M, van der Ploeg A, Reuser AJJ (2012) The genotype-phenotype correlation in Pompe disease. *Am J Med Genet C Semin Med Genet* 160C:59–68.

Lim J-A, Li L, Raben N (2014) Pompe disease: from pathophysiology to therapy and back again. *Front Aging Neurosci* 6: 177.

Lim J-A, Li L, Shirihai OS, Trudeau KM, Puertollano R, Raben N (2017) Modulation of mTOR signaling as a strategy for the treatment of Pompe disease. *EMBO Mol Med* 9: 353–370.

Llerena Junior JC, Nascimento OJ, Oliveira AS, Dourado Junior ME, Marrone CD, Siqueira HH et al. (2016) Guidelines for the diagnosis, treatment and clinical monitoring of patients with juvenile and adult Pompe disease. *Arq Neuropsiquiatr* 74: 166–176.

Lollert A, Stihl C, Hötker AM, Mengel E, König J, Laudemann K et al. (2018) Quantification of intramuscular fat in patients with late-onset Pompe disease by conventional magnetic resonance imaging for the long-term follow-up of enzyme replacement therapy. *PLoS One* 13:e0190784.

Montagnese F, Granata F, Musumeci O, Rodolico C, Mondello S, Barca E et al. (2016) Intracranial arterial abnormalities in patients with late onset Pompe disease (LOPD). *J Inherit Metab Dis* 39: 391–398.

Mori M, Haskell G, Kazi Z, Zhu X, DeArmey SM, Goldstein JL et al. (2017) Sensitivity of whole exome sequencing in detecting infantile- and late-onset Pompe disease. *Mol Genet Metab* 122: 189–197.

Pascarella A, Terracciano C, Farina O, Lombardi L, Esposito T, Napolitano F et al. (2018) Vacuolated PAS-positive lymphocytes as an hallmark of Pompe disease and other myopathies related to impaired autophagy. *J Cell Physiol* 233: 5829–5837.

Puzzo F, Colella P, Biferi MG, Bali D et al. (2017) Rescue of Pompe disease in mice by AAV-mediated liver delivery of secretable acid α-glucosidase. *Sci Transl Med* 9(418). doi: 10.1126/scitranslmed.aam6375.

Rairikar MV, Case LE, Bailey LA, Kazi ZB, Desai AK, Berrier KL et al. (2017) Insight into the phenotype of infants with Pompe disease identified by newborn screening with the common c.-32-13T>G "late-onset" GAA variant. *Mol Genet Metab* 122: 99–107.

Remiche G, Ronchi D, Magri F, Lamperti C, Bordoni A, Moggio M et al. (2014) Extended phenotype description and new molecular findings in late onset glycogen storage disease type II: a northern Italy population study and review of the literature. *J Neurol* 261: 83–97.

Schänzer A, Kaiser A-K, Mühlfeld, C, Kulessa M, Paulus W, von Pein H et al. (2017) Quantification of muscle pathology in infantile Pompe disease. *Neuromuscul Disord* 27: 141–152. doi: 10.1016/j.nmd.2016.10.010

Schoser B, Laforêt P, Kruijshaar ME, Toscano A, van Doorn PA, van der Ploeg AT et al. (2015) 208th ENMC International Workshop: formation of a European Network to develop a European data sharing model and treatment guidelines for Pompe disease Naarden, The Netherlands, 26–28 September 2014. *Neuromuscul Disord* 25: 674–678.

Tarnopolsky M, Katzberg H, Petrof BJ, Sirrs S, Sarnat HB, Myers K et al. (2016) Pompe Disease: Diagnosis and Management. Evidence-Based Guidelines from a Canadian Expert Panel. *Can J Neurol Sci* 43: 472–485.

Ünver O, Hacifazlioglu NE, Karatoprak E, Güneş AS, Sağer G, Kutlubay B et al. (2016) The frequency of late-onset Pompe disease in pediatric patients with limb-girdle muscle weakness and nonspecific hyperCKemia: A multicenter study. *Neuromuscul Disord* 26: 796–800. doi: 10.1016/j.nmd.2016.09.001.

van Capelle CI, van der Meijden JC, van den Hout JM, Jaeken J, Baethmann M, Voit T et al. (2016) Childhood Pompe disease: clinical spectrum and genotype in 31 patients. *Orphanet J Rare Dis* 11: 65.

van den Hout HMP, Hop W, van Diggelen OP, Smeitink JA, Smit GP, Poll-The BT et al. (2003) The natural course of infantile Pompe's disease: 20 original cases compared with 133 cases from the literature. *Pediatrics* 112: 332–340.

van der Ploeg AT, Kruijshaar ME, Toscano A, Laforêt P, Angelini C, Lachmann RH et al. (2017) European consensus for starting and stopping enzyme replacement therapy in adult patients with Pompe disease: a 10-year experience. *Eur J Neurol* 24: 768–e31.

van der Ploeg AT, Reuser AJ (2008) Pompe's disease. *Lancet* 372: 1342–1353.

van der Wal E, Bergsma AJ, Pijnenburg JM, van der Ploeg AT, Pijnappel WWMP (2017) Antisense Oligo-nucleotides Promote Exon Inclusion and Correct the Common c.-32-13T>G GAA Splicing Variant in Pompe Disease. *Mol Ther Nucleic Acids* 7: 90–100.

Vissing J, Lukacs Z, Straub V (2013) Diagnosis of Pompe disease: muscle biopsy vs blood-based assays. *JAMA Neurol* 70: 923–927.

Winchester B, Bali D, Bodamer OA, Caillaud C, Christensen E, Cooper A et al. (2008) Methods for a prompt and reliable laboratory diagnosis of Pompe disease: report from an international consensus meeting. *Mol Genet Metab* 93: 275–281.

# 17
# MITOCHONDRIAL DISORDERS

*Rudy Van Coster*

For an introduction to Metabolic Myopathies, please see Chapter 16 (page 240).

## Introduction

The prevalence of mitochondrial diseases is estimated to be around 1 in 5 000. Mitochondrial diseases are among the most frequent causes of metabolic myopathies and encephalopathies. Mitochondrial diseases usually affect multiple organs. Skeletal muscle and brain are most often involved. The term mitochondrial myopathy is used when skeletal muscle is predominantly affected. Mitochondrial myopathy is characterized clinically by weakness, hypotonia and intolerance to physical effort. Some patients also suffer from muscle pain or muscle cramps. Rarely, rhabdomyolysis can occur, which is a sign of acute energy crisis in myofibers. Clinical examination typically reveals amyotrophy of skeletal muscles. In most cases, a proximal myopathy is seen. Preferential involvement of a specific muscle group is not seen, except for the extra-ocular muscles. When affected it results in external ophthalmoplegia. The term mitochondrial disease is used when two or more tissues are involved. Mitochondrial syndromes were reported in the literature describing typical combinations of signs and symptoms. Overt signs of myopathy are seen in several of these mitochondrial syndromes, including MELAS (Mitochondrial Encephalopathy and Stroke-like episodes) (Pavlakis et al. 1984), MERRF (Myoclonic epilepsy and ragged-red-fibers) (Fukuhara et al. 1980), Kearns-Sayre syndrome (Kearns and Sayre 1958), Leigh syndrome (Leigh 1951), mitochondrial DNA depletion syndromes (for example, thymidine kinase 2 deficiency) (Saada et al. 2001), CPEO (Chronic Progressive External Ophthalmoplegia) (Moraes et al. 1989) and MNGIE (Mitochondrial neurogastro-intestinal encephalopathy) (Bardosi et al. 1987). The latter is characterized by chronic abdominal dysfunction, pseudo-obstruction, diarrhea, vomiting and external ophthalmoplegia. In individuals with NARP (Neuropathy, Ataxia and Retinitis Pigmentosa) (Holt et al. 1990) neuromuscular involvement is mainly caused by the underlying peripheral neuropathy.

## Clinical features

In patients with mitochondrial myopathy, the onset of symptoms can be either insidious, slowly progressive, or subacute as in acute rhabdomyolysis. In general, the affected individuals typically show exacerbations of symptoms during intercurrent infections, fever, physical or psychological stress. This can be explained by the fact that affected cells are able to produce a sufficient amount of energy needed under resting conditions. When more energy is needed, as in periods of illness, physical stress or emotional stress, energy production fails. The affected individuals then become weak and hypotonic. The more severe the defect, the younger the age at onset of symptoms. The most severely affected patients already present in the neonatal period and their clinical picture is characterized by generalized hypotonia, weakness and respiratory insufficiency (Honzik et al. 2012 Jonckheere et al. 2013; De Praeter et al. 2015). In blood, an overwhelming hyperlactacidemia is detected. Milder defects become symptomatic at later age (infantile age, childhood, adolescence or adulthood). The oxidative phosphorylation capacity decreases progressively with age which explains that very mild defects can become ultimately symptomatic in the fifth or sixth decade (Dermaut et al. 2010).

Brain involvement is not rare in patients with mitochondrial defects and can vary from minimal to severe. For this reason, whenever a mitochondrial cause is suspected cerebral abnormalities should be searched for. Clinical features of cerebral involvement can vary and include fluctuating symptoms of general encephalopathy, seizures (Desguerre et al. 2014), dementia, migraine, stroke-like episodes, ataxia, spasticity or dystonia. The presence of external ophthalmoplegia is suggestive of a mitochondrial defect. Only a few other diseases are associated with external ophthalmoplegia such as ocular myasthenia gravis and congenital fibrosis of extra-ocular muscles. Ptosis of the eyelids is also a common finding in individuals with a mitochondrial defect (myasthenia gravis must again be excluded).

Additional clinical findings in individuals with mitochondrial myopathy can be cardiomyopathy, sensorineural deafness, optic atrophy, pigmentary retinopathy, hepatopathy (microvesicular steathosis, fibrosis, cirrhosis), diabetes mellitus and tubulopathy.

Family history can be informative. Mitochondrial DNA mutations follow a maternal type of inheritance. Only women transmit the disease, but daughters and sons can be affected which distinguishes it from X-linked diseases. Besides maternal inheritance other types of inheritance can be seen in mitochondrial myopathies, including autosomal recessive, autosomal dominant and X-linked.

**Radiological features**

Radiological investigations are helpful in the diagnosis of mitochondrial myopathies. Magnetic resonance imaging (MRI) of the affected skeletal muscles shows atrophy of skeletal muscles, without increase of fat or connective tissue. MRI of the brain is highly recommended (Mascalchi et al. 2018; Finsterer and Zarrouk-Mahjoub 2018). Some abnormalities detected in the brain can provide additional arguments for a mitochondrial defect, such as, for example, bilateral symmetrical signal abnormalities in the striatum or in the posterior part of mesencephalon/pons, cerebellar atrophy and cerebral cortical atrophy. Stroke-like lesions not corresponding to a vascular territory are typical for MELAS.

**Diagnosis**

In case a mitochondrial defect is suspected, lactate measurements are very useful. Lactate can be measured in blood (normal <2mM) and in cerebrospinal fluid (CSF) (normal <1.7mM). In individuals with a severe defect in skeletal muscle and possibly in other organs, lactate is increased continuously in blood. When the mitochondrial defect is less severe, lactate is only intermittently increased in blood. Therefore, it is preferable to perform repeated measurements in the course of one day (for example, under fasting conditions, two hours after breakfast, before lunch, two hours after lunch and one in the evening), also called a "lactate day profile". An intravenous catheter is placed to avoid repeated punctures. It is important not to create too much pressure when garroting before taking blood to avoid artificial pre-analytical increases of lactate. Arterial lactate measurements are more reliable, but are difficult to perform in daily practice. Measurement of lactate in CSF is indicated in case of concomitant encephalopathy. Measurements of lactate in urine are also informative. Lactate can be measured in urine enzymatically or by gas chromatography/mass spectrometry (GC/MS) which is routinely used for determining the organic acid profile. Determination of lactate in urine is sometimes more reliable than in blood. Even when lactate is only intermittently increased in blood, the threshold concentration for reabsorption of lactate by the renal tubuli at peak moments will be exceeded which will result in an increased lactate concentration in urine.

Lactate can be normal in blood under resting conditions but can become significantly increased after physical effort. In healthy individuals, lactate in blood increases after physical effort but in the individual with mitochondrial myopathy lactate increases are seen even after a minor physical effort and the increases are higher and last longer than in nonaffected individuals. Cyclo-ergometry can be used for this purpose, although not in very young children.

In cases in which an individual is suspected of having a mitochondrial myopathy, additional investigations are indicated for detection of involvement of other organs. An echocardiogram and electrocardiogram are performed for detection of signs of cardiomyopathy and heart rhythm abnormalities. In most cases, a hypertrophic type will be seen, but other forms of cardiomyopathy also can be detected (dilated cardiomyopathy, non-compaction cardiomyopathy). Examination of the eye is necessary to see whether there are abnormalities of the retina (retinopathy, retinitis pigmentosa), or optic atrophy. Also, audiometry and/or brainstem evoked response audiometry (BERA) for detection of sensorineural deafness is indicated. Measurement of transaminases is useful to detect possible underlying liver abnormalities (high aspartate aminotransaminase (AST) and alanine aminotransaminase (ALT), normal creatine kinase) and also ultrasound examination of liver (detection of steatosis). An increase of creatine kinase is not seen in most patients with mitochondrial defects. Only in the patients in whom rhabdomyolysis occurs will creatine kinase will be increased significantly.

Until recently, the criterion standard for the diagnosis of a mitochondrial myopathy was a skeletal muscle biopsy. The finding of ragged-red-fibers (in more than 1% of fibers) is suggestive for a mitochondrial DNA (mtDNA) defect (point mutation, depletion or deletion of mtDNA) (Fig. 17.1). Also, an abnormal increase of lipid droplets in the myofibers (accumulation of neutral lipids) or an increased amount of glycogen can be seen. Histochemically, complex IV (COX) deficient fibers are suggestive of a mitochondrial defect. A general decrease of COX staining in myofibers suggests a nuclear defect, or a homoplasmic pathogenic mtDNA mutation. A mosaic staining with COX-negative fibers along with COX-positive fibers pleads more for a mtDNA abnormality; most frequently a point mutation in one of the mitochondrial genes coding for mitochondrial tRNA, or for mtDNA depletion (Roels et al. 2009). Electron microscopic findings can be informative

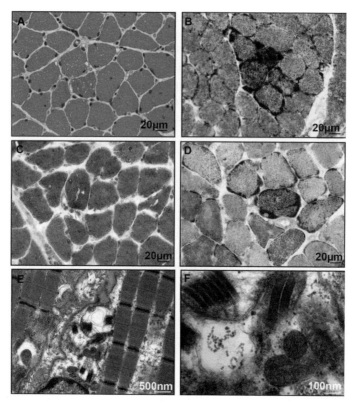

**Fig. 17.1.** Muscle biopsy from a 16-year-old girl with childhood onset myopathy and developmental delay. Biochemical analysis showed a combined complex I+IV deficiency. In the hematoxylin eosin (HE) stained section, the muscle fibers show a moderately increased variability of muscle fiber size and increased internalized nuclei. Some fibers show irregular contours and sarcoplasm. (A). Accumulation of mitochondria with characteristic ragged-red-fibers is visible as dark blue at SDH (B), and red at Gomori Trichrome staining (C). COX-negative fibers stain blue in the COX/SDH staining (D). At ultrastructural sections, mitochondria are swollen with abnormal structures of the cristae and crystalloid inclusions (E, F). (Images with courtesy of P.D. Dr Anne Schänzer, Gießen).

and swelling of mitochondria, together with an electron non-dense matrix, can be seen as a result of severe mitochondrial distress. In more chronic situations, abnormal structures of the cristae and crystalloid inclusions can be detected (Fig. 17.1).

The activities of the five oxidative phosphorylation complexes can be measured in a skeletal muscle biopsy specimen (50–100mg). Usually, the biopsy is taken from the M. quadriceps. Some centers will measure activities only in freshly taken muscle (not frozen). Other diagnostic labs also accept fresh-frozen biopsy specimens. In affected individuals, most frequently an isolated complex I deficiency is seen. Numerous gene defects can cause isolated complex I deficiency (Table 17.1). Less frequently seen is an isolated complex IV deficiency. The number of underlying gene defects causing isolated complex IV deficiency is also large (Table 17.1). Only rarely seen are isolated complex II deficiency (Sonam et al.

**TABLE 17.1**
**List of genes reported to be associated with mitochondrial myopathy[a]**

| Complex I | Mitochondrial tRNAs | Maintenance and transcription of mtDNA | Intramitochondrial translation |
|---|---|---|---|
| *TMEM126B* | | | *YARS2* |
| *ACAD9* | *MT-TE* | *POLG* | *TARS2* |
| *NUBPL* | *MT-TK* | *POLG2* | *MARS2* |
| *FOXRED1* | *MT-TG* | *TK2* | *FARS2* |
| *NDUFA1* | *MT-TL1* | *TWNK* | *VARS2* |
| *NDUFAF4* | *MT-TQ* | *RRM2B* | *AARS2* |
| *NDUFAF5* | *MT-TH* | *SUCLG1* | *CARS2* |
| *NDUFA13* | *MT-TW* | *SUCLA2* | *EARS2* |
| *NDUFB3* | *MT-TF* | *TYMP* | *NARS2* |
| *NDUFS2* | *MT-TA* | *DGUOK* | *GTPBP3* |
| *NDUFS3* | *MT-TC* | *TRIT1* | *PUS1* |
| *NDUFS4* | *MT-TS1* | *MPV17* | *MTFMT* |
| *NDUFS8* | *MT-TS2* | *NCPH* | *COXPD12* |
| *NDUFV2* | *MT-TY* | *OPA1* | *COXPD23* |
| *MT-ND1* | *MT-TT* | *SLC25A4* | *COXPD25* |
| *MT-ND2* | **Iron-sulfur** | *FBXL4* | *COXPD28* |
| *MT-ND4* | **cluster biosynthesis** | *TFAM* | *COXPD29* |
| *MT-ND5* | *ISCU* | *SCAE* | *COXPD33* |
| *MT-ND6* | *IBA57* | *DNA2* | *TRMT10C* |
| **Complex II** | *LYRM4* | *RNASEH1* | *MRPL3* |
| *SDHA* | *FDX1L* | | *MRPL44* |
| *SDHD* | *FDXL2* | **Other** | *MRPS2* |
| *SDHAF1* | *FDX2* | *AGK* | *MRPS7* |
| **Complex IV** | *ALR* | *TAZ* | *MRPS16* |
| *SCO1* | | *GFER* | *MRPS34* |
| *SCO2* | | *MSTO1* | *ATP5A1* |
| *COA5* | | *CHCHD10* | *SLC25A26* |
| *COA6* | | *PNPLA8* | *GFM1* |
| *COX6B1* | | | *MTO1* |
| *COA7* | | | *RMND1* |
| *COX8A* | | | *SFXN4* |
| *COX20* | | | *TSFM* |
| *COX10* | | | *C12ORF65* |
| *COX15* | | | *MIPEP* |
| *FASTKD2* | | | *KIAA1393* |
| *APOPT1* | | | *TUFM* |
| *PET100* | | | *C1QBP* |
| *MT-CO3* | | | *ELAC2* |
| *MT-CO2* | | | *C1QBP* |
| **Complex III** | | | *AIFM1* |
| *MT-CYB* | | | |
| **Complex V** | | | |
| *MT-ATP6* | | | |

[a]Defects in these genes can give either a clinical phenotype predominated by myopathy or a clinical phenotype not predominantly myopathic but with at least some myopathic involvement.

2014), isolated complex III deficiency (Andreu et al. 2000) and isolated complex V deficiency. The most common cause of mitochondrial myopathy associated with isolated complex III deficiency is a pathogenic mutation in *MT-CYB*, and the most common cause of isolated complex V deficiency is a pathogenic mutation in *MT-ATP6*. A combined complex I+IV deficiency (with or without complex III deficiency) is also a frequent cause of mitochondrial myopathy. This type of combined deficiency is suggestive of a pathogenic mutation in a mitochondrial encoded tRNA (Carelli and La Morgia 2018) or a nuclear defect in the protein machinery needed for intramitochondrial transcription or translation (D'Souza and Minczuk 2018; Vanlander et al. 2015; Vantroys et al. 2018) (Table 17.1). However, to make it more complicated, in these cases a combined I+IV deficiency is not always seen, but an isolated I or isolated complex IV deficiency. A combined complex I+II deficiency can be found in the individuals with an iron/sulfur cluster biosynthesis defect (Vanlander and Van Coster 2018; Ajit Bolar and Vanlander et al. 2013) (Table 17.1). In the latter, in addition to the combined complex I and II deficiency, a defect in pyruvate dehydrogenase complex can also be found, as the synthesis of subunit E2 of the pyruvate dehydrogenase complex is dependent upon iron/sulfur clusters.

In patients with one of the better defined syndromes, such as MELAS, MERRF or NARP, biochemical assays are not necessary as the possible underlying mtDNA defect can be detected directly in blood (WBC).

When an open skeletal muscle biopsy is performed, a skin biopsy can also be taken for culturing skin fibroblasts. Activities can be tested in cultured skin fibroblasts too, and the cells can be used as source of DNA.

Blue native polyacrylamide gel electrophoresis (BN-PAGE) followed by activity staining of the five complexes are helpful to confirm enzyme deficiency (Van Coster et al. 2001). In addition, this technique allows detection of sub-complexes of complex V which is suggestive of a defect in intramitochondrial transcription or translation caused by a pathogenic mtDNA mutation or by a pathogenic mutation in one of the genes encoding proteins needed for intramitochondrial transcription or translation (Smet et al. 2009).

The use of next generation sequencing has changed the diagnostic strategy. Mitochondrial gene panels are increasingly used for detection of the underlying molecular defect. Panels using specific primers for genes known to cause mitochondrial diseases can be used. Even more frequently used nowadays is whole exome sequencing (WES) followed by "in silico" selection of genes associated with mitochondrial disorders (Stenton and Prokisch 2018). Panels testing around 1 500 mitochondrial genes are available now. The advantage of the latter is that when no pathogenic mutations are found in the selected genes, the data from WES can be used to search for pathogenic mutations in genes that have not been reported yet, and in this way new gene defects can be detected. Functional testing will be necessary to prove pathogenicity when variants of unknown significance are detected.

**Treatment**

The treatment for mitochondrial diseases is disappointing. To date, only supportive therapy has been offered to the patient (El-Hattab et al. 2017). Rare exceptions are the vitamin-responsive defects like for example, riboflavine-responsive ACAD9 deficiency (Table 17.1). Mitochondrial disorders caused by a defect in biosynthesis of coenzyme Q can be treated by daily administration of coenzyme Q. Nowadays, many mitochondrial patients are given riboflavin (100mg/d), thiamine (50mg/d), L-arginine (3 000mg/d), citrulline (3 000mg/d), creatine (100mg/kg/d) and coenzyme Q (300mg/d) in varying combinations (Valero 2014). Both L-arginine and L-citrulline act as nitric oxide precursors. The benefits of daily administration of these nutritional supplements have not been demonstrated by placebo-controlled studies. The patients with diabetes mellitus due to a mitochondrial defect in the pancreas can be treated by daily administration of oral anti-diabetic medication or subcutaneous insulin. In patients with cardiac conduction disorders a pacemaker can be installed. For patients with severe ptosis, a surgical correction of the ptosis can be considered. For patients suffering from sensorineural hearing loss a cochlear implantation is a possibility. A physical exercise training program helps to train the anaerobic fibers to increase muscle power. Recently, new molecular therapies are being developed (Hirano et al. 2018).

**Key points**
- Mitochondrial myopathies are not rare and should be suspected in individuals suffering from intolerance of physical effort or abnormal fatigability.
- Lactate measurements are an important diagnostic tool (blood, urine, CSF), although a mitochondrial defect cannot be excluded when lactate is normal. Partial defects can be accompanied by normal lactate concentrations.
- Classification of mitochondrial diseases can be made based on clinical characteristics, on biochemical results, or on the underlying molecular defect. The goal is to find the underlying molecular defect as it provides important information on the hereditary aspects of the disease (maternal, autosomal recessive or dominant, X-linked). The outcome of the individuals affected by a mitochondrial defect is variable, although not good in the majority of the affected individuals. New treatment strategies are currently being developed.

**Clinical vignette**

A 6-year-old girl was seen by the paediatrician because of recurrent vomiting. Gastrointestinal investigations were negative. Apparently, vomiting occurred only after physical exercise. Lactate concentration in blood was 7mM (normal <2mM) after a moderate physical effort. The lactate day profile in blood confirmed significant increases of lactate during the day. Urinary organic acid profile was characterized by an increase of lactate and of Krebs cycle intermediates. Echocardiogram showed left ventricle hypertrophy. Eye fundus was normal. Microscopic examination of the skeletal muscle revealed the presence of ragged-red-fibers and biochemical examination a combined complex I+IV deficiency. Subcomplexes of complex V were detected using BN-PAGE. Cerebral MRI was normal. The m.3243A>G mutation in the gene coding for tRNA$^{Leu}$ was detected in skeletal muscle in a heteroplasmic state (90%) suggestive for the diagnosis of MELAS. In blood, m.3243A>G was present in 45% of WBC. The mother was heteroplasmic for the mutation in WBC (40%) as were the two brothers of the proband, although the mother and the two brothers were asymptomatic. Despite daily treatment with coenzyme Q, L-arginine, thiamine and riboflavin she deteriorated neurologically. MRI of the brain initially showed cortical lesions in the left occipital lobe. Subsequent MRIs revealed extensive lesions bilaterally involving the cerebral cortex, cerebral white matter and basal ganglia. She died at the age of 15 years.

## REFERENCES

Ajit Bolar N, Vanlander AV, Wilbrecht C, Van der Aa N, Smet J, De Paepe B et al. (2013) Mutation of the iron-sulfur cluster assembly gene IBA57 causes severe myopathy and encephalopathy. *Hum Mol Genet* 22(13): 2590–2602. doi: 10.1093/hmg/ddt107.

Andreu AL, Checcarelli N, Iwata S, Shanske S, DiMauro S (2000) A missense mutation in the mitochondrial cytochrome b gene in a revisited case with histiocytoid cardiomyopathy. *Pediatr Res* 48(3): 311–314. doi:10.1203/00006450-200009000-00008.

Bardosi A, Creutzfeldt W, DiMauro S, Felgenhauer K, Friede RL, Goebel HH et al. (1987) Myo-, neuro-, gastrointestinal encephalopathy (MNGIE syndrome) due to partial deficiency of cytochrome-c-oxidase. A new mitochondrial multisystem disorder. *Acta Neuropathol* 74: 248–258.

Carelli V, La Morgia C (2018) Clinical syndromes associated with mtDNA mutations: where we stand after 30 years. *Essays Biochem* 62(3): 235–254. doi: 10.1042/EBC20170097.

D'Souza AR, Minczuk M (2018) Mitochondrial transcription and translation: overview. *Essays Biochem* 62(3): 309–320. doi: 10.1042/EBC20170102.

De Praeter C, Vanlander A, Vanhaesebrouck P, Smet J, Seneca S, De Sutter P et al. (2015) Extremely high mutation load of the mitochondrial 8993 T>G mutation in a newborn: implications for prognosis and family planning decisions. *Eur J Pediatr* 174(2): 267–270. doi: 10.1007/s00431-014-2370-y.

Dermaut B, Seneca S, Dom L, Smets K, Ceulemans L, Smet J et al. (2010) Progressive myoclonic epilepsy as an adult-onset manifestation of Leigh syndrome due to m.14487T>C. *J Neurol Neurosurg Psychiatry* 81(1): 90–93. doi: 10.1136/jnnp.2008.157354.

Desguerre I, Hully M, Rio M, Nabbout R (2014) Mitochondrial disorders and epilepsy. *Rev Neurol (Paris)* 170(5): 375–380. doi: 10.1016/j.neurol.2014.03.010.

El-Hattab AW, Zarante AM, Almannai M, Scaglia F (2017) Therapies for mitochondrial diseases and current clinical trials. *Mol Genet Metab* 122(3): 1–9.

Finsterer J, Zarrouk-Mahjoub S (2018) Cerebral imaging in paediatric mitochondrial disorders. *Neuroradiol J* 31(6):596–608. doi: 10.1177/1971400918786054.

Fukuhara N, Tokiguchi S, Shirakawa K, Tsubaki T (1980) Myoclonus epilepsy associated with ragged-red fibres (mitochondrial abnormalities ): disease entity or a syndrome? Light-and electron-microscopic studies of two cases and review of literature. *J Neurol Sci* 47: 117–133.

Hirano M, Emmanuele V, Quinzii CM (2018) Emerging therapies for mitochondrial diseases. *Essays Biochem* 62(3): 467–481. doi: 10.1042/EBC20170114.

Holt IJ, Harding AE, Petty RK, Morgan-Hughes JA (1990) A new mitochondrial disease associated with mitochondrial DNA heteroplasmy. *Am J Hum Genet* 46(3): 428–433.

Honzik T, Tesarova M, Magner M, Mayr J, Jesina P, Vesela K et al. (2012) Neonatal onset of mitochon-drial disorders in 129 patients: clinical and laboratory characteristics and a new approach to diagnosis. *J Inherit Metab Dis* 35(5): 749–759.

Jonckheere AI, Renkema GH, Bras M, van den Heuvel LP, Hoischen A, Gilissen C et al. (2013) A complex V ATP5A1 defect causes fatal neonatal mitochondrial encephalopathy. *Brain* 136(Pt 5): 1544–1554. doi: 10.1093/brain/awt086.

Kearns TP, Sayre GP (1958) Retinitis pigmentosa, external ophthalmophegia, and complete heart block: unusual syndrome with histologic study in one of two cases. *AMA Arch Opthalmol* 60: 280–289.

Leigh D (1951) Subacute necrotizing encephalomyelopathy in an infant. *J Neurol Neurosurg Psychiatry* 14: 216–221.

Mascalchi M, Montomoli M, Guerrini R (2018) Neuroimaging in mitochondrial disorders. *Essays Biochem* 62(3): 409–442. doi: 10.1097/RMR.

Moraes CT, DiMauro S, Zeviani M, Lombes A, Shanske S, Miranda AF et al. (1989) Mitochondrial DNA deletions in progressive external ophthalmoplegia and Kearns-Sayre syndrome. *N Engl J Med* 320: 1293–1299.

Pavlakis SG, Phillips PC, DiMauro S, De Vivo DC, Rowland LP (1984) Mitochondrial myopathy, encephalopathy, lactic acidosis, and strokelike episodes: a distinctive clinical syndrome. *Ann Neurol* 16(4): 481–488. doi:10.1002/ana.410160409.

Roels F, Verloo P, Eyskens F, François B, Seneca S, De Paepe B et al. (2009) Mitochondrial mosaics in the liver of 3 infants with mtDNA defects. *BMC Clin Pathol* 9: 4. doi: 10.1186/1472-6890-9-4.

Saada A, Shaag A, Mandel H, Nevo Y, Eriksson S, Elpeleg O (2001) Mutant mitochondrial thymidine kinase in mitochondrial DNA depletion myopathy. *Nat Genet* 29(3): 342–344. doi:10.1038/ng751.

Smet J, Seneca S, De Paepe B, Meulemans A, Verhelst H, Leroy J et al. (2009) Subcomplexes of mitochondrial complex V reveal mutations in mitochondrial DNA. *Electrophoresis* 30(20): 3565–3572. doi:10.1002/elps.200900213.

Sonam K, Bindu PS, Taly AB, Nalini A, Govindaraju C, Aravinda HR et al. (2014) Mitochondrial myopathy, cardiomyopathy, and pontine signal changes in an adult patient with isolated complex II deficiency. *J Clin Neuromuscul Dis* 16(2): 69–73. doi: 10.1097/CND.0000000000000046.

Stenton SL, Prokisch H (2018) Advancing genomic approaches to the molecular diagnosis of mitochondrial disease. *Essays Biochem* 62(3): 399–340. doi: 10.1042/EBC20170110.

Valero T (2014) Mitochondrial biogenesis: pharmacological approaches. *Curr Pharm Des* 20: 5507–5509.

Van Coster R, Smet J, George E, De Meirleir L, Seneca S, Van Hove J et al. (2001) Blue native polyacrylamide gel electrophoresis: a powerful tool in diagnosis of oxidative phosphorylation defects. *Pediatr Res* 50(5): 658–65. doi:10.1203/00006450-200111000-00020.

Vanlander AV, Van Coster R (2018) Clinical and genetic aspects of defects in the mitochondrial iron-sulfur cluster synthesis pathway. J *Biol Inorg Chem* 23(4): 495–506. doi: 10.1007/s00775-018-1550-z.

Vanlander AV, Menten B, Smet J, De Meirleir L, Sante T, De Paepe B et al. (2015) Two siblings with homozygous pathogenic splice-site variant in mitochondrial asparaginyl-tRNA synthetase (NARS2). *Hum Mutat* 36(2): 222–31. doi: 10.1002/humu.22728.

Vantroys E, Smet J, Vanlander AV, Vergult S, De Bruyne R, Roels F et al. (2018) Severe hepatopathy and neurological deterioration after start of valproate treatment in a 6-year-old child with mitochondrial tryptophanyl-tRNA synthetase deficiency. *Orphanet J Rare Dis* 13(1): 80. doi: 10.1186/s13023-018-0822-6.

# 18
# CHANNELOPATHIES

*Nicolas Deconinck*

## Introduction

Muscle channelopathies, although very rare in prevalence, form a group of disorders with a frequent pediatric presentation. They typically involve the genetic dysfunction of an ionic channel at the level of the sarcolemmal membrane, impacting its excitability, either making it hypo- or inexcitable in the case of the periodic paralysis or hyperexcitable in the case of the non-dystrophic myotonias.

THE PERIODIC PARALYSIS

The inherited periodic paralyses consist of three disorders that may appear during childhood: hypokalemic periodic paralysis, hyperkalemic periodic paralysis, and Andersen–Tawil syndrome. Their relative exact incidence is unknown but hypokalemic periodic paralysis is thought to be the most common with an estimated incidence of 1 in 100 000 (Fontaine 1994; Venance et al. 2006). They are all autosomal dominant disorders.

Fluctuations in serum potassium levels during paralytic attacks were originally at the basis for the distinction of hypokalemic periodic paralysis and hyperkalemic periodic paralysis. Since their original description it is now becoming clear that rising or decreasing serum potassium levels do occur but these can be mild and the absolute value may be in the normal range, and do not exclude the diagnosis. With the availability of genetic testing many cases of reported normokalemic periodic paralysis has been demonstrated in patients suffering from genetically determined hyperkalemic periodic paralysis (Chinnery et al. 2002).

Hereafter we provide a short description of the three disorders.

*Hypokalemic periodic paralysis*

Hypokalemic periodic paralysis is caused in a majority of cases by a mutation in the dihydropyridine receptor, *CACNA1S*, and more rarely in the *SCN4A* gene. The disorder is characterized by episodes of flaccid skeletal muscle paralysis associated with low serum potassium levels during the attack. As a result precipitators to attacks include factors that will lower serum potassium; for example, eating a large carbohydrate meal or rest after physical exercise. It can present at any age from the first to the third decade (Miller et al. 2004) but typically presents in the teenage years. The paralysis affects skeletal muscle, predominantly the limb muscles, although occasionally respiratory muscles may be involved

(Arzel-Hézode et al. 2010). Attacks usually take place during the night or early morning and last for several hours even days.

*Hyperkalemic periodic paralysis*

Hyperkalemic periodic paralysis is caused by a mutation in the *SCN4A* gene. It is characterized by episodes of skeletal muscle weakness generally in association with high serum potassium levels. Precipitating factors include ingestion of potassium-rich foods, particularly fruits; for example, tomatoes and bananas. Most frequently, it starts during the first decade (typically at a younger age than in hypokalemic periodic paralysis) (Miller et al. 2004). Attacks of skeletal muscle weakness are also shorter, commonly lasting minutes to hours, and occurring at any time of the day.

As with hypokalemic periodic paralysis, hyperkalemic periodic paralysis does not directly impact the heart but arrthythmia may be precipitated by an acute phase of raised serum potassium.

### Andersen–Tawil syndrome

Andersen–Tawil syndrome is caused by mutations in the *KCNJ2* gene. Typically, the syndrome is characterized by a triad of episodic skeletal muscle paralysis, dysmorphic features, and cardiac conduction defects (Andersen et al. 1971; Tawil et al. 1994). It is the only skeletal muscle channelopathy to directly affect organs other than skeletal muscle. The paralysis most commonly resembles the one observed in the case of hypokalemic periodic paralysis (Davies et al. 2005). The dysmorphic features can include mandibular micrognathia, short stature, clinodactyly, hypertelorism or hypotelorism, low-set ears, a broad forehead, and a high arched palate (Tawil et al. 1994; Haruna et al. 2007).

Likewise there are often no cardiac symptoms, and unless an electrocardiogram (ECG) is performed for unrelated circumstances or for a suspected diagnosis of Andersen–Tawil syndrome the cardiac conduction defects are often undetected. This can have significant consequences because, although rare, sudden death may occur (Davies et al. 2005; Zhang L et al. 2005). Conduction defects described include abnormal U waves, a prolonged QUc interval, a prolonged QTc interval, bigeminy, and bidirectional VT.

### Diagnosis

In children differential diagnosis may include epilepsy or other causes of malaises (hypoglycemia, etc.). A careful recording of the sequence of events and the timing of the attacks as well as the potential triggers is essential for establishing the diagnosis. Genetic testing is currently considered the cornerstone for diagnosis. Diagnosis can be helped by some electrophysiological investigations including exercise tests not detailed in this chapter (Tan et al. 2011). Provocative tests or a muscle biopsy are not any more required in the diagnostic work up.

### Treatment

PREVENTION OF ATTACKS

Symptom severity is very variable in the periodic paralyses. If mild, patients may opt to manage their symptoms by lifestyle modification and the avoidance of precipitating factors alone. None of the treatments used in the periodic paralyses have been subjected to large-scale randomized controlled trials (Sansone et al. 2008). However, if treatment is considered necessary, available therapies for hypokalemic periodic paralysis include potassium supplements or potassium-sparing diuretics such as spironolactone. Thiazide diuretics may be beneficial in hyperkalemic periodic paralysis. Inhaled salbutamol, if taken at the onset of a hyperkalemic attack, may help to abort it or limit its duration (Hanna et al. 1998).

Although their exact mechanism of action is still not so well described, carbonic anhydrase inhibitors, including acetazolamide or dichlorphenamide, are the mainstay of treatment for all the periodic paralyses. They reduce the severity, duration, or frequency of paralyptic attacks (Tawil et al. 2000). The natural history of these disorders, however, is that the frequency of attacks does tend to diminish with increasing age making the treatment unnecessary. An annual renal ultrasound screening should be performed when using carbonic anhydrase inhibitors.

TREATMENT OF ACUTE ATTACKS OF PARALYSIS

Total body potassium during an attack of muscle weakness is normal but the distribution between the intracellular and the extracellular space is displaced. This is an important consideration as equilibrium will be restored by the body when the attack diminishes. As a consequence, if potassium supplementation is given in an attack of hypokalemic periodic paralysis a subsequent high serum potassium level may be induced and could have adverse cardiac consequences (Ahmed and Chilimuri 2010).

Replacing or attempting to reduce serum potassium levels should only be considered if there are detrimental ECG changes during an attack of muscle weakness, or if there is weakness of respiratory muscles leading to respiratory failure (a rare event). ECG and serum potassium monitoring are mandatory.

## The non-dystrophic myotonias

The exact incidence of the non-dystrophic myotonias is unknown but estimates range from 1 in 10 000 to 7 in 10 000 (Matthews et al. 2010). Three classic disorders have been described: paramyotonia congenital, sodium channel myotonia (including potassium and cold-aggravated myotonias), and myotonia congenital. The predominant symptom in each is myotonia, although variable muscle weakness or paralysis can additionally occur. Importantly in the context of diagnosis reasoning, none of these disorders have systemic features unlike myotonic dystrophy (Table 18.1, Fig. 18.1). We will also describe the rare Schwartz–Jampel syndrome involving generalized muscle stiffness/ myotonia and chondrodysplasia.

PARAMYOTONIA CONGENITA

Paramyotonia congenita is a sodium channel disorder due to mutations in the *SCN4A* gene but is considered separately from the sodium channel myotonias due to the presence of episodic muscle weakness, which differentiates it from this group. Symptoms can be present from birth and parents may note facial myotonia, especially if the infant is washed with cool water (Eulenberg 1886). Symptoms are generally noted by the patient themselves within their first decade (Matthews et al. 2008; Trip et al. 2009), often when they attend primary

**TABLE 18.1**

**Non-dystrophic myotonia categories: clinical symptoms and electrodiagnostic features**

| | Recessive myotonia congenita | Dominant myotonia congenita | Paramyotonia congenita | Sodium channel myotonia |
|---|---|---|---|---|
| Inheritance | Recessive | Dominant | Dominant | Dominant |
| Causative gene | CLCN1 | CLCN1 | SCN4A | SCN4A |
| Myotonia distribution | Lower limbs more than upper limbs | Upper limbs more than lower limbs. Facial muscles may be involved | Upper limbs and face more than lower limbs | Upper limbs, face, extraocular, more than lower limbs |
| Myotonia cold sensitivity | None or minimal | None or minimal | Yes – often dramatic | Variable – ranging from none to severe |
| Warm-up phenomenon | Present | Present | Absent | May be present |
| Paradoxical myotonia | Absent | Absent | Present | May be present |
| Delayed onset myotonia after exercise | Absent | Absent | Absent | May be present. Characteristic of myotonia fluctuans |
| Episodic muscle weakness | Common, develops on initiation of movement but transient and improves rapidly | Uncommon | Common, often exacerbated by cold and/or exercise and frequently prolonged for several hours | Not reported |
| Eyelid myotonia | Infrequent | Infrequent | Common | Common |
| SET without cooling | Early decrement in CMAP with rapid recovery. Decrement reduces with repetition | Little or no decrement in CMAP | Gradual and persistent reduction in CMAP enhanced by repetition | No significant change of the CMAP from baseline |
| SET with cooling | Cooling has little further effect | Early decrement with rapid recovery and reduction with repetition may be seen | Gradual and persistent reduction in CMAP enhanced further by cooling | No significant change of the CMAP from baseline |

SET: short exercise test; CMAP: compound muscle action potential.

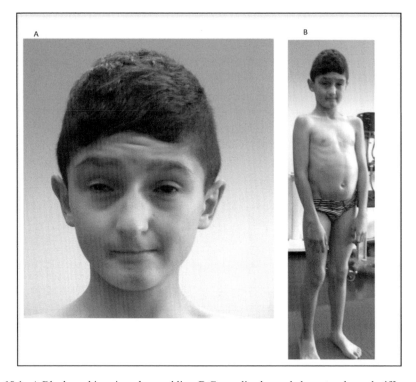

**Fig. 18.1. A** Blepharophimosis and pursed lips. **B** Generalized muscle hypertrophy and stiffness.

school. Characteristic symptoms are myotonia, especially of the hand and facial muscles, that is exacerbated by a cold environment or by repetitive muscle action. A common story is facing difficulties to changing clothes in a cold atmosphere after swimming in a cool pool because of stiff hands (due to myotonia).

SODIUM CHANNEL MYOTONIAS

The sodium channel myotonias can be the hardest group of the non-dystrophic myotonias to characterize. The key feature is that they are purely myotonic disorders and muscle weakness or paralysis does not occur. They are due to mutations of the same gene as paramyotonia congenita (the *SCN4A* gene). Symptoms also can be present from birth and usually within the first decade. The myotonia predominantly affects the face and hand muscles as with paramyotonia congenita, but the legs are more frequently affected than in paramyotonia congenita (Matthews et al. 2008).

MYOTONIA CONGENITA

The age at onset of myotonia congenita is commonly also in the first decade (Thomsen 1876). Overall there is a relatively wide spectrum from the first to the fourth decade. The distribution of myotonia also varies, and lower limbs tend to be most severely affected. Affected patients may appear very athletic because of muscle hypertrophy, particularly in the calves (Fialho et al. 2007). It is important to enquire about physical activity because the significance of a muscular physique may be overlooked in young patients if it is assumed that it reflects an active lifestyle. The typical feature of the myotonia is the warm-up phenomenon where it can be seen to improve with repetitive muscle action. The myotonia is often worst when attempting to move after a period of rest.

A cold environment may exacerbate the myotonia of myotonia congenita but this is variable and it is not prominent as in paramyotonia congenita.

Myotonia congenita can be inherited in either a dominant (Thomsen 1876) or recessive manner (Becker disease) (Becker 1977), both involving the voltage-gated chloride channel CLCN1.

NEONATAL COMPLICATIONS OF PARAMYOTONIA CONGENITA AND SODIUM CHANNEL MYOTONIA
In recent years more significant neonatal presentations of paramyotonia congenita have been reported. Fatal myotonia of respiratory muscles, but also severe laryngospasm and stridor have been described, often responding well to mexiletine (Lion-François et al. 2010).

It is important to be aware of neonatal or infantile presentations of non-dystrophic myotonia in order to advise expectant mothers appropriately and to provide essential information to the relevant pediatric and obstetric teams who may be involved. Overall, labor in skeletal muscle channelopathy should be considered of relatively high risk and managed in a tertiary center with multidisciplinary experience.

MAKING THE DIAGNOSIS
When suspecting myotonia, the first step is trying to confirm the presence of myotonic discharges with needle examination during an electromyography (EMG) examination, always bearing in mind that the first cause of abnormal myotonic discharges is myotonic dystrophy type 1 (DM1). It is also very important to check how myotonia is influenced by temperature and/or exercise, particularly in the case of paramytonia congenita (Table 18.1). In the hands of a specialized neurophysiologist, a repeat short effort protocol performed at room temperature and afterwards in iced water may be very useful to orient to one of the three forms of the non-dystrophic myotonias. Nowadays, genetic testing has taken a prominent role in the diagnostic work up.

**Management**
As with the periodic paralyses, some patients will opt for lifestyle modification and the avoidance of factors that provoke myotonia rather than choosing pharmacological therapies. There are no currently available drugs that directly target the dysfunctional CLCN1 channel in myotonia congenita. There is a lack of evidence from randomized controlled trials for any of the available therapies and recommendations are based upon case reports and clinical experience (Trip et al. 2006). The most effective and tolerated drug seems to be mexiletine. Although it is a sodium channel blocker it is also reported to have benefit in myotonia congenita (Leheup et al. 1986). A randomized double-blind placebo-controlled clinical trial of mexiletine in non-dystrophic myotonia demonstrated positive effects on muscle stiffness and is now frequently used by patients, although the accessibility of the drug may prove difficult in some countries (Statland et al. 2012).

As with all anti-arrhthymics, mexiletine can also be pro-arrhythmic and an ECG and cardiac history should be taken prior to commencing treatment. If there is any uncertainty over its safe use in an individual, cardiological review should be sought.

In the future, finding new compounds able to target the CIC-1 channel and the finding of new safer analogues of tocainide may prove very efficient in the field.

SCHWARTZ–JAMPEL SYNDROME

Schwartz–Jampel syndrome (SJS) is a rare condition characterized by permanent muscle stiffness (myotonia) and bone abnormalities known as chondrodysplasia (Viljoen and Beighton 1992). The signs and symptoms of this condition become apparent sometime after birth, usually in early childhood. Either muscle stiffness or chondrodysplasia can appear first. The muscle and bone abnormalities worsen in childhood, although most affected individuals have a normal lifespan. The specific features of SJS vary widely.

Myotonia involving continuous contraction of muscles causes stiffness that interferes with eating, sitting, walking, and other movements (Fig. 18.2). Sustained contraction of muscles in the face leads to a fixed, "mask-like" facial expression with narrow eye openings (blepharophimosis) and pursed lips (Fig. 18.1). This facial appearance is very specific to

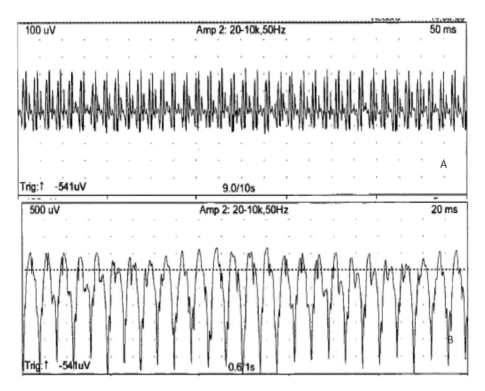

**Fig. 18.2.** Electromyography of the right quadriceps demonstrating continuous activity at resting state with **A** pseudomyotonic discharges and **B** complex repetitive discharges.

SJS (Arya et al. 2013). Affected individuals may also be nearsighted and experience abnormal blinking or spasms of the eyelids (blepharospasm).

Chondrodysplasia affects the development of the skeleton, particularly the long bones in the arms and legs and the bones of the hips. These bones are shortened and unusually wide at the ends, so affected individuals have short stature. The long bones may also be abnormally curved (bowed). Other bone abnormalities associated with SJS include a protruding chest (pectus carinatum), abnormal curvature of the spine, flattened bones of the spine (platyspondyly), and joint abnormalities called contractures that further restrict movement.

SJS is caused by mutations in the *HSPG2* gene. This gene encodes the SJS perlecan protein, which consists of a core protein to which three long chains of glycosaminoglycans (heparan sulfate or chondroitin sulfate) are attached. Perlecan is found in the extracellular matrix, specifically in the basal membrane, found in cartilage but also at the neuromuscular junction.

Most individuals with SJS have a good long-term outlook (prognosis) with a nearly normal life expectancy. Patients may be at risk of malignant hyperthermia.

Treatment of SJS aims to reduce muscle stiffness and cramping and may include massage, muscle warming, and gradual strengthening exercises. Medications might also be used and may include muscle relaxants and anti-seizure medications, particularly carbamazepine. Botox might additionally be used to relieve eye symptoms such as blepharospasm. When considering surgery as an option, an important consideration is malignant hyperthermia, an associated complication, that can increase the risk of adverse outcomes

**Key points**
- The muscle channelopathies in children are a group of disorders caused by mutations of various voltage-gated ion channel genes, including non-dystrophic myotonia and periodic paralysis.
- Within the group of non-dystrophic myotonias, chloride channelopathy (Becker disease and Thomsen disease) form a first sub group in which warm-up phenomenon and muscle hypertrophy are common clinical manifestations. Sodium channelopathy (paramyotonia congenita and other sodium channel myotonia) form a second subgroup. Stiffness of the facial muscles is an important presenting symptom, and eyelid myotonia is a common clinical finding in this subgroup. Electrical myotonia is very often observed and mexiletine is effective in controlling symptoms in patients.
- Patients suffering from periodic paralysis fall under three groups, either hyperkalemic periodic paralysis, hypokalemic periodic paralysis, and finally Andersen–Tawil syndrome. Acetazolamide is commonly used to prevent paralytic attacks.
- Altogether, non-dystrophic muscle channelopathies present with diverse clinical manifestations including myotonia, muscle hypertrophy, proximal weakness, swallowing difficulties, and periodic paralysis.
- Cardiac arrhythmias are potentially life threatening in Andersen–Tawil syndrome.
- Timely identification of these disorders is helpful for effective symptomatic management and genetic counseling.

**Clinical vignette**

A 10-year-old boy patient was referred to the neurology department for assessment of an episode of global muscle weakness after a 100m sprint. There was no loss of consciousness. Proximal hip muscles and shoulder girdle weakness was noted raising the possibility of a myopathy with a very slow progression. A muscle biopsy was normal.

Medical background was unremarkable. Physical examination revealed short stature, mandibular hypoplasia, hypertelorism and a broad nasal root. Neurological assessment demonstrated a waddling gait, with inability to rise from a sitting position without assistance. No fasciculation or myotonia was evident. Marked proximal upper and lower limb girdle weakness (MRC 3/5) was found associated with hypotonia. Distal strength was largely preserved. Reflexes were symmetrically depressed.

At the age of 15 the patient experienced several episodes of transient loss of consciousness over a 5-week period. The episodes were always followed by a period of confusion but without any no urinary incontinence or tongue biting. No trigger was identified. A work up including electroencephalography (EEG) and MRI brain were normal. A cardiac monitoring showed a marginally prolonged QTc. Echocardiogram showed no evidence of structural heart disease. An Holter monitor confirmed the background rhythm was sinus, with the recording of episodes of non-sustained bidirectional ventricular tachycardia and frequent multi-morphological left ventricular ectopy with a 30% ectopic burden.

A channelopathy for the cause of his frequent ventricular ectopy and syncope was postulated. Brugada syndrome and arrhythmogenic right ventricular cardiomyopathy were thought less likely as the ECG did not show features typically associated with these disorders. Because of the association of the proximal muscle weakness, some characteristic dysmorphic features and the recording of an episode of bidirectional ventricular tachycardia, the medical team suspected a diagnostic of Andersen–Tawil syndrome, although the baseline ECG did not demonstrate the classic prominent U waves. A missense mutation in *KCNJ2* (chromosome 17q23) was found confirming the diagnosis. This gene encodes the inward potassium rectifier channel $K_{ir}2.1$ ($I_{K1}$), leading to prolongation of the terminal phase of the cardiac action potential.

Metoprolol (a beta blocker), and flecainide were sequentially tried, but were either ineffective or produced intolerable side effects. Because of the attenuation of syncope episodes over time, the treatment with an implantable automatic cardioverter defibrillator or implantable cardioverter defibrillator (ICD) was not recommended.

## REFERENCES

Ahmed I, Chilimuri SS (2010) Fatal dysrhythmia following potassium replacement for hypokalemic periodic paralysis. *West J Emerg Med* 11: 57–59.

Andersen ED, Krasilnikoff PA, Overvad H (1971) Intermittent muscular weakness, extrasystoles, and multiple developmental anomalies. A new syndrome? *Acta Paediatr Scand* 60: 559–564.

Arya R, Sharma S, Gupta N, Kumar S, Kabra M, Gulati S (2013) Schwartz Jampel syndrome in children. *J Clin Neurosci* 20: 313–317.

Arzel-Hézode M, Sternberg D, Tabti N, Vicart S, Goizet C, Eymard B et al. (2010) Homozygosity for dominant mutations increases severity of muscle channelopathies. *Muscle Nerve* 41: 470–477.

Becker PE (1977) *Myotonia Congenita and Syndromes Associated with Myotonia.* Stuttgart: Georg Thieme Verlag.

Chinnery PF, Walls TJ, Hanna MG, Bates D, Fawcett PR (2002) Normokalemic periodic paralysis revisited: does it exist? *Ann Neurol* 52: 251–252.

Davies NP, Imbrici P, Fialho D, Herd C, Bilsland LG, Weber A et al. (2005) Andersen-Tawil syndrome: new potassium channel mutations and possible phenotypic variation. *Neurology* 65: 1083–1089.

Eulenberg A (1886) Ueber eine Familiäre, durch 6 Generationen Verfolbare form Congenitaler Paramyotonie. *Neurol Centralblatt* 12: 265–272.

Fialho D, Schorge S, Pucovska U, Davies NP, Labrum R, Haworth A et al. (2007) Chloride channel myotonia: exon 8 hot-spot for dominant-negative interactions. *Brain* 130: 3265–3274.

Fontaine B (1994) Primary periodic paralysis and muscle sodium channel. *Adv Nephrol Necker Hosp* 23: 191–197.

Hanna MG, Stewart J, Schapira AH, Wood NW, Morgan-Hughes JA, Murray NM (1998) Salbutamol treatment in a patient with hyperkalaemic periodic paralysis due to a mutation in the skeletal muscle sodium channel gene (SCN4A). *J Neurol Neurosurg Psychiatry* 65: 248–250.

Haruna Y, Kobori A, Makiyama T, Yoshida H, Akao M, Doi T et al. (2007) Genotype-phenotype correlations of KCNJ2 mutations in Japanese patients with Andersen-Tawil syndrome. *Hum Mutat* 28: 208.

Leheup B, Himon F, Morali A, Brichet F, Vidailhet M (1986) [Value of mexiletine in the treatment of Thomsen-Becker myotonia]. *Arch Fr Pediatr* 43: 49–50.

Lion-François L, Mignot C, Vicart S, Manel V, Sternberg D, Landrieu P et al. (2010) Severe neonatal episodic laryngospasm due to de novo SCN4A mutations: a new treatable disorder. *Neurology* 75: 641–645.

Matthews E, Tan SV, Fialho D, Sweeney MG, Sud R, Haworth A et al. (2008) What causes paramyotonia in the United Kingdom? Common and new SCN4A mutations revealed. *Neurology* 70: 50–53.

Matthews E, Fialho D, Tan SV, Venance SL, Cannon SC, Sternberg D et al. (2010) The non-dystrophic myotonias: molecular pathogenesis, diagnosis and treatment. *Brain* 133: 9–22.

Matthews E, Manzur AY, Sud R, Muntoni F, Hanna MG (2011) Stridor as a neonatal presentation of skeletal muscle sodium channelopathy. *Arch Neurol* 68: 127–129.

Miller TM, Dias da Silva MR, Miller HA, Kwiecinski H, Mendell JR, Tawil R et al. (2004) Correlating phenotype and genotype in the periodic paralyses. *Neurology* 63: 1647–1655.

Sansone V, Meola G, Links TP, Panzeri M, Rose MR (2008) Treatment for periodic paralysis. *Cochrane Database Syst Rev* 1:CD005045.

Statland JM, Bundy BN, Wang Y, Rayan DR, Trivedi JR, Sansone VA et al. (2012) Mexiletine for symptoms and signs of myotonia in nondystrophic myotonia: a randomized controlled trial. *JAMA* 308: 1357–1365.

Tan SV, Matthews E, Barber M, Burge JA, Rajakulendran S, Fialho D et al. (2011) Refined exercise testing can aid DNA-based diagnosis in muscle channelopathies. *Ann Neurol* 69: 328–340.

Tawil R, Ptacek LJ, Pavlakis SG, DeVivo DC, Penn AS, Ozdemir C et al. (1994) Andersen's syndrome: potassium-sensitive periodic paralysis, ventricular ectopy, and dysmorphic features. *Ann Neurol* 35: 326–330.

Tawil R, McDermott MP, Brown R Jr, Shapiro BC, Ptacek LJ, McManis PG et al. (2000) Randomized trials of dichlorphenamide in the periodic paralyses. *Ann Neurol* 47: 46–53.

Thomsen J (1876) Tonische Krampfe in Willkurlich beweglichen Muskeln in Folge von ererbter psychischer Disposition. *Arch Psychiatr Nervenkr* 6: 702–718.

Trip J, Drost G, van Engelen BG, Faber CG (2006) Drug treatment for myotonia. *Cochrane Database Syst Rev* 1:CD004762.

Trip J, Drost G, Ginjaar HB, Nieman FH, van der Kooi AJ, de Visser M et al. (2009) Redefining the clinical phenotypes of non-dystrophic myotonic syndromes. *J Neurol Neurosurg Psychiatry* 80: 647–652.

Venance SL, Cannon SC, Fialho D, Fontaine B, Hanna MG, Ptacek LJ et al. (2006) The primary periodic paralyses: diagnosis, pathogenesis and treatment. *Brain* 129: 8–17.

Viljoen D, Beighton P (1992) Schwartz-Jampel syndrome (chondrodystrophic myotonia). *J Med Genet* 29(1): 58–62.

Zhang L, Benson DW, Tristani-Firouzi M, Ptacek LJ, Tawil R, Schwartz PJ et al. (2005) Electrocardiographic features in Andersen-Tawil syndrome patients with KCNJ2 mutations: characteristic T-U-wave patterns predict the KCNJ2 genotype. *Circulation* 111: 2720–2726.

# 19
# INFLAMMATORY MYOPATHIES

*Nicolas Deconinck and Laurence Goffin*

## Introduction

The Juvenile idiopathic inflammatory myopathies (JIIMs) are heterogeneous, systemic autoimmune diseases characterized by muscular weakness related to chronic inflammation of skeletal muscles, and accompanied by typical skin rashes (Gottron papules or heliotrope rash) with early onset during childhood. The criteria established by Bohan and Peter (1975) based on these features, together with the presence of elevated serum levels of muscle enzymes or increased electrical activity in the muscle detected by electromyography (EMG), have been used to diagnose these disorders. However, new classification criteria have recently been developed and validated (Tjärnlund et al. 2012).

The most common clinical phenotype of myositis in children is juvenile dermatomyositis (JDM), which makes up approximately 80% of all patients with JIIMs. Patients with JDM are often the youngest among those with JIIMs, as JDM has a median age at onset of 7.4 years (Rider and Miller 2011; Rider and Nistala 2016).

JDM is a systemic vasculopathy characterized by symmetrical proximal muscle weakness, raised serum concentrations of muscle enzymes, and pathognomonic skin rashes that include the heliotrope rash over the eyelids and Gottron papules over the extensor joint surfaces (Rider and Miller 2011; Rider and Nistala 2016). This disease is classified in the group of the idiopathic inflammatory myopathies; the adult forms being the most common.

## Epidemiology

The incidence of JDM in the USA is 3.2 per million children per year, which is similar to the incidence in the UK. The average age at onset is 7 years, but 25% of patients are younger than 4 years at onset. In the USA, the ratio of girls to boys is 2.3 to 1, compared with 5 to 1 in the UK. The rash is the first symptom to be recognized in half of all children diagnosed and weakness is the first symptom in a quarter (Miller et al. 2013).

## Etiology and pathogenesis

Both genetic and environmental risk factors seem to be involved in the pathogenesis of JDM, and genome–environment interactions raise complexity in the pathogenesis of this disease (Pachman et al. 2005). This disease is thought to be the result of environmental triggers in genetically susceptible children, resulting in immune dysfunction and specific tissue responses. The international Myositis Genetics Consortium (Myogen) recently published the first genome-wide analysis of idiopathic inflammatory myopathies (IIM), confirming that the HLA region was the strongest locus linked to both adult and juvenile dermatomyositis, in particular the HLA B8-DRB1*0301 ancestral haplotype. A few new genetic loci were found to be associated with myositis although further data are required for many of them: *CCL21* (chemokine [C-C motif] ligand 21), *PLCL1* (phospholipase C-like 1), and *BLK* (B lymphoid kinase) (Rider and Miller 2011; Liu et al. 2012).

Previous infections and birth seasonality suggest that environmental stimuli might also increase the risk for JDM (Pachman et al. 2005). Prior upper respiratory, or gastro-intestinal infection are frequently observed within the 3 months before the onset of JDM symptoms.

One of the most consistent observations in JDM is the activation of plasmacytoid dendritic cells (most probably by viral nucleic acids or self-DNA) that goes together with the release of large amounts of type I interferon (IFNs) (IFNα and IFNβ), leading to immune cell activation and vasculopathy (Lee et al. 2007). The expression of genes induced by IFN, termed IFN-responsive elements, is often used as a surrogate measure of excessive IFN signaling in vivo, and has been shown to partially correlate with disease activity in JDM (Bilgic et al. 2009). Both humoral and cellular immunity contribute to the pathogenesis.

**Pathological changes and pathophysiology**

Juvenile dermatomyositis is a vasculopathic condition. Typical histological changes in the muscle include swelling of the capillary endothelium with obliteration of the lumen, perifascicular atrophy, perivascular inflammation, muscle degeneration and regeneration and the presence of tubuloreticular inclusions (which are visible by electron microscopy). An international consensus working group has developed a scoring system for juvenile dermatomyositis muscle biopsies (Wedderburn et al. 2007; Miles et al. 2007).

The score examines four domains: (1) endomysial, perivascular, and perimysial inflammation; (2) vascular changes; (3) changes to muscle fiber including MHC class I overexpression, atrophy of perifascicular and degeneration or regeneration of other muscle fibers, and presence of neonatal myosin; and (4) endomysial and perimysial fibrosis (Ramanan and Feldman 2002). A similar score shows that more diffuse early changes seen in biopsy samples could predict a chronic course for the disease (Sato et al. 2009).

The vasculopathy of juvenile dermatomyositis affects skeletal muscle, skin, the gastro-intestinal tract, and other tissues such as lungs, kidneys, eyes and heart.

**Clinical features**

The onset of JDM is often characterized by an insidious muscle weakness, malaise, easy fatigue, fever and rash over a few months before the diagnosis is made. Muscle weakness is symmetric, predominantly proximal, and can be associated with myalgia or stiffness. Functional impairment can lead the child to stop walking. On clinical examination, symmetrical weakness in the proximal muscles of the shoulders and hips can be associated with an involvement of the abdominal musculature and the neck flexors. Affected muscles are sometimes tender and edematous. Gowers' sign is usually present, as well as Trendelenburg sign. Distal muscle can be affected in later stages of the disease. Difficult swallowing and dysphonia can arise as a result of pharyngeal, hypopharyngeal and palatal muscles. Validated myositis assessment tools, such as the Childhood Myositis Assessment Scale (CMAS), can help the clinician in evaluating muscle strength impairment.

Most of the children have pathognomonic cutaneous abnormalities at presentation, including heliotrope discoloration of the upper eyelids, Gottron papules over the extensor surfaces of joints (interphalangeal and metacarpophalangeal joints, elbows, knees) and peri-ungueal erythema. Cutaneous ulceration can occur in children with severe and prolonged disease (Fig. 19.1).

In addition to muscle weakness and characteristic skin signs, the presenting features of juvenile dermatomyositis are multiple (Miles et al. 2007):

• Dystrophic calcification occurs in up to 30% of patients (Ramanan and Feldman 2002; Rider 2003). The sites most frequently affected are the pressure points: elbows, knees, digits and buttocks (Fig. 19.1). Calcinosis most often begins 1–3 years after onset of illness, but might begin at illness onset or as late as 20 years after onset. Four subtypes have been described (Bohan and Peter 1975): cutaneous or subcutaneous plaques

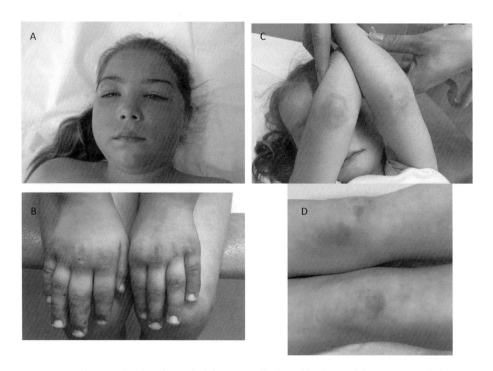

**Fig. 19.1.** Heliotrope discoloration and violaceous suffusion with edema of the upper eyelids in a girl with acute dermatomyositis. Erythematous, scaly rash in a malar distribution (**A**); Gottron papules: symmetrical, scaly, erythematous papules over the metacarpophalangeal and interphalangeal joints of the hands (**B**); Gottron papules on the elbows (**C**) and knees (**D**). A colour version of this figure can be seen in the plate section at the end of the book.

or nodules (Tjärnlund et al. 2012); deposits that extend to muscle; calcinosis along fascial planes that might lead to contractures; and widespread calcium exoskeleton (Rider and Nistala 2016). Calcinosis can result in skin ulceration; functional disability from joint contractures, pain because of nerve entrapment: or local inflammation with local erythema, tenderness, and drainage that should be distinguished from cellulitis. Calcinosis is associated with delayed diagnosis and long duration of untreated disease, a chronic disease course, and inadequate corticosteroid therapy. It can result in severe disability. Cutaneous ulcerations are pathologically the result of complement deposition with occlusive endarteropathy of dermal vessels.

- Vasculopathy of the mucosa of the gastro-intestinal tract occurs in a minority of children and signifies a poor prognosis. It can result in tissue ischemia or acute mesenteric infarction with ulceration, hemorrhage, pneumatosis intestinalis or perforation. Abdominal pain that is persistent, progressive or severe should be carefully assessed clinically and radiologically, and stool should be tested for occult blood (Mamyrova et al. 2007).
- Vasculopathy sometimes causes other acute and potentially life-threatening manifestations, such as widespread edema or anasarca (Mitchell et al. 2001), and involvement of the gallbladder, urogenital tract, liver or pancreas. Pulmonary manifestations are mostly due to respiratory muscle weakness resulting in restrictive pulmonary disease but vasculopathies can induce spontaneous pneumothorax or pneumomediastinum, which are often associated with cutaneous ulceration (De Souza Neves et al. 2007).
- 10–40% of patients with JDM have acquired lipodystrophy, which might involve all, a part, or a localized region of the body. Insulin resistance with acanthosis nigricans, diabetes and dyslipidemia accompanies this progressive subcutaneous or visceral fat loss in many of these patients. Other sequelae include hyperpigmentation, hepatomegaly, hypertension and menstrual irregularity (Pope et al. 2006).

**Diagnostic criteria**

The diagnosis of juvenile dermatomyositis is mainly made through a constellation of clinical and laboratory tests, as applied in the 1975 criteria by Bohan and Peter (1975).

Criteria for a diagnosis of juvenile dermatomyositis:

- Symmetrical weakness of the proximal musculature.
- Characteristic cutaneous changes consisting of heliotrope discoloration of the eyelids, which may be accompanied by periorbital edema and erythematous papules over the extensor surfaces of joints, including the dorsal aspects of the metacarpophalangeal and proximal interphalangeal joints, elbows, knees or ankles (i.e., Gottron papules).
- Elevation of the serum level of one or more of the following skeletal muscle enzymes: creatine kinase, aspartate aminotransferase, lactate dehydrogenase, and aldolase.
- Electromyographic demonstration of the characteristics of myopathy and denervation, including the triad of polyphasic, short, small motor-unit potentials; fibrillations, positive sharp waves, increased insertional irritability; and bizarre, high-frequency repetitive discharges.

- Muscle biopsy documenting histological evidence of necrosis; fiber size variation, particularly perifascicular atrophy; degeneration and regeneration; and a mononuclear inflammatory infiltrate, most often in a perivascular distribution.

Patients with characteristic rashes and two other criteria are considered to have probable juvenile dermatomyositis, and those with rashes and three other criteria have definite juvenile dermatomyositis. Because children with muscle weakness but without rash frequently have other myopathies, it is recommended that they undergo a muscle biopsy.

Only two-thirds of affected children will have high creatine kinase enzyme activity in the sera, so other myositis-associated enzymes, including aldolase, transaminases, and lactate dehydrogenase, should be tested and followed up.

Although a biopsy sample and electromyography give specific information about the inflammatory response, they are invasive procedures (Wedderburn et al. 2007). Because of their invasive nature, alternative tests are frequently sought to aid in diagnosis (Brown et al. 2006). In clinical practice, magnetic resonance imaging (MRI) of the thigh muscles demonstrating symmetrical muscle edema on fat-suppressed T2-weighted sequences seems to be very sensitive to confirm a diagnosis of JDM. In a prevalence sample (all stages of the disease), 76% patients with childhood myositis had an abnormal MRI (McCann et al. 2006). The sensitivity and specificity at diagnosis are not yet well defined, and MRI can localize muscle edema, but cannot ascertain its cause as some dystrophies might also show muscle edema inflammation (Brown et al. 2006). However, many rheumatologists use MRI to establish a diagnosis of IIM; the pediatric rheumatologists who were surveyed rated MRI as one of the most important diagnostic tools to be added to the revised criteria.

Even if the MRI were to become preferred over EMG, a muscle biopsy is, however, considered requisite to confirm a diagnosis of polymyositis in the absence of the characteristic skin rash.

Nailfold capillaroscopy is highly sensitive for diagnosis of JDM. It is helpful for differentiating dermatomyositis from muscular dystrophies, but might not always distinguish it from other connective-tissue diseases, such as scleroderma, overlap myositis or mixed connective-tissue disease (Ingegnoli et al. 2005).

HETEROGENEITY OF THE CHILDHOOD IDIOPATHIC INFLAMMATORY MYOPATHIES

*A clinical classification*

The JIIMs can be divided into more homogeneous clinico-pathological or serological subsets with distinctive epidemiologies and clinical, pathological or prognostic features (Tjärnlund et al. 2012). Juvenile dermatomyositis is the most common subset, representing up to 85% of childhood IIM (Ramanan and Feldman 2002).

The three other major subsets of IIM are:

- **Juvenile polymyostitis** (JPM) (5% of JIIM patients), in which the characteristic rashes are absent. Weakness is often both proximal and distal and muscle atrophy is frequent. JPM has a more severe disease onset than JDM, often with weight loss and Raynaud phenomenon; cardiac involvement occurs in 35% of patients.

Furthermore, patients with JPM do not have Gottron papules or heliotrope rash. The pathologic findings also differ from those of JDM, typically with endomysial infiltrates in affected muscles (McCann et al. 2006; Sato et al. 2009; Lorenzoni et al. 2011). Because JPM is often misdiagnosed with other non-inflammatory myopathies, particularly the muscular dystrophies, a muscle biopsy is required for diagnosis (Mamyrova et al. 2013).

- **Overlap myositis** (3–10%), in which juvenile dermatomyositis is associated with another autoimmune disease; for example, lupus erythematosus or scleroderma, the latter being the most frequent association form. In this subgroup of disorders, Raynaud phenomenon, interstitial lung disease (ILD), arthritis, and malar rash are frequently observed, as well as sclerodactyly and dysphagia. Patients with overlap myositis are more frequently not white and generally have myositis-associated autoantibodies (MAAs).
- **Clinically amyopathic dermatomyositis** (CADM) is occasionally observed in children; skin rashes are present for at least 6 months in patients who have no detectable weakness but who have laboratory evidence of muscle inflammation (e.g. elevated serum muscle enzyme levels or abnormal EMG, muscle biopsy, or MRI results) (Mukamel and Brik 2001).

*Classification based on autoantibodies*

JIIMs can also be classified based on the presence of two classes of myositis autoantibodies (Table 19.1):

- Myositis-specific autoantibodies (MSAs), which are present almost exclusively in patients with myositis;
- Myositis-associated autoantibodies (MAAs), which are present in patients with myositis but also in other autoimmune diseases.

These myositis autoantibodies define more homogeneous groups of patients with similar clinical features, responses to therapy, and prognoses. At least one myositis autoantibody can be identified in approximately 70% of JIIM patients (Rider et al. 2013). Of the autoantibodies studied in both children and adults, generally the same myositis autoantibodies are present, but they differ in frequency between children and adults. Detailing the complete set of antibodies is out of the scope of this chapter, and we refer to the excellent review of Lisa G. Rider and Kiran Nistala (Rider and Nistala 2016).

**Management**

The aim of treatment in JDM is to induce and maintain complete remission of all symptoms, in order to allow the child to achieve normal growth and development.

Criteria for clinically inactive disease, with evidence-based cut-offs for muscle strength/endurance, muscle enzymes and physical global evaluation of disease activity, have been established by the Pediatric Rheumatology International Trial Organization (PRINTO). These criteria can be used in clinical trials, in research and in clinical practice (Lazarevic et al. 2013).

**TABLE 19.1**
**Autoantibodies with juvenile idiopathic inflammatory myopathies**

| Autoantibody | Autoantigen target | Frequency in juvenile patients (%) | Clinical features and associations in JIMMs |
|---|---|---|---|
| **Myositis-specific autoantibodies** | | | |
| Anti-Aminoacyl-tRNA synthetases: | | 1–5 | Typically associated with those with moderate to severe weakness and creatine kinase levels, also frequently have non-erosive small joint arthritis, mechanics hands, Raynaud phenomenon, fevers, interstitial lung disease |
| Anti-Jo-1 | Histidyl-tRNA synthetase | 2–5 | |
| Anti-PL-12 | Alanyl-tRNA synthetase | 1–3 | |
| Anti-PL-7 | Threonyl-tRNA synthetase | <1 | |
| Anti-EJ | Glycyl-tRNA synthetase | <1 | |
| Anti-OJ | Isoleucy-tRNA synthetase | <1 | |
| Anti-MI-2 | NuRD helicases: MI-2α and Mi-2β, histone deacetylases | 1–7 | Mild JDM, classic rashes, responsive to treatment |
| Anti-SRP | Signal recognition particle (6 polypeptides and 7SLRNA) | 1–3 | Associated with severe refractory polymyositis, acute onset, proximal and distal weakness |
| **Myositis-associated autoantibodies** | | | |
| Anti-p155 | Transcriptional Intermediary factor (TIF)-1g | 23–29 | More severe cutaneous involvement, generalized lipodystrophy |
| Anti-p140 (MJ) | Nuclear matrix protein NXP2 | 13–23 | Calcinosis, contractures |
| Anti-Ro | 52-or 60-kD ribonucleoproteins (hYRNA) | 2–8 | |
| Anti-PM-5cl | Exosome protein: 100 and 75kD | 3–7 | Associated with sclerodermatous overlap features; scleroderma usually limited cutaneous |
| Anti-U1-RNP | U1 small nuclear ribonucleoprotein (snRNP) | 5–6 | Associated with sclerodermatous overlap features |
| Anti-U3-RNP | U3 ribonucleoprotein (fibrillarin) | 1 | Associated with sclerodermatous overlap features |
| Anti-La | Ribonucleoprotein | 1 | Associated with Anti-R0 |
| Anti-Ku | DNA binding complex: 70 and 80kDa heterodimer | 1 | |
| Anti-Topo | DNA topoisomerase 1 | 1 | |

JIMMS: juvenile idiopathic inflammatory myopathies ; JDM: juvenile dermatomyositis.

Early pharmacological and non-pharmacological treatment is mandatory to prevent irreversible organ damage and to maintain quality of life. Until recently, very few randomized-controlled trials had been done and therapeutic strategies were mainly based on anecdotal evidence from case reports and retrospective studies. The mainstay of therapy is high-dose corticosteroid. An immunosuppressive drug was often added as a steroid-sparing agent in steroid-resistant or steroid-dependent cases. The two most common immunosuppressants used in this indication are methotrexate and ciclosporin, the choice of which relies mostly on the experience of the clinician. It had been suggested that combining steroids with an immunosuppressive drug at disease onset could result in a better outcome than with monotherapy. Recently, an international multicenter, randomized, open-label trial was performed by PRINTO for newly diagnosed patients with JDM. It compared three commonly used protocols: prednisone alone, or in combination with either methotrexate or ciclosporin. This trial demonstrated that combined treatment with prednisone and an immunosuppressant at disease onset was more effective than prednisone alone. The safety profile and steroid-sparing effect was in favor of the combination with methotrexate. This protocol could become the reference standard treatment for JDM (Ruperto et al. 2016).

Different corticosteroid regimens have been proposed for the initial treatment of JDM. Most commonly, children receive oral prednisolone (2mg/kg/day in the induction phase, with slow tapering over a period of 2 years, according to the clinical response). Pulses with high-dose of intravenous methylprednisolone (3 pulses of 30mg/kg/day) may be considered at induction, followed by oral prednisone. This regimen could allow lower subsequent oral steroid doses, reducing the effects on the hypothalamic–pituitary–adrenal function and growth. Oral absorption of drugs can be reduced, as a consequence of gastro-intestinal vasculopathy.

Methotrexate is given at a dose of 15–20mg/m$^2$/week, orally or subcutaneously. Its administration has been associated with gastro-intestinal side-effects, including oral ulceration, nausea, and vomiting. Anticipatory gastro-intestinal adverse effects experienced before methotrexate administration are also common. Serious side-effects such as bone marrow suppression and hepatotoxicity are less frequently reported and usually transient.

Ciclosporin could be proposed to patients who have failed to respond adequately to steroids and other immunosuppressive agents. It is usually given in divided doses of 3–5mg/ kg/day. Its use is more difficult, necessitating careful monitoring during the first few months of trough serum level, kidney and liver functions and complete blood count because of its potential toxicity. Hirsutism, arterial hypertension and neurotoxicity occur commonly as adverse events.

Mycophenolate mofetil (MMF) is emerging as an additional therapeutic modality for the treatment of children with JDM. Both skin and muscle manifestations respond to MMF in children with JDM, but the skin inflammation, which is often resistant to therapy, responds especially well. It appears to be well-tolerated, but clinicians should judiciously monitor patients for infectious and hematologic complications. It could be recommended as the second-line immunosuppressant, in case of failure or intolerance of methotrexate (Rouster-Stevens et al. 2010).

Treatments used for refractory disease include intravenous immunoglobulins, cyclophosphamide, azathioprine, hydroxychloroquine, tacrolimus, rituximab, infliximab and autologous stem cell transplantation. No head-to-head or superiority trial has been carried out (Enders et al. 2017).

Published data suggest that early aggressive treatment may decrease incidence of calcinosis.

There is no high-level evidence regarding when to stop immunosuppressive therapy. Withdrawal of methotrexate (or an alternative disease-modifying drug) could be considered once the patient is in remission and off steroids for a minimum of 1 year.

**Key points**

• The juvenile idiopathic inflammatory myopathies (JIIMs) are heterogeneous, systemic autoimmune diseases characterized by weakness, chronic inflammation of skeletal muscles, and typical skin rashes with onset during childhood. New classification criteria have recently been developed and validated.

• Recently, JIMMs could be divided into more homogeneous clinico-pathological or serological subsets with distinctive epidemiology and clinical, pathological or prognostic features.

• Juvenile dermatomyositis (JDM) is by far the most prevalent form (approximately 85% of all patients with JIIMs), followed by juvenile polymyositis and overlap syndrome.

• The myositis autoantibodies seen most frequently in children with juvenile idiopathic inflammatory myopathies (JIIMs) are anti-p155, anti-p140 (MJ), and anti-MI-2 autoantibodies. These differ from the autoantibodies seen most frequently in adults.

• The aim of treatment in JDM is to induce and maintain complete remission of all symptoms as early as possible, in order to allow the child to achieve normal growth and development.

• The recent prospective PRINTO trial demonstrated that combined treatment with prednisone and an immunosuppressant at disease onset (either methotrexate or ciclosporin) was more effective than prednisone alone. The safety profile and steroid-sparing effect was in favor of the combination with methotrexate. This protocol could become the reference standard treatment for JDM.

REFERENCES

Bilgic H, Ytterberg SR, Amin S, McNallan KT, Wilson JC, Koeuth T et al. (2009) Interleukin-6 and type I interferon-regulated genes and chemokines mark disease activity in dermatomyositis. *Arthritis Rheum* 60: 3436–3446. PubMed: 19877033

Bohan A, Peter JB (1975) Polymyositis and dermatomyositis. Parts 1 and 2. *N Engl J Med* 292: 344–347; 3403–3407.

Brown VE, Pilkington CA, Feldman BM, Davidson JE, Network for Juvenile Dermatomyositis, Paediatric Rheumatology European Society (PReS). (2006) An international consensus survey of the diagnostic criteria for juvenile dermatomyositis (JDM). *Rheumatology (Oxford)* 45: 990–993.

Enders FB, Bader-Meunier B, Baildam E, Constantin T, Dolezalova P, Feldman BM et al. (2017) Consensus-based recommendations for the management of juvenile dermatomyositis. Ann Rheum Dis 76(2): 329–340.

Ingegnoli F, Zeni S, Gerloni V, Fantini F (2005) Capillaroscopic observations in childhood rheumatic diseases and healthy controls. *Clin Exp Rheumatol* 23: 905–911.

Lazarevic D, Pistorio A, Palmisani E, Miettunen P, Ravelli A, Pilkington C et al. (2013) The PRINTO criteria for clinically inactive disease in juvenile dermatomyositis. *Ann Rheum Dis* 72: 686–693.

Lee PY, Li Y, Richards HB, Chan FS, Zhuang H, Narain S et al. (2007) Type I interferon as a novel risk factor for endothelial progenitor cell depletion and endothelial dysfunction in systemic lupus erythematosus. *Arthritis Rheum* 56: 3759–3769. PubMed: 17968925

Liu Y, Ramot Y, Torrelo A, Paller AS, Si N, Babay S et al. (2012) Mutations in proteasome subunit β type 8 cause chronic atypical neutrophilic dermatosis with lipodystrophy and elevated temperature with evidence of genetic and phenotypic heterogeneity. *Arthritis Rheum* 64: 895–907.

Lorenzoni PJ, Scola RH, Kay CS, Prevedello PG, Espíndola G, Werneck LC (2011) Idiopathic inflammatory myopathies in childhood: a brief review of 27 cases. *Pediatr Neurol* 45: 17–22.

Mamyrova G, Kleiner DE, James-Newton L, Shaham B, Miller FW, Rider LG (2007) Late-onset gastrointestinal pain in juvenile dermatomyositis as a manifestation of ischemic ulceration from chronic endarteropathy. *Arthritis Rheum* 57: 881–884.

Mamyrova G, Katz JD, Jones RV, Targoff IN, Lachenbruch PA, Jones OY et al. (2013) Clinical and laboratory features distinguishing juvenile polymyositis and muscular dystrophy. *Arthritis Care Res (Hoboken)* 65: 1969–1975.

McCann LJ, Juggins AD, Maillard SM, Wedderburn LR, Davidson JE, Murray KJ et al. (2006) The Juvenile Dermatomyositis National Registry and Repository (UK and Ireland) – clinical characteristics of children recruited within the first 5 yr. *Rheumatology (Oxford)* 45: 1255–1260.

Miles L, Bove KE, Lovell D, Wargula JC, Bukulmez H, Shao M et al. (2007) Predictability of the clinical course of juvenile dermatomyositis based on initial muscle biopsy: a retrospective study of 72 patients. *Arthritis Rheum* 57: 1183–1191.

Miller FW, Cooper RG, Vencovský J, Rider LG, Danko K, Wedderburn LR et al. (2013) Genome-wide association study of dermatomyositis reveals genetic overlap with other autoimmune disorders. *Arthritis Rheum* 65: 3239–3247.

Mitchell JP, Dennis GJ, Rider LG (2001) Juvenile dermatomyositis presenting with anasarca: A possible indicator of severe disease activity. *J Pediatr* 138: 942–945.

Mukamel M, Brik R (2001) Amyopathic dermatomyositis in children: a diagnostic and therapeutic dilemma. *J Clin Rheumatol* 7(3):191–193.

Neves FS, Shinjo SK, Carvalho JF, Levy-Neto M, Borges CT (2007) Spontaneous pneumomediastinum and dermatomyositis may be a not so rare association: report of a case and review of the literature. Clin Rheumatol 26: 105–107.

Pachman LM, Lipton R, Ramsey-Goldman R, Shamiyeh E, Abbott K, Mendez EP et al. (2005) History of infection before the onset of juvenile dermatomyositis: results from the National Institute of Arthritis and Musculoskeletal and Skin Diseases Research Registry. *Arthritis Rheum* 53(2): 166–172.

Pachman LM, Veis A, Stock S, Abbott K, Vicari F, Patel P et al. (2006) Composition of calcifications in children with juvenile dermatomyositis: association with chronic cutaneous inflammation. *Arthritis Rheum* 54: 3345–3350.

Pope E, Janson A, Khambalia A, Feldman B (2006) Childhood acquired lipodystrophy: a retrospective study. *J Am Acad Dermatol* 55: 947–950.

Ramanan AV, Feldman BM (2002) Clinical features and outcomes of juvenile dermatomyositis and other childhood onset myositis syndromes. *Rheum Dis Clin North Am* 28: 833–857.

Rider LG (2003) Calcinosis in JDM: pathogenesis and current therapies. *Pediatr Rheumatol Online J* 1: 119–133.

Rider LG, Miller FW (2011) Deciphering the clinical presentations, pathogenesis, and treatment of the idiopathic inflammatory myopathies. *JAMA* 305: 183–190. PubMed: 21224460

Rider LG, Nistala K (2016) The juvenile idiopathic inflammatory myopathies: pathogenesis, clinical and autoantibody phenotypes, and outcomes. *J Intern Med* 280: 24–38.

Rider LG, Shah M, Mamyrova G, Huber AM, Rice MM, Targoff IN et al. (2013) The myositis autoantibody phenotypes of the juvenile idiopathic inflammatory myopathies. *Medicine (Baltimore)* 92: 223–243.

Rouster-Stevens KA, Morgan GA, Wang D, Pachman LM (2010) Mycophenolate mofetil: a possible therapeutic agent for children with juvenile dermatomyositis. *Arthritis Care Res (Hoboken)* 62: 1446–1451.

Ruperto N, Pistorio A, Oliveira S, Zulian F, Cuttica R, Ravelli A et al. (2016) Prednisone versus prednisone plus ciclosporin versus prednisone plus methotrexate in new-onset juvenile dermatomyositis: a randomised trial.Paediatric Rheumatology International Trials Organisation (PRINTO). *Lancet* 387(10019): 671–678.

Sato JO, Sallum AM, Ferriani VP, Marini R, Sacchetti SB, Okuda EM et al. (2009) A Brazilian registry of juvenile dermatomyositis: onset features and classification of 189 cases. *Clin Exp Rheumatol* 27: 1031–1038. PubMed: 20149327

Symmons DP, Sills JA, Davis SM (1995) The incidence of juvenile dermatomyositis: results from a nation-wide study. *Br J Rheumatol* 34: 732–736.

Tjärnlund A, Bottai M, Rider LG, Werth VP, Pilkington C, de Visser M, Alfredsson L et al. (2012) Progress report on development of classification criteria for adult and juvenile idiopathic inflammatory myopathies. *Arthritis Rheum* 64(Suppl):S323–S324.

Wedderburn LR, Varsani H, Li CK, Newton KR, Amato AA, Banwell B et al. (2007) International consensus on a proposed score system for muscle biopsy evaluation in patients with juvenile dermatomyositis: a tool for potential use in clinical trials. *Arthritis Rheum* 57: 1192–1201.

# Section 4
## Physical Rehabilitation and Orthopaedic Management

# 20
# LIFELONG PHYSIOTHERAPY: STAYING ACTIVE

*Imelda de Groot*

## Introduction

In the past, often the advice to parents with a child with a neuromuscular disorder would be: "Try not to overload your child as it can be harmful for the muscles". Parents, therefore, often restricted their child in participating in age-related daily activities, a wheelchair was soon used and/or parents took over all types of daily activities, such as dressing or grooming. Thus, potentially there is a disuse of the capabilities that the child stills has, and, more importantly, the restriction in age-related daily activities can lead to less social participation. Having a sedentary lifestyle, however, can lead to secondary problems such as increased risk of overweight, osteoporosis, and cardiovascular events. Furthermore, maintaining functional abilities is important as this is beneficial for quality of life and social participation (Shields et al. 2015; Woodmansee et al. 2016). Nevertheless, physical inactivity is fairly common in children with a disability (Murphy et al. 2008; Heutinck et al. 2017). While the World Health Organization (WHO) advises that healthy children should be active in a moderate or vigorous way for at least 60 minutes per day (WHO 2016), this is not always achieved by children with disabilities especially if they are wheelchair confined.

Increasingly the awareness of disuse becomes apparent, which in itself can cause secondary muscle atrophy. Muscle atrophy is defined as a decrease in muscle mass leading to a loss of muscle strength and increased muscular fatigability (Bodine 2013). Thus, disuse can introduce secondary functional loss leading to increased disability. Disuse can also lead to increased fatigability and to the assumption that performing daily activities causes disease-related deterioration as the child experiences increased fatigue. In other words a vicious circle! (Fig. 20.1) The important question is can this circle be broken? One of the options is to be more active, either by training or by performing activities during daily life.

Nowadays, we know more about the effects of staying active or training in neuromuscular disorders. For adults, there is scientific evidence that shows that aerobic training is effective in several neuromuscular disorders (Voet et al. 2013). Apart from aerobic and strength training, cognitive behavior training is also effective (Voet et al. 2014), indicating that the way a person thinks of the disease is of influence. It is obvious that this could also be of influence in children with neuromuscular disorders and their parents. For children with neuromuscular disorders, there are studies, mostly non-randomized, that show benefits for strength training

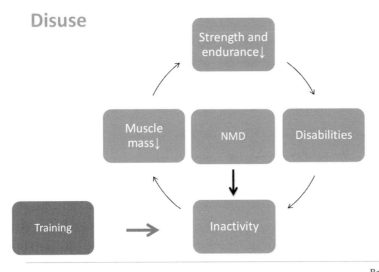

**Fig. 20.1.** Vicious circle introduced by disuse: neuromuscular disorder leading to inactivity, leading to reduced muscle mass, leading to decreased strength and endurance, leading to (further) disabilities, leading to more inactivity. Possible intervention is training or performing daily activities. NMD: neuromuscular disorder. Used with the permission of Imelda de Groot and Merel Jansen, Radboundumc.

(Burns et al. 2009; Sjögreen et al. 2010; Jones et al. 2014; Lewelt et al. 2015; Alemdaroğlu et al. 2015,) or endurance training (Alemdaroğlu et al. 2015; Jansen et al. 2015). The first randomized controlled training trial with endurance training in boys with Duchenne muscular dystrophy (DMD) showed a slowing down of disease progression at the functional level (Jansen et al. 2013). In this study boys with DMD cycled with their arms and with their legs on an electrical supported ergometer bicycle showing beneficial effects on functional level. No adverse events were found in any of these studies. More studies are needed to establish evidence-based advice on how to maintain activity level and/or develop training programs, especially as most aerobic training programs that are available are aimed at children that are still able to walk or to cycle using their own strength. For children who are wheelchair confined, adjusted training options should be developed, such as the one that was applied in the study on assisted cycling in boys with DMD (Jansen et al. 2013).

**Potential working mechanisms for staying active**

Neuromuscular system

In children, it is hard to study the pathophysiological changes in the neuromuscular system, as has been done in adults by using biopsies. Indicative studies with laboratory animals that performed exercise point to (temporary) enhancement of muscle regeneration and repair in early disease stages (Okano et al. 2005). Also, animal studies point to the fact that low-intensity exercises increase antioxidant activity, thus reducing oxidative stress, which is a well-known phenomenon in neuromuscular disorders (Kaczor et al. 2007). Biomarkers that are under development for these phenomena would make it possible in future to study these mechanisms in children.

CARDIOVASCULAR SYSTEM

In healthy children the advice is that an aerobic training that improves the cardiovascular system should be performed with approximately 80% of the maximum heart rate (American Academy of Pediatrics et al. 2016). However, in children with neuromuscular disorders the muscle weakness and muscle fatigability are often limiting factors meaning that the child is not able to reach the requested level of training intensity. Furthermore, the heart is often involved in the disease, leading to cardiomyopathy. Medications, such as beta-blockers used for cardiomyopathy, can also restrict the achievable heart rate. However, it is possible to perform exercise in children with cardiomyopathies using specific programs (Somarriba et al. 2008) in dialogue with the pediatric cardiologist.

JOINT MOBILITY

There is much advice for stretching joints in children with neuromuscular disorders with many types of orthoses or splinting. However, there is hardly evidence that staying active has a positive influence on the joints. Indications for positive effects of exercise on joint mobility of the elbow are shown in two arm training studies carried out with boys with DMD (Jansen et al. 2013; Heutinck et al. 2016). In one study the boys used an arm-support thus increasing the range of movement of the arm and performed daily activities including gaming. In the other study, the boys were trained with a sling (hanging up the arm to make it weightless) to play a three-dimensional video game.

CEREBRAL SYSTEM

In healthy children, there is increasing evidence that exercise improves cognitive functioning and academic achievement (Lees and Hopkins 2013; Donnelly et al. 2016; Jackson et al. 2016). There are pediatric neuromuscular disorders ( e.g. DMD) that have comparable cognitive impairments, such as attention-deficit–hyperactivity disorder. These impairments can be influenced by exercise or exercise breaks in classroom activities in healthy children and it is possible that these interventions could work for children with NMDs; however, the evidence is lacking for neuromuscular disorder patients.

IN PRACTICE

The positive effects (described in the Potential working mechanisms for staying active section) are not necessarily exclusive to the one type of neuromuscular disorder for which they have been studied. The possible working mechanisms are generic, although the effects may differ in magnitude.

GENERAL

In general it is advised not to perform eccentric exercise, as in most neuromuscular disorders in childhood the muscle membrane is regarded as unstable. Stretch could therefore be deteriorating. In healthy boys there are indications that eccentric muscle damage is dependent on the age, with increasing damage while growing up (Chen et al. 2014). This should be kept in mind when designing the composition of the training or activity types being considered.

**Ambulant children**

Physiotherapists are well aware of how to provide functional training in ambulant children with neuromuscular disorders. It is advisable to have physiotherapy close to once or twice per week and also some moderate load activities each day (moderate load means somewhat tiring). The involvement of a child in playing physically demanding games would differ according their developmental needs. Parents tend to be somewhat (over)protective. It is necessary to educate the parents that exercise or other activities are not causing deteriorating of the disease and that they should allow children to play. Adjustments in the play are sometimes necessary, which can be made with the advice of a physiotherapist or occupational therapist. Daily activities can be regarded as moments of exercise. Many parents are involved in caretaking of their child and tend to take over activities that a child is still able to do (although the child might take longer to perform the activity). Being aware as a parent of these activities and how to integrate them into daily family life is another educational issue for parents.

**Children in wheelchairs**

For children who are wheelchair confined, the activities available depends on whether they are having residual strength in the arms to perform three-dimensional activities. Playing wheelchair sports, such as wheelchair hockey using a hand-stick, or wheelchair table tennis, or wheelchair basket ball using lighter balls, can be tried. If children are too weak to perform these activities, training with devices that support movement is possible. In Jansen et al.'s study (2013) (Fig. 20.2), training the arms and legs for 15 min, 3–4 times a week using electrically assisted home-ergometer bicycles showed a positive effect in boys with DMD: during the 6 month training period, the boys remained stable on the motor function measurement, while the comparison group who received usual care showed a significant decrease in motor function measurement. This type of training is not disease specific, and although its effectiveness for other neuromuscular disorders is not yet established there are no contra-indications to applying it.

Another way to increase active life is integrating assistive devices in daily life activities. For example, in another of Jansen et al.'s (2015) studies, non-ambulant boys with DMD, who had limited arm function, used an arm-support (Top help, Focal Meditech, The Netherlands) to use the non-dominant arm to eat and also play a video game. The dominant arms of the boys were used as the comparison group in this study. The results show that the arm function in the supported arm decreased less at the functional level than the arm without a support.

If a child becomes wheelchair confined, a choice can be made between an electric wheelchair or a wheelchair with electrical motion wheels which assist the wheeling of the

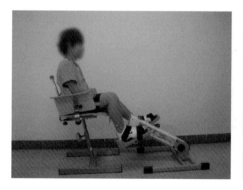 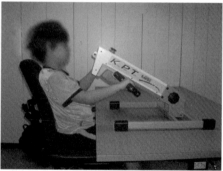

**Fig. 20.2.** Posture during dynamic leg and arm training (Jansen et al. 2013).

chair. By using the latter wheelchair, children train their arms during the day. Thus, when thinking about advising on an aid or assistive device to support an activity, one should consider what the residual capabilities of the child are and how the device could be used to train the joints and muscles. Also, the ability to allow the child to experience positive physical performances should also be considered.

**Advice**

Overall, in accordance with the guidelines for healthy children, activities should be stimulated which have a moderate physical demand on the child for at least 30 minutes per day. Activity can be achieved either by playing or by performing daily activities that give a moderate physical demand (somewhat tiring), with or without the support of assistive devices. To evaluate if an activity is moderately demanding, a fatigue scale can be used, such as the Faces scale or the OMNI scale (Utter et al. 2002), to evaluate the level of fatigue of the child. Sport activities should be encouraged, as even powered wheelchair sports gives a physical demand (Barfield et al. 2016). Furthermore, sport also is important for social contact, participation, and provides a learning process in collaborating as a team, and in winning and losing. Sport can help children to develop positive self-esteem (Sahlin and Lexell 2015) as well as a better physical condition.

**Key points**
- The awareness of the importance of staying active in children with neuromuscular disorders is increasing as there are indications that it can retard progression of the disorder and prevent secondary complications such as overweight or cardiovascular complications.
- Individualized programs for all children are possible with the use of assisted devices.
- Daily activities can be regarded as opportunities to stay active, and parents need to be educated to understand this.
- Staying active, including getting involved in sports, has positive influence on participation and quality of life.

## REFERENCES

Alemdaroğlu J, Karaduman A, Yilmaz ÖT, Topaloğlu H (2015) Different types of upper extremity exercise training in Duchenne muscular dystrophy: effects on functional performance, strength, endurance, and ambulation. *Muscle Nerve* 51(5): 697–705. doi 10.10002/mus.24451.

American Academy of Pediatrics (2016) Aerobic training. https://www.healthychildren.org/English/healthy-living/fitness/Pages/Aerobic-Training.aspx.

Barfield JP, Newsome L, Malone LA (2016) Exercise intensity during power wheelchair soccer. *Arch Phys Med Rehabil* 97(11):1938–1944. doi: 10.1016/j.apmr.2016.05.012.

Bodine SC (2013) Disuse-induced muscle wasting. *Int J Biochem Cell Biol* 45(10):2200–2208. doi: 10.1016/j.biocel.2013.06.011.

Burns J, Raymond J, Ouvrier R (2009) Feasibility of foot and ankle strength training in childhood Charcot–Marie–Tooth disease. *Neuromuscul Disord* 19(12):818–21. doi: 10.1016/j.nmd.2009.09.007.

Chen TC, Chen HL, Kuy YC, Nosaka K (2014) Eccentric exercis-induced muscle damage of pre-adolescent and adolescent boys in comparison to young men. *Eur J Appl Physiol* 114(6):1183–1195. doi: 10.1007/s00421–014–2848–3.

Donnelly JE, Hillman CH, Castelli D, Etnier JL, Lee S, Tomporowski P et al. (2016) Physical activity, fitness, cognitive function, and academic achievement in children: a systematic review. *Med Sci Sports Exerc* 48(6): 1197–222. doi 10.1249/MSS.0000000000000901.

Heutinck L, Jansen M, van den Elzen Y, van der Pijl D, de Groot IJ (2016) Virtual reality computer gaming with dynamic arm support in boys with Duchenne muscular dystrophy: the Gainboy study. *Neuromusc Dis* 26(Suppl 2): S125.

Heutinck L, van Kampen N, Jansen M, de Groot IJ (2017) Physical activity in boys with Duchenne muscular dystrophy is lower and less demanding compared to healthy boys. *J Child Neurol* 32(5): 450–7 doi: 10.1177/0883073816685506.

Jackson WM, Davis N, Sands SA, Whittington RA, Sun LS (2016) Physical activity and cognitive development: a meta-analysis. *Neurosurg Anesthesiol* 28(4): 373–380.

Jansen M, van Alfen N, Geurts ACH, de Groot IJ (2013) Assisted bicycle training delays functional deterioration in boys with Duchenne muscular dystrophy: the randomized controlled trial "No Use Is Disuse". *Neurorehabil Neural Repair* 27(9):816–27. doi: 10.1177/1545968313496326.

Jansen M, Burgers J, Jannink M, van Alfen N, de Groot IJ (2015) Upper limb training with dynamic arm support in boys with Duchenne muscular dystrophy: a feasibility study. *Int J Phys Med Rehabil* 3: 2. doi: 10.4172/2329–9096.1000256.

Jones HN, Crisp KD, Moss T, Strollo K, Robey R, Sank J et al. (2014) Effects of respiratory muscle training (RMT) in children with infantile-onset Pompe disease and respiratory muscle weakness. *J Pediatr Rehabil Med* 7(3):255–65. doi: 10.3233/PRM-140294.

Kaczor JJ, Hall JE, Payne E, Tarnopolsky MA (2007) Low intensity training decreases markers of oxidative stress in skeletal muscle of mdx mice. *Free Radic Biol Med* 43(1):145–54.

Lees C, Hopkins J (2013) Effect of aerobic exercise on cognition, academic achievement, and psychosocial function in children: a systematic review of randomized control trials. *Prev Chronic Dis* 10:E174. doi: 10.5888/pcd10.130010.

Lewelt A, Krosschell KJ, Stoddard GJ, Weng C, Xue M, Marcus RL et al. (2015) Resistance strength training exercise in children with spinal muscular atrophy. *Muscle Nerve* 52(4):559–67. doi: 10.1002/mus.24568.

Murphy NA, Carbone PS, American Academy of Pediatrics Council on Children With Disabilities (2008) Promoting the participation of children with disabilities in sports, recreation, and physical activities. *Pediatrics* 121(5):1057–1061. doi: 10.1542/peds.2008–0566.

Okano T, Yoshida K, Nakamura A, Sasazawa F, Oide T, Takeda S et al. (2005) Chronic exercise accelerates the degeneration-regeneration cycle and downregulates insulin-like growth factor-1 in muscle of mdx mice. *Muscle Nerve* 32(2):191–9.

Sahlin KB, Lexell J (2015) Impact of organized sports on activity, participation, and quality of life in people with neurologic disabilities. *PMR* 7(10):1081–1088. doi: 10.1016/j.pmrj.2015.03.019.

Shields N, Synnot A, Kearns C (2015) The extent, context and experience of participation in out-of-school activities among children with disability. *Res Dev Disabil* 47: 165–74. doi: 10.1016/j.ridd.2015.09.007.

Sjögreen L, Tulinius M, Kiliaridis S, Lohmander A (2010) The effect of lip strengthening exercises in children and adolescents with myotonic dystrophy type 1. *Int J Pediatr Otorhinolaryngol* 74(10):1126–1134. doi: 10.1016/j.ijporl.2010.06.013.

Somarriba G, Extein J, Miller TL (2008) Exercise rehabilitation in pediatric cardiomyopathy. *Prog Pediatr Cardiol* 25(1):91–102.

Utter AC, Robertson RJ, Nieman DC, Kanq J (2002) Children's OMNI scale of perceived exertion: walking/running evaluation. *Med Sci Sport Exerc* 34(1): 139–44.

Voet NB, van der Kooi EL, Riphagen II, Lindeman E, van Engelen BG, Geurts AC (2013) Strength training and aerobic exercise training for muscle disease. *Cochrane Database Syst Rev* CD003907. doi: 10.1002/14651858.CD003907.pub3.

Voet NB, Bleijenberg G, Hendriks J, de Groot IJ, Padberg G, van Engelen B et al. (2014) Both aerobic exercise and cognitive-behavioral therapy reduce chronic fatigue in FSHD: an RCT. *Neurology* 83(21):1914–1922. doi: 10.1212/WNL.0000000000001008.

WHO (2016) Global Strategy on Diet, Physical Activity and Health. Geneva: World Health Organization. http://www.who.int/dietphysicalactivity/factsheet_young_people/en/.

Woodmansee C, Hahne A, Imms C, Shields N (2016) Comparing participation in physical recreation activities between children with disability and children with typical development: A secondary analysis of matched data. *Res Dev Disabil* 49–50: 268–76. doi: 10.1016/j.ridd.2015.12.004.

# 21
# MANAGEMENT OF CONTRACTURES: STRETCHING, POSITIONING AND SPLINTING

*Tina Duong and Kristy Rose*

## Introduction

Contracture is a term used to describe the abnormal shortening of muscles, skin or connective tissue causing restrictions in active and passive range of motion (ROM) (Archibald and Vignos 1959; McDonald 1998). Contractures are prevalent and inevitably developed in many pediatric neuromuscular disorders (Johnson et al. 1992). While the etiology of contracture development varies depending on the neuromuscular disease (NMD), regardless of the disorder, joint contractures can result in a number of disabling complications such as orthopedic deformity, pain, decreased function and mobility with direct impact on activities of daily living (ADL) and quality of life (QOL). Knowledge of the underlying pathology of the NMD is essential in understanding the nature of muscle weakness, contracture development and progression that is key in clinical management. This chapter will therefore focus on understanding contracture development and management in pediatric NMDs.

## Pathophysiology of contracture development in pediatric neuromuscular disease

Contractures are typically categorized as physiological or myostatic based on the etiology of development. Most physiologically based contractures result from upper motor neuron defects, physiological processes, or electrolyte imbalances. Myostatic contractures, most common in NMD, result from immobilization or muscle weakness/imbalances.

Myostatic contractures in NMD are typically caused by neuropathic or myopathic processes. Contractures are more prevalent in myopathic disease as individuals typically have proximal weakness compared with neuropathic diseases which have more distal weakness (Johnson et al. 1992). Loss of joint range of motion (ROM) in NMDs usually occur due to fibrosis and fatty tissue infiltration of the muscle occurring in tandem with progressive muscle weakness and imbalance. This causes increased passive resistance and non-contractility in the endomysium, perimyseium and epimysium contributing to shortened muscle fibers (Cornu et al. 1998). A study of dystrophic muscle found the non-contractile component highly correlated with strength and function (Akima et al. 2012). Increased stiffness within the muscle fibers reduced contractile force while stiffness in passive structures such as tendons and connective tissues was associated with severity of contractures (Cornu et al. 1998; Cornu et al. 2001; Magnusson et al. 1997). The reduction in sarcomeres as a result of the pathological process changes the force tension curve causing shortened muscles and contracture formation.

Contractures may be a critical clinical marker with significant value in diagnosing and tracking clinical progression. For example, contractures at birth with associated fetal akinesia such as in arthrogryposis, congenital myopathies and myotonic dystrophies tend to be the primary feature of the disease and develop prior to muscle weakness while others are secondary features resulting from muscle imbalances. With these progressive muscular dystrophies, contractures appear to develop alongside weakness patterns. Contractures in weight-bearing joints such as knees and ankles appear to be most debilitating as they affect walking. The inability to actively move a joint through the full available range of motion (ROM) is one of the leading causes for fixed contractures as it results in a static positioning of limbs, shortening of muscle fibers and decreased sarcomeres.

Muscles that cross multiple joints are at higher risk of contractures as these muscles must have sufficient flexibility to allow both joints to move through full range. These bi-articular muscles have origins and insertions crossing different joints and have greater risk of change within the length tension curve for muscle force production. These bi-articular muscles serve multiple roles in movement especially in closed chain activities which constitutes most functional mobility. With isometric contractions, bi-articular muscles assist in controlling movement through the ROM. Examples of muscles that fall into this category are pectoralis major, biceps brachii, pronator teres, rectus femoris, semitendinosus, semimembranosus, long head biceps, femur, and gastrocnemius. As a result of muscle weakness, these muscles are not stretched to their full functional range across both joints inhibiting appropriate biomechanics for movement and tissue shortening.

While individuals are still ambulatory, lower extremity contractures are less prevalent and severe. However, as weakness progresses, the biomechanics of walking change making for a less efficient gait pattern with increased energy demands. For example, as boys with Duchenne muscular dystrophy (DMD) develop plantarflexion contractures, the ankle contracture and anterior pelvic tilt shifts their center of gravity posterior to the hip joint and anterior to the knee and ankle joint (Barrett et al. 1988). This leads to the adoption of compensatory strategies with a more inefficient gait pattern and postural abnormalities of equinus posture and excessive lumbar lordosis. This type of posture allows them to stay upright but results in decreased gait velocity and associated loss of ambulation (Hsu and Fufumasu 1993; D'Angelo et al. 2009; Sienko Thomas et al. 2010; Doglio et al. 2011). Table 21.1 lists the contractures associated with specific NMDs.

**Duchenne muscular dystrophy and Becker muscular dystrophy**

Duchenne muscular dystrophy (DMD) is the most common muscular dystrophy in childhood and is characterized by the absence of dystrophin; the less severe form, Becker muscular dystrophy (BMD), retains some functional dystrophin (Hoffman et al. 1987). Dystrophin provides strength and resilience to the muscle fiber membrane. When dystrophin is absent the muscle fiber is more susceptible to degradation and is broken down at a rapid rate.

**TABLE 21.1**
**Muscle groups prone to contracture**

| Neuromuscular disease | Contracture prevalence |
|---|---|
| Duchenne and Becker muscular dystrophy | Ankle plantar flexors, hip flexors, abductors, wrist flexors, supinators, finger flexors |
| Emery-Dreifus muscular dystrophy | Posterior cervical spine, elbow flexors, ankle plantar flexors |
| Ullrich muscular dystrophy | Hyperlaxity distal interphalangeal joints, Contractures: hip, knee and elbow flexors, kyphoscoliosis, torticollis, equinovarus, |
| Bethlem myopathy | Distal contractures of fingers and ankle plantar flexors. Hyperlaxity of interphalangeal joints with proximal contractures, equinovarus/pes cavus |
| Spinal muscular atrophy | Ankle plantar flexors, hip, knee, wrist, elbow flexors, forearm supinators |
| Charcot–Marie–Tooth disease | Ankle plantar flexors, intrinsic muscles of the hands and feet, long finger flexors |

Overtime, muscle is replaced by fatty and scar tissue resulting in muscle weakness and contracture formation (Cornu et al. 1998; Akima et al. 2012; Cornu et al. 2001).

Boys with DMD have a more severe phenotype, while BMD has marked heterogeneity in disease progression but tends to follow the same weakness and contracture patterns as DMD (McDonald et al. 1995a; 1995b). To better understand contracture management, it is important to understand the patterns of weakness and imbalance unique to the disease. Muscle weakness is initially seen in proximal muscles of the hip flexors/extensors and knee extensor muscles (McDonald 1998). However, contractures typically develop first in the ankles followed by hip flexors, hip abductors and knee flexors (McDonald 1998). This is largely owing to the fact that boys with BMD and DMD make a number of biomechanical adaptations to maintain standing and ambulation. The unique combination of contracture development and weakness leads to a standing posture of increased plantar-flexion, hyper-lordosis, and an anterior pelvic tilt. This alignment allows for a biomechanical advantage that is limited by dorsiflexion range and quadriceps weakness causing an extensor moment arm that allows for maintenance of upright standing. This is a stabilizing mechanism to shift the center of gravity behind the greater trochanter and anterior to the knee resulting in toe walking. Although initially a functional adaptation, with time muscle weakness and contractures become so severe that individuals with DMD are unable to rely on these compensations to preserve ambulation. If not treated with corticosteroids, boys with DMD typically lose independent ambulation by the age of 9 years (McDonald et al. 2018). If treated, boys can remain ambulant into their teens.

**Congenital muscular dystrophy and congenital myopathies**

Congenital muscular dystrophy is a term describing a group of disorders associated with a similar phenotype of contractures and joint hypermobility being more prominent than muscle weakness. Onset of symptoms range from hypotonia at birth, prominent proximal joint contractures, distal finger hyperlaxity and generally slowly progressive muscle weakness (Flanigan et al. 2000; Mercuri et al. 2002; Mercuri et al. 2005; Eymard et al. 2013). These individuals tend to have prominent contractures that are present at birth due to fetal akinesia. These may include congenital myotonic dystrophies, congenital muscular dystrophies/myopathies and congenital myasthenic syndromes (Eymard et al. 2013). Contracture onset ranges from congenital to later onset. In arthrogryposis multiplex congenital, non-progressive contractures affect at least two or more joints. In this chapter, we will focus on genetic myopathy, Emery–Dreifus muscular dystrophy (EDMD) and collagen VI-related myopathies (Col 6 RM); collagen VI-related myopathies encompass a range of severities from the more severe phenotype with Ullrich (UCMD) and milder Bethlem myopathy (BM) and a range of intermediate phenotypes.

EMERY–DREIFUS MUSCULAR DYSTROPHY

Emery–Dreifus muscular dystrophy (EDMD) is characterized by contractures evolving in adolescence/early adulthood, slowly progressive muscle weakness and cardiac disease. Unlike other dystrophic disorders, contracture development precedes muscle weakness. Muscle weakness and wasting initially affects the humeroperoneal muscles progressing to scapular and pelvic girdle muscles. Contractures typically develop in the posterior cervical muscles, elbow and ankle at the Achilles tendon (Goncu et al. 2003). Spinal rigidity may also develop later in the disease causing rigid spine syndrome (RSS) (Kubo et al. 1998; Madej-Pilarczyk and Kochański 2016).

COLLAGEN VI-RELATED MYOPATHIES

*Ullrich*

Symptoms for Ullrich (UCMD) typically occur in the neonatal period with patterns of hyperlaxity and contractures. Proximal contractures develop at the hips, knees and elbows alongside severe hyperlaxity of the distal hands, fingers and feet (Bönnemann 2011). Infants may be born with such severe hyperlaxity that hands may be extended to the forearm or feet dorsiflexed to tibia. A key feature in UCMD include a prominent calcaneus. Tightness around the pelvis is also associated with congenital hip dislocation, talipes equinovarus, torticollis and kyphoscoliosis (Bönnemann 2011). Congenital contractures revert during childhood and progress during the second decade of life, primarily due to positioning and muscle weakness affecting the elbow, finger, hip, knee flexors and ankles resulting in loss of function and continued hyperlaxity at the interphalangeal joints. Individuals vary in clinical presentation from delayed ambulation to non-ambulatory. Due to spinal kyphosis, there may be associated respiratory decline that may require ventilatory support.

*Bethlem myopathy*

Bethlem myopathy (BM) has a very heterogeneous presentation ranging from mild distal contractures of the fingers and Achilles tendon to debilitating contractures and weakness that results in the inability to ambulate. Most individuals with Bethlem myopathy have mild weakness and symptoms are not prominent until the first or second decade of life; however, many cases indicate that early signs were evident such as torticollis, hypotonia and equinovarus deformities during the neonatal period (Eymard et al. 2013). Contractures develop proximally during the teenage years in the neck and shoulder with possible progression to the temporomandibular joint followed by long finger flexors, wrists, elbows and Achilles tendon. A hallmark feature of the disease is the hyperlaxity at the interphalangeal joints along with the more proximal contractures. Equinovarus or pes cavus foot deformity may develop. Muscle weakness becomes significant after the fourth decade.

Spinal muscular atrophy

Spinal muscular atrophy (SMA) is an autosomal recessive disease resulting in the degeneration of anterior horn cells, causing hypotonia, hyporeflexia and generalized weakness with the proximal and lower extremities muscles most severely affected historically. Three different phenotypes are usually documented (SMA types 1, 2 and 3) based on age of onset the maximum motor milestone achieved by the patient. SMA1, or infantile onset SMA is the most severe form and is characterized by disease onset within the first few months of life. Children with SMA1 never achieve sitting and typically succumb to respiratory failure by the age of 2. There are other subtypes such as SMA0 where contractures are prevalent at birth due to utero movement. Individuals with SMA2 generally present with symptoms between 6–18 months of age. They usually gain the ability to sit but never walk unaided. There is considerable heterogeneity in disease progression and symptomology for individuals with SMA2. Life expectancy is reduced but varies widely. Individuals with SMA3 are the least affected across the spectrum. They are able to sit and walk, although the majority lose the ability to stand and walk unaided in adolescence or early adulthood. With the advances in therapeutic treatments for SMA, the phenotype and contracture development is rapidly changing.

Individuals with SMA2 typically develop the most severe contractures due to their longer life expectancy compared with SMA1 and reduced motor function when compared with type 3 individuals. Muscles most at risk of contracture are ankle plantarflexors, hip and knee flexors and wrist and elbow flexors (Wang et al. 2004; Willig et al. 1995). These contractures may occur as early as 2 years of age (Johnson et al. 1992; Fujak et al. 2011; Wang et al. 2004). Hip abduction and external rotation may become restricted with disease progression (Fujak et al. 2011; Wang et al. 2004). Hip subluxation and dislocations may also be an issue due to overall weakness of hip stabilizers. Neuromuscular scoliosis can rapidly develop due to generalized axial weakness. Upper extremity contractures may be seen as early as 3 years of age and often occur in combination with lower extremities contractures. Most prevalent restrictions in the upper limbs start with elbow flexors and forearm supinators with nearly 80% having some degree of contracture by 3 years of age (Wang et al. 2004; Fujak et al. 2010; Benady 1978). Other upper limb restrictions include shoulder abduction with less involvement of the shoulder rotators, restriction of radial abduction and wrist and finger extensors (Carter et al. 1995; Wang et al. 2004). Severity of contractures have been associated with level of function; therefore, prevention should be key in management. Salazar et al. (2018) found that hip and knee flexion contracting were associated with decreased gross motor function. Due to the prevalence of contracture development in SMA, understanding of muscle imbalances, positioning for appropriate prevention and management of contracture development are crucial to maintain the appropriate musculoskeletal length to obtain the most benefit from exercise and therapies that may contribute to strength and function gains.

CHARCOT–MARIE–TOOTH DISEASE

Charcot–Marie–Tooth disease (CMT) describes a group of clinically and genetically hetero-geneous neuropathies characterized by a common phenotype of abnormal electrophysiol-ogy, absent tendon reflexes, distal sensory loss and progressive distal muscle weakness and atrophy (Barisic et al. 2008). The underlying genetic defect responsible for CMT results in distal demyelination and axonal loss (Lupski et al. 1991). Selective involvement of these nerves causes weakness and wasting of the supplied muscles resulting in an imbalance of force about the distal joints. This imbalance has been proposed to contribute to the develop-ment of contracture of the ankle plantar flexors, which in turn is thought to contribute to the development of orthopedic deformities which are the hallmark of CMT such as pes cavus (Burns et al. 2009). The situation is similar in the upper limbs whereby the larger muscles of the forearm and hand retain greater strength than the smaller intrinsic muscles of the hand resulting in hyperextension of the metacarpophalangeal (MCP) joints and flexion of the proximal and distal interphalangeal joints. The long finger extensors act unopposed across the MCP joints and stronger long flexors across the interphalangeal joints, resulting in the characteristic claw hand deformity.

Joint contracture in CMT can have a number of disabling consequences for upper and lower limb function such as impaired motor function, inefficient gait as well poor functional dexterity resulting in difficulties with activities of daily living such as handwriting and self care (Burns et al. 2010). There is an emerging body of literature suggesting these problems have a negative impact on quality of life and health status in children and adults with CMT (Burns et al. 2010; Padua et al. 2006; Padua et al. 2008; Redmond et al. 2008).

**Measurement of contractures**

The assessment of joint ROM in pediatric NMD is important for monitoring joint flexibility and response to interventions. While a variety of methods for quantifying joint ROM have been described, goniometry is by far the most popular in the clinical setting. It is important to note the quality and reliability of joint range measurement relies largely on the practitioner's knowledge of anatomy and physiology for proper alignment of the axis of the goniometer to the fulcrum of the joint and positioning. Additional factors affecting measurement error include, the force applied to the end range, end range feel, test position and instrumental dif-ferences (Johnson et al. 2015; Gajdosik and Bohannon 1987; Bohannon et al. 1989; Konor et al. 2012; Kim et al. 2011). A practitioners ability to assess quality of resistance within the range of motion is important to identify the pathology underlying the joint tightness.

Besides goniometry, other methods to measure joint range include tape measures, incli-nometers and smartphone apps which have similar functionality to inclinometers. Most of these methods have an equitable reliability to goniometry with intraclass correlations between 0.085–0.990 (Konor et al. 2012). Further, joint range may be measured in non-weight-bearing or weight-bearing positions in which the later is believed to best translate to functional activities such as walking and stair climbing. Joints to prioritize for ROM assessment are those that lack antigravity strength and are prone to contracture in that particular NMD.

## Stretching physiology

Stretching interventions refer to techniques or modalities that apply tension to soft tissues (Harvey et al. 2002). Physical therapists use a number of techniques that elicit short (active and passive stretches) and long duration (positioning, night splinting and serial casting) stretches to maintain or improve joint flexibility.

Stretching interventions are thought to increase soft tissue extensibility via two different mechanisms of initial viscous deformation of the muscle (dynamic phase) and through structural adaptations within the muscle and surrounding soft tissues (static phase) (Herbert 1988). Viscous deformation refers to the initial mechanical response of soft tissue such as muscle, ligament and tendon to sustained stretching that may initiate the stretch reflex. It is a transient response that is thought to last as long as the actual stretch time followed by the static phase that allows for viscoelastic stress relaxation (Doung et al. 2001; Sobolewski et al. 2014; McHugh et al. 1992). If a muscle is immobilized in a lengthened position, longer lasting changes in muscle length occur as a result of structural adaptations taking place within the muscle (Herbert 1988). Via this mechanism, increases in muscle length occur as sarcomeres are added in series and can occur within 48 hours of a muscle being immobilized in a lengthened position (Goldspink et al. 1974; Tabary et al. 1972; Tardieu et al. 1977; Lieber 2009). This suggests that the duration of the stretch is an important factor in achieving molecular changes in muscle length. The intensity of the stretch appears to be another important factor in achieving increases in muscle length. Studies of muscular adaptations following limb lengthening surgery in which up to 10cm in bone length can be gained in a matter of months has provided evidence that large increases in muscle length are possible with an intense stretch (Pontén et al. 2007).

The physiology of increased flexibility is unclear. Many have theorized autogenic inhibition may be a possible mechanism where a muscle relaxes with time, dampening the stretch reflexive or other neuro-reflexive mechanisms (Magnusson et al. 1996; Klinge et al. 1997). Many studies have shown that improved stretch tolerance with a daily stretch routine is the primary factor in improved ROM (Magnusson et al. 1997; Harvey et al. 2002; Magnusson 1998; Halbertsma et al. 1999; Ben and Harvey 2010). Structures associated with stretch tolerance are unknown but has been hypothesized that it is related to nociceptive nerve endings in the muscle; hence, the reason for active stretch techniques, activating agonist muscle to stretch antagonist, appear to have improved short-term ROM from tolerance to stretch rather than actual muscle extensibility (Magnusson et al. 1997; Harvey 2002; Ben and Harvey 2010; Went et al. 2009).

## Rehabilitative management of contractures

Contracture management in pediatric NMD requires a multifaceted approach requiring considerations from a multidisciplinary team with distinct functional goals. Clinicians should prioritize muscle groups most prone to contractures by first understanding the phenotypical presentation of the NMD. Secondly, a thorough strength exam identifying

**Table 21.2**
**Types of stretch therapies**

| *Short duration (stretching between 15 sec–30 min)* | *Long duration (stretching >30min)* |
| --- | --- |
| • Methods of Stretching<br>  • Standing wedge, Standing Frame, Nada chair and manual stretches<br>• Types of manual stretches<br>  • Active and passive: recommend rotating between both types<br>• Evaluate joint range end feel<br>• Utilize massage or heat to increase tolerance to passive stretch<br>• Slowly passively move the limb towards a firm end feel and hold for 90 seconds.<br>• Standing board/Standing device: Up to tolerance. Goal is 30 minutes.<br>• Perform regularly: Make it a routine | • Methods of Stretching<br>  • Positioning: adaptive equipment, Wheelchair lower extremity abductor guards, abductor ties in sitting<br>  • Orthosis/splints: static or hinged AFOs, KAFOs, custom hand/wrist/finger splints, wrist cock up splints<br>  • Standing board: prone or supine<br>• Perform regularly:<br>  • Braces: Work up to 6–8 hours. May be worn at night.<br>  • Positioning: Best if positioned in optimal posture throughout the day |

muscles that lack full antigravity strength provides insight on muscles prone to contracture development (Table 21.2).

STRETCHING: SHORT DURATION

Passive stretching involves an external force to passively lengthen muscles but active assisted force by the agonist muscle is required to maintain ROM (Cherry 1980). Passive stretches of 15 seconds to 2 minute intervals have been reported in the literature (Ben and Harvey 2010; Bandyopadhyay and Brawerman 1992; Bandy and Irion 1994; Bandy et al. 1997; 1998; Ayala and Branda Andújar 2010). A study of the optimal duration of static stretching indicated no difference between 30 and 90 seconds in improving stretch tolerance (Bandy et al. 1997). Passive lengthening tends to activate the stretch reflex; therefore, methods to inhibit the stretch reflex would result in a greater stretch (Eldred 1967; Tanigawa 1972). These methods include activation of the agonist to inhibit the antagonist muscle. However, this may not be possible in very weak individuals; therefore, passive lengthening would be the optimal treatment. With passive lengthening, the joint must be slowly moved to the maximum tolerated range and held for a prolonged period of time to desensitize the stretch receptors. Ballistic or rapid maneuvers with the intention of removing adhesions are contra-indicated. To affect muscle physiology, viscoelastic accommodation of the muscle has been shown at 90 seconds resulting in a stress relaxation response to stretching (Magnusson et al. 1997). Additionally, in review of the viscoelastic response, early stretching would be beneficial in younger individuals because their muscles are more pliable to maintain extensibility. For maximum impact of change in the muscle physiology and stretch tolerance, a stretch of 90 seconds is recommended. Regular passive and active range is recommended to counter complications that may arise from muscle imbalances and immobilization both in the muscle and joints along with possible downstream influences on cellular and biomechanical processes of tissue repair (Frank et al. 1984). Immobilization may lead to chemical changes consistent with osteoarthritis (Videman et al. 1976) in extra-articular tissue alignment (Salter et al. 1980; Videman et al. 1979) and degradation of collagen mass that may be further complicated by inflammation or fibrosis typically seen in many NMD thus inhibiting normal joint gliding motion (Akeson et al. 1980).

Two systematic reviews have provided evidence that manual stretching of the hamstrings (Harvey 2002) and gastrocnemius/soleus (Radford et al. 2006) increases joint ROM while other studies support evidence of improved range with stretching but no evidence of long term changes in muscle extensibility with fiber or sarcomere length (Halbertsma et al. 1999; Ben and Harvey 2010; Magnusson et al. 1996; Halbertma and Göeken 1994). The improvement in ROM is hypothesized to improve due to tolerance of the stretch by patients rather than actual improvement of muscle fiber length. The studies reviewed included otherwise healthy individuals with limitations in joint ROM. While these results are promising, individuals with pathological changes in the structure and function of their muscle, such as those with NMD, are unlikely to respond to stretch in a similar way.

Other systematic reviews have investigated stretching interventions for individuals with neuromuscular (Rose et al. 2010) and other neurological disorders (Harvey et al. 2002, 2017 and Craig et al. 2016). One systematic review specifically investigated interventions for increasing ankle ROM in individuals with NMD (Rose et al. 2010). Although stretching interventions aiming to improve ankle dorsiflexion ROM are widely employed for individuals with NMD, only four studies involving 149 participants met inclusion criteria for the review. Three of these studies pertained to stretching interventions or surgery in individuals with neuromuscular conditions. Systematic reviews investigating stretch for the treatment and prevention of contracture in people with neurological and non-neurological conditions (Harvey et al. 2017) found that night splints have minimum support. Casts show short term improvements in ROM and insufficient evidence for stretching. In individuals, it is highly likely that stretching interventions of greater intensity and duration may not improve joint ROM but may contribute to improved quality of movement, flexibility and joint integrity.

STRETCHING: LONG DURATION

Animal studies support management with long duration stretching (Tsujimura et al. 2006; Williams et al. 1998). These studies have shown that even dystrophic or denervated muscle fibers are capable of adding sarcomeres in series when immobilized in a lengthened position. The major difference between diseased muscle and unaffected muscle is that addition of sarcomeres occurs at a slower rate (Williams and Goldspink 1976). It is also likely that response to stretching interventions differs depending on the type of neuromuscular disorder. While similarities in muscle morphology are seen in some disorders, the response to stretching interventions may be better in some disorders than others. For example, dystrophic muscle, is characterized by a high percentage of fat and scar tissue that increases with disease progression (Mercuri 2009). Collagen, which comprises a large portion of scar tissue has a greater modulus of stiffness than muscle thus reducing muscle tissue extensibility requiring greater force to stretch it (Herbert 1988). By comparison, muscle in neuropathic diseases is characterized by fatty infiltration of selectively denervated muscles (Mercuri 2009; Gallardo et al. 2006). While some scar tissue is present it is not as abundant as seen in DMD, which might indicate that individuals with CMT may respond better to stretch and require a stretch of a lesser intensity and duration than boys with DMD. A systematic review of neurological conditions noted moderate evidence of short-term effect of joint mobility and no effect on functional activities (Glanzman et al. 2011).

Long duration stretches are defined as stretches lasting more than 30 minutes. There are numerous ways to achieve stretches of a long duration: positioning, splinting, bracing and orthoses and serial casting. Orthoses are a popular choice for maintaining range in the lower limb. They can be made static or dynamic. The static ankle foot orthoses (AFOs) maintains the current ROM while the dynamic AFO has the ability to provide added force for a more intensive stretch. Two studies investigated night splinting for individuals with CMT (Refshauge et al. 2006) and the other investigated serial night casting (Rose et al. 2010) for individuals with CMT showing improvements in ROM. In a small randomized comparative study of boys with DMD, they found that strength was a significant variable in degree of contractures and concluded that individuals who performed both manual stretches and night time splints had 23% less chance of developing contractures compared to stretching alone (Hyde et al. 2000). Hyde et al. (2000) and Seeger et al. (1985) found decreases in plantar flexion contractures; Nihizawa et al. (2018) found ROM maintenance with the use of night time braces, while Brooke et al. (1989) did not find any differences with night time splints. Possible explanations for the differences would be small sample sizes and lack of standardization in the methodology of assessing contractures. Most of these studies measured ROM with a goniometer without standard force applied to the measurement and since elastic deformation of soft tissue is directly proportional to velocity of stretch and force of application (Sobolewski et al. 2014; McHugh et al. 1992), the amount of force placed on the limb by the evaluator could vary resulting in differences in measurement of ROM.

Other bracing used for stretching and weight-bearing are knee-ankle-foot orthoses (KAFOs). KAFOs have been used in studies of upright stretching of the lower extremities and assisted gait in DMD and SMA (Fujak et al. 2011). Considerations for KAFOS should focus on light weight polypropylene material, drop-locked knee joints, solid neutral ankle and ischial weight-bearing. Ischial height is important for appropriate trunk support and upright positioning. If the ischial height is too high, it may push the patient forward shifting the center of gravity posteriorly. Additionally, individuals must have some truncal strength in order to use KAFOs. These studies did not focus on ROM and only noted minimal to poor evidence of the use of KAFOs in DMD (Bakker et al. 2000). A few case studies in SMA found that early fitting of KAFOs have been beneficial for gait (Granata et al. 1987). KAFOs are primarily not recommended for ambulation due to safety concerns and the increased energy cost associated with walking in them but may have indirect benefits to bone health and joint ROM. However, they are infrequently prescribed in DMD. With progressive weakness, individuals with DMD tend to lock out their knees and use a circumducted gait pattern along with momentum to ambulate; therefore, the added weight of KAFOs would not make independent ambulation possible. For SMA, KAFOs maybe prescribed mainly for weight-bearing or stretching but the overall weakness and fatigue would prevent functional use of KAFOs for ambulation.

Serial casting is another method that may improve ROM. This is typically indicated for ankle contractures where less intensive stretching has been ineffective. Considerations include weight of cast effects on function, atrophy due to immobilization, tolerance and sensory impairment, as seen in some types of CMT. Serial casting has been studied in DMD (Glanzman et al. 2011; Main et al. 2007; Carroll et al. 2017) with a mean of 12 degrees improvement in ROM without effects on timed function tests (Glanzman et al. 2011). Main et al. (2007) also found serial casting reduced contractures and was well tolerated but noted the considerable psychological impact of the procedure. A study of four weeks of serial night casting in CMT showed a mean improvement of 4 degrees of ankle dorsiflexion and improvement on some timed function tests (Rose et al. 2010). Serial casting may be a viable option for individuals with NMD. Careful consideration with a multidisciplinary team must be given to individuals biomechanics, strength and functional status.

## Other modalities including surgical intervention

Heat and massage

Heat has been commonly used to increase flexibility of muscles and tendons but with limited evidence of actual improvement in ROM. Heat has been used to increase tissue extensibility but mdx mice research indicates that there was increased muscle fatigue and decreased activity with higher tissue temperature (35°C) while a lower temperature of 20°C did show differences in activity (Wineinger et al. 1998). There is no literature supporting the use of heat in individuals with DMD.

Massage has been used for relaxation, to increase muscle circulation, decrease fascial adhesions and to stimulate the anti-inflammatory response (Crane et al. 2012). This modality maybe considered in conjunction with stretching for muscular health and to improve tolerance of stretching but further research is needed to understand the possible anti-inflammatory or anti-fibrotic effects of massage on dystrophic muscle.

Surgery

For rigid/fixed contractures that cannot be managed by conservative approaches, surgery may be an option, particularly if the contractures are causing pain, inhibiting function or causing orthopedic deformity. Improvement in pain or function should be the primary surgical goal. Lengthening a muscle results in immediate pseudo decrease in strength from lengthening of the lever arm to produce force at the joint. It is essential to understand the possible advantages of a shortened muscle for function. Additionally, after surgery, the patient will need to be immobilized which may contribute to muscle atrophy in already weak muscles.

Some studies have shown Achilles tendon lengthening prophylactically has improved maintenance of ambulation in DMD (Forst and Forst 2012), while others report no difference or loss of function (Leitch et al. 2005; Garralda et al. 2006; Manzur et al. 1992). For instance, individuals with DMD who are in the transitional phase of walking may not improve walking efficiency after a tendon lengthening due to the change in biomechanics and proximal weakness that may result in loss of ambulation. Surgery should

**TABLE 21.3**
**Minimal ROM requirements for activities of daily living**

| Joint | Range of Motion (ROM) | Function |
|---|---|---|
| Ankle Dorsiflexion | 10° | Late midstance and foot clearance (Manzur et al. 1992) |
| Ankle Dorsilflexion | 30° | Stairs (D'Amico et al. 2017) |
| Shoulder abduction | 130° | Place containers on shelf. Wash backside. Place hand on head (Leitch et al. 2005, Garralda et al. 2006) |
| Shoulder flexion | 100°–120° | Reaching over head, comb hair (Leitch et al. 2005, Garralda et al. 2006) |
| Elbow flexion | 80° | Hand to mouth/head (Leitch et al. 2005) |
| Wrist flexion/extension | 40° | Perineal care, picking up objects, donning/doffing pants, drinking from a cup (Leitch et al. 2005) |
| Forearm supination | 50° | Perineal care (Leitch et al. 2005) |

DF: dorsiflexion; ROM: range of movement.

only be considered for boys with DMD who have quadriceps strength of at least a Medical Research Counccil (MRC) grade of 4 or better and bracing should be planned in advanced to ensure proper positioning post-operatively. Surgery may also be considered for individuals who are non-ambulatory with severe equinovarus with pain due to lateral weight-bearing on the foot or inability to wear shoes.

**Upper extremity rehabilitation management of contractures**
Most of the literature regarding management of contractures focuses on the lower extremities as this is most prevalent in NMD and most debilitating. Upper limb contractures hindering function develop later in the disease progression along with associated weakness. Common upper limb contractures include wrist flexion, forearm supination and elbow flexion. Shoulder tightness of the adductors/ internal rotators is evident but less problematic. Upper body and trunk positioning is important for function and respiratory health. Individuals who are contracted in a flexed position will have a harder time breathing. Mild elbow contractures of less than 20 degrees tend to not inhibit function while contractures greater than that may inhibit functional use of walking devices. Severe elbow contractures of more than 80 degrees may inhibit reachable workspaces and the ability to feed oneself or with dressing (D'Amico et al. 2017). Wrist flexion and extension of 35 degrees is required for appropriate donning and doffing of clothes and perineal care (Gates et al. 2016). A study looking at required ROM for upper limb self-care ADLs indicated that the minimum necessary range required a shoulder flexion of 120 degrees, abduction of 130 degrees, horizontal adduction of 115 degrees and 60 degrees of external rotation (Namdari et al. 2012). Splinting and stretches maybe combined such as elbow flexors may be stretched along with forearm supinators, wrist and finger flexors (Table 21.3). Similar to lower extremity contractures, management should consist of regular passive stretching, appropriate positioning with assistive devices or bracing to maintain independence with ADLs and fine motor skills. Due to frequency of re-occurrence, surgical release is rarely

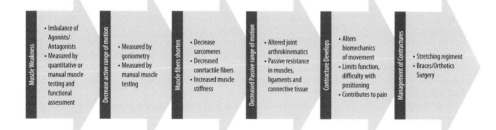

**Fig. 21.1.** Evolution of the development of contractures.

recommended performed only when it hinders ability to maintain proper hygiene ie: ability to open hands.

## Conclusion

Development of contractures is disabling and inevitable with the multifaceted pathogenesis in NMDs. Physiological changes aggravate the effects of muscle weakness and joint malalignment. The most effective conservative management include a combination of short and long duration stretches. Stretches should be performed prophylactically while muscles are pliable, and for indirect benefits of enhancing blood circulation to the muscle and joints, and reducing muscle tension/stiffness and pain. Even though the evidence behind some of the principles of contracture management are conflicting, the physiological benefits of early passive range and positioning support stretch interventions as an effective tool to minimize the impact of contractures on function and disability. The key to management is prevention (Fig. 21.1). For specific joint management, clinicians should have a thorough understanding of muscle weaknesses, progression and imbalances to prescribe early appropriate prophylactic stretch therapies.

## Key points
- Evaluate overall strength for muscle imbalances.
  - Strengthen weak agonist based muscle integrity of NMD.
  - Stretch the antagonist.
- Identify muscle groups at risk for contracture development.
  - Muscles with MRC of <3− (not full active range of motion)
  - Extensors are at greater risk than flexors .
- Prescribe regularly short duration manual stretching home exercise program.
  - Stretches should be performed slowly towards end range and held for 30–90 sec.
  - Consider contract-relax and active assisted stretches.
- Prescribe  regularly long duration management .
  - This could be a combination of appropriate positioning, standing frame and/or braces.
  - Increased duration of stretch is preferable over intensity of stretch.

## REFERENCES

Akeson WH, Amiel D, Woo SL (1980) Immobility effects on synovial joints the pathomechanics of joint contracture. *Biorheology* 17: 95–110.

Akima H, Lott D, Senesac C, Deol J, Germain S, Arpan I et al. (2012) Relationships of thigh muscle contractile and non-contractile tissue with function, strength, and age in boys with Duchenne muscular dystrophy. *Neuromuscul Disord* 22: 16–25.

Archibald KC, Vignos PJ Jr (1959) A study of contractures in muscular dystrophy. *Arch Phys Med Rehabil* 40: 150–157.

Ayala F, de Baranda Andújar PS (2010) Effect of 3 different active stretch durations on hip flexion range of motion. *J Strength Cond Res* 24: 430–436.

Bakker JP, de Groot IJ, Beckerman H, de Jong BA, Lankhorst GJ (2000) The effects of knee-ankle-foot orthoses in the treatment of Duchenne muscular dystrophy: review of the literature. *Clin Rehabil* 14: 343–359.

Bandy WD, Irion JM (1994) The effect of time on static stretch on the flexibility of the hamstring muscles. *Phys Ther* 74: 845–850, discussion 850–852.

Bandy WD, Irion JM, Briggler M (1997) The effect of time and frequency of static stretching on flexibility of the hamstring muscles. *Phys Ther* 77: 1090–1096.

Bandy WD, Irion JM, Briggler M (1998) The effect of static stretch and dynamic range of motion training on the flexibility of the hamstring muscles. *J Orthop Sports Phys Ther* 27: 295–300.

Bandyopadhyay R, Brawerman G (1992) Secondary structure at the beginning of the poly(A) sequence of mouse beta-actin messenger RNA. *Biochimie* 74: 1031–1034.

Barisic N, Claeys KG, Sirotković-Skerlev M, Löfgren A, Nelis E, De Jonghe P et al. (2008) Charcot-Marie-Tooth disease: a clinico-genetic confrontation. *Ann Hum Genet* 72: 416–441.

Barrett R, Hyde SA, Scott OM, Dubowitz V. (1988) Changes in center of gravity in boys with Duchenne muscular dystrophy. *Muscle & Nerve*, 11(11): 1157–1163.

Ben M, Harvey LA (2010) Regular stretch does not increase muscle extensibility: a randomized controlled trial. *Scand J Med Sci Sports* 20: 136–144.

Benady SG (1978) Spinal muscular atrophy in childhood: review of 50 cases. *Dev Med Child Neurol* 20: 746–757.

Bohannon RW, Tiberio D, Zito M (1989) Selected measures of ankle dorsiflexion range of motion: differences and intercorrelations. *Foot Ankle* 10: 99–103.

Bönnemann CG (2011) The collagen VI-related myopathies Ullrich congenital muscular dystrophy and Bethlem myopathy. *Handb Clin Neurol* 101: 81–96.

Brooke MH, Fenichel GM, Griggs RC, Mendell JR, Moxley R, Florence J et al. (1989) Duchenne muscular dystrophy: patterns of clinical progression and effects of supportive therapy. *Neurology* 39: 475–481.

Burns J, Ryan MM, Ouvrier RA (2009) Evolution of foot and ankle manifestations in children with CMT1A. *Muscle Nerve* 39: 158–166.

Burns J, Ryan MM, Ouvrier RA (2010) Quality of life in children with Charcot-Marie-Tooth disease. *J Child Neurol* 25: 343–347.

Carroll K, de Valle K, Kornberg A, Ryan M Kennedy R (2017) Evaluation of Serial Casting for Boys with Duchenne Muscular Dystrophy: A Case Report. *Phys Occup Ther Pediatr* 38(1):88–96.

Carter GT, Abresch RT, Fowler WM Jr, Johnson ER, Kilmer DD, McDonald CM (1995) Profiles of neuromuscular diseases. Spinal muscular atrophy. *Am J Phys Med Rehabil* 74(Suppl):S150–S159.

Cherry DB (1980) Review of physical therapy alternatives for reducing muscle contracture. *Phys Ther* 60: 877–881.

Cornu C, Goubel F, Fardeau M (1998) Stiffness of knee extensors in Duchenne muscular dystrophy. *Muscle Nerve* 21: 1772–1774.

Cornu C, Goubel F, Fardeau M (2001) Muscle and joint elastic properties during elbow flexion in Duchenne muscular dystrophy. *J Physiol* 533: 605–616.

Craig J, Hilderman C, Wilson G, Misovic R, et al. (2016) Effectiveness of stretch interventions for children with neuromuscular disabilities: evidence-based recommendations. *Pediatr Phys Ther*. 28: 262–275.

Crane JD, Ogborn DI, Cupido C, Melov S, Hubbard A, Bourgeois JM et al. (2012) Massage therapy attenuates inflammatory signaling after exercise-induced muscle damage. *Sci Transl Med* 4: 119ra13.

D'Amico A, Catteruccia M, Baranello G, Politano L, Govoni A, Previtali SC et al. (2017) Diagnosis of Duchenne Muscular Dystrophy in Italy in the last decade: critical issues and areas for improvements. *Neuromuscul Disord* 27: 447–451.

D'Angelo MG, Berti M, Piccinini L, Romei M, Guglieri M, Bonato S et al. (2009) Gait pattern in Duchenne muscular dystrophy. *Gait Posture* 29: 36–41.

Doglio L, Pavan E, Pernigotti I, Petralia P, Frigo C, Minetti C (2011) Early signs of gait deviation in Duchenne muscular dystrophy. *Eur J Phys Rehabil Med* 47: 587–594.

Duong B, Low M, Moseley AM, Lee RY, Herbert RD (2001) Time course of stress relaxation and recovery in human ankles. *Clin Biomech (Bristol, Avon)* 16: 601–607.

Eldred E (1967) Functional implications of dynamic and static components of the spindle response to stretch. *Am J Phys Med* 46: 1290140.

Eymard B, Ferreiro A, Ben Yaou R, Stojkovic T (2013) Muscle diseases with prominent joint contractures: main entities and diagnostic strategy. *Rev Neurol (Paris)* 169: 546–563.

Eymard B, Ferreiro A, Ben Yaou R Stojkovic T (2013) Muscle disease with prominent joint contractures: main entities and diagnostic strategy. *Rev Neurol (Paris)* 169: 546–563.

Fishman FG, Goldstein EM, Peljovich AE (2017) Surgical treatment of upper extremity contractures in Emery-Dreifuss muscular dystrophy. *J Pediatr Orthop B* 26: 32–35.

Flanigan KM, Kerr L, Bromberg MB, Leonard C, Tsuruda J, Zhang P et al. (2000) Congenital muscular dystrophy with rigid spine syndrome: a clinical, pathological, radiological, and genetic study. *Ann Neurol* 47: 152–161.

Forst J, Forst R (2012) Surgical treatment of Duchenne muscular dystrophy patients in Germany: the present situation. *Acta Myol* 31: 21–23.

Frank C, Akeson WH, Woo SL, Amiel D, Coutts RD (1984) Physiology and therapeutic value of passive joint motion. *Clin Orthop Relat Res* &NA;113–125.

Fujak A, Kopschina C, Gras F, Forst R, Forst J (2010) Contractures of the upper extremities in spinal muscular atrophy type II. Descriptive clinical study with retrospective data collection. *Ortop Traumatol Rehabil* 12: 410–419.

Fujak A, Kopschina C, Gras F, Forst R, Forst J (2011) Contractures of the lower extremities in spinal muscular atrophy type II. Descriptive clinical study with retrospective data collection. *Ortop Traumatol Rehabil* 13: 27–36.

Gajdosik RL, Bohannon RW (1987) Clinical measurement of range of motion. Review of goniometry emphasizing reliability and validity. *Phys Ther* 67: 1867–1872.

Gallardo E, García A, Combarros O, Berciano J (2006) Charcot-Marie-Tooth disease type 1A duplication: spectrum of clinical and magnetic resonance imaging features in leg and foot muscles. *Brain* 129: 426–437.

Garralda ME, Muntoni F, Cunniff A, Caneja AD (2006) Knee-ankle-foot orthosis in children with Duchenne muscular dystrophy: user views and adjustment. *Eur J Paediatr Neurol* 10: 186–191.

Gates DH, Walters LS, Cowley J, Wilken JM, Resnik L (2016) Range of motion requirements for upper-limb activities of daily living. *Am J Occup Ther* 70(1): 7001350010p1–7001350010p10.

Glanzman AM, Flickinger JM, Dholakia KH, Bönnemann CG, Finkel RS (2011) Serial casting for the management of ankle contracture in Duchenne muscular dystrophy. *Pediatr Phys Ther* 23: 275–279.

Goldspink G, Tabary C, Tabary JC, Tardieu C, Tardieu G (1974) Effect of denervation on the adaptation of sarcomere number and muscle extensibility to the functional length of the muscle. *J Physiol* 236: 733–742.

Goncu K, Guzel R, Guler-Uysal F (2003) Emery-Dreifuss muscular dystrophy in the evaluation of decreased spinal mobility and joint contractures. *Clin Rheumatol* 22: 456–460.

Granata C, Cornelio F, Bonfiglioli S, Mattutini P, Merlini L (1987) Promotion of ambulation of patients with spinal muscular atrophy by early fitting of knee-ankle-foot orthoses. *Dev Med Child Neurol* 29: 221–224.

Halbertsma JP, Göeken LN (1994) Stretching exercises: effect on passive extensibility and stiffness in short hamstrings of healthy subjects. *Arch Phys Med Rehabil* 75: 976–981.

Halbertsma JP, Mulder I, Göeken LN, Eisma WH (1999) Repeated passive stretching: acute effect on the passive muscle moment and extensibility of short hamstrings. *Arch Phys Med Rehabil* 80: 407–414.

Harvey L, Herbert R, Crosbie J (2002) Does stretching induce lasting increases in joint ROM? A systematic review. *Physiother Res Int* 7: 1–13.

Harvey LA, Katalinic OM, Herbert RD, et al. (2017) Stretch for the treatment and prevention of contractures (review). *Cochrane Database of Syst Rev*.

Herbert R (1988) The passive mechanical properties of muscle and their adaptations to altered patterns of use. *Aust J Physiother* 34: 141–149.

Hoffman EP, Brown RH Jr, Kunkel LM (1987) Dystrophin: the protein product of the Duchenne muscular dystrophy locus. *Cell* 51: 919–928.

Hsu JD, Furumasu J (1993) Gait and posture changes in the Duchenne muscular dystrophy child. *Clin Orthop Relat Res* &NA;122–125.

Hyde SA, FlŁytrup I, Glent S, Kroksmark AK, Salling B, Steffensen BF et al. (2000) A randomized comparative study of two methods for controlling Tendo Achilles contracture in Duchenne muscular dystrophy. *Neuromuscul Disord* 10: 257–263.

Johnson LB, Sumner S, Duong T, Yan P, Bajcsy R, Abresch RT et al. (2015) Validity and reliability of smartphone magnetometer-based goniometer evaluation of shoulder abduction – A pilot study. *Man Ther* 20: 777–782.

Johnson ER, Fowler WM Jr, Lieberman JS (1992) Contractures in neuromuscular disease. *Arch Phys Med Rehabil* 73: 807–810.

Kim PJ, Peace R, Mieras J, Thoms T, Freeman D, Page J (2011) Interrater and intrarater reliability in the measurement of ankle joint dorsiflexion is independent of examiner experience and technique used. *J Am Podiatr Med Assoc* 101: 407–414.

Klinge K, Magnusson SP, Simonsen EB, Aagaard P, Klausen K, Kjaer M (1997) The effect of strength and flexibility training on skeletal muscle electromyographic activity, stiffness, and viscoelastic stress relaxation response. *Am J Sports Med* 25: 710–716.

Konor MM, Morton S, Eckerson JM, Grindstaff TL (2012) Reliability of three measures of ankle dorsiflexion range of motion. *Int J Sports Phys Ther* 7: 279–287.

Kubo S, Tsukahara T, Takemitsu M, Yoon KB, Utsumi H, Nonaka I et al. (1998) Presence of emerinopathy in cases of rigid spine syndrome. *Neuromuscul Disord* 8: 502–507.

Leitch KK, Raza N, Biggar D, Stephen D, Wright JG, Alman B (2005) Should foot surgery be performed for children with Duchenne muscular dystrophy? *J Pediatr Orthop* 25: 95–97.

Lieber RL (2009) Skeletal muscle adaptation to decreased use, p. 183–228. *In* Lieber RL (ed), *Skeletal muscle structure, function and plasticity. The physiological basis of rehabilitation*. Lippincott Williams and Wilkins, Baltimore.

Lupski JR, de Oca-Luna RM, Slaugenhaupt S, Pentao L, Guzzetta V, Trask BJ et al. (1991) DNA duplication associated with Charcot-Marie-Tooth disease type 1A. *Cell* 66: 219–232.

Madej-Pilarczyk A, Kochański A (2016) Emery-Dreifuss muscular dystrophy: the most recognizable laminopathy. *Folia Neuropathol* 54: 1–8.

Magnusson SP (1998) Passive properties of human skeletal muscle during stretch maneuvers. A review. *Scand J Med Sci Sports* 8: 65–77.

Magnusson SP, Simonsen EB, Aagaard P, Sørensen H, Kjaer M (1996) A mechanism for altered flexibility in human skeletal muscle. *J Physiol* 497: 291–298.

Magnusson SP, Simonsen EB, Aagaard P, Kjaer M (1996) Biomechanical responses to repeated stretches in human hamstring muscle in vivo. *Am J Sports Med* 24: 622–628.

Magnusson SP, Simonsen EB, Aagaard P, Boesen J, Johannsen F, Kjaer M (1997) Determinants of musculoskeletal flexibility: viscoelastic properties, cross-sectional area, EMG and stretch tolerance. *Scand J Med Sci Sports* 7: 195–202.

Main M, Mercuri E, Haliloglu G, Baker R, Kinali M, Muntoni F (2007) Serial casting of the ankles in Duchenne muscular dystrophy: can it be an alternative to surgery? *Neuromuscul Disord* 17: 227–230.

Manzur AY, Hyde SA, Rodillo E, Heckmatt JZ, Bentley G, Dubowitz V (1992) A randomized controlled trial of early surgery in Duchenne muscular dystrophy. *Neuromuscul Disord* 2: 379–387.

McDonald CM (1998) Limb contractures in progressive neuromuscular disease and the role of stretching, orthotics, and surgery. *Phys Med Rehabil Clin N Am* 9: 187–211.

McDonald CM, Abresch RT, Carter GT, Fowler WM Jr, Johnson ER, Kilmer DD (1995) Profiles of neuromuscular diseases. Becker's muscular dystrophy. *Am J Phys Med Rehabil* 74(Suppl): S93–S103.

McDonald CM, Abresch RT, Carter GT, Fowler WM Jr, Johnson ER, Kilmer DD et al. (1995) Profiles of neuromuscular diseases. Duchenne muscular dystrophy. *Am J Phys Med Rehabil* 74(Suppl): S70–S92.

McDonald CM, Henricson EK, Abresch RT, Duong T, Joyce NC, Hu F et al. (2018) Long-term effects of glucocorticoids on function, quality of life, and survival in patients with Duchenne muscular dystrophy: a prospective cohort study. *Lancet*, 391(10119): 451–461.

McHugh MP, Magnusson SP, Gleim GW, Nicholas JA (1992) Viscoelastic stress relaxation in human skeletal muscle. *Med Sci Sports Exerc* 24: 1375–1382.

Mercuri E (2009) New methods for assessing disease progression in neuromuscular disorders: assessment of strength and function. *Neuromuscul Disord* 19: 543.

Mercuri E, Yuva Y, Brown SC, Brockington M, Kinali M, Jungbluth H, Feng L, Sewry CA, Muntoni F (2002) Collagen VI involvement in Ullrich syndrome: a clinical, genetic, and immunohistochemical study. *Neurology* 58: 1354–1359.

Mercuri E, Bushby K, Ricci E, Birchall D, Pane M, Kinali M et al. (2005) Muscle MRI findings in patients with limb girdle muscular dystrophy with calpain 3 deficiency (LGMD2A) and early contractures. *Neuromuscul Disord* 15: 164–171.

Namdari S, Yagnik G, Ebaugh DD, Nagda S, Ramsey ML, Williams GR Jr et al. (2012) Defining functional shoulder range of motion for activities of daily living. *J Shoulder Elbow Surg* 21: 1177–1183.

Nishizawa H, Matsukiyo A, Shiba N, Koinuma M, Nakamura A (2018) The effect of wearing night splints for one year on the standing motor function of patients with Duchenne muscular dystrophy. *J Phys Ther Sci* 30: 576–579.

Padua L, Aprile I, Cavallaro T, Commodari I, La Torre G, Pareyson D et al. (2006) Variables influencing quality of life and disability in Charcot Marie Tooth (CMT) patients: italian multicentre study. *Neurol Sci* 27: 417–423.

Padua L, Shy ME, Aprile I, Cavallaro T, Pareyson D, Quattrone A et al. (2008) Correlation between clinical/neurophysiological findings and quality of life in Charcot-Marie-Tooth type 1A. *J Peripher Nerv Syst* 13: 64–70.

Pontén E, Gantelius S, Lieber RL (2007) Intraoperative muscle measurements reveal a relationship between contracture formation and muscle remodeling. *Muscle Nerve* 36: 47–54.

Radford JA, Burns J, Buchbinder R, Landorf KB, Cook C, Rome K (2006) Does stretching increase ankle dorsiflexion range of motion? A systematic review. *Br J Sports Med* 40: 870–875, discussion 875.

Redmond AC, Burns J, Ouvrier RA (2008) Factors that influence health-related quality of life in Australian adults with Charcot-Marie-Tooth disease. *Neuromuscul Disord* 18: 619–625.

Refshauge KM, Raymond J, Nicholson G, van den Dolder PA (2006) Night splinting does not increase ankle range of motion in people with Charcot-Marie-Tooth disease: a randomised, cross-over trial. *Aust J Physiother* 52: 193–199.

Rose KJ, Burns J, Wheeler DM, North KN (2010) Interventions for increasing ankle range of motion in patients with neuromuscular disease. *Cochrane Database Syst Rev* 2: CD006973.

Rose KJ, Raymond J, Refshauge K, North KN, Burns J (2010) Serial night casting increases ankle dorsiflexion range in children and young adults with Charcot-Marie-Tooth disease: a randomised trial. *J Physiother* 56: 113–119.

Salazar R, Montes J, Dunaway Young S, McDermott MP, Martens W, Pasternak A et al. (2018) Quantitative Evaluation of Lower Extremity Joint Contractures in Spinal Muscular Atrophy: Implications for Motor Function. *Pediatr Phys Ther.* 30(3): 209–215.

Salter RB, Simmonds DF, Malcolm BW, Rumble EJ, MacMichael D, Clements ND (1980) The biological effect of continuous passive motion on the healing of full-thickness defects in articular cartilage. An experimental investigation in the rabbit. *J Bone Joint Surg Am* 62: 1232–1251.

Seeger BR, Caudrey DJ, Little JD (1985) Progression of equinus deformity in Duchenne muscular dystrophy. *Arch Phys Med Rehabil* 66: 286–288.

Sienko Thomas S, Buckon CE, Nicorici A, Bagley A, McDonald CM, Sussman MD (2010) Classification of the gait patterns of boys with Duchenne muscular dystrophy and their relationship to function. *J Child Neurol* 25: 1103–1109.

Skalsky AJ, McDonald CM (2012) Prevention and management of limb contractures in neuromuscular diseases. *Phys Med Rehabil Clin N Am* 23: 675–687.

Sobolewski EJ, Ryan ED, Thompson BJ, McHugh MP, Conchola EC (2014) The influence of age on the viscoelastic stretch response. *J Strength Cond Res* 28: 1106–1112.

Tabary JC, Tabary C, Tardieu C, Tardieu G, Goldspink G (1972) Physiological and structural changes in the cat's soleus muscle due to immobilization at different lengths by plaster casts. *J Physiol* 224: 231–244.

Tanigawa MC (1972) Comparison of the hold-relax procedure and passive mobilization on increasing muscle length. *Phys Ther* 52: 725–735.

Tardieu C, Tabary JC, Tabary C, Huet de la Tour E (1977) Comparison of the sarcomere number adaptation in young and adult animals. Influence of tendon adaptation. *J Physiol (Paris)* 73: 1045–1055.

Tsujimura T, Kinoshita M, Abe M (2006) Response of rabbit skeletal muscle to tibial lengthening. *J Orthop Sci* 11: 185–190.

Videman T, Michelsson JE, Rauhamäki R, Langenskiöld A (1976) Changes in 35S-sulphate uptake in different tissues in the knee and hip regions of rabbits during immobilization, remobilization the development of osteoarthritis. *Acta Orthop Scand* 47: 290–298.

Videman T, Eronen I, Candolin T (1979) Effects of motion load changes on tendon tissues and articular cartilage. A biochemical and scanning electron microscopic study on rabbits. *Scand J Work Environ Health* 5(suppl 3):56–67.

Wang HY, Ju YH, Chen SM, Lo SK, Jong YJ (2004) Joint range of motion limitations in children and young adults with spinal muscular atrophy. *Arch Phys Med Rehabil* 85: 1689–1693.

Weng MC, Lee CL, Chen CH, Hsu JJ, Lee WD, Huang MH et al. (2009) Effects of different stretching techniques on the outcomes of isokinetic exercise in patients with knee osteoarthritis. *Kaohsiung J Med Sci* 25: 306–315.

Williams PE, Goldspink G (1976) The effect of denervation and dystrophy on the adaptation of sarcomere number to the functional length of the muscle in young and adult mice. *J Anat* 122: 455–465.

Williams P, Kyberd P, Simpson H, Kenwright J, Goldspink G (1998) The morphological basis of increased stiffness of rabbit tibialis anterior muscles during surgical limb-lengthening. *J Anat* 193: 131–138.

Wineinger MA, Walsh SA, Abresch RT (1998) The effect of age and temperature on mdx muscle fatigue. *Muscle Nerve* 21: 1075–1077.

# 22
# OCCUPATIONAL THERAPY AND ROBOTICS

*Imelda de Groot*

## Introduction

A child with a neuromuscular disorder is likely to (slowly) encounter loss of functional ability or activity due loss of muscle strength with progression of the disease. The loss of the ability to rise from the floor, for example, means the child needs help if the child plays on the floor or falls, the loss of the ability to walk means the child needs a mobility device, the loss of the ability to reach means either help or the use of some arm support device. The functional limitations of the child due to muscle weakness make the child at risk for participation restrictions. Furthermore, a child also needs experiences, both physical and social, to mature at the cognitive level (Woodmansee et al. 2016; Donnelly et al. 2016; Jackson et al. 2016). Not every neuromuscular disorder in childhood leads to the same limitation patterns in activities, as this is not even the case within one neuromuscular disorder. It can be dependent on the stage of the disease, but is also dependent on the preferences of the child, the environment of the child and the child's family life. This is best illustrated by the World Health Organization's scheme of the International Classification of Functioning, Disability and Health (WHO 2016) (Fig. 22.1). In this scheme, one can see that impairments in body function, such as muscle weakness, or body structure, such as contractures or scoliosis, can lead to limitations in basic activities such as walking, sitting, reaching, grasping, but also to complex activities such as grooming, toileting, eating, drinking, etc. These limitations can restrict a child's participation in social life, such as going to school, doing sports or leisure activities. Contextual factors may have influence on the extend of the limitations of activities or restrictions in participation as in some countries schools are easily accessible by wheelchair while in other countries even sidewalks are not wheelchair friendly. Also, family factors can play a role; it is not always easy to organize all the care for your child in the local area and visiting a special school with all therapies available in school is more convenient.

Thus, child-centered care is necessary aiming at the preferences of the child and the child's family. This implies that only general recommendations can be given, but the composition of all occupational interventions or advice for a child are individually specific. If a child or parent considers a device not useful in practice, the device will not be used (Peredo et al. 2010). For several disorders, such as for Duchenne muscular dystrophy, spinal muscular atrophy and congenital muscular dystrophy, guidelines for rehabilitation management

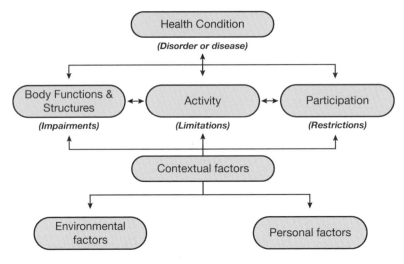

**Fig. 22.1.** International Classification of Functioning, Disability and Health of WHO. Reprinted from WHO (2016) pg 18, with permission from WHO.

are available, including occupational interventions, on the Treat-NMD site (www.Treat-NMD.eu). These guidelines are also useful for other neuromuscular disorders.

**Home adjustments**

Adjustments in a home, or even moving to an adjusted house, takes time, not only to complete all adjustments but also to give the parents time to thoroughly think over all the adjustments that might be needed. As most of the neuromuscular disorders in childhood are progressive, either due to the disorder or due to growth and the child becoming bigger and heavier, a plan for house adjustments should be anticipatory to all changes in functioning that can be expected during the next 10 or 20 years. This is not only necessary to make optimal caring for a child possible, such as having an accessible shower and toilet, but the necessity to develop adjusted autonomy for the child is as important. Autonomy is more than being functionally independent with assisted devices; it also means that a child or adolescent is able to make their own decisions. An adjusted environment can help a child to mature in decision making, as being always dependent can lead to learned dependency in more than the physical aspects alone. Being dependent can lead to symbiotic binding with the caregivers, which are mostly the parents. As many children with neuromuscular disorders reach adulthood nowadays, it is important to let them grow up to become people who are able to live by themselves in adjusted environments with professional caregivers. This is, of course, limited if a child has cognitive impairments, but to some extend each child can make their own choices. The process of learning autonomy starts with giving the child the chance to live as their healthy peers in suitable house and environment. Getting in or out the house by themselves with automatic doors with a remote control to manage the doors themselves is for example one of the prerequisites.

The numbers of technical solutions available is increasing and, due to the fact that the growing elderly population and not only children with neuromuscular disorders need adjustments of their environment, the devices will become cheaper and more available. Although they are not available yet everywhere in the world.

## Mobility aids and wheelchair

Type of mobility aid or wheelchair

As ambulation becomes more difficult, several options are there. The easiest is to start using a wheelchair; however, as staying active can prevent disuse to a certain extent, mobility aids should be considered to make use of the child's residual capacities. If a child has enough strength in their legs, a bicycle or tricycle is an option or even a walking-bicycle (such as the racerunner: www.racerunning.org). Tricycles are more stable to get on and off than bicycles. Motorized (electrical) bicycles or tricycles are available and sometime have starting assistance to get the bi/tricycle moving.

When a child is non-ambulant but still has enough strength in his/her arms, a wheelchair with electrical wheels is an option (for example, e-motion wheels, Alber GmBH[R]). Thus. the arms are trained during the day and disuse of the arms can be prevented. Importantly, a symmetrical movement is made which could prevent asymmetrical sitting positions and asymmetrical contracture formation. There are several assistance levels possible in the electrical wheels thus making it possible to use this type of wheelchair for a long time.

If a child is non-ambulant and has not enough strength in the arms to propel a wheelchair, even with assistance, then an electrical wheelchair is needed. Often a central joy-stick within a table-top is chosen to promote a symmetrical position of the arms on the top and thus promoting a midline position of the back. However, this prevents a child in getting close to a normal table, desk or other children. For this reason, a joy-stick placed at the side of the wheelchair could also be chosen. One should be aware of the possibility a child could lean more on the side of the steering arm, thus introducing an asymmetrical load on the trunk. The sitting position and the extend of support needed for the trunk is an additional factor in the choice of the type of wheelchair.

## Sitting position

In choosing the support for sitting, a distinction should be made between the ability to perform active sitting or passive sitting; the second consideration should be whether or not there is a deformity of the back; and the third is whether or not the trunk can still be corrected (structural deformity) (Strobl 2013). A weak trunk can either be supported by a corset or brace or a seating shell, depending how active the child is to be able to change their position by flexion or extension in the pelvis. In general, a slightly tilted position is recommended (Michael et al. 2007). Several instruments exist to evaluate children's sitting capacities and these can be used to make a choice between the different seating supports (Field and Livingstone 2013).

The options to support a seating position are increasing. Nowadays, a seating shell with side lateral support patches and a shaped back support is often chosen for a support as braces are often not well tolerated due to pain or pressure with skin reactions. This type of seating restricts the child's ability, however, to reach and decreases the workspace. There are new developments in designing support systems for the trunk that allow bending and thus reaching. Also, braces of soft tissue that are still stiff enough to deliver support to the trunk have been designed and tested (for example: www.spioworks.com).

## Arm supports

Most daily activities are performed by the arms either sitting or standing and/or walking. Proportionally, standing and/or walking occupy much less in time. Limitations in arm activities lead to decrease of participation or increase in dependence on other persons. For this reason, many supportive arm devices have been developed (van der Heide et al. 2014).

ASSISTING ARM DEVICES

Assisted arm devices can either be passive or active. A passive arm support can be actuated or non-actuated. An non-actuated passive arm support helps the arm to move around in the space by balancing the weight of the arm and can be mounted on a table or wheelchair (Fig. 22.2A). An actuated passive arm support balances the weight of the arm, but can also support arm movements in different directions using springs (Fig. 22.2B).

Active arm supports have externally driven supports to move the support in different directions. This is mostly done using electrical motors, placed on the wheelchair or placed within the arm support, that need input by pushing a button or a joy-stick movement. However, intuitive active supports are being developed in which force sensors are used to determine the direction a person wants to move to.

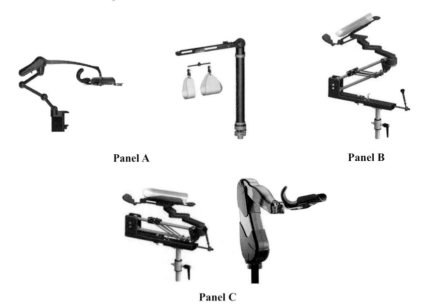

Panel A                                           Panel B

Panel C

**Fig. 22.2.** **A** Examples of non-actuated passive arm supports (Focal MeditechTM and Dowing and Sling). **B** Example of actuated passive arm supports by sprints (Focal MeditechTM Top-Help). **C.** Example of active arm support and intuitive arm support (Focal MeditechTM and Top-Help electrical and ExoArm).

The choice between a balancing arm support or an actuated arm support depends on the remaining strength of the shoulder and arm muscles. The active range of motion is a good predictor for functional ability (Janssen et al. 2017). A choice of the type of arm support (only balanced or actuated) can be made to use a device as a sling (Fig. 22.2A ) and asking the child to perform tasks. The use of arm supports can prevent disuse (Jansen et al. 2015) and can reduce the extent of the help needed; however, more medical technology assessment research is needed. The arm supports are increasingly available in different countries. With all the arm supports, it is necessary to explore the desired tasks the child wants to perform, and prioritize these tasks next to the options an arm support can give. An individual match should be made keeping in mind that there is no perfect match possible. If expectations do not match what is delivered, the supports will not be used (van der Heide et al. 2015a; 2015b).

Robot arms

A robot arm is a type of mechanical arm with similar functions to a human arm. A robot arm takes over the function of the arm and is applicable if there is no or very little arm and/ or hand function left. The use of robot arms can decrease the need of help from caregivers significantly (Maheu et al. 2011). Examples of robot arms can be found on: http://kinovaro-botics.com or http://www.exactdynamics.nl.

**Robotics**

All kind of robotics are introduced increasingly in healthcare, ranging from apps on mobile phones to monitor your activity level or mood, to telemedicine devices monitoring vital signs, to environmental control (lights, doors, heating etc.), to humanoid robots helping in daily activities, to exoskeletons (www.medicalfuturist.com). With the development of new kind of robotics, such as soft robotics, a new world is developing (Laschi et al. 2017). In elderly care, robotics are being tested and improved and it is to be expected that many of the robotics developed for the elderly will be applicable for persons with motoric impairments.

The development of exoskeletons is especially interesting as a wearable assistive device for daily tasks. At the moment, many supportive devices need an attachment to a wheelchair; for example, either as they are too huge to attach to the body or they need electrical actuation. This is restricting and does not allow children to reach a workspaces. Alternatively, the device can only be used in a wheelchair. Furthermore, these devices are conspicuous and affect social interaction (Dunning and Herder 2013). Exoskeletons in principle are attached to the body; leg exoskeletons are well known for assisted walking, but arm exoskeletons are also being developed (Kooren et al. 2015). Although this seems like science fiction, development is fast and in the future it will be possible for children with neuromuscular disorders to be more independent by means of the use of high technology devices and aids.

**Key points**
• Children with neuromuscular disorders lose functional abilities due to muscle strength loss with progression of disease.

- To preserve the ability to interact in their social environment, assisted devices are necessary, either to support the activity (such as arm supports) or to replace the bodily function such as wheelchairs for mobility or, in the future, exoskeletons for the whole body.
- Technology is developing rapidly and will provide new options for preserving autonomy, not only functional autonomy but also social.

## REFERENCES

Donnelly JE, Hillman CH, Castelli D, Etnier JL, Lee S, Tomporowski P, Lambourne K et al. (2016) Physical activity, fitness, cognitive function, and academic achievement in children: a systematic review. *Med Sci Sports Exerc* 48: 1197–1222.

Dunning AG, Herder JL (2013) A review of assistive devices for arm balancing. *IEEE Int Conf Rehabil Robot* 2013: 6650485.

Field D, Livingstone R (2013) Clinical tools that measure sitting posture, seated postural control or functional abilities in children with motor impairments: a systematic review. *Clin Rehabil* 27: 994–1004.

Jackson WM, Davis N, Sands SA, Whittington RA, Sun LS (2016) Physical activity and cognitive development: a meta-analysis. *Neurosurg Anesthesiol* 28(4):373–380.

Jansen M, Burgers J, Jannink M, van Alfen N, de Groot IJM (2015) Upper limb training with dynamic arm support in boys with Duchenne muscular dystrophy: A feasibility study. *Int J Phys Med Rehabil* 3: 2.

Janssen MMHP, Harlaar J, Koopman B, de Groot IJM (2017) Dynamic arm study: quantitative description of upper extremity function and activity of boys and men with Duchenne muscular dystrophy. *J Neuroeng Rehabil* 14: 45.

Kooren PN, Dunning AG, Janssen MM, Lobo-Prat J, Koopman BF, Paalman MI et al. (2015) Design and pilot validation of A-gear: a novel wearable dynamic arm support. *J Neuroeng Rehabil* 12: 83. Erratum in: *J Neuroeng Rehabil* 12: 111

Laschi C, Mazzolai B, Cianchetti M (2017) Soft robotics: technology and systems pushing the boundaries of robot abilities. *Sci Robot* 1: 1–11.

Maheu V, Frappier J, Archambault PS, Routhier F (2011) Evaluation of the JACO robotic arm: clinico-economic study for powered wheelchair users with upper-extremity disabilities. *IEEE Int Conf Rehabil Robot* 2011: 5975397.

Michael SM, Porter D, Pountney TE (2007) Tilted seat position for non-ambulant individuals with neurological and neuromuscular impairment: a systematic review. *Clin Rehabil* 21: 1063–1074.

Peredo DE, Davis BE, Norvell DC, Kelly PC (2010) Medical equipment use in children with disabilities: A descriptive survey. *J Pediatr Rehabil Med* 3: 259–267.

Strobl WM (2013) Seating. *J Child Orthop* 7: 395–399.

van der Heide LA, van Ninhuijs B, Bergsma A, Gelderblom GJ, van der Pijl DJ, de Witte LP (2014) An overview and categorization of dynamic arm supports for people with decreased arm function. *Prosthet Orthot Int* 38: 287–302.

van der Heide LA, Gelderblom GJ, de Witte LP (2015a) Effects and effectiveness of dynamic arm supports: a technical review. *Am J Phys Med Rehabil* 94: 44–62.

van der Heide LA, de Witte LP (2015b) Daily activity patterns of people provided with a dynamic arm support. *Stud Health Technol Inform* 217: 819–824.

WHO (2016) *International Classification of Functioning, Disability and Health: ICF*. Geneva: World Health Organization.

Woodmansee C, Hahne A, Imms C, Shields N (2016) Comparing participation in physical recreation activities between children with disability and children with typical development: A secondary analysis of matched data. *Res Dev Disabil* 49–50: 268–276.

# 23
## ORTHOPEDIC COMPLICATIONS IN NEUROMUSCULAR DISORDERS

*Maarten Van Nuffel and Pierre Moens*

### Introduction

The role of the orthopedic surgeon in the treatment of neuromuscular disorders (NMD) involves more than decision making on surgical interventions. Orthopedic management is embedded in a multidisciplinary approach of the problems in the upper and lower limbs and spine. In the early stages of the disease, this mostly includes physiotherapy, orthotics and environmental adaptation. In more progressive stages, surgical interventions may be warranted.

With the increase in life expectancy due to improving knowledge and treatment modalities in some of the NMDs, previously unseen orthopedic complications may develop and pose new challenges to the multidisciplinary team. Nowadays, the comprehensive management of the upper and lower limb functioning in NMD will require a detailed functional assessment; this will be illustrated in this chapter.

This chapter aims to give a description of the approach for both the lower and the upper limbs in different pathologies where specific orthopedic problems develop: motor neuron diseases, hereditary neuropathies, Duchenne muscular dystrophy, facioscapulohumeral muscular dystrophy and congenital myopathies and dystrophies. Where appropriate, specific surgical interventions will be discussed.

### Spinal muscular atrophy and other motor neuron diseases

The clinical features and natural histories of the different spinal muscular atrophy (SMA) subtypes has been provided in Chapter 6, highlighting the broad spectrum of the disease, ranging from the early lethal SMA type I to the milder, adult form, type IV.

LOWER LIMB INVOLVEMENT

Lower limb problems in SMA are mostly linked to the type of disease. Contractures of the hip and knee joint occur regularly and talipes equino varus is also a common feature in SMA type II patients whereas ambulatory patients have only mild orthopedic disturbance (Haaker and Fujak 2013). Physiotherapy, serial casting and orthosis are part of the treatment to control those contractures ( Haaker and Fujak 2013; Wang et al. 2007; Skalsky and McDonald 2012). Surgical treatment for lower extremity contractures can be effective for patients with type II or type IIIa. Tenotomy and tendon transfer have shown to be effective in some cases (Haaker and Fujak 2013).

Although there is a higher rate of hip subluxation in SMA, few are painful. Surgical reduction and osteotomies are frequently followed by redislocation; therefore. a conservative attitude is warranted in SMA hip subluxation (Wang et al. 2007). In our SMA population, in 24 years we have performed three hip surgeries in SMA patients because of pain resistant to classic treatment (positioning and analgesics); twice, a proximal femur resection was done because of poor bone quality making a reconstruction impossible in two SMA II patients, and once, a varus derotation osteotomy was done in a type III ambulatory patient, with relief of pain for all the three children.

The severe physical impairment associated with SMA results in an impaired bone mineralization and an increased risk of fractures, particularly of the lower extremities (Markowitz et al. 2012; Haaker and Fujak 2013).

UPPER LIMB INVOLVEMENT

SMA results in diffuse muscle weakness and atrophy with a specific disease progression pattern, from proximal to distal. Due to the severe nature and early mortality of SMA type I (Werdnig–Hoffmann disease), the evaluation and management of upper limb dysfunction has not been considered a priority. However, with changing standards of care and the development of new therapies for this disease, early and preventive management of the orthopedic aspects will have a more important role. In type II (Intermediate type – Dubowitz disease) and in type III (Kugelberg–Welander disease), contractures may develop in the upper limbs from an age of between 3–5 years. These contractures tend to become worse with age (Haaker and Fujak 2013).

Elbow contractures especially are perceived by the patients to hinder their daily functions and seem to be associated with greater discomfort. As well as elbow flexion contractures with limited supination, shoulder and wrist contractions can also occur, but hypermobile joints have also been described, especially in the wrist (Skalsky and McDonald 2012).

The role of surgery is limited in the management of upper limb orthopedic complications in SMA. Most often orthoses are fitted with a likely positive effect, although the scientific evidence for this is low. Physiotherapy and occupational therapy remain essential throughout life to preserve remaining capabilities and range of motion by decreasing contracture progression.

Because of the severe muscle weakness, upper limb function is not always easily evaluated. However, specific upper limb modules have been developed even for use in non-ambulatory patients. These can be used in addition to more general assessment scales such as the Hammersmith Functional Motor Scale (HMFS) and the Motor Function Measure (MFM), especially in type II or very weak type III patients. These scales can be used from the age of 30 months and have been proven to capture even subtle functional changes in non-ambulant spinal muscular atrophy patients. (Mazzone et al. 2011; Sivo et al. 2015). Hand-held dynamometry is another easy method to evaluate upper limb function: elbow flexion, handgrip and three-point pinch can be reliably measured using this method. (Seferian et al. 2015).

Further description of assessment tools to assess upper and lower limb function is provided in Chapter 5.

## Hereditary neuropathies (Charcot–Marie–Tooth)

In the different subtypes of Charcot–Marie–Tooth disease (CMT), the clinical features include mostly distal muscle weakness, impaired sensation and diminished deep tendon reflexes.

LOWER LIMB INVOLVEMENT

Regarding lower limb and in particular foot management we also refer to Chapter 7 (inherited neuropathies). The classic lower limb complication in CMT is the cavo varus foot with clawing toes. In a study of 148 children with cavus feet, 78% had CMT (Nagai et al. 2006). Whereas adolescents present with cavo varus feet, one should bear in mind that plano valgus foot is not uncommon in young children with CMT (Jani-Acsadi et al. 2015).

Because CMT represents a spectrum of clinical phenotypes with substantial variability of gait patterns from child to child, a single treatment recommendation is not possible (Jani-Acsadi et al. 2015). Those gait patterns are best documented by three-dimensional gait analysis (Ferrarin et al. 2012) to provide prognostic information on ambulation, to assist in surgical decision making and to evaluate results of treatment.

Non-operative treatments of foot deformities include physiotherapy (stretching) and bracing (Skalsky and McDonald 2012). There is no evidence that bracing of the foot in CMT patient can prevent progression of deformities; however, it can be used to manage drop foot and ankle instability, and facilitate the gait (Phillips et al. 2012; Yagerman et al. 2012).

Surgical treatment is indicated in case of progression of the foot deformities with increasing gait difficulties. The aim of surgery is to restore the foot ankle alignment and the stability of the joint. Different procedures are described: soft-tissue releases (fascia plantaris); tendon transfer (peroneus longus to brevis, tibial posterieur tendon to dorsum of the foot, Jones transfer, etc.); osteotomies to re-align the foot (calcaneus osteotomy, extension osteotomy of the first ray); arthrodesis (triple arthrodesis: re-alignment and fusion of the calcaneo-cuboid and talo-navicular joints) (Pareyson and Marchesi 2009).

If foot and ankle problems are well known in CMT patient, hip dysplasia should not be underestimated. In a study of 74 CMT patients, 8.1% were found with a dysplastic hip (Walker et al. 1994). For Chan et al. (2006) the dysplasia in CMT patients is from the neuromuscular nature; it is not present at birth, but is a consequence of the weakness of the hip muscles (abductors and extensors) resulting in the development of a shallow acetabulum and femoral increased anteversion with growth. A dysplastic hip present from birth in CMT patients should be considered and treated as a development dysplasia of the hip (DDH). Most of the CMT dysplasias are asymptomatic and there is lack of evidence-based decision-making literature on treatment (Yagerman et al. 2012).

For Chan, CMT hip dysplasia, even asymptomatic, requires treatment and the only modality is surgical. He advocates to first correct the acetabulum and if necessary, in a second time if the femoral head lateralizes, to perform an osteotomy of the proximal femur (Chan et al. 2006). In our institution we prefer to address both femur and acetabulum in one surgery.

UPPER LIMB INVOLVEMENT

There is variable penetrance in most subtypes, but limited hand function and manual dexterity is commonly found in one-half to two-thirds of patients, starting at a young age (Cornett et al. 2016).

Especially in type 1 and 3, the hand intrinsics are the second group of muscles showing weakness, after the foot intrinsics, resulting in a (mild) clawing position of the fingers, loss of thumb opposition, and impaired grip and pinch strengths. There seems to be a logarithmic relationship between the duration of the hand symptoms and the decline in strength. Despite the severe functional impairment, patients tend to develop adaptation mechanisms.

Specifically in CMT type 1A, it has been demonstrated that hand weakness and dysfunction are present from the earliest stages of the disease. However, due to the emphasis on lower limb problems in the early stages, the hand dysfunction may remain unnoticed initially, thus delaying therapy.

Tripod pinch strength and thumb opposition have been shown to be the major determinants of manual dexterity in CMT1A. Sensory impairments appear to have some, but limited, consequences for manual dexterity (Videler et al. 2010b). For this reason, the use of a thumb opposition splint worn during activities can significantly improve upper limb function in these patients. Even though it cannot compensate for a weak pinch strength, there seems to be a positive effect on the whole hand, including the clawing of the fingers, possibly due to a positive influence on the imbalance of intrinsic and extrinsic hand muscles (Videler et al. 2012). There is a strong relationship between reduced hand function and upper limb disability. A reduced hand function compared to healthy controls was reported in CMT, corresponding to about 60% of normal function, causing various degrees of limitations in daily life measured with DASH scores (Disabilities of the Arm, Shoulder and Hand). The DASH score may however show a better score than expected, because of adaptation mechanisms developed by the patients confronted with a slowly progressive disease (Eklund et al. 2009). The majority of patients in CMT type 1A perceive limitations in upper limb functioning that are strongly related to restricted participation and autonomy, whereas lower limb disability seems not as related (Videler et al. 2009). Problems with handwriting, weakness, pain and sensory symptoms in the hand tend to worsen with age. Despite increasing hand strength and function measures throughout childhood, they never reach normal values. With ageing, the strength starts to decrease again (Burns et al. 2008). Additionally, patients with CMT seem to manifest so-called overwork weakness, according to certain authors: a phenomenon in which muscles are permanently weakened through exercise. This results in the dominant hand becoming weaker than the non-dominant hand. Thus, patients with CMT are sometimes advised not to exercise to exhaustion and to be aware of signs such as feeling weak 30min after exercise or excessive muscle soreness 24–48hours following exercise (van Pomeren et al. 2009).

TREATMENT

A recent review from 2015 on exercise in CMT showed that most studies reported some changes in outcome in different exercise modalities. However, the quality of the studies included was low: none of them reached statistical significance and only two of them actually contained exercises of the upper limbs (Sman et al. 2015). Given the frequent enlargement of peripheral nerves (mostly in CMT1), compression problems are frequent and can worsen the paresthesias and weakness or give pain. For this reason, peripheral nerve decompression in the carpal tunnel or cubital tunnel can be considered when these symptoms quickly worsen. Nerve decompression, however, is not always helpful and often gives only partial improvement. Since all patients, especially those with CMT1, have aberrant nerve conduction studies, it is difficult to determine who will benefit from nerve decompression (Chalekson et al. 1999).

The atrophy of intrinsic hand muscles and thenar muscles can cause inability to perform fine manipulations, especially by diminishing thumb opposition. This can be restored by tendon transfer of the flexor digitorum superficialis (FDS) of the 4th finger to the thumb (Bunnell's opponensplasty). A modification of this technique, specifically reported in CMT patients, is demonstrated in Fig. 23.1. Other donor tendons have been proposed as well such as the extensor carpi ulnaris (ECU) or the extensor indicis proprius (EIP), connected to the extensor pollicis brevis (PB).

Historically, these procedures were most commonly performed at an adult age (Brown et al. 1992). However, there is increasing evidence that these transfers can already be performed during childhood with satisfactory functional results. Since there is a gradual decrease in strength over 5–7 years followed by a relative stability, is has been suggested that surgical intervention should be postponed until a reliable and durable transfer can be performed. A similar technique using the FDS of the 3rd finger has shown to be effective in children from the age of 6 (Estilow et al. 2012).

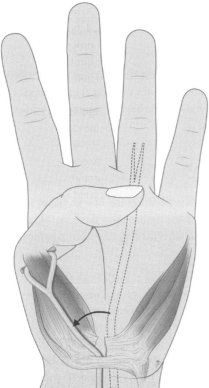

**Fig. 23.1.** Michelinakis and Vourexakis described a technique using the proximal part of the flexor retinaculum as a fulcrum for the flexor tendon of the fourth finger. Illustration by Myrthe Boijmans, www.myrtheboymans.nl. A colour version of this figure can be seen in the plate section at the end of the book.

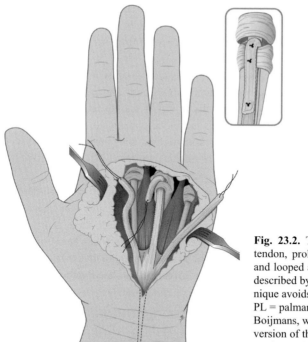

**Fig. 23.2.** Transfer of the palmaris longus tendon, prolonged with palmar aponeurosis and looped around the A1 flexor pulley, was described by Ochiai et al. in 1992. This technique avoids the need for a free tendon graft. PL = palmaris longus. Illustration by Myrthe Boijmans, www.myrtheboymans.nl. A colour version of this figure can be seen in the plate section at the end of the book.

Lastly, the clawing of the fingers, especially the 4th and 5th, can be corrected in different ways. These techniques are largely similar to the ones used for correction of clawing after ulnar palsy from other causes (Wood et al. 1995). One of these lasso procedures, specifically appealing for CMT disease, is demonstrated in Fig. 23.2.

### Duchenne muscular dystrophy

Duchenne muscular dystrophy (DMD) is another condition where the lower limb problems precede the upper limb symptoms and ambulation becomes the first problem. Hence, most of the orthopedic research and treatment target the problems in the legs. Please see Chapter 7 (inherited neuropathies) for further information regarding lower limb, particularly foot, management.

LOWER LIMB INVOLVEMENT

Contractures of Achilles tendons, iliotibial bands, knee and hip flexors are the classic lower limb involvements in DMD patients leading to characteristic gait (hyperlordosis, flexion abduction of the hips, flexion of the knees, equino varus feet). Later on, patients will lose the ability to stand and finally become wheelchair bound, with a high risk of developing scoliosis. A major aim of the treatment in DMD is to prolong the independent walking and standing abilities.

Treatment with corticosteroid is nowadays part of the standard care for DMD. Both prednisone and deflazacort have shown to slow the disease progression and delay the loss of important milestones, such as ambulation (McDonald et al. 2018). Preventive physiotherapy by mobilization and regular passive stretching of the Achilles tendon, hamstrings, hip flexors and abductors is advocated to prevent contractures (Birnkrant et al. 2018).

Serial casting of the ankles can be performed in DMD patients with moderate Achilles tendon contractures and without iliotibial band shortening, although the long-term results are less convincing in maintaining correction than surgical release (Main et al. 2007).

Surgery is able to correct the deformities, but has no effect on strength or function. At the contrary some operated patients showed more rapid deterioration of function (Manzur et al. 1992). For others lower limb surgery leads to a prolongation of independent ambulation of 1.25 years on average (Forst and Forst 1999). Surgery is indicated, to preserve the assisted standing position, when contractures become severe and impair standing ability. Release of contractures and rehabilitation in knee-ankle-feet orthoses (KAFO) is an option in DMD patients in the transitional stage, offering the possibility to prolong standing and limited household ambulation, facilitating transfers and other activities of daily living. This provides also more stability in the sitting position. This requires however an intensive, coordinated, postoperative rehabilitation program and a full understanding of the patient's ability and motivation (Goemans and Buyse 2014).

Hip subluxation or dislocation is a common feature in the non-ambulant DMD but the prevalence is lower than in other neuromuscular disorders. Hip subluxation, particularly unilateral, can play a role in the progression of scoliosis (Patel and Shapiro 2015); for this reason, pelvic asymmetry has to be taken into account in spinal surgery decision-making to avoid further deterioration of the sitting balance and the hip migration.

UPPER LIMB INVOLVEMENT

Weakness is an early and generalized sign, but still the pelvic girdle weakness predates the shoulder girdle weakness by several years. Hand strength tends to increase with age in the first decade, although it never reaches normal values as compared to healthy controls. Decrease of muscle strength in the wrist extensors has been noted to occur by age 8. In patients older than 10 years, both grip strength and pinch grip decrease again, which is associated with a decrease in the functional capacity in the hand (Mattar and Sobreira 2008). Between the ages of 8 to 14 years, patients generally develop extrinsic and intrinsic digital muscle shortness, boutonniere and swan neck deformities, hyperextension of the digital interphalangeal joints and flexion and ulnar deviation contractures of the wrist. Prophylactic active and passive stretching exercises for wrist and fingers, and encouraging the patients with DMD to sit with the wrist and fingers in a neutral or slightly extended position without wrist ulnar deviation, should be considered. After the age of 14, more and more motor tasks become difficult or even impossible. The muscle strength of the wrist extensors, and the radial deviation range of motion at the wrist, seems strongly correlated with wrist and hand function. Wrist flexion strength and range of motion do not seem to be correlated (Wagner et al. 1993).

To evaluate upper limb function in Duchenne muscular dystrophy, specifically developed scales can be used, such as the Brooke Upper Extremity Functional Scale. This scale

319

scores the upper extremity function from "0" (full range) to "6" (no use of hands) and has been frequently used as an outcome measure in DMD (Brooke et al. 1989). However, this scale limits the upper extremity functional rating of the DMD patient to one of six possible levels of function and may not adequately follow DMD disease progression with respect to hand function. Patients maintain the ability to perform motor tasks that require little proximal strength while having more difficulties with lifting objects against gravity.

Therefore, alternatives have been developed, such as the Egan Klassifikation (EK) Scale or the Performance of Upper Limb (PUL) assessment and the UL–PROM (see Chapter 5). These scores showed a steady deterioration after 5 years of age, compared to normal developing boys. They also showed that the shoulder function worsens first, while the changes in elbow and forearm appear at a later age (Mayhew et al. 2013; Pane et al. 2014).

Problems in the upper limb may initially be difficult to detect since patients tend to use so-called trick movements. By unknowingly using alternative movement patterns, they compensate for movements that are difficult or impossible, thus masking muscle weakness. A typical example is flexing the elbow when abducting the shoulder to decrease the force needed from the lateral deltoid, compared to shoulder abduction with the elbow extended.

While the hand function itself may be reasonably preserved, correct positioning of the hand will become the first main difficulty in the upper limb. Wasting of the shoulder muscles causes an inability to lift the arms by the age of 13–15 years. Attaching a special dynamic support for the arm to the wheelchair to eliminate the effects of gravity may aid in this problem. This dynamic arm support can even be used safely for upper limb training in order to retain motor function in the arms (Jan Burgers 2015).

Later in the disease, contractures usually develop. This occurs first in the lower limbs as well, but elbow flexion and later wrist flexion contractures generally follow. The elbow contractures frequently appear soon after full-time wheelchair dependency, probably due to prolonged static positioning with the arm in flexion. Also, the shoulders tend to be retracted with mild scapular winging (Skalsky and McDonald 2012). Since these contractures develop rather late in the disease and do not necessarily preclude wheelchair use, they seldom require surgical treatment.

Throughout childhood, the distal muscle groups of the upper extremities are those best preserved. With an ongoing improvement in life expectancy, upper limb function also deserves specific attention in rehabilitation programs and research.

Preserving muscle strength and range of motion may be relevant for a better outcome of distal motor function of the upper limbs in these patients. The remaining distal upper limb function generally only consists of isolated finger movements, such as flexion of the index finger and adduction of the thumb. Patients often rely on these small finger and thumb movements for manipulation of assisting devices, such as an electric wheelchair. This explains why a small loss of distal motor function in the hand can have a devastating effect on daily life (Bartels et al. 2011).

Adapting the conventional joystick to an easier to handle system (mini-joystick, isometric mini-joystick, finger joystick or pad) and changing the position to different fingers can help to regain driving ability for the power wheelchair. This seems true even for mechanical ventilation-dependent patients or those with a tracheostomy. When hand function decreases further, the design of a call bell may also need to be adapted to a more sensitive key-pinch interrupter or, eventually, to a mouth operated device instead of a push-button device (Pellegrini et al. 2007).

## Facioscapulohumeral muscular dystrophy

As its name suggests, facioscapulohumeral muscular dystrophy (FSHD) affects mostly the face and the proximal part of the upper limb, especially in the early stages of the disease. Weakness is in most cases relatively mild and the rate of strength loss is quite slowly progressive. An early age at onset is associated with greater likelihood of more severe and progressive weakness. Progression is descending, with subsequent involvement of either the distal anterior leg or hip-girdle muscles. The muscles that are most severely affected in patients with FSHD are the muscles that abduct the shoulder above 90° (deltoid), the shoulder anteflexors (deltoid, pectoralis major and subscapularis) and the shoulder extensors (deltoid and latissimus dorsi). The extensor muscles are weaker than the flexors, the external rotators are more severely affected than the internal rotators, and the forearm muscles are largely spared. In general, FSHD patients experience difficulty elevating their upper extremities and the execution of tasks takes a considerably longer time. At times the deltoids are, surprisingly, spared if tested with the scapulae stabilized. The biceps and triceps may both be more affected than the deltoids. Late in the disease course of early-onset FSHD, patients may show marked wrist extension weakness.

The involvement of shoulder girdle musculature in FSHD can be quite asymmetric, with some authors reporting greater weakness of selected dominant limb muscle groups. Due to the clinical heterogeneity of the disease, there is a wide variation in disability with FSHD, but motor weakness uniformly translates to impaired motor performance skills.

Contractures are normally rare and mild, but attention is needed for pain and stiffness experienced in the upper extremity, as these are frequently present in patients with FSHD (Bergsma et al. 2016).

In FSHD, involvement of the latissimus dorsi, lower trapezius, rhomboids and serratus anterior result in a characteristic appearance of the shoulders with the scapula positioned more laterally and superiorly, giving the shoulders a forward-sloped appearance. FSHD patients have a unique combination of winging at rest, persistence of winging throughout the range of motion and elevation of scapulae (Khadilkar et al. 2015).

There is limited scope for surgery in this condition. The only well-established surgical intervention in the upper limbs seems to be stabilization of the scapula to the chest wall. This can be performed as a scapulopexy, using muscle tor fascia transfers to the spinous process of the vertebrae. However, since these structures can stretch over time, the scapula becomes instable again. The other alternative is scapulodesis, or thoracoscapular arthrodesis: fixation of the scapula to the chest wall with wires or screws and bone grafting. This stabilizes the winging scapula and creates a stable fulcrum so the deltoid muscle can lift the humerus. This obviously means that patients considering surgery should have reasonable residual upper arm strength, especially in the deltoid and supraspinatus, and sufficient passive range of motion in the shoulder. An example case is described in the clinical vignette.

Several observational studies and case series have documented improvement in shoulder function, shoulder range of motion, or improvement in scapular pain after this procedure. Forward elevation gains of 10–40° and abduction gains of 10–60° have been reported. Even complaints of shoulder instability and subluxation have been noted to improve, as well as improvement of the cosmetic appearance. Of course, abduction over 90°, adduction, internal and external rotation will decrease after this operation (Goël et al. 2014).

This remains major surgery and the most important risks during the operation are fractures of the ribs or the scapula, pneumothorax, hemothorax and pleural effusion, which can be safely managed according to the literature. Other drawbacks are the prolonged postoperative immobilization of the shoulder and the need for intensive physiotherapy postoperatively (Cooney et al. 2014).

Despite good effects on short and long-term shoulder function, there is a significant failure rate associated with this procedure, with studies reporting a revision rate of between 10 and 20%. Also, hardware removal is frequently necessary; up to 50% of the cases in some series ( Goël et al. 2014; Van Tongel et al. 2013).

Children with FSHD start walking at a normal age; however, the gait progressively deteriorates due to weakness of the glutei muscles (maximus and medius) and the anterior abdomen muscles. The combination with strong hip flexors and spinal extensors leads to a striking hyperlordotic posture. Progressive weakness of foot dorsi-flexors and evertors is also a common feature in children with FSHD.

Release of the hip flexors and bracing the lordosis are not options as long as the child is able to walk (risk of compete loss of ambulation); ankle foot orthosis can support the drop foot.

## Congenital myopathies and dystrophies

The term congenital myopathy refers to a heterogeneous group of disorders based on genetic defects, usually presenting with infantile hypotonia, without any structural abnormality of the central nervous system or peripheral nerves. In early infancy, there can be hypotonia and delayed motor milestones. Later the patients develop a nonprogressive muscle weakness. This weakness is predominantly proximal, symmetric and in a limb-girdle distribution.

This group of disorders is quite heterogeneous, as are the repercussions on lower and upper limb function. The treatment for these conditions still remains purely supportive. Regular physiotherapy is recommended to preserve muscle power and function and prevent contractures. In cases where surgical treatment is warranted, postoperative mobilization should be initiated as soon as possible to avoid the adverse effects of prolonged immobilization such as muscle atrophy (Jungbluth et al. 2008).

Congenital muscular dystrophy

Congenital muscular dystrophy is a group of clinical entities. Infants present with hypotonia, muscle weakness at birth or within the first few months of life. They often also demonstrate contractures. These early flexion contractures mostly occur in the ankles, knees and hips. Involvement of the upper limbs is far less frequent, but there can be tightness of the wrist flexors and long finger flexors. Over time, these contractures become more severe, especially with prolonged static positioning and without adequate passive mobilization and splinting. Surgery, however, is seldom needed for these upper limb problems, in contrast to the lower limb.

ULLRICH CONGENITAL MUSCULAR DYSTROPHY

Ullrich congenital muscular dystrophy, is a rare early-onset and usually severe collagen VI-related myopathy (Gilbreath et al. 2014), characterized by muscle weakness, a unique combination of distal ligamentous laxity with hypermobile joints and proximal contractures. These children most often have an early-onset scoliosis, congenital hip dislocation and torticollis (Yonekawa et al. 2013).

The hip dislocation is treated like a developmental dysplasia with a flexion abduction brace, but as those children are prompt to develop contractures the brace immobilization may not exceed 10 to 12 weeks (Wang et al. 2012).

EMERY–DREIFUSS MUSCULAR DYSTROPHY

Early elbow flexion contractures are the hallmark of Emery–Dreifuss muscular dystrophy (EMD1). Release of elbow flexion contractures in Emery–Dreifuss muscular dystrophy is not usually performed due to the high rate of contracture recurrence (Skalsky and McDonald 2012).

**Key points**
- Neuromuscular disorders are commonly associated with a wide range of orthopedic issues including limb contractures, joint dislocations and scoliosis.
- The management of orthopedic issues requires a multidisciplinary approach including physiotherapy, surgery, orthotics and environmental adaptation aiming at preserving or improving functional capacities.
- Decision-making processes should take into consideration the specific aspects of the underlying neuromuscular disease as each disease has its own characteristics and carries specific risks, and should include expert input from the multidisciplinary team.
- Pre-, peri and postoperative management of orthopedic surgery deserves specific multidisciplinary and coordinated attention considering the complexity of medical problems in patients with neuromuscular disorders, such as increased risks associated with anesthesia, cardio-respiratory issues and nutritional aspects.

**Clinical vignette**
A 14-year-old boy had a confirmed diagnosis of facioscapulohumeral dystrophy. He reported a decrease in shoulder function, especially elevating the arm above shoulder level. Initially, only certain activities, such as table tennis, were troublesome, but over the years more and more activities became gradually more difficult. A conservative treatment of bracing was tried, but showed very little benefit. The shoulder function became more and more impaired and he started developing pain from the age of 22.

On clinical examination at that time, he manifested posterior muscle wasting around the shoulder with scapular winging. Palpation was painful over the anterior capsule, long tendon of the biceps brachii and the acromioclavicular joint. Active abduction and anterior elevation of the shoulder were 55° and 70°, respectively. Exorotation in the glenohumeral joint and rotation of the scapula on shoulder abduction were severely weakened.

Since the symptoms interfered with his professional activities, hobbies and sleep, the decision to perform a scapulothoracic fusion was taken.

Through a longitudinal incision midway between the medial border of the scapula and the spinous processes, the scapula was approached. The medial 2/3 of the subscapularis muscle was detached from the scapula and a fixation of the scapula against the posterior surface of the fourth, fifth, and sixth rib was performed using a plate and cerclage wires with bone grafts.

The second day after the operation, the patient was short of breath, demonstrated decreased breath sounds and dullness on percussion of the right hemithorax. A radiography of the thorax demonstrated a pleural effusion on the right side. This was treated with a chest drain for 4 days and had no further negative effects on his rehabilitation.

Postoperatively, the arm was immobilized in a standard shoulder immobilizer with a small abduction pillow. The first 6 weeks, no shoulder movement was permitted, only elbow and hand movements were encouraged. After this period, the passive range of motion was gradually increased until active range of motion was permitted 10 weeks postoperatively. Radiographies and CT scan showed a good bony healing 3 months postoperatively (Fig. 23.3).

At 8 months postoperatively, his symptoms were significantly improved. His shoulder was pain free and showed an abduction of 100° and anterior elevation of 120°. He was also pleased with the improved cosmetic appearance of his shoulder and even had the impression that his gait and posture had somewhat improved.

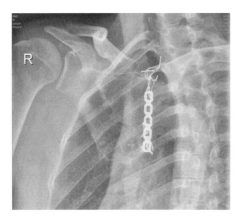 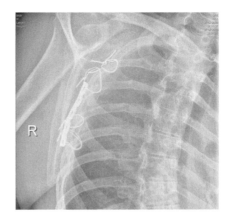

**Fig. 23.3.** Anterior and lateral radiography at 8 months postoperatively demonstrating the position of the scapula, the bony fixation and the osteosynthesis. (Images courtesy of Dr Bart Van de Meulebroucke).

CONCLUSION

Scapulothoracal arthrodesis is an effective treatment for symptomatic scapular winging in FSHD, whereas conservative treatment and soft-tissue procedures usually yield disappointing results. Since this procedure has an important complication rate, it is only considered in severe cases and usually performed after skeletal maturity.

REFERENCES

Bartels B, Pangalila RF, Bergen MP, Cobben NA, Stam HJ, Roebroeck ME (2011) Upper limb function in adults with Duchenne muscular dystrophy. *J Rehabil Med* 43: 770–775.

Bergsma A et al. (2016) Upper limb function and activity in people with facioscapulohumeral muscular dystrophy: a web-based survey. *Disabil Rehabil* 8288: 1–8.

Birnkrant DJ, Bushby K, Bann CM, Apkon SD, Blackwell A, Brumbaugh D et al. (2018) Diagnosis and management of Duchenne muscular dystrophy, part 1: diagnosis, and neuromuscular, rehabilitation, endocrine, and gastrointestinal and nutritional management. *Lancet Neurol* 17: 251–267.

Brooke MH, Fenichel GM, Griggs RC, Mendell JR, Moxley R, Florence J et al. (1989) Duchenne muscular dystrophy: patterns of clinical progression and effects of supportive therapy. *Neurology* 39: 475–481.

Brown RE, Zamboni WA, Zook EG, Russell RC (1992). Evaluation and management of upper extremity neuropathies in Charcot-Marie-Tooth disease. *J Hand Surg* 17(3): 523–530.

Burns J, Bray P, Cross LA, North KN, Ryan MM, Ouvrier RA (2008). Hand involvement in children with Charcot-Marie-Tooth disease type 1A. *Neuromuscul Disord* 18: 970–973.

Chalekson CP, Brown RE, Gelber DA, Haws MJ (1999). Nerve decompression at the wrist in patients with Charcot-Marie-Tooth disease. *Plast Reconstr Surg* 104(4): 999–1002.

Chan G, Bowen JR, Kumar SJ (2006). Evaluation and treatment of hip dysplasia in Charcot-Marie-Tooth disease. *Orthop Clin North Am* 37: 203–209, vii.

Cooney AD, Gill I, Stuart PR (2014). The outcome of scapulothoracic arthrodesis using cerclage wires, plates, and allograft for facioscapulohumeral dystrophy. *J Shoulder Elbow Surg* 23:e8–e13.

Cornett KM, Menezes MP, Bray P, Halaki M, Shy RR, Yum SW, et al. (2016). Phenotypic Variability of Childhood Charcot-Marie-Tooth Disease. *JAMA Neurol* 73: 645–651.

Eklund E, Svensson E, Häger-Ross C (2009). Hand function and disability of the arm, shoulder and hand in Charcot-Marie-Tooth disease. *Disabil Rehab* 31(23): 1955–1962.

Estilow T, Kozin SH, Glanzman AM, Burns J, Finkel RS (2012). Flexor digitorum superficialis opposition tendon transfer improves hand function in children with Charcot-Marie-Tooth disease: case series. *Neuromuscul Disord* 22: 1090–1095.

Ferrarin M, Bovi G, Rabuffetti M, Mazzoleni P, Montesano A, Pagliano E, et al. (2012). Gait pattern classification in children with Charcot–Marie–Tooth disease type 1A. *Gait Posture* 35(1): 131–137.

Forst J, Forst R (1999). Lower limb surgery in Duchenne muscular dystrophy. *Neuromuscul Disord* 9: 176–181.

Gilbreath HR, Castro D, Iannaccone ST (2014). Congenital myopathies and muscular dystrophies. *Neurol Clin* 32: 689–703, viii.

Goël DP, Romanowski JR, Shi LL, Warner JJ (2014). Scapulothoracic fusion: outcomes and complications. *J Shoulder Elbow Surg* 23: 542–547.

Goemans N, Buyse G (2014). Current treatment and management of dystrophinopathies. *Curr Treat Options Neurol* 16: 287.

Haaker G, Fujak A (2013). Proximal spinal muscular atrophy : current orthopedic perspective. *Appl Clin Genet* 6(11): 113–120.

Jan Burgers MJ (2015) Upper limb training with dynamic arm support in boys with Duchenne muscular dystrophy: a feasibility study. *Int J Phys Med Rehabil* 5(3):359–372.

Jani-Acsadi A, Ounpuu S, Pierz K, Acsadi G (2015) Pediatric Charcot-Marie-Tooth disease. *Pediatr Clin North Am* 62: 767–786.

Khadilkar SV, Chaudhari CR, Soni G, Bhutada A (2015) Is pushing the wall, the best known method for scapular winging, really the best? A comparative analysis of various methods in neuromuscular disorders. *J Neurol Sci* 351(1-2): 179–183.

Main M, Mercuri E, Haliloglu G, Baker R, Kinali M, Muntoni F (2007) Serial casting of the ankles in
    Duchenne muscular dystrophy: can it be an alternative to surgery? *Neuromuscul Disord* 17: 227–230.
Manzur AY, Hyde SA, Rodillo E, Heckmatt JZ, Bentley G, Dubowitz V (1992) A randomized controlled trial
    of early surgery in Duchenne muscular dystrophy. *Neuromuscul Disord* 2: 379–387.
Markowitz JA, Singh P, Darras BT (2012) Spinal muscular atrophy: a clinical and research update. *Pediatr
    Neurol* 46: 1–12.
Mattar FL, Sobreira C (2008) Hand weakness in Duchenne muscular dystrophy and its relation to physical
    disability. *Neuromuscul Disord* 18: 193–198.
Mayhew A, Mazzone ES, Eagle M, Duong T, Ash M, Decostre V et al. (2013) Development of the
    Performance of the Upper Limb module for Duchenne muscular dystrophy. *Dev Med Child Neurol*
    55: 1038–1045.
Mazzone E, Bianco F, Martinelli D, Glanzman AM, Messina S, De Sanctis R et al. (2011) Assessing upper
    limb function in nonambulant SMA patients: development of a new module. *Neuromuscul Disord* 21:
    406–412.
McDonald CM, Henricson EK, Abresch RT, Duong T, Joyce NC, Hu F et al. 2018 Long-term effects of glu-
    cocorticoids on function, quality of life, and survival in patients with Duchenne muscular dystrophy: a
    prospective cohort study. *Lancet* 391(10119):451–46. doi.10.1016/S0140-6736(17)32160-8.
Nadeau A, Kinali M, Main M, Jimenez-Mallebrera C, Aloysius A, Clement E et al. (2009) Natural history of
    Ullrich congenital muscular dystrophy. *Neurology* 73(1): 25–31.
Nagai MK, Chan G, Guille JT, Kumar SJ, Scavina M, Mackenzie WG (2006) Prevalence of Charcot-
    Marie-Tooth disease in patients who have bilateral cavovarus feet. *J Pediatr Orthop* 26: 438–443.
Pane M, Mazzone ES, Fanelli L, De Sanctis R, Bianco F, Sivo S et al. (2014) Reliability of the Performance
    of Upper Limb assessment in Duchenne muscular dystrophy. *Neuromuscul Disord* 24: 201–206.
Pareyson D, Marchesi C (2009) Diagnosis, natural history, and management of Charcot-Marie-Tooth disease.
    *Lancet Neurol* 8: 654–667.
Patel J, Shapiro F (2015) Simultaneous progression patterns of scoliosis, pelvic obliquity, and hip sublux-
    ation/dislocation in non-ambulatory neuromuscular patients: an approach to deformity documentation.
    *J Child Orthop* 9: 345–356.
Pellegrini N, Pelletier A, Orlikowski D, Lolierou C, Ruquet M, Raphaël JC et al. (2007) Hand versus mouth
    for call-bell activation by DMD and Becker patients. *Neuromuscul Disord* 17: 532–536.
Phillips MF, Robertson Z, Killen B, White B (2012) A pilot study of a crossover with randomized use of
    ankle-foot orthoses for people with Charcot-Marie-tooth disease. *Clin Rehabil* 26: 534–544.
Seferian AM, Moraux A, Canal A, Decostre V, Diebate O, Le Moing AG et al. (2015) Upper limb evaluation
    and one-year follow up of non-ambulant patients with spinal muscular atrophy: an observational multi-
    center trial. *PLoS One* 10:e0121799.
Sivo S, Mazzone E, Antonaci L, De Sanctis R, Fanelli L, Palermo C et al. (2015) Upper limb module in non-
    ambulant patients with spinal muscular atrophy: 12 month changes. *Neuromuscul Disord* 25: 212–215.
Skalsky AJ, McDonald CM (2012) Prevention and management of limb contractures in neuromuscular
    diseases. *Phys Med Rehabil Clin N Am* 23: 675–687.
Sman AD, Hackett D, Fiatarone Singh M, Fornusek C, Menezes MP, Burns J (2015) Systematic review of
    exercise for Charcot-Marie-Tooth disease. *J Peripher Nerv Syst* 20: 347–362.
van Pomeren M, Selles RW, van Ginneken BT, Schreuders TA, Janssen WG, Stam HJ (2009) The hypothesis
    of overwork weakness in Charcot-Marie-Tooth: a critical evaluation. J Rehabil Med 41: 32–34.
Van Tongel A, Atoun E, Narvani A, Sforza G, Copeland S, Levy O (2013) Medium to long-term outcome
    of thoracoscapular arthrodesis with screw fixation for facioscapulohumeral muscular dystrophy. *J Bone
    Joint Surg Am* 95: 1404–1408.
Videler AJ, Beelen A, van Schaik IN, de Visser M, Nollet F (2009) Limited upper limb functioning has
    impact on restrictions in participation and autonomy of patients with hereditary motor and sensory neu-
    ropathy 1a. J Rehabil Med 41: 746–750.
Videler AJ, Beelen A, Nollet F (2010a) Verifying the hypothesis of overwork weakness in Charcot-Marie-
    Tooth. J Rehabil Med 42: 380–381, author reply 380–381.
Videler AJ, Beelen A, van Schaik IN, Verhamme C, van den Berg LH, de Visser M et al. (2010b) Tripod pinch
    strength and thumb opposition are the major determinants of manual dexterity in Charcot-Marie-Tooth
    disease type 1A. J Neurol Neurosurg Psychiatry 81: 828–833.
Videler A, Eijffinger E, Nollet F, Beelen A (2012) A thumb opposition splint to improve manual dexterity and
    upper-limb functioning in Charcot-Marie-Tooth disease. *J Rehabil Med* 44: 249–253.

Wagner MB, Vignos PJ Jr, Carlozzi C, Hull AL (1993) Assessment of hand function in Duchenne muscular dystrophy. *Arch Phys Med Rehabil* 74: 801–804.

Walker J, Nelson K, Heavilon JA, Stevens DB, Lubicky JP, Ogden JA et al. (1994) Hip abnormalities in children with Charcot–Marie–Tooth. *J Pediatr Orthop* 14: 54–59.

Wang CH, Finkel RS, Bertini ES, Schroth M, Simonds A, Wong B et al. (2007) Consensus statement for standard of care in spinal muscular atrophy. *J Child Neurol* 22: 1027–1049.

Wang CH, Dowling JJ, North K, Schroth MK, Sejersen T, Shapiro F et al. (2012) Consensus statement on standard of care for congenital myopathies. *J Child Neurol* 27: 363–382.

Wood VE, Huene D, Nguyen J (1995) Treatment of the upper limb in Charcot-Marie-Tooth disease. *J Hand Surg [Br]* 20: 511–518.

Yagerman SE, Cross MB, Green DW, Scher DM (2012) Pediatric orthopedic conditions in Charcot-Marie-Tooth disease: a literature review. *Curr Opin Pediatr* 24: 50–56.

Yonekawa T, Komaki H, Okada M, Hayashi YK, Nonaka I, Sugai K et al. (2013) Rapidly progressive scoliosis and respiratory deterioration in Ullrich congenital muscular dystrophy. *J Neurol Neurosurg Psychiatry* 84: 982–988.

# 24
# NEUROMUSCULAR SCOLIOSIS

*Pierre Moens*

## Introduction

The development of spine deformities is a major problem in the disease course of neuromuscular disorders in children and require a comprehensive, multidisciplinary approach.

It is generally accepted that neuromuscular scoliosis behaves differently from the idiopathic curve (Patel and Shapiro 2015). Although this is true, it is not possible to describe one curve pattern that is suitable for all neuromuscular scoliosis. Each disease has its own characteristics and is associated with its specific risk and evolution of scoliosis and its specific curve pattern. In the same neuromuscular disorder (NMD), the curve can behave differently depending on the age at onset of the disease. One study, however, assumes that curve patterns of neuromuscular scoliosis are similar to what is seen in typical adolescent idiopathic scoliosis (Kouwenhoven et al. 2006).

In NMD, between birth and the age of 5, screening of the spine is mandatory every 6 months, until the prepubertal growth spurt once a year and during the growth spurt again every 6 month.

The neuromuscular scoliosis described in this chapter is divided into two groups: myopathic (muscular dystrophies, congenital myopathies) and neuropathic (Friedreich ataxia, hereditary motor sensory neuropathies and spinal muscular atrophy).

The typical curve pattern in NMD is a long, C-shaped collapsing kyphoscoliosis with pelvic obliquity, which means that the pelvis is not in a perfect horizontal position in the frontal plane. However, an S-shaped type is also observed in some patients (some Duchenne curves, late onset Friedreich ataxia, Charcot–Marie–Tooth).

The management of scoliosis in NMD carries specific challenges due to the important comorbidities associated with NMD and therefore requires a multidisciplinary approach. The therapeutic options, medication, bracing, spinal fusion and growing rods (implants without fusion allowing lengthening of the spine during growth) will be discussed with each NMD.

The goal of treatment of scoliosis in NMD is to prevent progression, to restore sitting balance and the use of upper limbs and to improve quality of life (Cervellati et al. 2004; Mercado et al. 2007; Van Opstal et al. 2011).

## Duchenne muscular dystrophy

Duchenne muscular dystrophy (DMD) patients are at risk of developing scoliosis (68 to 90% have scoliosis by the age of 20) (Kinali et al. 2007). This scoliosis develops generally after the loss of ambulation, although scoliosis has been observed in 15% to 25% of ambulant DMD patients.

According to Oda et al. (1993), DMD scoliosis can be divided into three subtypes, which have a prognostic value.

- Type 1 curves are long, C-shaped collapsing kyphoscoliosis which have a high evolutive potential.
- Type 2 curves show a transition from kyphosis to lordosis. In case of an S-shaped curve, there is a low risk of progression. On the contrary, the C-shaped type will most likely progress.
- Type 3 curves are minimal (never >30°), are associated with good pulmonary function (vital capacity >2 000ml) and are unlikely to progress.

TREATMENT OF SCOLIOSIS

*Nonsurgical*

There is no evidence that bracing will control the curve (Harvey et al. 2014). Moreover, in the few ambulatory patients developing a curve, bracing carries the risk of impairing the ambulatory capacities.

Treatment with corticosteroids has been effective in delaying the onset of the scoliotic curve (Lebel et al. 2013; Goemans and Buyse 2014; Matthews et al. 2016) but has well-known adverse effects such as osteoporosis with vertebral collapses and other fractures (Perera et al. 2016), significant weight gain (Goemans and Buyse 2014; Matthews et al. 2016), and short stature, resulting in additional risks to be monitored in the orthopedic management of the spine.

*Surgical*

Surgical intervention of a progressive scoliosis is indicated should the curve evolve to a Cobb angle greater than 35° (Cervellati et al. 2004) to 50°(Kinali et al. 2006; Master et al. 2011).

Surgery will not lengthen life expectancy, and for some, surgery will not influence the deterioration of pulmonary function (Alexander et al. 2013). Others, however, have found a trend in slowing down the alteration of respiratory function (Van Opstal et al. 2011) or a significant decrease in the rate of respiratory decline following surgery (Velasco et al. 2007).

Posterior spinal fusion is the treatment of choice. There is still some controversy concerning pelvic fixation, since there is a 35% risk of failure (Myung et al. 2015), increased blood loss, longer operation time (Sengupta et al. 2002), and higher risk for infections (McCall and Hayes 2005).

For curves with a pelvic obliquity of less than 15°, fusions can stop on level L5 (Takaso et al. 2010; McCall and Hayes 2005) and maintain correction in the long term. In case of long, C-shaped curves with pelvic obliquity greater than 15°, spinal fusion will

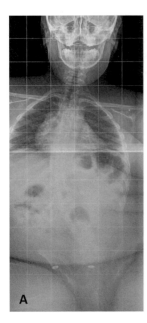
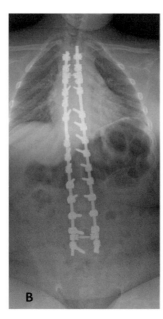

**Fig. 24.1.** Scoliosis surgery in Duchenne muscular dystrophy: posterior spinal fusion without pelvic fixation. A Pre-operative status. B Postoperative status.

include the pelvis in order to restore sitting balance. Various techniques are available, such as Luque Galveston (Van Opstal et al. 2011), pedicle screw constructs, which would provide better stability allowing for a better correction of the curve (Modi et al. 2010) as well as making pelvic fixation unnecessary in small curves (Mehta et al. 2009) (Figs. 24.1 and 24.2).

Surgery must be performed by a trained team who understand the possible intra-operative and postoperative complications such as excessive blood loss (Labarque et al. 2008), malignant hyperthermia (Bamaga et al. 2016) and cardiomyopathy (Kamdar and Garry 2016).

**Other inherited diseases of the muscle**

These are a heterogenic group of rare diseases, presenting a wide spectrum of severity, including muscular dystrophies (Becker, Limb-Girdle, Fascioscapulohumeral, etc.), con-genital muscular dystrophies (merosine deficient or positive, Fukuyama, etc.) and congenital myopathies (core myopathies, Bethlem, etc.) (see Section 3).

Some are associated with early-onset evolutive scoliosis, with respiratory impairment and weakness while others are associated with rigid spine syndrome (see Section 3), which is characterized by a difficulty in bending the neck and, with time, the entire spine. In some cases it is associated with an evolutive scoliosis which requires surgical treatment.

In this group of diseases, and in the case of early-onset scoliosis, there can be a thera-peutic indication for bracing. This, however, will unlikely be able to control the deformity, and in some cases will impair walking ability. In some cases, bracing does provide the opportunity to develop a sitting position and to improve upper limb function.

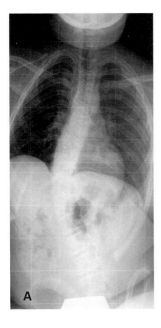

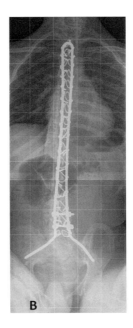

**Fig. 24.2.** Scoliosis surgery in Duchenne muscular dystrophy: Posterior spinal fusion with pelvic fixation. A Pre-operative status. B Postoperative status.

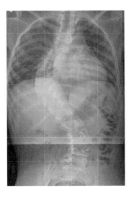
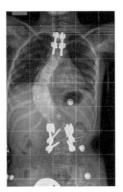
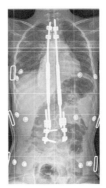
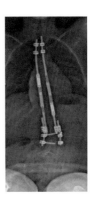

**Fig. 24.3.** Scoliosis management in a young, prepubertal girl with *RYR1* congenital muscular dystrophy developing a severely progressive scoliosis. Non-fusion surgery: use of magnetic growing rods. A Pre-treatment. B Implantation of anchors. C/D Surgical tensioning of rods.

In this type of early-onset scoliosis, when the curve cannot be controlled, there is a place for non-fusion surgery (growing rods), allowing control of the curve during growth. In this surgery, anchors are implanted at the extremities of the curve and are connected with rods without grafting. A surgical tensioning of the rod every 6 to 9 months is necessary to control the curve during growth (Tobert and Vitale 2013).

Recently, magnetic growing rods have been introduced, allowing an external tensioning with a magnet, thus avoiding repetitive anesthesia (Brooks and Sponseller 2016) (Fig. 24.3).

## Friedreich ataxia

The incidence of scoliosis in patients with Friedreich ataxia ranges from 63% (Milbrandt et al. 2008) to 91.5% (McCabe et al. 2000) and almost 100% (Cady and Bobechko 1984). These differences may be due to the fact that in the study of Milbrandt, the diagnosis is based on clinical features and genetic testing, when available. On the contrary, the incidence of 91.5% comes from a population of typical homozygotes.

There is continued debate concerning the pattern of the curve, and also regarding its evolution. Late onset would be less progressive than early onset. The problem remains in the criteria for diagnosis. Older studies only have a clinical diagnosis while no study is available with genetic diagnosis and curve pattern or evolution.

In recent literature it is clear that scoliosis in Friedreich ataxia does not have an idiopathic pattern. Numerous scoliosis are S-shaped, associated with hyperkyphosis (Milbrandt et al. 2008; Tsirikos and Smith 2012), and left sided (Milbrandt et al. 2008). The classic C-shaped collapsing type is not common in Friedreich ataxia (Tsirikos and Smith 2012; Milbrandt et al. 2008).

TREATMENT OF SCOLIOSIS

*Nonsurgical*

One-third of scoliosis is non-evolutive (Tsirikos and Smith 2012). Bracing has not been proven to control the curve (Cady and Bobechko 1984; Milbrandt et al. 2008; Tsirikos and Smith 2012); however, some recommend a brace in young patients with early-onset scoliosis in order to delay surgery (Corben et al. 2014; Milbrandt et al. 2008). The parents must be informed about the limitations of this therapy.

*Surgical*

Surgical treatment must be considered for a scoliosis reaching a Cobb angle of 40° (Corben et al. 2014), 50° (Milbrandt et al. 2008) and 40° to 60° (Tsirikos and Smith 2012).

Posterior instrumentation and arthrodesis is the treatment of choice. Segmental fixation with hybrid constructs (Caekebeke et al. 2013) gives good control of sagittal balance; these day all screw constructs are more frequently used (Tsirikos and Smith 2012). Selective fusion is not indicated in Friedreich ataxia scoliosis because of the risk of junctional kyphosis (Friedreich ataxia has frequent hyperkyphosis) and the risk of progression of the non-instrumented curve (Milbrandt et al. 2008).

A multidisciplinary management should address the cardio-respiratory issues associated with Friedreich ataxia and include specific cardiac and pulmonary pre-operative evaluation and coordinated postoperative care.

## Spinal muscular atrophy

Spinal muscular atrophy (SMA) is a recessively inherited disease characterized by a degeneration of spinal cord motor neurons resulting in a wide spectrum of clinical severity. SMA has been classified into four subtypes, SMA types I–IV, according to the age at onset and the maximum motor function achieved. Within those types are subtypes which may add to prognostic significance (see Chapter 6).

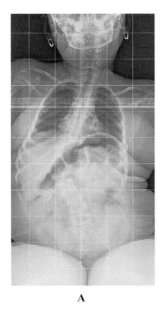
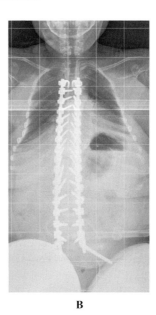

A                                                         B

**Fig. 24.4.** Scoliosis surgery in spinal muscular atrophy type II. A Pre-operative curve. B Post operative correction.

Scoliosis is more likely to develop and to worsen in early-onset SMA, which has a high degree of muscle weakness (Fujak et al. 2013; Granata et al. 1989). The majority of curves have a C-shaped collapsing pattern with pelvic obliquity (Allam and Schwabe 2013; Fujak et al. 2013) (Fig. 24. 4).

TREATMENT OF SCOLIOSIS
*Nonsurgical*
Bracing is not able to control the deformity (Granata et al. 1989); however, it can play a role in positioning and stabilizing the sitting position (Allam and Schwabe 2013). It may, however, impair walking ability and respiratory function (Tangsrud et al. 2001).

*Surgical*
As previously discussed for DMD and Friedreich ataxia scoliosis, posterior spinal instrumentation and fusion is a solution, but in young patients (type 2) this treatment is questionable because of the early-onset of scoliosis and remaining growth.

In these patients, non-fusion surgery (growing rods) is an alternative, allowing growth in height and avoiding thoracic deformity (Tobert and Vitale 2013). As discussed for the treatment of scoliosis in young children with congenital dystrophies, the new instrumentation using magnetic growing rods (Brooks and Sponseller 2016) allows a non-invasive approach for lengthening of the rods during growth.

**Hereditary motor and sensory neuropathies: Charcot–Marie–Tooth disease**

Charcot–Marie–Tooth disease (CMT) includes a wide variety of inherited sensory and/or motor neuropathies and is the most common hereditary NMD in the pediatric population (Chapter 7). Spinal deformity was observed in 26% of a mixed group of children and adults (Horacek et al. 2007) to 37% to 50% in a group limited to a pediatric population (Walker et al. 1994b). The types of deformity are quite consistent among both studies with scoliosis (54%), kyphoscoliosis (38%) and kyphosis (8%) (Walker et al. 1994) to 58%, 31%, and 11%, respectively (Horacek et al. 2007).

The curve patterns range from a majority of double curves with more dextro convex thoracic curves (45%) (Horacek et al. 2007) to a majority of single thoracic curves with an equal dextro and sinistro convex (Walker et al. 1994b). In both studies the ratio of dextro sinistro convex is greater than in idiopathic scoliosis. In Walker's study (1994b) females are at greater risk.

Most of the time the curves in CMT are not very evolutive and rarely require treatment, but routine screening is mandatory (Horacek et al. 2007; Walker et al. 1994b; Yagerman et al. 2012). Early-onset type of CMT are more at risk of developing scoliosis. In these patients, the curve severity and the rapidity of evolution are higher (Horacek et al. 2007).

TREATMENT OF SPINAL DEFORMITY

The treatment modalities depend on the curve. Bracing can be used for curves greater than 20°. A few patients will need surgery, such as evolutive curves of more than 40° and early-onset scoliosis as observed in the Dejerine Sottas subgroup.

**Key points**
- Neuromuscular disorders are commonly associated with a wide range of orthopedic issues including limb contractures, joint dislocations and scoliosis.
- The management of orthopedic issues requires a multidisciplinary approach including physiotherapy, surgery, orthotics and environmental adaptation aiming at preserving or improving functional capacities.
- Decision-making processes should take into consideration the specific aspects of the underlying neuromuscular disease as each disease has its own characteristics and carries specific risks, and should include expert input from the multidisciplinary team.
- Pre-, peri and postoperative management of orthopedic surgery deserves specific multidisciplinary and coordinated attention considering the complexity of medical problems in patients with neuromuscular disorders, such as increased risks associated with anesthesia, cardio-respiratory issues and nutritional aspects.

**Clinical vignette**

This 29-year-old man was referred at the age of 6 with a clinical suspicion of Duchenne muscular dystrophy (DMD), which was confirmed by genetic testing (Del 47–50).

Deflazacort was started at 21mg daily (0.9mg/kg/d) and further increased to a maximum of 30mg daily, his current dose. He has been followed in the multidisciplinary clinic on a 6 monthly basis, including regular orthopedic assessments. A minimal dextroconvex thoracal scoliosis was noted for the first time at the age of 19 years (Cobb angle 10°). This curve however progressed to a curve of 30° in 6 months time and reached a curve of 45° at the age of 21. The decision-making process to propose scoliosis surgery included all medical and paramedical disciplines: a posterior fusion and arthrodesis was performed 6 months later. The peri- and postoperative course was uneventful despite the underlying cardio-respiratory status characterized by a dilated cardiomyopathy (fractional shortening 23%) and a restricted respiratory function with nocturnal hypoventilation, treated by non-invasive ventilatory support.

CONCLUSION

The prescription of corticosteroids in DMD has been associated with a striking reduction in the occurrence of scoliosis in adolescents with DMD. However, with increasing age, there is still a risk of developing a progressive scoliosis. Scoliosis surgery in older patients should be undertaken cautiously, taking into consideration all cardiac, respiratory and anesthetic risks that are characteristic to this progressive disease.

## REFERENCES

Alexander WM, Smith M, Freeman BJC, Sutherland LM, Kennedy JD, Cundy PJ (2013) The effect of posterior spinal fusion on respiratory function in Duchenne muscular dystrophy. *Eur Spine J* 22: 411–416.

Allam AM, Schwabe AL (2013) Neuromuscular scoliosis. *PM R* 5: 957–963.

Bamaga AK, Riazi S, Amburgey K, Ong S, Halliday W, Diamandis P et al. (2016) Neuromuscular conditions associated with malignant hyperthermia in paediatric patients: A 25-year retrospective study. *Neuromuscul Disord* 26: 201–206.

Brooks JT, Sponseller PD (2016) What's new in the management of neuromuscular scoliosis. *J Pediatr Orthop* 36:627–633

Cady RB, Bobechko WP (1984) Incidence, natural history, and treatment of scoliosis in Friedreich's ataxia. *J Pediatr Orthop* 4: 673–676.

Caekebeke P, Moke L, Moens P (2013) Sublaminar devices for the correction of scoliosis: metal wire versus polyester tape. *Acta Orthop Belg* 79: 216–221.

Cervellati S, Bettini N, Moscato M, Gusella A, Dema E, Maresi R (2004) Surgical treatment of spinal deformities in Duchenne muscular dystrophy: a long term follow-up study. *Eur Spine J* 13: 441–448.

Corben LA, Lynch D, Pandolfo M, Schulz JB, Delatycki MB, Clinical Management Guidelines Writing Group (2014) Consensus clinical management guidelines for Friedreich ataxia. *Orphanet J Rare Dis* 9: 184.

Dubowitz V (1995) Chaos in the classification of SMA: a possible resolution. *Neuromuscul Disord* 5: 3–5.

Fujak A, Raab W, Schuh A, Richter S, Forst R, Forst J (2013) Natural course of scoliosis in proximal spinal muscular atrophy type II and IIIa: descriptive clinical study with retrospective data collection of 126 patients. *BMC Musculoskelet Disord* 14: 283.

Goemans N, Buyse G (2014) Current treatment and management of dystrophinopathies. *Curr Treat Options Neurol* 16: 287.

Granata C, Merlini L, Magni E, Marini ML, Stagni SB (1989) Spinal muscular atrophy: natural history and orthopaedic treatment of scoliosis. *Spine* 14: 760–762.

Harvey A, Baker L, Williams K (2014) Non-surgical prevention and management of scoliosis for children with Duchenne muscular dystrophy: what is the evidence? *J Paediatr Child Health* 50:E3–E9.

Horacek O, Mazanec R, Morris CE, Kobesova A (2007) Spinal deformities in hereditary motor and sensory neuropathy: a retrospective qualitative, quantitative, genotypical, and familial analysis of 175 patients. *Spine* 32: 2502–2508.

Kamdar F, Garry DJ (2016) Dystrophin-Deficient Cardiomyopathy. *J Am Coll Cardiol* 67: 2533–2546.

Kinali M, Messina S, Mercuri E, Lehovsky J, Edge G, Manzur AY et al. (2006) Management of scoliosis in Duchenne muscular dystrophy: a large 10-year retrospective study. *Dev Med Child Neurol* 48: 513–518.

Kinali M, Main M, Eliahoo J, Messina S, Knight RK, Lehovsky J et al. (2007) Predictive factors for the development of scoliosis in Duchenne muscular dystrophy. *Eur J Paediatr Neurol* 11: 160–166.

Kouwenhoven J-WM, Van Ommeren PM, Pruijs HEJ, Castelein RM (2006) Spinal decompensation in neuromuscular disease. *Spine* 31:E188–E191.

Labarque V, Freson K, Thys C, Wittevrongel C, Hoylaerts MF, De Vos R et al. (2008) Increased Gs signalling in platelets and impaired collagen activation, due to a defect in the dystrophin gene, result in increased blood loss during spinal surgery. *Hum Mol Genet* 17: 357–366.

Lebel DE, Corston JA, McAdam LC, Biggar WD, Alman BA (2013) Glucocorticoid treatment for the prevention of scoliosis in children with Duchenne muscular dystrophy: long-term follow-up. *J Bone Joint Surg Am* 95: 1057–1061.

Master DL, Son-Hing JP, Poe-Kochert C, Armstrong DG, Thompson GH (2011) Risk factors for major complications after surgery for neuromuscular scoliosis. *Spine* 36: 564–571.

Matthews E, Brassington R, Kuntzer T, Jichi F, Manzur AY (2016) Corticosteroids for the treatment of Duchenne muscular dystrophy. *Cochrane Database Syst Rev* (5):CD003725.

McCabe DJ, Ryan F, Moore DP, McQuaid S, King MD, Kelly A, Daly K, Barton DE, Murphy RP (2000) Typical Friedreich's ataxia without GAA expansions and GAA expansion without typical Friedreich's ataxia. *J Neurol* 247: 346–355.

McCall RE, Hayes B (2005) Long-term outcome in neuromuscular scoliosis fused only to lumbar 5. *Spine* 30(18): 2056–2060. doi.10.1097/01.brs.0000178817.34368.16.

Mehta SS, Modi HN, Srinivasalu S, Suh S-W, Yi J-W, Cho J-W et al. (2009) Pedicle screw-only constructs with lumbar or pelvic fixation for spinal stabilization in patients with Duchenne muscular dystrophy. *J Spinal Disord Tech* 22: 428–433.

Mercado E, Alman B, Wright JG (2007) Does spinal fusion influence quality of life in neuromuscular scoliosis? *Spine* 32(Suppl): S120–S125.

Milbrandt TA, Kunes JR, Karol LA (2008) Friedreich's ataxia and scoliosis: the experience at two institutions. *J Pediatr Orthop* 28: 234–238. pii

Modi HN, Suh SW, Hong JY, Cho JW, Park JH, Yang JH (2010) Treatment and complications in flaccid neuromuscular scoliosis (Duchenne muscular dystrophy and spinal muscular atrophy) with posterior-only pedicle screw instrumentation. *Eur Spine J* 19: 384–393.

Myung KS, Lee C, Skaggs DL (2015) Early pelvic fixation failure in neuromuscular scoliosis. *J Pediatr Orthop* 35: 258–265.

Oda T, Shimizu N, Yonenobu K, Ono K, Nabeshima T, Kyoh S (1993) Longitudinal study of spinal deformity in Duchenne muscular dystrophy. *J Pediatr Orthop* 13: 478–488.

Pareyson D, Marchesi C (2009) Diagnosis, natural history, and management of Charcot–Marie–Tooth disease. *Lancet Neurol* 8: 654–667.

Patel J, Shapiro F (2015) Simultaneous progression patterns of scoliosis, pelvic obliquity, and hip subluxation/dislocation in non-ambulatory neuromuscular patients: an approach to deformity documentation. *J Child Orthop* 9: 345–356.

Perera N, Sampaio H, Woodhead H, Farrar M (2016) Fracture in Duchenne muscular dystrophy: natural history and vitamin d deficiency. *J Child Neurol* 31: 1181–1187.

Sengupta DK, Mehdian SH, McConnell JR, Eisenstein SM, Webb JK (2002) Pelvic or lumbar fixation for the surgical management of scoliosis in duchenne muscular dystrophy. *Spine* 27(18): 2072–2079.

Takaso M, Nakazawa T, Imura T, Okada T, Toyama M, Ueno M et al. (2010) Two-year results for scoliosis secondary to Duchenne muscular dystrophy fused to lumbar 5 with segmental pedicle screw instrumentation. *J Orthop Sci* 15: 171–177.

Tangsrud SE, Carlsen KC, Lund-Petersen I, Carlsen KH (2001) Lung function measurements in young children with spinal muscle atrophy; a cross sectional survey on the effect of position and bracing. *Arch Dis Child* 84: 521–524.

Tobert DG, Vitale MG (2013) Strategies for treating scoliosis in children with spinal muscular atrophy. *Am J Orthop (Belle Mead NJ)* 42:E99–E103.

Tsirikos AI, Smith G (2012) Scoliosis in patients with Friedreich's ataxia. *J Bone Joint Surg Br* 94: 684–689.

Van Opstal N, Verlinden C, Myncke J, Goemans N, Moens P (2011) The effect of Luque-Galveston fusion on curve, respiratory function and quality of life in Duchenne muscular dystrophy. *Acta Orthop Belg* 77: 659–665.

Velasco MV, Colin AA, Zurakowski D, Darras BT, Shapiro F (2007) Posterior spinal fusion for scoliosis in duchenne muscular dystrophy diminishes the rate of respiratory decline. *Spine* 32(4) 459–465. doi: 10.1097/01.brs.0000255062.94744.52.

Walker JL, Nelson KR, Heavilon JA, Stevens DB, Lubicky JP, Ogden JA et al. (1994a) Hip abnormalities in children with Charcot–Marie–Tooth disease. J Pediatr Orthop 14:54–59.

Walker JL, Nelson KR, Stevens DB, Lubicky JP, Ogden JA, VandenBrink KD (1994b) Spinal deformity in Charcot–Marie–Tooth disease. *Spine* 19: 1044–1047.

Yagerman SE, Cross MB, Green DW, Scher DM (2012) Pediatric orthopedic conditions in Charcot–Marie–Tooth disease: a literature review. *Curr Opin Pediatr* 24: 50–56.

# Section 5
## Respiratory Management

# 25
# ASSESSMENT AND MANAGEMENT OF RESPIRATORY FUNCTION IN CHILDREN WITH NEUROMUSCULAR DISORDERS

*Oscar Mayer, Hemant Sawnani, and Michel Toussaint*

## Introduction

People working in the field of pediatric neuromuscular disease (NMD) have long been hoping for a cure or a disease-modifying therapy, while focusing on symptom management and quality of life. Over the last decade the field has advanced to the point where there are now a variety of pharmacotherapies with disease-modifying potential that are being evaluated and should soon come to market. This has changed the dynamics of those involved in the care of NMD to one of hope and a positive outlook for the future that will add to the clinical support that has been the hallmark of care.

While many are familiar with respiratory symptoms and their management in Duchenne muscular dystrophy (DMD) and spinal muscular atrophy (SMA), there are a variety of less common myopathies and neuropathies whose natural history and evolution are less well known. The challenge is then understanding and prognosis, and when to offer specific clinical interventions, in particular regarding respiratory management. It is exceptionally difficult to do this individually for each disease process, but there is a tremendous amount of overlap between certain events within the natural history of each disease. There is potential for a broad management strategy based on certain events in the natural history of disease progression, with the timing of each management decision being based on each specific disease in a principle-based approach to care.

This review will start by discussing natural history principles in managing patients with NMD, and then looks into options for clinical assessment and testing, and management options including both ventilation and airway clearance.

## Natural history

At its essence, natural history is the progression of a condition without intervention. There are fairly well defined stages of disease from pre-symptomatic, to early clinical progression, to a more rapid rate of decline, to the end stage of disease (Mayer et al. 2015). Within these are a variety of clinically meaningful events that, based on this natural history, have been shown to occur at set times, or within a range of times, and herald the onset of a more severe stage of disease progression. These events are typically easy to track and as such are often used as outcome measurements to demonstrate a positive impact on disease progression.

However, true natural history is a concept that is becoming more abstract than real to the extent that it is a moving target (Dubowitz 2015). With many NMDs, natural history or disease progression has been significantly altered or improved by the introduction of clinical support (Eagle et al. 2007; Passamano et al. 2012) and will likely be affected further with disease-modifying pharmacotherapies. As these treatments become the standard of care and are widely used, the concept of true "natural history" is abandoned and instead one considers current disease progression with use of the current standard of care (Dubowitz 2015). Of course, this means that the natural history from one epoch of time will not be applicable in a later epoch.

In addition, in comparing disease progression between patients it is critical to compare patients in similar stages of disease progression to minimize the impact of the natural history itself (Humbertclaude et al. 2012; Mayer et al. 2015). For instance, if one is looking to demonstrate the efficacy of an intervention in altering rate of decline of forced vital capacity (FVC) and the study population is in a more advanced stage of disease, perhaps with a FVC predicted as less than 30%, then the "progression" and loss of function may be governed more by the progression of disease than the intervention itself. In addition within each disease there are patients with different disease progression (Humbertclaude et al. 2012) and whether this is taken into account or not can have an impact in how well one can resolve clinical progression. The solution either is to choose a study cohort in an earlier stage of progression or chose an outcome measurement that is still changing measurably.

Whether a neuropathy or myopathy, all progressive NMD causes skeletal muscle failure and since the skeletal muscles govern movement of all joints and ultimately functional output, progression of disease can be measured by the impact on this functional output. While the standard pulmonary outcomes are typically volume (FVC), respiratory pressure (maximal inspiratory and expiratory pressure), and gas exchange (carbon dioxide removal), it is important to consider the "upstream" determinants of each of these factors.

While both the rate of progression and the type of progression can vary widely among different neuromuscular conditions, there are common pathways of deterioration that remain the same. This progression causes clinical dysfunction within three inter-related categories: diaphragm dysfunction, chest wall dysfunction and spinal dysfunction (Fig. 25.1). The ultimate downstream outcome is respiratory failure which is determined by the balance between the load on the respiratory system and the respiratory pump or diaphragm.

DIAPHRAGM/ABDOMINAL MUSCLES

The diaphragm is the primary respiratory muscle and is the primary muscular determinant of depth of breathing during restful tidal breathing. With more forceful breathing there are additional contributions from the external intercostal muscles, pectoralis muscles and the anterior neck muscles. While at rest, exhalation is largely due to passive recoil of the chest and lungs, but with exertion or coughing the anterior abdominal musculature drives increased expiratory effort.

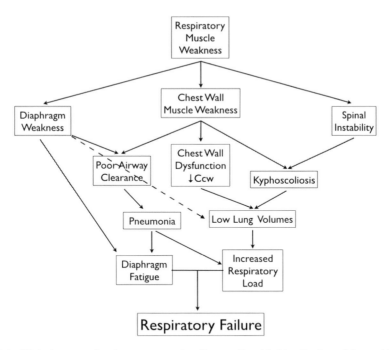

**Fig. 25.1.** Clinical progression in neuromuscular disease. (Provided by Dr Oscar Mayer. All rights reserved.)

The depth of inspiration (inspiratory capacity) is critical in both recruiting more lung capacity during exertion, but more importantly during rest, in opening up atelectatic lung units and filling the lungs fully, as is the case with a cough. As inspiratory capacity falls there is a progressive loss of lung volume and a decrease in lung compliance and, therefore, an increase in the inspiratory pressure (diaphragm work) required to breathe. Furthermore, a submaximal inspiration, even with a forceful exhalation, will limit airway clearance and put a patient at risk for lower respiratory tract illnesses. The combination of a progressive increase in the work of breathing or respiratory load and weaker respiratory muscles leads to respiratory muscle fatigue. Then, with worsening airway clearance, the frequency and duration of respiratory illnesses increases and puts further load on the respiratory system and can overwhelm the capacity of the respiratory pump and cause respiratory failure.

CHEST WALL

In normal circumstances the chest wall complements the contraction of the diaphragm pushing the lower rib cage outward, by the fulcrum effect, and the external intercostal muscles and pectoralis and neck muscles elevating the ribs. However, in many neuromuscular conditions, especially spinal muscular atrophy (SMA) type 1, the chest wall musculature is profoundly weak and the chest wall becomes flaccid and moves in paradoxically during inspiration. This occurs because the negative intrathoracic pressure developed by the diaphragm cannot be resisted by the chest wall thereby causing inward motion. The compensation is increased caudal expansion of the lungs by greater diaphragm contraction and if not effective the patient will increase his/her respiratory rate. The problem, of course, is that both mechanisms of compensation are very energy intensive.

With the progressive loss of muscle function and a decrease in the amount of chest expansion the muscles and joints (costovertebral) of the respiratory system can become stiff and poorly compliant, which adds further to the work of breathing. In more extreme situations, such as SMA types 1 and 2 there can be substantial bilateral or unilateral caudal rotation of the ribs often with scoliosis which narrows the chest wall and further limits inspiration and FVC.

SPINE

The spine is an integral component of the thorax in supporting both the ribs and respiratory musculature. As is the case with the chest wall, it is also a complex dynamic structure with multiple joints, the alignment of which is governed by the perispinal and axial skeletal muscles. With weak spinal and chest wall support it is difficult to maintain an erect posture, which then leads to the spine tilting to one side often with asymmetric spinal rotation. In DMD this often presents as a somewhat two-dimensional curve in the coronal plane, occasionally with additional rotation at the hip causing pelvic obliquity. In SMA type 2 the curve can also be more complex with an S-shaped curve in the coronal plane, also with a kyphotic curve in the sagittal plane.

Because the abdominal contents are effectively incompressible, a spinal curve decreasing the effective length of the thorax or abdomen will directly limit lung volume. In addition, this spinal curve can distort diaphragm contour and put it in a less favorable position for contraction; then, the concave thorax may compress the chest and abdomen enough to limit diaphragm excursion during contraction. This process in parallel with the chest wall deformity can create a stiff poorly compliant thorax at an already low volume which can substantially increase the load on the respiratory system.

In summary, the pathophysiologic endpoint of NMD is respiratory failure or the point beyond which the respiratory pump can no longer overcome the load on it. Management, however, is focused on intervening proactively in an attempt to minimize the load on the respiratory system. Doing so is based both on clinical assessment, testing and management, which will be the topic of the remainder of this chapter.

**Assessment of respiratory function**

Though the ultimate outcome of NMD is respiratory failure, there is a substantial loss of function and capacity before a patient develops respiratory failure. The changes leading to this loss can be assessed longitudinally to identify early respiratory function decline and to intervene with appropriate supportive care.

LUNG VOLUME

NMD causes restrictive respiratory disease with a low total lung capacity (TLC), forced vital capacity FVC and residual volume (RV), but a high RV/TLC (Fig. 25.2). However, in

## Normal

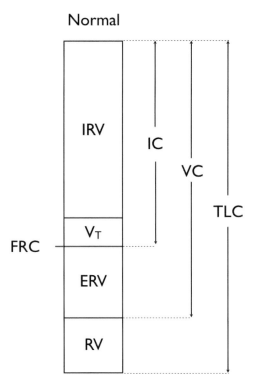

**Fig. 25.2.** Partitioned lung volumes. FRC: functional residual capacity; IRV: inspiratory reserve volume; IC: inspiratory capacity; VC: vital capacity; TLC: total lung capacity; $V_T$: tidal volume; ERV: expiratory reserve volume; RV: residual volume; FVC: forced vital capacity. (Provided by Dr Oscar Mayer. All rights reserved.)

contrast with interstitial lung disease, the pattern of volume loss in NMD is a decrease in TLC and FVC, but with a residual volume that is similarly low relative to TLC, with a normal RV/TLC (Estenne et al. 1993). The restrictive defect occurs for two important reasons, the inability to inhale fully (low inspiratory capacity [IC]) and then exhale fully (low expiratory reserve volume [ERV]), thereby leaving a higher residual volume relative to TLC (RV/TLC). Since the ability to inhale deeply is determined by the inspiratory muscles (primarily diaphragm) and the ability to exhale fully is determined by the expiratory muscles (primarily abdominal muscles), FVC can be used as an integrated measurement of inspiratory and expiratory muscle function. For this reason it is the primary outcome measurement of many recently reported intervention studies in NMD (Buyse et al. 2015; 2016) and the longitudinal trend has been shown to be an accurate reflection of clinical decline in both DMD and SMA (Khirani et al. 2013a; 2013b; Foley et al. 2013).

There is also meaning in TLC and the functional residual capacity (FRC) or resting lung volume. FRC is directly measured either by body plethysmography ("body box") or by either helium dilution or nitrogen washout techniques. It is the resting lung volume where there no energy is required to maintain lung volume and is the point where the outward elastic recoil of the chest wall is balanced by the inward recoil of the lungs. When the lungs become less compliant (less elastic or stiffer) due to atelectasis, the FRC is brought to a lower lung volume, and when the chest wall becomes more compliant the FRC is brought to a higher lung volume. In NMD the FRC does decline (Khirani et al. 2013a; 2013b) and respiratory system compliance (Crs) is lower (Estenne et al. 1993), but interestingly that difference is much more related to low lung compliance (Cl) as opposed to low chest wall compliance (Ccw) (Estenne et al. 1983; 1993). However, while this progression is clear, the FRC changes later in disease progression and at a lower rate than FVC and, therefore, is not felt to be as useful as FVC in longitudinal tracking of lung volume (Estenne et al. 1983; 1993; Khirani et al. 2013a; 2013b).

INSPIRATORY MUSCLE FUNCTION

There are two general categories of respiratory muscle function testing, invasive measurements requiring the passage of an esophageal and/or gastric pressure catheter and non-invasive measurements that are made at the mouth or nose. The invasive measurements allow for a direct assessment of diaphragm contractile force (transdiaphragmatic pressure [Pdi]) by recording the change in gastric pressure relative to esophageal pressure during a maximal inspiration. Non-invasive measurements of diaphragm contractile force are the maximum inspiratory pressure (MIP) and the sniff inspiratory pressure (SNIP). MIP is measured at the mouth and is the maximal pressure sustained for 1 second during a maximal inspiration from either FRC or residual volume and the SNIP is the same maneuver but measured at a naris through an occlusive pressure catheter while the patient performs a sniffing maneuver. While all three measurements are only as accurate as the effort the patient gives, the SNIP maneuver is felt to be the easiest to perform because sniffing is a common maneuver, which makes it easier to get reliable data in younger patients less willing to follow directions (Anderson et al. 2012; Nève et al. 2013). Because Pdi requires placement of a bipolar esophageal and gastric catheter, it is largely within the realm of research testing and is not widely used clinically. Interestingly, SNIP has been shown to have a lower coefficient of variability than MIP (Nève et al. 2013) and is superior to both MIP and Pdi in demonstrating decline in respiratory function in cohorts of patients with DMD or SMA (Khirani et al. 2013a; 2013b).

Inspiratory flow reserve (IFR) is the ratio of the maximal flow generated during a tidal inspiration to the maximal flow generated during a maximal inspiratory effort (De Bruin et al. 2001). IFR is significantly worse (higher) in patients with DMD, but is only weakly correlated with FVC percentage and MIP (De Bruin et al. 2001; Buyse et al. 2016). In a recent pharmacotherapy intervention study in DMD there was a significant treatment effect demonstrated by IFR in addition to FVC and peak expiratory flow, but not by MIP (Buyse et al. 2015; 2016), which was in part felt to be due to the variability of the measurement (Buyse et al. 2015).

EXPIRATORY MUSCLE FUNCTION

At rest exhalation is passive, relying on the recoil of the respiratory system to FRC, but with maximal effort the abdominal muscles give the primary force of exhalation. The most widely used measurement of expiratory muscle function is the maximal inspiratory pressure (MEP), which is the maximal pressure sustained for 1 second on a forceful exhalation from TLC. As is the case with MIP, the MEP can be hard to perform reproducibly because of the effort needed to produce a full maneuver (Buyse et al. 2015). Furthermore, MEP is not as reliable as either SNIP or FVC in demonstrating loss of function in patients with DMD and SMA (Khirani et al. 2013a; 2013b).

Interestingly, however, peak expiratory flow (PEF), which has most commonly been used an assessment of airway obstruction in asthma, has been applied in NMD as a measurement of peak expiratory effort in flow as opposed to pressure (Buyse et al. 2015). Perhaps because of the less sustained pressure that MEP requires, PEF has been shown to have a smaller coefficient of variability than MEP and has been shown in the Cooperative International Neuromuscular Research Group (CINRG) DMD database (McDonald et al. 2018) and in a recent DMD intervention study, to more closely parallel the rate of decline of FVC (Buyse et al. 2015).

Finally, peak cough flow (PCF) has the advantage of being a "normal" maneuver, like the sniff in SNIP, and in adults has been shown to be a predictor of success in extubation and of having an ineffective cough (<160L/m) (Bach and Saporito 1996), with later extrapolation to a different threshold to identify patients who are likely to have airway clearance difficulties (<270L/m) (Boitano 2006). While these determinations were made in adult patients with NMD, the thresholds may not apply in children, especially in the first decade of life where both lung volumes and expiratory flows will be lower (Bianchi and Baiardi 2008).

GAS EXCHANGE

Arguably the most important outcome measurement is gas exchange with inhalation of oxygen to support the body's metabolic needs and removal of carbon dioxide produced during metabolic activity. In NMD there is gradual progression toward respiratory failure and in NMD this first occurs during sleep. Respiratory insufficiency starts during rapid eye movement (REM) sleep and eventually progresses further into non-REM sleep, and then into daytime. However, daytime normocapnia is no indication of nocturnal ventilatory capacity with 70% of patients having sleep disordered breathing (SDB), 39% nocturnal hypoxemia and 44% hypercapnia (Bersanini et al. 2012). Others found that a $PaCO_2$ of more than 40mmHg while awake was predictive of nocturnal hypoventilation with a sensitivity of 92% and specificity of 72% (Mellies et al. 2003b).

Interestingly, there are variable data on the predictive value of pulmonary function parameters on SDB, with some showing no correlation (Bersanini et al. 2012). However, Mellies et al. showed that an inspiratory capacity (IC) of less than 60% had a 97% sensitivity and an 87% specificity for identifying SDB, while an inspiratory capacity of less than 40% had a 96% sensitivity and a specificity of 88% for SDB and hypoventilation (Mellies et al. 2003b).

**Predictors of sleep disordered breathing**

Sleep symptoms are often poorly perceived and articulated by children with NMD only to be under-reported by themselves and their parents (Barbé et al. 1994; Sawnani et al. 2015;

Mellies et al. 2003b). This underscores the importance of an objective measure of sleep quality and hypoventilation and polysomnogram (PSG) evaluations are the most reliable. In adults, nocturnal hypoventilation is defined as an increase in end tidal $CO_2$ ($EtCO_2$) to more than 55mmHg for 10 or more minutes, or increase in $EtCO_2$ by at least 10mmHg over baseline awake values. In children, nocturnal hypoventilation is considered if there is an $EtCO_2$ of greater than 50mmHg for over 25% of total sleep time (Berry et al. 2012). Because of the overlap in PSG findings in patients with NMD and patients with intact muscle strength and upper airway obstruction, modified criteria for interpretation are needed.

In a cohort of NMD patients in which non-invasive ventilation (NIV) was started only after there was both diurnal and nocturnal hypoventilation, most patients had diurnal hypoventilation within 1 year of the onset of nocturnal hypoventilation (Ward et al. 2005). Therefore, waiting to start NIV until a patient has daytime hypercapnia is inappropriate and by the time patients have daytime hypercapnia, most have severely limited pulmonary reserve and higher risk of acute respiratory failure.

Paiva et al. showed that 42% of children on long-term NIV experienced nocturnal hypercapnia without hypoxemia and that daytime capillary $CO_2$ ($PcCO_2$) levels were normal in 85% of these patients (Paiva et al. 2009). Thus, the absence of capnography monitoring in a PSG can delay identifying respiratory failure until it becomes severe. Therefore, capnography is a critical and necessary component of a PSG and not having it can produce results that do not accurately reflect the true severity of a patient's respiratory status.

Home pulse oximetry testing is cheaper and easier to obtain, but substantially limited by giving information only on oxygenation and heart rate and no information on ventilation. While one consensus group suggested that an $SpO_2$ below 90% for more than 10% of study time indicates respiratory failure and need for mechanical ventilation (Robert et al. 1993), others feel that this definition is too liberal and that an $SpO_2$ less than 90% for 2% of sleep time is significant. Because of this, home pulse oximetry should not be used as the sole test to assess for nocturnal hypoventilation and instead a PSG should be used to properly assess for hypoventilation (Arens and Muzumdar 2010; Hull et al. 2012b).

**Sleep disordered breathing: polysomnogram features and challenges**

In patients without NMD, during sleep there are changes in respiratory mechanics, with increased airway resistance due to a decrease in FRC and decreased tone in the intercostal and upper airway muscles. During sleep there can be a decrease in tidal volume and minute ventilation, which along with changes in central chemoreceptor sensitivities, results in a slight physiologic rise of $PCO_2$ by about 3–5mmHg. These changes are magnified during REM sleep when there is marked reduction in skeletal muscle tone, with the exception of the diaphragm (Tabachnik et al. 1981). During REM sleep, breathing is irregular with periods of decreased rib cage motion and decreased tidal volume, and increased respiratory rate and diaphragm activity (Gould et al. 1988).

In patients with NMD, sleep architecture can be different, with reduced total sleep time, reduced sleep efficiency, increased sleep fragmentation, and increased stage 1 (light) sleep. In addition, there is REM sleep suppression that is felt to be adaptive in reducing exposure to the period of sleep associated with respiratory instability.

On polysomnography, SDB can include obstructive sleep apnea or hypopnea due to upper airway obstruction and central apnea or hypopnea due to respiratory muscle fatigue. Obstructive apnea can occur in patients with a high BMI or relative macroglossia and can be worsened by relaxation of upper airway muscles in REM sleep. Central (non-obstructive) hypopneas are the more frequent respiratory events in patients with NMD (Ferguson et al. 1996; Barbé et al. 1994; Smith et al. 1988). These events, like most others, are more frequent and prolonged during REM sleep, particularly during phasic REM. During REM sleep, the degree of muscle suppression and alveolar hypoventilation is proportional to the amount of phasic REM sleep and the degree of hypoxemia is proportional to the severity of diaphragmatic weakness (White et al. 1995). Related to this, obstructive apnea may be misclassified as central when respiratory muscles are too weak to move the chest wall against a collapsed pharynx. Respiratory muscle weakness causes thoracoabdominal asynchrony in the absence of upper airway obstruction, which can further confuse classification of respiratory events on polysomnogram studies.

MANAGEMENT

Once a deficiency in ventilation or airway clearance is identified it is critical that it be managed expediently and effectively. There are, however, a variety of different approaches to doing so that are based on both the age and needs of the patient.

*Nocturnal ventilation*

The goals of initiation of NIV are to normalize ventilation, reduce the work of breathing, improve sleep architecture by reducing sleep fragmentation, and to treat SDB. Timing of initiating NIV in NMD is not clearly defined and agreed upon.

Patients may be treated with pressure or volume-cycled modes of ventilation. In pressure-cycled ventilation a higher inspiratory positive airway pressure (IPAP) is delivered above the end expiratory pressure (EPAP) until the airway pressure reaches the designated pressure, at which point the IPAP cycles off. In volume-cycled ventilation, flow is delivered until a specific tidal volume is reached and the flow then cycles off and pressure returns to the EPAP. For NIV, pressure cycled ventilation is used because of the single limb "open" ventilator circuits needed to give the pressure, but also to allow exhalation of $CO_2$. Using an open ventilator circuit with volume ventilation will limit effective ventilation because of the loss of the applied tidal volume through the open exhalation port; however, leak compensation software is being used to overcome this problem.

The EPAP increases resting lung volume above FRC, which can improve peripheral ventilation by preventing airway collapse and atelectasis, but it also can treat obstructive apneas by preventing upper airway collapse at the end of expiration. The IPAP treats the obstructive hypopneas and hypoventilation by increasing tidal volume and improving minute ventilation. In addition, it is important to always set a back-up rate in order to insure a minimum number of breaths are administered irrespective of a patient's capacity to trigger or initiate a breath. Optimal tidal volumes may produce reflex central apneas and the use of a back-up rate insulates against these events, and allows for improved control over the patient's ventilation and sleep continuity. The level of positive pressure required to treat

SDB and normalize gas exchange should be determined during polysomnography or by a bedside evaluation and monitoring of carbon dioxide and oxygen levels.

Continuous positive airway pressure (CPAP) should never be used to support ventilation in patients with NMD since it does not augment the tidal volume, nor does it provide respiratory muscle rest. On the other hand, it can be used in select situations where there is clear evidence of obstructive sleep apnea in the presence of preserved respiratory muscle strength. It may be considered in situations where a young or very weak NMD patient may be unable to trigger IPAP and may benefit from maintain resting lung volume above FRC. In a situation, such as in a young SMA type 1 patient, this can be a viable support to eliminate the wasted inspiratory work to raising the lung volume up to FRC from which an effective breath can start.

In patients with a variety of different NMDs, initiation of NIV has been associated with enhanced quality of life and functional status, and at the same time, prolonging survival (Mellies et al. 2003a). Long-term NIV use in NMD has been shown to improve sleep quality and normalize gas exchange, and in some patients attenuate the loss of FVC (Mellies et al. 2003a). It is then important to evaluate the clinical efficacy of NIV longitudinally, and when there is a concern about disease progression or a change in body habitus consider getting a follow-up PSG to assess whether NIV settings need to be further titrated.

While the focus of NIV is on finding the proper settings to support the patient's respiratory needs, arguably the most important component is the interface. There are a variety of different nasal masks and cannula interfaces, which are the most common type of interface used. For patients unable to keep his/her mouth closed an oronasal or full face mask is another option, though there is a potential concern about aerophagia.

*Diurnal ventilation*

About 3–5% of patients with NMDs using effective nocturnal NIV require diurnal ventilation (Chailleux et al. 1996). In slowly progressive forms of NMD, this extension occurs several years after initiation of nocturnal NIV. In severe pediatric forms of NMD, such as congenital myopathies or SMA type I, patients may be 24 hour-ventilator dependent from birth.

Current guidelines from the American Thoracic Society (ATS) recommend starting diurnal ventilation after the onset of hypercapnia (Finder et al. 2004). In the light of current knowledge, this criterion appears to be obsolete. Patients would benefit from daytime ventilatory support before becoming hypercapnic. A study reported that 95% of patients with DMD complain about daytime dyspnea before hypercapnia occurs (Toussaint et al. 2006; Khirani et al. 2014). Clinical observations suggest that patients maintain normal PCO$_2$ by altering their position and breathing pattern to maintain ventilation, which causes increased work of the respiratory muscles by 92% and an increased risk for respiratory muscle fatigue (Toussaint et al. 2008). This may in turn lead to dyspnea, general fatigue, anorexia and loss of weight. In other words, there is respiratory failure compensated for by increased work of breathing before there is clear diurnal respiratory failure and hypercapnia. This is why nocturnal respiratory failure precedes diurnal respiratory failure, since while asleep the daytime ventilatory compensation is less and certainly absent in REM sleep. Diurnal ventilation improves dyspnea and associated symptoms by compensating for the load on

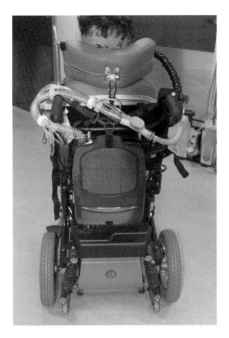

respiratory muscle and then reducing the risk for fatigue (Chatwin et al. 2011; Garuti et al. 2014; Toussaint et al. 2008).

Adequate ventilators and interfaces must be chosen carefully to ensure the best compromise between optimal quality of life and ventilation. In practice, equipment for daytime ventilation is compatible with sitting in a wheelchair. Smart carrying bags including external batteries and chargers are available and can easily be mounted on a wheelchair (Fig. 25.3).

Interfaces for ventilation

There are a variety of different interfaces available for daytime ventilation such as the nasal mask, the mouthpiece and tracheostomy.

*Nasal interface*   A nasal mask can be a clever alternative to a mouthpiece. Nasal mask can be used by those patients unable to sit upright, by some young patients not able to use the mouthpiece and by mouthpiece users who prefer the nasal mask when wheelchair-riding outdoors on unstable ground, and during travelling in the car, van or plane. Finally, some patients prefer the nasal mask during meals. There are nasal masks with contact points just on the nose or balanced between the nose and forehead and there are cannula interfaces with contact points just at the nares. Both of them have headgear to insure proper positioning and stability with movement. With care to maintaining skin integrity, sometimes by altering interfaces to alternate nasal contact points, nasal interfaces can be used for continuous ventilation (Chatwin et al. 2011). Nasal masks can also interfere with comfortable binocular vision, which may be lessened by using a cannula interface (Fig. 25.4).

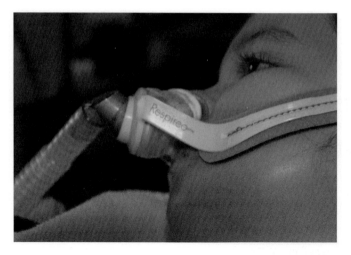

**Fig. 25.4.** Pediatric nasal mask with pillows. (Provided by Dr Michel Toussaint. All rights reserved.)

*Mouthpiece*  Mouthpiece ventilation (MPV) during the daytime can be used from approximately 5 years of age. The MPV interface is a plastic or silicone mouthpiece that is held between the lips and teeth. MPV has been used in the USA from 1968 in a large cohort of patients needing continuous ventilation (Bach et al. 1993). It was initially proposed as an alternative to tracheostomy but is now emerging as the first mode of ventilation for daytime support. Indeed, 90% of patients using NIV for more than 23/24h chose the mouthpiece interface for daytime ventilation (Lofaso et al. 2014). MPV is initially prescribed for 2 hours after lunch until dyspnea is relieved. If dyspnea is not relieved, MPV settings can be adjusted until dyspnea disappears (Toussaint et al. 2008). MPV is an inexpensive interface, easy to use and is safe and effective. Nasal ventilation is generally used in bed during sleep, while individual combinations of mouthpiece and nasal mask in the wheelchair during the daytime are possible. Some patients exclusively use MPV or nasal masks in the daytime but others may prefer to switch to the nasal mask during meals or during journeys and prefer the mouthpiece in stable circumstances, such as when watching television and using the computer, or when in a wheelchair.

There are two types of mouthpieces available on the market for daytime use. The first consists of a 22mm diameter plastic angled piece (Philips Respironics®) (Fig. 25.5a) and the second is a cylindrical silicone mouthpiece called a "straw" (Philips Respironics®) (Fig. 25.5b), which is felt to be less likely to cause orthodontic deformities.

*Tracheostomy*  With the wide variety of nasal interfaces and MPV, tracheostomy is no longer the only option for continuous ventilation. MPV and nasal ventilation in children and adolescents, and the use of nasal ventilation in infants and children under the age of 5 years may be effective to ensure daytime ventilation. In conditions where a nasal interface cannot be maintained, such as skin integrity or facial deformity, or when bulbar dysfunction

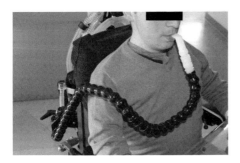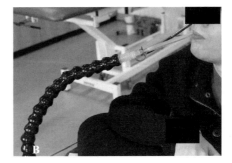

**Fig. 25.5.** Daytime ventilation via mouthpiece with articulating support arm with integrated ventilator circuit using: **A** a plastic angled mouthpiece, **B** a silicone straw mouthpiece. (Provided by Dr Michel Toussaint. All rights reserved.)

precludes the use of an oral interface, a tracheostomy is a very reasonable option. However, tracheostomy tubes require focused care and maintenance. Mucus hypersecretion and tracheal injuries, especially granuloma and tracheomalacia, are the most common complications (Soudon et al. 2008).

*Mouthpiece ventilation*   Single limb ventilator circuits with an integral exhalation valve and volume-control mode of ventilation are generally used for MPV (Boitano and Benditt 2005; Garuti et al. 2014; Ogna et al. 2016). MPV requires a specific management of low pressure alarms since with the mouth open or when taking breaks from using the circuit the low pressure alarm will engage and alarm almost incessantly (Khirani et al. 2014; Boitano and Benditt 2005). In order to avoid low pressure alarms, but also to increase the chances of easily triggering inspiration, a new mode of MPV with a "kiss trigger" and signal flow detection has been developed (Trilogy 100® ventilator, Philips Respironics®). This system allows on-demand ventilation via a single tube without an exhalation valve. This MPV mode with a back-up rate at zero is suggested as a promising mode to deliver MPV in NMD (Nardi et al. 2016).

Any ventilator for MPV should include a volume-cycled mode with few or no leak compensation and without an EPAP, since it cannot be maintained anyway. Furthermore the EPAP will be attempted by the ventilator by producing continuous air flow, which in a ventilatory system with a leak, as is the case with MPV, air will be flowing continuously out of the mouthpiece. It should provide a guaranteed volume with a fixed inspiratory time. The pressure modes are usually not effective, because they compensate for the leak in the circuit by delivering a higher flow when the patient is disconnected to the mouthpiece and do not allow air-stacking to clear out secretions.

The ideal ventilator should have a high-quality internal battery with more than 3 hours of use and an external battery ensuring more than 10 hours of autonomy in the wheelchair. Finally, the ventilator circuit needs to be attached to the wheelchair via a clamp that allows proper positioning of the mouthpiece to make it accessible to the patient (Toussaint et al. 2006; Boitano and Benditt 2005; McKim et al. 2013) (Figs. 25.5a and 25.5b).

Individualization of settings and accessories is important for patient comfort and compliance to the technique (Ogna and Lofaso 2016). Experience suggests using no back-up rate and higher tidal volume than those used at night; however, it is important to customize the interface, equipment arrangement and settings to meet each patient's need. Patients often do not inspire the whole tidal volume delivered by the ventilator. In addition patients manage leaks around the lips following their needs for air, and, therefore, it is important that the ventilator delivers stable tidal volumes with no leak compensation (Ogna et al. 2016).

Challenging situations including young age, macroglossia, intellectual disability or dysphagia are not exclusion criteria for receiving MPV. Effective MPV should correct $pCO_2$ and may alter the rate of decline of vital capacity (VC) (Toussaint et al. 2006). It has been shown to reduce fatigue (in 93% of cases), dyspnea (70%) and associated symptoms, and improves speech (43%) and eating (27%) in various NMDs (Khirani et al. 2014).

RESPIRATORY PHYSIOTHERAPY

In the absence of symptoms of airway encumbrance, sessions of preventive airway clearance are not systematically recommended. However, if mechanical insufflation–exsufflation (MI–E) devices are available, it is useful to train patients in case of respiratory emergency. Regular respiratory physiotherapy by intrapulmonary percussive ventilation (IPV) or intermittent positive pressure (IPPB) devices can be proposed at a rate of one session of 15 minutes a day in those patients with recurrent infections, even between infections.

There are several non-instrumental and instrumental airway clearance techniques (ACT), which used alone or in combination, may be considered according to the severity of respiratory muscle weakness. During chest infections, children with NMDs become weaker and instrumental techniques are used as the first choice with PCF is less than 150L/min, while non-instrumental techniques may be used when PCF is more than 150L/min. Patients under 2 years of age will be offered MI–E as a first choice to clear up secretions.

Non-instrumental ACT include cough augmentation techniques by (1) inspiratory assistance via glossopharyngeal "frog" breathing or by (2) expiratory assistance via chest compression.

Instrumental ACT include (1) all cough augmentation techniques by assisted inspiration via air-stacking, manual ventilator circuit or positive pressure generator, or by combining assisted inspiration/expiration via mechanical insufflation–exsufflation and (2) secretion mobilization via intrapulmonary percussive ventilation or high-frequency chest wall oscillations.

*Non-instrumental airway clearance techniques*
Inspiratory assistance
Inspiratory assistance may be achieved by glossopharyngeal breathing (GPB) with which, by self-insufflation using the oropharyngeal muscles, one can push small volumes of air into the lungs and, with a series of these breaths, can increase the air they inhale. It can be, however, a difficult technique for patients to understand and then master. In patients with SMA type 2, almost 45% of children were able to learn GPB and increase their vital capacity and

peak PCF without causing discomfort (Nygren-Bonnier et al. 2009). In contrast, only 27% of patients with DMD were able to learn GPB while 95% were able to learn air-stacking (AS), which requires external assistance and glottis control (Bach et al. 2007). GPB seems to have no limits of effectiveness; the weaker patients have the largest benefits.

Expiratory assistance

Expiratory assistance may be achieved by a self-induced abdominal thrust from a table to increase upward movement of the diaphragm and exhalation (Bianchi et al. 2014) or by manual assisted abdominal and/or chest compression (Toussaint et al. 2009). Expiratory assistance is felt to be feasible in patients with a vital capacity more than 1 030mL and an MEP more than 34cm $H_2O$ (Toussaint et al. 2009). The effectiveness of expiratory and inspiratory assistance is felt to be similar but can vary with patient and disease type (Bach et al. 2007; Nygren-Bonnier et al. 2009). For example, children with SMA type 2 generally have greater benefit from expiratory than inspiratory assistance (Toussaint et al. 2009).

*Instrumental airway clearance techniques*

Assisted inspiration

The deeper one inhales the greater the expiratory flow one can generate. There a variety of ways to augment inspiratory volumes prior to coughing using single or multiple mechanical insufflations.

Single insufflation

Inspiratory assistance to improve PCF can be delivered via any device producing intermittent positive pressure breathing (IPPB) such as a manual ventilator circuit, a ventilator or an insufflation device. The aim of single breath inspiratory assistance is to raise inspiratory volume well above the volume one can generate manually and therefore increase expiratory volume and flow beyond that which can be obtained unassisted. A single insufflation can increase the unassisted volume of air by 54% and unassisted expiratory flow by 64% in children (Toussaint et al. 2015). The patient triggered lung insufflation assist maneuver (LIAM) has been shown to be effective in both increasing inspiratory volume and augmenting cough (Trebbia et al. 2005).

Multiple insufflations

IPPB devices can be used for air-stacking (AS) for multiple, successive and "stacked" submaximal insufflations without expiration between. Children take two or three insufflations to obtain their maximal insufflation capacity. The British Thoracic Society (BTS) guidelines support air-stacking as an effective method of improving cough efficiency (Hull et al. 2012a).

The manual ventilation circuit includes a ventilation bag, a one-way-valve, to allow inflation but not exhalation, which is then applied to the airway opening. In this case, glottis control is not mandatory. If there is no valve, glottis control is mandatory to retain inspiratory air in the lungs beyond the vocal cords between two insufflations. This technique is easily taught to children with NMD (Bach et al. 2007) and air-stacking is useful in those children with mild degree of respiratory muscle weakness (Jenkins et al. 2014).

A ventilator or any other positive pressure generator may be used to provide inspiratory assistance (Hull et al. 2012a). Positive pressures between 30 and 40cm $H_2O$ improve the inspiratory capacity by 120% and expiratory flows during cough by 85%. A submaximal insufflation (lower than the maximal insufflation capacity) is ideal for generating the best expiratory flows during cough (Mellies and Goebel 2014).

*Combination of inspiratory and expiratory assistance*
The highest expiratory flows and best secretion clearance result from combining inspiratory/expiratory assistance and non-instrumental/instrumental techniques simultaneously (Toussaint et al. 2009; Ishikawa et al. 2008; Lacombe et al. 2014).

Assisted inspiration/expiration (mechanical insufflation–exsufflation)
Instrumental support to assist inspiration/expiration, known as mechanical insufflation–exsufflation (MI–E), is a very popular airway clearance therapy (Fig. 25.6). MI–E devices deliver a deep inspiration (insufflation by positive pressure) followed by a rapid expiration (exsufflation by negative pressure) to enhance airway clearance (Homnick 2007). Timing and pressures are set individually for each patient based on optimal visual expansion of the chest during insufflation and a cough sound during exsufflation. Positive and negative pressures range from 0 to 70cm $H_2O$ and inspiratory, expiratory and pause times range from 0 to 5 seconds. In children, positive pressures between 20 to 40cm $H_2O$ and negative pressures from 30 to 50 are often used. Low pressures are set initially and they are progressively increased based on chest expansion and patient comfort.

The initial setting of the timing in infants and children may be 2–3 seconds insufflation based on the time it takes to reach the prescribed pressure and then a 1 second hold of

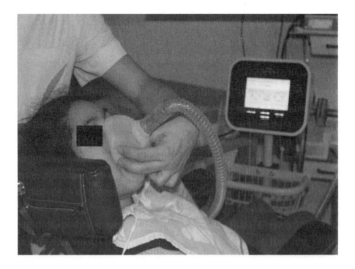

**Fig. 25.6.** Mechanical insufflation-exsufflation via an oronasal mask. (Provided by Dr Michel Toussaint. All rights reserved.)

that pressure and then an exsufflation of about the same time. The timing can be adjusted according to the comfort of patients and cough effectiveness. A treatment session usually lasts about 10–30 seconds (5 to 10 cough maneuvers) followed by 30 seconds of rest. An additional manual thrust on the chest/stomach can be provided during exsufflation. Sessions are repeated until secretions are cleared (Homnick 2007). The session should end with a last insufflation to avoid lung deflation after treatment (Hull et al. 2012a).

MI–E is possible, although, challenging to implement in infants with NMD based on how well one can synchronize insufflation during patient inspiration and then cycling to exsufflation during patient exhalation. Caregivers or members of the family provide MI–E timed to diaphragm movement via a face (oral–nasal) mask. Regular treatments can help to accommodate children to MI–E so that they will use MI–E effectively during respiratory tract infections (RTIs). Bearing in mind how often one coughs during a respiratory illness, during a RTI a patient with NMD may need very frequent MI–E treatments or a prolonged treatment until the secretions have been cleared and/or gas exchange is normal again.

Secretion mobilization

Secretion mobilization includes those techniques that aim to improve regional ventilation homogenization and enhance mucus transport from the peripheral airways to the central airways. Sessions of cough assistance must follow sessions of secretion mobilization since these techniques still require a cough to remove secretions. For this reason these procedures are accessory airway clearance techniques. Secretion mobilization techniques do not require patient co-operation and are possible to use in infants and children, even in the presence of a tracheostomy and/or bulbar failure or intellectual impairment. They include (1) intrapulmonary percussive ventilation and (2) high-frequency chest wall oscillations.

*Intrapulmonary percussive ventilation*

Intrapulmonary percussive ventilation (IPV) consists of pneumatic devices producing high-frequency pulsatile airflow during nebulization of normal saline or hypertonic saline (Percussionaire Corporation, USA and Pegaso, Dima, Italy). Mini volumes of air are delivered into the lungs at rates of 100 to 400 cycles per minute at peak pressures from 5 to 40cm $H_2O$. The high-frequency vibration helps to free secretions from the peripheral airways and move them from the peripheral bronchial tree toward the central airways. IPV has been shown to improve airway clearance in children with NMD (Riffard and Toussaint 2012a), with lower antibiotic usage and shorter hospitalization (Reardon et al. 2005), and to improve persistent pulmonary consolidation in patients with NMD (Birnkrant et al. 1996).

In order to obtain the optimal effect, high-frequency and short inspiration are recommended (Riffard and Toussaint 2012b). The length of the IPV session depends on the comfort of patients. With oro-nasal masks, patients cannot tolerate IPV ventilation for longer than 1 or 2 consecutive minutes. However, the use of a nasal interface increases comfort and allows sessions of 15 minutes or longer in children with neurologic disorders (Toussaint et al. 2015)

*High-frequency chest wall oscillations*

High-frequency chest wall oscillation (HFCWO) provides compressive oscillation of the chest at frequencies between 5 and 20Hz (King et al. 1983). This oscillation produces oscillatory airflow in the airways presumably similar to IPV which mobilizes secretions toward the central airways (Homnick 2007). Settings should be titrated to patient comfort and effect. A treatment of 20–30 minutes includes frequencies between 6 and 25Hz. In children with NMDs, HFCWO is proposed for short sessions of 5 minutes or until the patient feels the need to cough. HFCWO is safe and is suggested to be better tolerated than other ACT (Yuan et al. 2010). IPV and HFCWO are recommended by guidelines in those children who have difficulty mobilizing secretions or who have persistent atelectasis, despite using other ACT (Hull et al. 2012a). HFCWO should only be used in addition to MI–E or other airway clearance to expectorate mucus.

THE SPECIFIC SITUATION OF RESPIRATORY MANAGEMENT IN SMA TYPE 1

In more severe NMD, such as SMA type 1 respiratory interventions, both airway clearance and ventilatory assistance have been seen by some as futile and inappropriate since neither can prevent progression. However, with the exciting advances in SMA and in other NMDs with disease-modifying therapies having the potential to significantly alter the course of disease active and aggressive intervention can be seen as a more reasonable approach to therapy.

**Key points**

- There are a variety of1 different progressive NMDs that can cause significant respiratory morbidities.
- While there is overlap among many in having abnormalities in airway clearance and respiratory failure, these and the preceding symptoms can happen at varying times during progression of disease.
- With that in mind, it is important to recognize the progression of disease that leads to problems with airway clearance and respiratory failure and considering these issues one can take a proactive and effective approach in managing respiratory morbidity and ultimately improve quality of life in patients with NMD.

**Clinical vignette**

The overarching purpose of respiratory therapy and support is to augment or replace what a patient with NMD should be able to do. As discussed above the two main components of this support are airway clearance and ventilation. The level of support through a full day and night is obviously dependent on the severity of the neuromuscular weakness. We can use the following examples: a 12-month-old with SMA type 1, a 15-year-old with collagen-6 deficient (Ullrich) myopathy, and a 10-year-old with DMD.

12-MONTH-OLD WITH SPINAL MUSCULAR ATROPHY TYPE 1

The typical natural history of an infant with SMA type 1, in the absence of some of the newer disease-modifying therapies, will have an exceptionally weak cough, perhaps having led to multiple hospitalizations for lower respiratory tract illnesses, and chronic respiratory failure. This child when well will typically use mechanical airway clearance with mechanical in-exsufflation (e.g. Cough Assist®) twice a day and then as needed up to hourly at the earliest stages of an acute illness. The quality of this assessment and aggressiveness of therapy will largely determine the severity of an acute illness between home management, inpatient hospitalization with NIV and inpatient hospitalization with invasive ventilation. This is largely based on the quality of the assessment of the caregivers. In addition, a child this age with SMA type 1 will often require nocturnal NIV, with increase into diurnal support during acute illnesses.

### 15-YEAR-OLD WITH ULLRICH CONGENITAL MUSCULAR DYSTROPHY

A typical 15-year-old with Ullrich congenital muscular dystrophy (CMD) will have a weak cough, requiring mechanical in-exsufflation, and chronic respiratory failure, requiring nocturnal NIV. Beyond the difference in functional capacity and muscle strength the 15-year-old child with Ullrich CMD will have two practical advantages over the infant with SMA type 1: the ability to self-assess and communicate and substantially larger airways which are less prone to mucus impaction. While this does not eliminate the potential for needing inpatient hospitalization during an acute illness, with these advantages and good care providers the likelihood of inpatient hospitalization is much lower. However, as with the younger child with SMA type 1, the nocturnal NIV can transition to diurnal support during acute respiratory illness because of the related respiratory muscle fatigue.

### 10-YEAR-OLD WITH DUCHENNED MUSCULAR DYSTROPHY

The typical 10-year-old child with DMD will be ambulant or having recently lost the ability to ambulate and will have pulmonary function (FVC) that is at or just below the lower limit of normal. With this, during periods of wellness, this child will typically be asymptomatic when well and with no routine need for assisted airway clearance or NIV. However, it would be wrong to assume that that applies during acute respiratory illnesses. During these periods of acute illness with further fatigue, coughing may become ineffective and without airway clearance support at home may then require inpatient hospitalization to manage an illness that in the past had been manageable at home.

Therefore, while the principles of assisted airway clearance and ventilation can be applied across all types of NMD, the type and stage of disease will determine the need for support. The recognition is based both on data, such as pulmonary function testing and assessment of gas exchange, but most important is a high-quality clinical assessment.

## REFERENCES

Anderson VB, Mckenzie JA, Seton C, Fitzgerald DA, Webster RI, North KN et al. (2012) Sniff nasal inspiratory pressure and sleep disordered breathing in childhood neuromuscular disorders. *Neuromusc Dis* 22 (6): 528–33.

Arens R, Muzumdar H (2010) Sleep, sleep disordered breathing, and nocturnal hypoventilation in children with neuromuscular diseases. *Paediatr Respir Rev* 11: 24–30.

Bach JR, Alba AS, Saporito LR (1993) Intermittent positive pressure ventilation via the mouth as an alternative to tracheostomy for 257 ventilator users. *Chest* 103: 174–182.

Bach JR, Saporito LR (1996) Criteria for extubation and tracheostomy tube removal for patients with ventilatory failure. A different approach to weaning. *Chest* 110: 1566–1571.

Bach JR, Bianchi C, Vidigal-Lopes M, Turi S, Felisari G (2007) Lung inflation by glossopharyngeal breathing and "air stacking" in Duchenne muscular dystrophy. *Am J Phys Med Rehabil* 86: 295–300.

Barbé F, Quera-Salva MA, McCann C, Gajdos P, Raphael JC, de Lattre J et al. (1994) Sleep-related respiratory disturbances in patients with Duchenne muscular dystrophy. *Eur Respir J* 7: 1403–1408.

Berry RB, Budhiraja R, Gottlieb DJ, Gozal D, Iber C, Kapur VK et al. (2012) Rules for scoring respiratory events in sleep: update of the 2007 AASM Manual for the Scoring of Sleep and Associated Events. *J Clin Sleep Med* 8: 597–619.

Bersanini C, Khirani S, Ramirez A, Lofaso F, Aubertin G, Beydon N et al. (2012) Nocturnal hypoxaemia and hypercapnia in children with neuromuscular disorders. *Eur Respir J* 39: 1206–1212.

Bianchi C, Baiardi P (2008) Cough peak flows: standard values for children and adolescents. *Am J Phys Med Rehabil* 87: 461–467.

Bianchi C, Carrara R, Khirani S, Tuccio MC (2014) Independent cough flow augmentation by glossopharyngeal breathing plus table thrust in muscular dystrophy. *Am J Phys Med Rehabil* 93: 43–48.

Birnkrant DJ, Pope JF, Lewarski J, Stegmaier J, Besunder JB (1996) Persistent pulmonary consolidation treated with intrapulmonary percussive ventilation: a preliminary report. *Pediatr Pulmonol* 21: 246–249.

Boitano LJ (2006) Management of airway clearance in neuromuscular disease. *Respir Care* 51: 913–922, discussion 922–924.

Boitano LJ, Benditt JO (2005) An evaluation of home volume ventilators that support open-circuit mouthpiece ventilation. *Respir Care* 50: 1457–1461.

Buyse GM, Voit T, Schara U, Straathof CSM, D'Angelo G, Bernert G et al. (2015) Efficacy of idebenone on respiratory function in patients with Duchenne muscular dystrophy not using glucocorticoids (DELOS): a double-blind randomised placebo-controlled phase 3 trial. *Lancet* 385 (9979): 1748–1757.

Buyse GM, Voit T, Schara U, Straathof CSM, D'Angelo MG, Bernert G et al. (2016) Treatment effect of idebenone on inspiratory function in patients with Duchenne muscular dystrophy. *Pediatr Pulmonol* 52 (4): 508–515.

Chailleux E, Fauroux B, Binet F, Dautzenberg B, Polu JM (1996) Predictors of survival in patients receiving domiciliary oxygen therapy or mechanical ventilation. A 10-year analysis of ANTADIR Observatory. *Chest* 109: 741–749.

Chatwin M, Bush A, Simonds AK (2011) Outcome of goal-directed non-invasive ventilation and mechanical insufflation/exsufflation in spinal muscular atrophy type I. *Arch Dis Child* 96: 426–432.

De Bruin PF, Ueki J, Bush A, Y Manzur A, Watson A, Pride NB (2001) Inspiratory flow reserve in boys with Duchenne muscular dystrophy. *Pediatr Pulmonol* 31: 451–457.

Dubowitz V (2015) Unnatural natural history of Duchenne muscular dystrophy. *Neuromusc Dis* 25 (12): 936. doi.10.1016/j.nmd.2015.11.005.

Eagle M, Bourke J, Bullock R, Gibson M, Mehta J, Giddings D et al. (2007) Managing Duchenne muscular dystrophy – The additive effect of spinal surgery and home nocturnal ventilation in improving survival. *Neuromusc Dis* 17 (6): 470–475. doi.10.1016/j.nmd.2007.03.002.

Estenne M, Heilporn A, Delhez L, Yernault JC, De Troyer A (1983) Chest wall stiffness in patients with chronic respiratory muscle weakness. *Am Rev Respir Dis* 128: 1002–1007.

Estenne M, Gevenois PA, Kinnear W, Soudon P, Heilporn A, De Troyer A (1993) Lung volume restriction in patients with chronic respiratory muscle weakness: the role of microatelectasis. *Thorax* 48: 698–701.

Ferguson KA, Strong MJ, Ahmad D, George CF (1996) Sleep-disordered breathing in amyotrophic lateral sclerosis. *Chest* 110: 664–669.

Finder JD, Birnkrant D, Carl J, Farber HJ, Gozal D, Iannaccone ST et al. (2004) Respiratory care of the patient with Duchenne muscular dystrophy: ATS consensus statement. *Am J Respir Crit Care Med* 170: 456–465.

Foley AR, Quijano-Roy S, Collins J, Straub V, Mccallum M, Deconinck N et al. (2013) Natural history of pulmonary function in collagen VI-related myopathies. *Brain* 136 (Pt 12): 3625–33.

Garuti G, Nicolini A, Grecchi B, Lusuardi M, Winck JC, Bach JR (2014) Open circuit mouthpiece ventilation: concise clinical review. *Rev Port Pneumol* 20: 211–218.

Gould GA, Gugger M, Molloy J, Tsara V, Shapiro CM, Douglas NJ (1988) Breathing pattern and eye movement density during REM sleep in humans. *Am Rev Respir Dis* 138: 874–877.

Homnick DN (2007) Mechanical insufflation-exsufflation for airway mucus clearance. *Respir Care* 52: 1296–1305, discussion 1306–1307.

Hull J, Aniapravan R, Chan E, Chatwin M, Forton J, Gallagher J et al. (2012a). British Thoracic Society guideline for respiratory management of children with neuromuscular weakness. *Thorax* 67 (Suppl 1): 1–40.

Hull J, Aniapravan R, Chan E, Chatwin M, Forton J, Gallagher J et al. (2012b). British Thoracic Society guideline for respiratory management of children with neuromuscular weakness. *Thorax* 67 (Suppl 1): i1–i40.

Humbertclaude V, Hamroun D, Bezzou K Bérard C, Boespflug-Tanguy O, Bommelaer C et al. (2012) Motor and respiratory heterogeneity in Duchenne patients: Implication for clinical trials. *Eur J Paediatr Neurol* 16 (2): 149–60.

Ishikawa Y, Bach JR, Komaroff E, Miura T, Jackson-Parekh R (2008) Cough augmentation in Duchenne muscular dystrophy. *Am J Phys Med Rehabil* 87: 726–730.

Jenkins HM, Stocki A, Kriellaars D, Pasterkamp H (2014) Breath stacking in children with neuromuscular disorders. *Pediatr Pulmonol* 49: 544–553.

Khirani S, Colella M, Caldarelli V, Aubertin G, Boulé M, Forin V et al. (2013a). Longitudinal course of lung function and respiratory muscle strength in spinal muscular atrophy type 2 and 3. *Eur J Paediatr Neurol* 17 (6): 552–60.

Khirani S, Ramirez A, Aubertin G, Boulé M, Chemouny C, Forin V et al. (2013b). Respiratory muscle decline in duchenne muscular dystrophy. *Pediatr Pulmonol* 49 (5): 473–81.

Khirani S, Ramirez A, Delord V, Leroux K, Lofaso F, Hautot S, Toussaint M, Orlikowski D, Louis B, Fauroux B (2014) Evaluation of ventilators for mouthpiece ventilation in neuromuscular disease. *Respir Care* 59: 1329–1337.

King M, Phillips DM, Gross D, Vartian V, Chang HK, Zidulka A (1983) Enhanced tracheal mucus clearance with high frequency chest wall compression. *Am Rev Respir Dis* 128: 511–515.

Lacombe M, Del Amo Castrillo L, Boré A, Chapeau D, Horvat E, Vaugier I et al. (2014) Comparison of three cough-augmentation techniques in neuromuscular patients: mechanical insufflation combined with manually assisted cough, insufflation-exsufflation alone and insufflation-exsufflation combined with manually assisted cough. *Respiration* 88: 215–222.

Lofaso F, Prigent H, Tiffreau V, Menoury N, Toussaint M, Monnier AF et al. (2014) Long-term mechanical ventilation equipment for neuromuscular patients: meeting the expectations of patients and prescribers. *Respir Care* 59: 97–106.

Mayer OH, Finkel RS, Rummey C, Benton MJ, Glanzman AM, Flickinger J et al. (2015) Characterization of pulmonary function in Duchenne Muscular Dystrophy. *Pediatr Pulmonol* 50: 487–494.

McDonald CM, Gordish-Dressman H, Henricson EK, Duong T, Joyce NC, Jhawar S et al. (2018) CINRG investigators for PubMed. Longitudinal pulmonary function testing outcome measures in Duchenne muscular dystrophy: Long-term natural history with and without glucocorticoids. *Neuromuscul Disord* 28(11): 897–909. doi: 10.1016/j.nmd.2018.07.004.

McKim DA, Griller N, LeBlanc C, Woolnough A, King J (2013) Twenty-four hour noninvasive ventilation in Duchenne muscular dystrophy: a safe alternative to tracheostomy. *Can Respir J* 20: e5–e9.

Mellies U, Goebel C (2014) Optimum insufflation capacity and peak cough flow in neuromuscular disorders. *Ann Am Thorac Soc* 11: 1560–1568.

Mellies U, Ragette R, Dohna Schwake C, Boehm H, Voit T, Teschler H (2003a). Long-term noninvasive ventilation in children and adolescents with neuromuscular disorders. *Eur Respir J* 22: 631–636.

Mellies U, Ragette R, Schwake C, Boehm H, Voit T, Teschler H (2003b). Daytime predictors of sleep disordered breathing in children and adolescents with neuromuscular disorders. *Neuromuscul Disord* 13: 123–128.

Nardi J, Leroux K, Orlikowski D, Prigent H, Lofaso F (2016) Home monitoring of daytime mouthpiece ventilation effectiveness in patients with neuromuscular disease. *Chron Respir Dis* 13: 67–74.

Nève V, Cuisset JM, Edmé JL, Carpentier A, Howsam M, Leclerc O et al. (2013) Sniff nasal inspiratory pressure in the longitudinal assessment of young Duchenne muscular dystrophy children. *Eur Respir J* 42 (3): 671–80.

Nygren-Bonnier M, Markström A, Lindholm P, Mattsson E, Klefbeck B (2009) Glossopharyngeal pistoning for lung insufflation in children with spinal muscular atrophy type II. *Acta Paediatr* 98: 1324–1328.

Ogna A, Lofaso F (2016) Mouthpiece ventilation: individualized patient care is the key to success. *Chron Respir Dis* 13: 385–386; epub ahead of print.

Ogna A, Prigent H, Falaize L, Leroux K, Santos D, Vaugier I et al. (2016) Accuracy of tidal volume delivered by home mechanical ventilation during mouthpiece ventilation: A bench evaluation. *Chron Respir Dis* 13: 353–360; epub ahead of print.

Paiva R, Krivec U, Aubertin G, Cohen E, Clément A, Fauroux B (2009) Carbon dioxide monitoring during long-term noninvasive respiratory support in children. *Intensive Care Med* 35: 1068–1074.

Passamano L, Taglia A, Palladino A, Viggiano E, D'Ambrosio P, Scutifero M et al. (2012) Improvement of survival in Duchenne Muscular Dystrophy: retrospective analysis of 835 patients. *Acta Myol* 31: 121–125.

Reardon CC, Christiansen D, Barnett ED, Cabral HJ (2005) Intrapulmonary percussive ventilation vs incentive spirometry for children with neuromuscular disease. *Arch Pediatr Adolesc Med* 159: 526–531.

Riffard G, Toussaint M (2012a). [Indications for intrapulmonary percussive ventilation (IPV): a review of the literature]. *Rev Mal Respir* 29: 178–190.

Riffard G, Toussaint M (2012b). [Intrapulmonary percussion ventilation: operation and settings]. *Rev Mal Respir* 29: 347–354.

Robert D, Willig TN, Leger P, Paulus J (1993) Long-term nasal ventilation in neuromuscular disorders: report of a consensus conference. *Eur Respir J* 6: 599–606.

Sawnani H, Thampratankul L, Szczesniak RD, Fenchel MC, Simakajornboon N (2015) Sleep disordered breathing in young boys with Duchenne muscular dystrophy. *J Pediatr* 166: 640–5.e1. doi.10.1016/j.jpeds.2014.12.006.

Smith PE, Calverley PM, Edwards RH (1988) Hypoxemia during sleep in Duchenne muscular dystrophy. *Am Rev Respir Dis* 137: 884–888.

Soudon P, Steens M, Toussaint M (2008) A comparison of invasive versus noninvasive full-time mechanical ventilation in Duchenne muscular dystrophy. *Chron Respir Dis* 5: 87–93.

Tabachnik E, Muller NL, Bryan AC, Levison H (1981) Changes in ventilation and chest wall mechanics during sleep in normal adolescents. *J Appl Physiol* 51: 557–564.

Toussaint M, Steens M, Wasteels G, Soudon P (2006) Diurnal ventilation via mouthpiece: survival in end-stage Duchenne patients. *Eur Respir J* 28: 549–555.

Toussaint M, Soudon P, Kinnear W (2008) Effect of non-invasive ventilation on respiratory muscle loading and endurance in patients with Duchenne muscular dystrophy. *Thorax* 63: 430–434.

Toussaint M, Boitano LJ, Gathot V, Steens M, Soudon P (2009) Limits of effective cough-augmentation techniques in patients with neuromuscular disease. *Respir Care* 54: 359–366.

Toussaint M, Pernet K, Stagnara A (2015) Instrumental chest physiotherapy in central neurological child. *Motricité Cérébrale* 36: 66–71.

Trebbia G, Lacombe M, Fermanian C, Falaize L, Lejaille M, Louis A, Devaux C, Raphaël JC, Lofaso F (2005) Cough determinants in patients with neuromuscular disease. *Respir Physiol Neurobiol* 146: 291–300.

Ward S, Chatwin M, Heather S, Simonds AK (2005) Randomised controlled trial of non-invasive ventilation (NIV) for nocturnal hypoventilation in neuromuscular and chest wall disease patients with daytime normocapnia. *Thorax* 60: 1019–1024.

White JE, Drinnan MJ, Smithson AJ, Griffiths CJ, Gibson GJ (1995) Respiratory muscle activity and oxygenation during sleep in patients with muscle weakness. *Eur Respir J* 8: 807–814.

Yuan N, Kane P, Shelton K, Matel J, Becker BC, Moss RB (2010) Safety, tolerability, and efficacy of high-frequency chest wall oscillation in pediatric patients with cerebral palsy and neuromuscular diseases: an exploratory randomized controlled trial. *J Child Neurol* 25: 815–821.

# Section 6
## Feeding and Gastrointestinal Management

# 26
# GASTRO-INTESTINAL COMPLICATIONS AND NUTRITION

*Hasan Özen and Haluk Topaloglu*

## Introduction

Pediatric neuromuscular disorders (NMDs) cause complications in many organs and systems; musculoskeletal, respiratory, nutritional and gastro-intestinal complications. Sleep may also be compromised (Rönnblom and Danielsson 2004; Skalsky and Dalal 2015). Some of these complications may make life unbearable for the family and the patient. Although gastro-intestinal complications rarely cause life-threatening events, they lower the quality of life of the patients and their parents/care givers.

Feeding difficulties, such as difficulty getting the food to the mouth, opening the mouth and chewing, swallowing impairment and choking, are frequently seen in children with NMDs, and their prevalence increases with age. As overall survival has been prolonged with improved medical care, nutritional concerns have become more critical for these long-term survivors. While swallowing and feeding problems may cause underfeeding, immobility and weakness may cause obesity (Davidson and Truby 2009; Pane et al. 2006). Nutritional outcomes among neurologic disabilities have improved during the past three decades due to the development of new oral/enteral formulas and enteral access techniques such as endoscopic and radiologic gastrostomy placement.

In this chapter we shall review gastro-intestinal complications and feeding and nutrition problems. Feeding of patients with muscular dystrophy and spinal muscular atrophy (SMA) will be discussed in detail but the NMDs that have remissions or specific treatments such as the myasthenic syndromes or dermatomyositis are not discussed here in detail.

## Gastro-intestinal complications

Gastro-intestinal complications are common in patients with NMDs and almost half of patients have at least one gastro-intestinal problem (Table 26.1). In the upper digestive tract, dysphagia, heartburn, regurgitation and dyspepsia are the most common complaints, while in the lower tract, abdominal pain, bloating, dyschezia and constipation or diarrhea are. These clinical manifestations have generally been attributed to motility disorders caused by muscle damage. Digestive symptoms may be the first sign of some NMDs, particularly myotonic dystrophy type 1 (DM1), and may precede the musculo-skeletal features (Bellini et al. 2006; Rönnblom and Danielsson 2004).

| *Oral* | *Small and large intestines* |
|---|---|
| Oral motor impairment and oropharyngeal dysphagia | Antroduodenal dysmotility |
| Reduced mastication | Constipation |
| Poor lip closure and drooling | Diarrhea |
| Poor tongue coordination | Anorexia |
| Macroglossia | Pancreatitis |
| Malocclusion | Malabsorption |
| High arch palate | Meteorism |
| Dry mouth and poor oral hygiene | Dilatation of small intestines |
| Gingivitis and gingival hypertrophy | Megacolon |
| Periodontitis | Volvulus |
| Erosion of dental enamel, dental caries | Colitis |
| Delayed eruption of the permanent dentition | Colonic perforation |
| Dental agenesis, hypoplasia of premolars | Pseudoobstruction, ileus |
| Crowding of teeth | Fecal incontinans |
| Microdontia | Dyschezia |
| *Esophagus* | |
| Esophageal dysmotility and dysphagia | |
| Gastro-esophageal reflux disease | |
| Esophagitis | |
| Barret esophagus | |
| Stricture | |
| *Stomach* | |
| Gastric dysmotility/dysrhythmia | |
| Delayed gastric emptying | |
| Dyspepsia: early satiety, nausea, vomiting, epigastric pain | |
| Gastritis | |
| Peptic ulcer | |
| Gastric perforation | |
| Gastric dilatation | |

There is a positive correlation between the presence and severity of gastro-intestinal disturbances and the duration of the skeletal muscle disease. Because of the patients' more serious health problems, these gastro-intestinal disturbances are generally overlooked by caregiver and health professionals. Screening for and treating these common complications can lead to healthier children and a higher quality of life (Bellini et al. 2006; Rönnblom and Danielsson 2004; Wang et al. 2007).

ORAL MANIFESTATIONS

Patients with NMDs have significant oral healthcare problems, including gingivitis, peri-odontitis, and caries (Balasubramaniam et al. 2008). Risk factors for poor oral health are dependency for poor oral hygiene, oral aversions, medication side effects such as dry mouth or gingival overgrowth, dysphagia, prolonged bottle feeding, consumption of a liquid, pureed, or gastrostomy diet (Ptomey and Wittenbrook 2015).

Orofacial problems including malocclusion, facial deformities as a result of noninva-sive ventilation, and high arch palate are very common findings in children with congenital myopathy. Prevalence of malocclusion is high in patients with myotonic dystrophy and mandibular prognathism may be present in patients with Duchenne muscular dystrophy (DMD) (Sejerson et al. 2009). Malocclusion with crowding of teeth can make teeth cleaning difficult (Colombo et al. 2015; Wang et al. 2010; Wang et al. 2012). In patients with DMD, delayed eruption of the permanent dentition, agenesis, microdontia, and hypoplasia of pre-molars may occur (Balasubramaniam et al. 2008).

Gingival hyperplasia can occur due to prolonged "nothing by mouth" status and medi-cations such as phenytoin. Tricyclic antidepressants such as clomipramine and imipramine, and benzodiazepines may cause xerostomia and increase risk of caries. Mouth breathing can also lead to dry mouth and increased risk of oral infection, which can contribute to devel-opment of pneumonia (Balasubramaniam et al. 2008; Wang et al. 2010). Gastro-esophageal reflux can also cause erosion of dental enamel, caries and pain. Patients with myotonic dystrophy may have fewer teeth, higher frequency of plaque, and caries. Oral bacteria from dental caries or other infections can contribute to development of pneumonia. It is recom-mended that children with NMDs be referred to a pediatric dentist before 2 years of age.

Drooling is a common problem that can be a major issue for children with NMDs, particularly with congenital myopathies. This is often due to bulbar and facial weakness resulting in difficulties with lip closure and swallowing saliva. Suctioning, lip-strengthening exercises, anticholinergic drugs administered systemically (e.g. scopolamine, hyoscine) or topically (atropine), ligation of the ducts or excision of salivary glands, and L-tyrosine supplementation in children with nemaline myopathy have been suggested, but there is no consensus for the problem of drooling. Botulinum toxin injections and salivary gland ligation are not recommended for children with congenital myopathy (van den Engel-Hoek et al. 2015; Wang et al. 2012).

ESOPHAGUS AND GASTRO-ESOPHAGEAL REFLUX DISEASE

Esophageal motility may be affected in children with muscular dystrophies and SMA, and may be asymptomatic (Camelo et al. 1997; Karasick et al. 1982). Inflammatory myopathies may also cause esophageal dysmotility and esophagitis in children (Quartier and Gherardi 2013).

Vomiting, regurgitation, retching and gastro-esophageal reflux disease (GERD) are relatively common among children with neurologic disabilities. Gastric hypomotility and delayed gastric emptying, a long-term sitting position, progressive degradation of the dia-phragmatic muscular tone, abnormal esophageal and lower esophageal sphincter motility, increased abdominal pressure due to constipation and scoliosis can contribute to GERD

(Barohn et al. 1988; Bellini et al. 2006; Borrelli et al. 2005; Haensch et al. 2011; Wang et al. 2012). GERD is an important determinant of mortality and morbidity in patients with SMA (Wang et al. 2007). Although the majority of the patients with DMD complain occasional heartburn, only 4% of them required the use of medical treatment (Pane et al. 2006). GERD can lead to painful erosions, esophagitis, hemorrhage, peptic ulcer, Barrett esophagus and possible risks for aspiration. GERD may be evident through subtle signs such as early satiety or progressive lack of appetite and decreased food intake, placing them at risk for undernutrition.

In children old enough to describe their complaints reliably, the diagnosis of GERD can be made clinically. When it is necessary, evaluation by various diagnostic tests such as nuclear scintigraphy, pH monitoring, endoscopic examination and multichannel intraluminal impedance-pH monitoring (MII-pHM) are options for assessment. Currently, MII-pHM is accepted as the criterion standard. Barium studies may be required if there is suspicion of the development of esophageal stricture (Vandenplas et al. 2009).

Nutrition interventions, positioning and medications are treatment modalities. Prokinetics help facilitate gastro-intestinal motility. But, there is insufficient evidence of clinical efficacy to justify the routine use of metoclopramide, erythromycin, bethanechol, cisapride, or domperidone for GERD. Metoclopramide may cause extrapyramidal signs such as dystonic reactions. Erythromycin demonstrates some effect on gastric and intestinal motility; however, has not been a proven treatment for GERD. Cisapride use has been banned because of its cardiac side effects. Histamine-2 receptor antagonists such as famotidine and ranitidine decrease acid secretion and are common treatments for GERD. The rapid development of tachyphylaxis is a drawback to their chronic use. The usual dose of ranitidine is 5–10mg/kg/day (maximum 300mg), famotidine 1–2mg/kg/day (maximum 40mg), and nizatidine 5–10mg/kg/day (maximum 300mg), divided into 2–3 doses. They are not as effective in healing esophagitis as proton pump inhibitors (PPIs): omeprazole, lansoprazole, and esomeprazole. They maintain intragastric pH above 4 for longer periods and their effect does not diminish with chronic use. They must be taken once or twice a day and at least 30 minutes before meals. The most common side effects are headache, diarrhea, constipation, and nausea, each occurring in 2% to 7%. Prolonged hypochlorhydria may lead to gastric bacterial overgrowth and vitamin $B_{12}$ deficiency. Their usual doses are 1–2mg/kg body weight/day (maximum 40–60mg/day). Nissen fundoplication is the standard surgical therapy for GERD, but there are no randomized controlled trials testing its efficacy in children with neurological impairment. Indications include failure of optimized medical therapy, dependence on long-term medical therapy, significant nonadherence with medical therapy, or pulmonary aspiration of refluxate. When reflux treatment is not effective, eosinophilic esophagitis must be considered as a differential diagnosis (Vandenplas et al. 2009).

DYSPHAGIA

Between 6 and 12 months, infants learn to chew and swallow pureed or solid food. The complete swallowing mechanism develops thereafter, with the adult swallowing pattern being reached in puberty, after the pharynx has attained its adult length (van den Engel-Hoek et al. 2015).

The term dysphagia refers to difficulty with swallowing. Normal swallowing function has three successive phases: oral (bolus chewing and fragmentation), pharyngeal (bolus transition from the mouth to the upper esophageal sphincter), and esophageal (bolus progression towards the stomach). All of them may be affected and cause oropharyngeal dysphagia in patients with NMDs. Dysphagia in most NMDs results from progressive muscle weakness of the tongue, face, jaw, soft palate, and other related muscles. In SMA patients, the bulbar region may be affected. Poor head control may also be a factor in the development of feeding difficulties. In oculopharyngeal muscular dystrophy, dysphagia is a part of symptom complex and occurs, to some degree, in all patients. Oral dysphagia is more common in DMD than oropharyngeal dysphagia. Oropharyngeal incoordination may cause laryngeal penetration or aspiration (Davis et al. 2015; Jones et al. 2016, van den Engel-Hoek et al. 2015). The prevalence of swallowing difficulties in people with muscle disease is unknown and is different among children with different diagnoses. The prevalence of dysphagia in myotonic dystrophy type 1 has been reported between 25% to 80%. Although it has been hypothesized that both the pharynx and the striated and smooth muscles of the esophagus can be involved (Rönnblom and Danielsson 2004), the histologic data published to date has failed to demonstrate any alteration in the esophageal smooth muscle fibers. Manometric studies showed the presence of abnormal esophageal motility (Bellini et al. 2006). Dermatomyositis (Quartier and Gherardi 2013) and merosin deficient muscular dystrophy (Philpot et al. 1999) also may cause dysphagia and feeding problems. Although congenital myopathies or dystrophies are rarely revealed by pharyngeal troubles, myotonic dystrophy type 1 may be revealed by sucking/swallowing disorders causing pharyngeal obstruction with severe respiratory distress (Abadie and Couly 2013).

Different from central neurologic disorders, dysphagia in NMDs accompanies solid rather than liquid intake. Symptoms of dysphagia are several: prolonged meal times (>30 min) or meal times accompanied by fatigue, difficulty starting swallowing, discomfort during swallowing, sensation of food blocked in the throat, difficulty swallowing saliva, coughing during meals, loss of appetite, unintentional weight loss, increased occurrence of chest infections and choking episodes (Bushby et al. 2010b, Toussaint et al. 2016). These symptoms may not be clinically evident, may be unreported by the patients/parents unless they are systemically asked using a questionnaire such as the Sydney Swallowing Questionnaire (Wallace et al. 2000, van den Engel-Hoek et al. 2015). However, laryngeal food penetration, accumulation of food residue in the pharynx and/or true laryngeal food aspiration may occur. Silent aspiration is common in children with neurologic impairment and developmental delay. The prevalence of these issues in DMD is likely underestimated (Toussaint et al. 2016).

Dysphagia can be diagnosed on the basis of symptoms, clinical signs or diagnostic tests, such as esophageal manometry, video fluoroscopic swallow study (VFSS; modified barium swallow) and endoscopic examination. Esophageal manometry does not provide useful information regarding aspiration and technical problems limit its usefulness. Endoscopic examination of the larynx and hypopharynx provides a direct view of them and can identify related problems. Videofluoroscopy allows accurate assessment of all phases of swallowing, evaluation of therapeutic strategies, such as adapted food texture and positioning and detects silent aspiration more accurately (Bushby et al. 2010b, Wang et al. 2007). Surface electromyography may be used for diagnosis and monitoring (Archer et al. 2013b). The absence of a cough or overt clinical sign during swallowing in a child with respiratory problems suggests silent aspiration and it is difficult to detect during clinical evaluation.

Dysphagia associated with inflammatory NMDs can generally be effectively treated using immunosuppressant therapy. The treatment interventions for dysphagia include dietary manipulation (altering the consistency of food and liquids by adding appropriate dietary supplements), changing posture during swallowing, effortful swallowing, double swallows, increasing sensory input (altering bolus taste, flavor, temperature), exercises to increase oral motor function, pharmacological (baclofen, botox), surgical interventions and enteral feeding. In patients with muscular dystrophy, solid food causes the most oral phase problems and pharyngeal post-swallow residue. In this patient group, simple measures such as adjusting meals in terms of less solid food, and drinking water after meals to clear the oropharyngeal area can be taken. Treatment of dysphagia also includes the treatment of GERD if present, blood gas normalization, high-caloric diet for patients with unintentional weight loss, gastrostomy, noninvasive tracheal clearance techniques, and tracheostomy. Surgical options are cricopharyngeal myotomy, oesophageal dilatation and botulinum injection of the cricopharyngeus muscle. However, most of the evidence has been obtained from studies of neurogenic dysphagia. Unfortunately, there is currently no evidence from randomized controlled studies on these interventions for dysphagia in muscle disease (Davis et al. 2015; Jones et al. 2016; Toussaint et al. 2016, van den Engel-Hoek et al. 2013).

STOMACH

Delayed gastric emptying is common in children with NMDs, and may precede gastro-intestinal symptoms in children with progressive muscular dystrophy (Barohn et al. 1988; Haensch et al. 2011; Wang et al. 2012). Symptoms suggestive of slow gastric emptying are nausea, early satiety, epigastric pain and vomiting/regurgitation (Rönnblom and Danielsson 2004). Gastric emptying time is significantly more delayed in both DMD and Becker muscular dystrophy than in controls and worsens at the follow-up in DMD. Gastric dysrhythmias, mainly tachygastria, are also higher in muscular dystrophies compared to controls. Abnormalities in gastric motility are due to deranged regulatory mechanisms. Contractile activity of smooth muscle cells seems to be preserved (Borrelli et al. 2005).

Metoclopramide, 0.8mg/kg body weight divided into three doses (maximum 10mg three times a day), may improve gastric emptying of both liquid and solid food. Erythromycin has no effect on gastric emptying (Rönnblom and Danielsson 2004).

Dermatomyositis may cause gastritis (Quartier and Gherardi 2013). Concomitant use of nonsteroidal anti-inflammatory drugs with steroids may increase the risk of gastro-intestinal ulceration. It is a common practice to prescribe PPIs for patients receiving corticosteroid therapy to prevent complications including gastritis, peptic ulcers and to prevent reflux.

Although case reports on gastric dilatation were reported in the 1990s, there is no data in recent reports (Rönnblom and Danielsson 2004). Fig. 26.1 **A** shows a patient with SMA presenting with excess abdominal air. Gastric perforation due to gastric wall weakness has also been reported (Dinan et al. 2003).

CONSTIPATION

Constipation can be defined as infrequent and/or painful defecation, fecal incontinence, and abdominal pain. In healthy children, the normal frequency of defecation is more than two per week (Tabbers et al. 2014). Constipation is almost inevitable in children with mobility impairment. Factors responsible for constipation in NMDs are colonic hypomotility, immobility, weakness of abdominal wall muscles and inadequate fluid and fiber intake (Boland et al. 1996; Messina et al. 2008; Wang et al. 2007). The decreased physical activity results in prolonged gastro-intestinal transit time, which causes hard, dry stool and decreased frequency of defecation. Despite the findings of one study (Kraus et al. 2016), it is usually considered that risk of constipation increases with age and degree of immobility. More than 50% of children with DMD have constipation (Pane et al. 2006; Skalsky and Dalal 2015).

On abdominal examination, abdominal fullness or distention, hyperactive bowel sounds and palpable fecal mass can be detected. The presence of any abnormal finding on exam is specific, but not sensitive (Kraus et al. 2016). Plain abdominal X-ray may help to show fecal impaction (Fig. 26.1 **B**).

Constipation treatment should be individualized to each patient. The treatment of constipation starts with adequate fluid and fiber intake. But, extra fiber supplements and fluid intake more than the requirement are not recommended. The first step is fecal disimpaction. Poly-ethylene glycol and enemas are equally effective for fecal disimpaction. The use of poly-ethylene glycol with or without electrolytes orally or via a feeding tube 1 to 1.5g/kg/day for 3 to 6 days is recommended as the first-line treatment for children presenting with fecal impaction. An enema once per day for 3 to 6 days is recommended for children with

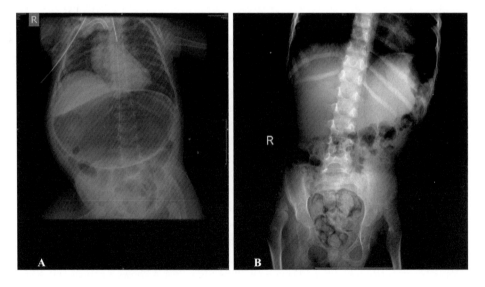

**Fig. 26.1. A** Excess air and gastric dilatation in a patient with spinal muscular atrophy. **B** Plain abdominal X-ray showing fecal impaction in a patient with Ullrich congenital muscular dystrophy

fecal impaction, if poly-ethylene glycol is not available or can not be administered. The usual recommended doses of rectal laxatives/enemas for children with functional constipation are 5mg once/day in children 2–10 years of age and 5–10mg once/day in children older than 10 years of age for bisacodyl, 60ml (<6 years) or 120ml (>6 years) for sodium docusate, 2.5ml/kg (maximum 133ml/dose) for sodium phosphate, and 30–60ml once day (2–11 years) or 60–150ml once/day (>11 years) for mineral oil. For maintenance therapy, poly-ethylene glycol (0.2–0.8g/kg/day) is more effective compared to lactulose (1–2g/kg, once or twice/day), milk of magnesia (0.4–1.2g/day for 2–5 years, 1.2–2.4g/day for 6–11 years, 2.4–4.8g/day for 12–18 years, once or divided), or mineral oil (1–3ml/kg/day, once or divided, maximum 90ml/day). Lactulose is considered to be safe for all ages. For these reasons, lactulose is recommended where poly-ethylene glycol is not available. But, lactulose may cause bloating. The use of milk of magnesia, mineral oil, and stimulant laxatives may be considered as an additional or second-line treatment. Evidence does not support the use of pre- or probiotics in the treatment of constipation (Tabbers et al. 2014). Bulk-forming agents, such as guar gum, bran, methycellulose, psyllium, should be used cautiously because they can lead to impaction in patients with decreased peristalsis. Most importantly, mineral oil may cause aspiration and pneumonia in patients with swallowing difficulty (Wang et al. 2010). Treatment with laxatives and enemas may cause severe metabolic acidosis resulting from the intestinal loss of bicarbonate (Lo Cascio et al. 2014).

OTHERS

Although constipation is more common in patients with NMDs, diarrhea, particularly in patients with myotonic dystrophy type 1, is seen more frequently than in comparison groups. Bile acid malabsorption, small bowel bacterial overgrowth due to reduced peristaltic activity and reduced levels of pancreatic isoamlylase may be the possible causes of diarrhea. Antibiotics and cholestyramine, a bile acid sequestrant, may be effective in treating diarrhea (Bellini et al. 2006; Rönnblom and Danielsson 2004). Dermatomyositis may cause pancreatitis, anorexia and malabsorption (Quartier and Gherardi 2013).

Meterorism may be seen in one-forth of the patients. Use of lactulose for constipation treatment may cause meteorism (Messina et al. 2008; Pane et al. 2006).

Loss of normal haustration in the colon, and jejunal and ileal dilatation have been reported (Karasick et al. 1982). All of them can be seen in muscular dystrophies, including myotonic dystrophy. In some patients with dermatomyositis colitis with a risk of perforation may develop (Quartier and Gherardi 2013). Megacolon, sigmoid volvulus and segmental narrowing have been reported in patients with myotonic dystrophy (Bellini et al. 2006). In episodes of gastro-enteritis, myotonic dystrophy patients may have recurrent intestinal pseudo-obstruction. Congenital myopathies may cause intestinal pseudo-obstruction a few days after birth and be dependent on parenteral nutrition (Giordano et al. 2009).

Anal incontinence, colonic dilatation and increased risk of gallstones have been reported associated with myotonic dystrophy type 1 (Rönnblom and Danielsson 2004). Dyschezia and fecal incontinence have frequently been reported in patients with myotonic dystrophy (Bellini et al. 2006).

## Feeding and nutrition

NUTRITIONAL ASSESSMENT

Nutritional assessment in children includes a thorough history and a complete physical examination. Laboratory evaluations are rarely used to assess nutritional status in daily practice.

History should include nutritional, medical and growth histories. The quantity and quality of food consumed and recent changes in intake of food, degree of dependency on a caregiver and the length of a typical meal must be asked. It is also very helpful to obtain a 3 to 5 day record of food intake. The child must be observed while eating and the amount of spilling, signs of oromotor dysfunction and dysphagia, symptoms of aspiration, should be recorded. Stress associated with meals and the interaction between the child and caregiver/family at meal times should be seen. Medical and family histories should also be taken: chronic respiratory problems, constipation, physical activity level, medications (child's and mother's if the child is breastfeeding), socio-economic condition of the family, sibling number, etc. (Wang et al. 2007).

Weight, length (<2 years of age)/height (>2 years of age) and head circumference (in children <3 years of age) must be measured at each visit and be plotted on appropriate growth charts. By using appropriate growth charts a child's growth is compared with population-based normative data.

In children with NMDs, measurement of height may be impossible due to spinal deformity, neuromuscular weakness, wheelchair dependency and lower limb deformities. Measurements of arm span, ulna height, tibial length, upper limb and knee height have been used to predict the height by using special prediction equations and growth charts (Davidson and Truby 2009).

After obtaining weight and length/height, weight for age, length/height for age, weight for length/height, body mass index (BMI: weight in kg ÷ squared length/height in meters), and Z-scores (standard deviation score) are calculated. BMI is now accepted as the best choice for assessing body weight relative to height in children over 2 years of age. For healthy children and adolescents, recommended BMI for age cutoffs are: ≥95th percentile; obese, 85th to <95th percentile; risk of obesity, 5th to <85th percentile; normal, and <5th percentile; underweight. However, there have been no anthropometric standards established for many disabling conditions. Although a specific growth chart for patients with DMD has been proposed (Griffiths and Edwards 1988), there are no widely accepted growth charts designed for patients with muscular dystrophies and SMA. World Health Organization (WHO) growth charts can be used for children aged 0–24 (or 60) months, and WHO or valid national growth charts can be used for older patients in clinical settings (Davis et al. 2015; Tinggaard et al. 2014).

The definition of failure to thrive (FTT) is still controversial. It is generally based on a decline in nutritional status that is related to clinical endpoints. In clinical practice, weight for age <5th percentile, weight for length/height <5th percentile, decreased growth velocity (a decrease of 2 or more weight percentile over 3–6 months), ≤80% ideal body weight can be used (Joosten and Hulst 2011).

Serum albumin, transthyretin, hemoglobin, iron and trace elements such as zinc are useful laboratory indicators and should be measured periodically or when needed. Acute phase proteins indicate inflammation. Most common methods used to measure body composition are dual-energy X-ray absorptiometry (DEXA), bioelectrical impedance analysis (BIA), and magnetic resonance imaging (MRI) (Wiskin et al. 2015).

GROWTH AND NUTRITIONAL STATUS

Observations of the natural evolution of weight status in SMA patients show that growth failure is nearly universal in type 1 and common in type 2. Age at disease onset determines the rapidity of the development of growth failure. Most late onset (>6 months) patients avoided growth failure (Sproule et al. 2012). Body weight and/or body weight Z-score is consistently low to normal (Moore et al. 2016) and one study demonstrated a significant decrease in weight Z-score, correlated with inadequacy of energy intake, over a 3-year time frame (Mehta et al. 2016). Standardized growth charts may overestimate FTT status in SMA type 1 (Poruk et al. 2012). The presence of feeding and swallowing difficulties in SMA type 3 is significantly related to low body weight. Reported length/height measurements are largely normal in SMA patients (Moore et al. 2016).

The results of BMI measures are controversial. BMI is not an adequate measure of obesity or underweight, and a normal BMI for age likely does not represent the ideal weight for children with SMA (Skalsky and Dalal 2015). The use of standard BMI percentiles obtained from cohorts of normal persons underestimates total body fat in these patients, and thus underestimates overweight, a potentially important modifiable source of morbidity (Sproule et al. 2009; Wang et al. 2007). The body composition in children with SMA is altered by decreased fat free mass (FFM), and they may have adequate fat mass (FM) despite being significantly underweight based on standard growth charts and percentiles.

Bone mineral density (BMD) is also reduced in SMA populations, although one study found that it was normal in 83% of participants. Ambulatory status significantly impacted on BMD (Moore et al. 2016).

At birth, weight and length in DMD are similar to healthy infants. A retrospective study describing the natural evolution of weight status in DMD patients born before 1992 showed that 73% were obese and 4% underweight at the age of 13 years. Obesity at the age of 13 years was associated with later obesity, whereas normal weight status and underweight predicted later underweight. BMI for age between the 10th and 85th percentile on national percentile charts or mild obesity (weight for age ratio between 120 and 150%) in 13-year old DMD patients should be encouraged because it prevents later underweight (Bushby et al. 2010b, Martigne et al. 2011).

Although overweight is already a phenomenon in DMD independent of steroid use (Davis et al. 2015), the early introduction of steroids has altered the natural course of the disease and can exacerbate weight gain (Davidson and Truby 2009). In a longitudinal study, the highest prevalence of obesity based on the BMI Z-score in children with DMD, 72% of whom currently or previously using steroids, was 50% at the age of 10 years. Longitudinally, BMI Z-scores from the age of 2 to 12 years were above the mean, after which there was a marked and progressive decline. BMI was associated with age, ambulatory status and lung function (Davidson et al. 2014). Weight loss and undernutrition becomes a greater concern around age 18 years (Davis et al. 2015).

BMI as a screen for obesity is not accurate in boys with DMD because it tends to be higher due to increased fat mass. Measurement of body composition may give information on whether weight gain is due to the increase of fat mass or muscle mass (Davidson and Truby 2009; Davis et al. 2015). In DMD patients, bioelectrical impedance analysis (BIA) is a more accurate way to estimate body composition compared to skin-fold thickness, which overestimates FFM and underestimates the percentage of fat mass (Mok et al. 2010). Lean body mass is correlated with muscle function. Steroid treatment increases not only weight but also muscle mass (Moxley et al. 2005). This finding suggests that body composition be measured as a routine part of nutrition assessment and monitoring.

The Z-scores for height for children with DMD are lower compared to healthy children and those receiving corticosteroid treatment are shorter than those who are not. From the ages 14 to 17 years, there is a marked decrease in height Z-scores (Biggar et al. 2006; Davidson et al. 2014; Davidson and Truby 2009). Although factors, such as low human growth hormone level and reduced muscle tone leading to poor bone turnover, have been suggested causes of short stature, the exact etiology of short stature is not known yet (Davis et al. 2015).

Boys with DMD have lower BMD measurements. The differences between DMD boys and typically developing children increase with age. DMD boys also have reduced bone turnover, low vitamin D levels but high leptin levels in comparison with the comparison group (Söderpalm et al. 2007).

Different from the muscular dystrophies, the ratio of being underweight in congenital myopathies at an early age is 25%. About one-forth of infants with congenital myopathy need nasogastric feeding at birth and about one-fifth of the patients, more than half of them with fundoplication, require gastrostomy tube placement at an average age of 9.5 months (Colombo et al. 2015; Maggi et al. 2013).

Many children with neurologic disabilities have comorbid conditions requiring medication that may affect nutritional status. Nutritional status may also affect the bioavailability and the metabolism of medications. Corticosteroids, combined with decreased mobility, may lead to the development of osteoprosis and may also cause increased appetite, fluid retention and hyperglycemia. Presence of vitamin D deficiency, independent from corticosteroid use, contributes to the development of decreased BMD (Bianchi et al. 2011). Antidepressants may cause weight gain and overweight/obesity by craving for carbohydrates and sweets. Anticonvulsants may decrease vitamin D levels. Diuretics may increase excretion of electrolytes. Mineral oil may interfere with absorption of fat-soluble vitamins and stimulants may cause decreased appetite and growth. Selective serotonin reuptake inhibitors appear less problematic (Serretti and Mandelli 2010).

NUTRITIONAL INTERVENTION STRATEGIES

The first step in the nutritional support spectrum is to increase the quality and quantity of the food consumed. Depending on the nature and the course of the underlying disease, patients may require mealtime support: from minimal, such as cutting up food, to full support by a caregiver. Changing head position may improve the efficiency of swallowing. Energy density of food is increased and taste/flavor of the food is improved. The consistency of food/drink can best be determined on the basis of the results of a swallow study. Simple measures such as adjusting meals in terms of providing less solid food and drinking water after meals to clear the oropharyngeal area can be taken. A collaboration among physicians, dietitians and the child and their parents is required. In selected case and situations, oral nutrition supplements may be prescribed. If oral strategies are unsuccessful or oral feeding is contra-indicated, the second step is enteral strategies, namely tube feeding. In some cases, a combination of oral and enteral feeding may be used (enteral nutrition at nights and oral nutrition at daytime). Parenteral nutrition is rarely required in children with NMDs (Braegger et al. 2010; Davis et al. 2015; Davoodi et al. 2012; Mehta et al. 2016; Moore et al. 2016; Ptomey and Wittenbrook 2015, van den Engel-Hoek et al. 2013; Wang et al. 2007).

ENTERAL NUTRITION (TUBE FEEDING)

Experts and guidelines recommend that a feeding tube be placed if (1) the child has an unsafe swallow and aspirates on the VFSS, (2) mealtimes are always longer than 30 minutes or 3–4 hours/day, (3) the child is not able to feed independently, (4) the child is unable to meet nutritional needs for growth and development, (5) there is weight loss or lack of weight gain for 1 month in children less than 2 years of age or for 3 months in children ≥2 years of age, or (6) there is a decrease of 2 or more weight or height percentiles (Braegger et al. 2010; Bushby et al. 2010b, Davis et al. 2015; Toussaint et al. 2016). Intellectual disability (IQ<70) is frequently seen among patients with DMD and these patients require tube feeding earlier (Mochizuki et al. 2008).

Enteral nutrition (EN) may be given into the stomach or into the jejunum. When the stomach is not preferred for tube feeding because of delayed gastric emptying, dysmotility or reflux symptoms, post-pyloric feeding is required. The placement of nasojejunal or gastrojejunal tubes generally requires fluoroscopy. Complications of jejunal tubes are common; for example, migration from the intestine back into the stomach, occlusion of the tube (Braegger et al. 2010; Roper et al. 2010).

Nasogastric tubes may supplement short-term nutritional needs (less than 2–3 months), or act as a trial for gastric feedings before gastrostomy tube placement. If the problems persist for longer, it is often decided to place a gastrostomy tube (Braegger et al. 2010, van den Engel-Hoek et al. 2015). However, no international guidelines are yet available for optimal timing of gastrostomy, the indication for simultaneous Nissen fundoplication, and optimal nutrition and supplementation in this patient population. There is also no consensus about the optimal time for performing percutaneous endoscopic gastrostomy (PEG) relative to tracheostomy. Tracheostomy may improve swallowing and may delay the need for gastrostomy (Terzi et al. 2010) and may protect the lungs from aspiration by inflating the cuff (Toussaint et al. 2016).

Gastrostomy tube insertion can be performed by laparotomy, laparascopically, endoscopically or radiologically. The most preferred method is insertion of a PEG because it can be placed at the bedside and may be more effective in reducing aspiration than a nasogastric feeding tube (Bushby et al. 2010b, Davis et al. 2015; Toussaint et al. 2016).

Patients and their family should be informed about PEG placement beforehand. Children and their parents may be resistant the idea of PEG feeding, and may refuse this intervention.

Insertion of a feeding tube can be considered as a "terminal event" and that once inserted it is permanent and that the individual can never feed orally again.

Improvement in growth and amelioration of malnutrition, swallowing difficulty and respiratory status are common after gastrostomy tube placement (Ramelli et al. 2007). Although gastrostomy may cause complications such as local infection, leakage, gastro-esophageal reflux (GER), vomiting, tube obstruction and dislodgement, respiratory failure and peritonitis, they are tolerable (Ramelli et al. 2007).

Gastrostomy placement at an appropriate time is advisable in patients with muscular dystrophy (Davidson and Truby 2009; Mizuno et al. 2012). About 20% of DMD children older than 18 years of age have gastrostomy (Pane et al. 2006). When a surgical procedure is needed, nutrition and hydration prior to and after surgery must be optimized (Wang et al. 2010).

All children with SMA type I will be dependent on tube feeding as they get older. The average age of feeding tube placement in SMA patients is 11 months. The benefits of gastrostomy for these infants must be balanced against the risks of anesthesia. Most of these children can be managed well with nasogastric feeds. Gastrostomy may be considered for some infants, but the benefits should be carefully weighed against the risks (Davis et al. 2014; Poruk et al. 2012; Roper et al. 2010; Sproule et al. 2012). There are striking international differences in nutrition support practices, particularly in the variability of feeding tube placement in infants with SMA type 1, which ranged from 0% to 98% (Moore et al. 2016).

Gastrostomy tube placement should be strongly considered in a child with a very severe myopathy in the newborn period. Nasojejunal or gastrojejunal tube may be helpful in the presence of GER. Excessive weight gain must be prevented in these children (Wang et al. 2012).

Although there are controversial reports (Thomson et al. 2011), it is generally considered that gastrostomy placement in children with neurological impairment does not increase the number of children with GERD and does not influence GER indices (Kawahara et al. 2014; Toporowska-Kowalska et al. 2011; Vandenplas et al. 2009). Some centers advocate a proactive simultaneous gastrostomy and Nissen fundoplication procedures, whereas others advocate simple percutaneous gastrostomy or jejunostomy without further procedures. Underlying respiratory problems, risk of aspiration, advice of the surgeon and pediatric anesthesiologist must be considered to chose the safest procedure in children with congenital dystrophies (Wang et al. 2010). With appropriate gastrostomy-delivered feed management, it is rare to require fundoplication in infants with severe SMA type 1. In patients with frequent chest infection and documented GERD, laparoscopic Nissen fundoplication during gastrostomy tube placement under noninvasive ventilation is well tolerated and improves patients' growth and decreases the number of chest infection in children with SMA type 1 and severe SMA type 2 (Durkin et al. 2008; Yuan et al. 2007). However, although Nissen is intended to reduce reflux symptoms, it is not always fully protective (Davis et al. 2014). There is no published literature to support gastrostomy over nasogastric feeding, although there is one report of a small series of infants with severe SMA type 1 having survived gastrostomy (Roper et al. 2010).

Tube feeds may be given as boluses, intermittent or continuous. The mode of infusion is dependent on the patient's clinical status. For ambulatory children who have scheduled daily activities, bolus feeds are preferred because they allow more freedom. A child with high-caloric needs or with significant respiratory impairment and poor tolerance to volume may benefit from a combination of daytime boluses and nocturnal continuous feeds. Feeds given via a naso-jejunal tube should always be given by continuous infusion, not by bolus (Braegger et al. 2010; Roper et al. 2010).

NUTRITIONAL REQUIREMENTS

The daily nutrient needs are fluid, electrolytes/minerals, energy (macronutrients; carbohydrate and fat), protein, and vitamins. Until more specific data are available, nutrient intake should meet the daily recommended intakes (DRI) for age. Daily fluid requirements of patients with DMD and SMA are no different from healthy children. Fluid requirement can be calculated based on the patient's weight (100ml/kg body weight for 1–10kg, 50ml/kg body weight for 11–20kg, and 20ml/kg body weight for >20kg) but may be individualized as needed (Davis et al. 2015). Fluid losses by sweating and excess salivary losses, particularly if there is frequent suctioning, increase in children with severe SMA and must be replaced (Roper et al. 2010).

It is fundamental to predict the required energy needs of patients with DMD prior to weight management, and energy requirement changes with age and the clinical situation of the patients. Dependence on mechanical ventilation and wheelchairs decrease energy need and the use of corticosteroids early makes its prediction complicated. Currently, the best method is indirect calorimetry, but it is not widely available and is not easily applicable in clinical settings. When measuring resting energy expenditure (REE) is not possible, predictive equations may be used. Currently, there are no any predictive equations to estimate energy needs in patients with DMD. It has been shown that the Schofield weight equation was the most accurate and precise equation in children with DMD (Elliott et al. 2012). Another alternative is to use 80% of the DRI (https://fnic.nal.usda.gov/dietary-guidance/dietary-reference-intakes) for ambulatory patients and 70% of the DRI for nonambulatory ones. Individual longitudinal monitoring of body weight helps to adjust energy supply (Davidson and Truby 2009; Davis et al. 2015). Individualized energy requirements can be predicted using the equation: total energy expenditure = REE (measured if possible) × physical activity level. The development of obesity is not primarily due to a low REE but to other causes such as a reduction in physical activity and or overfeeding. Excess weight gain must be prevented by providing adequate energy prior to prescribing steroid therapy. Reduction of energy intake may decrease muscle mass and must be done cautiously. As the patient with DMD ages, the aim of nutrition intervention changes from prevention of weight gain to prevention of undernutrition (Davidson and Truby 2009).

Similar to infants with DMD, predictive equations have not been validated for infants with SMA type 1, either. These children have reduced lean body mass and lower energy expenditure compared with other infants of similar age and weight. The caloric intake relative to age-matched recommended daily allowance (RDA) recommendations in kcal/kg decreases from infancy to 3 years and there is little increase in caloric need with increasing age. Caloric intake is not associated with FTT, normal, or obese status based on growth chart evaluation. Progressive weight gain across percentiles can occur even without any increase in calories in some children. Energy prescription in these children must be guided by indirect calorimetry where available. The energy needs of patients with SMA are significantly lower than those predicted by standard equations and even modest caloric increases may cause dramatic weight gain. The lack of association between growth percentile categories and daily caloric intake indicates that standardized growth charts may not be adequate for determining healthy weight status in this population (Mehta et al. 2016; Poruk et al. 2012; Roper et al. 2010; Sproule et al. 2012; Wang et al. 2007).

In healthy children, more than half of the daily energy expenditure must come from carbohydrates, with no more than 25% of calories derived from simple sugars/sweeteners. Energy from lipids should not exceed 35% (preferably 30%) of total energy. The remaining 15–20% of total energy must be received from protein. In children younger than 2 years of age, fat and cholesterol should not be restricted because of high energy requirements (IMMNA 2002). Unless a different composition of macronutrients is indicated, the composition of nutrients can be the same composition as that for healthy children.

There is no data suggesting that patients with DMD require additional protein. Protein intake must meet the DRI for age and 10–30% of total daily calories should be achieved from protein in patients 4–18 years of age (Davis et al. 2015). Many patients with SMA also exhibit metabolic abnormalities consistent with a secondary fatty acid oxidation disorder, which may be related to mitochondrial dysfunction. Dietary treatment such as a high-carbohydrate/low-fat diet or use of medium-chain triglycerides can ameliorate effects of this abnormality (Davis et al. 2014; Wang et al. 2007).

In children with SMA type 1, vitamin D, calcium and magnesium intakes are strong predictors of increased BMD while intakes of alpha-linolenic acid, linoleic acid, vitamin A, vitamin D, vitamin E, vitamin K, folate, calcium, iron, and magnesium are frequently below DRI recommended ranges. Thus, multivitamin and mineral supplementation to meet DRIs should be considered in children with SMA type I, especially for bone-related nutrients (Mehta et al. 2016; Moore et al. 2016; Poruk et al. 2012). Tube feeding increases the energy intake, but micronutrient intake such as vitamin D may be suboptimal. Future studies describing optimal nutrient requirements and body composition variables in this group are required. Assessment of nutritional intake by a dietitian or other healthcare provider proficient in nutrition is recommended at each visit. Analysis should target the adequacy of the macronutrient (including fiber intake) as well as micronutrient intake (Mehta et al. 2016; Poruk et al. 2012; Wang et al. 2007).

Vitamin D deficiency or insufficiency is prevalent in boys with DMD and the long-term use of corticosteroid treatment increases the risk of osteopeni/osteoprosis. Adequate vitamin D and calcium supplementation must be given to prevent the development of bone disease (Davis et al. 2015). Usual maintenance daily doses of 400–800IU may be insufficient and at least 1 000–1 500IU vitamin D and calcium (750mg/day) should be supplemented (Alshaikh et al. 2016; Davidson and Truby 2009). In patients with vitamin D deficiency, a 3-month replacement regimen of daily cholecalciferol 6 000IU before starting the maintenance regimen appeared to be effective in achieving optimal vitamin D levels without resulting in toxic levels (Alshaikh et al. 2016).

DIET TYPE

Before 12 months of age, an infant formula should be used. In patients with high-caloric needs or with poor tolerance to increased formula volume, the energy density of the formula may be increased by adding modular nutrients or a high-caloric commercial formula may be used. After 12 months of age, a pediatric 1kcal/ml formula is preferred. A 1.5kcal/ml formula may be used with careful monitoring of hydration status. Fiber-containing formulas are often used to alleviate constipation but may lead to abdominal bloating. Adult formulas should be avoided before 10 years of age because of inadequate calorie-to-nutrient ratio for children. Most children will tolerate a polymeric formula, but some children may require a semi-elemental or elemental formula. Despite its frequent use there are no well-designed prospective studies investigating the use of the elemental diet in children with NMDs. The benefits of the diet reported by parents were anecdotal (Moore et al. 2016; Poruk et al. 2012; Sproule et al. 2012, van den Engel-Hoek et al. 2016; Wang et al. 2007).

NUTRACEUTICALS AND PHARMACONUTRIENTS

Complementary and alternative medicine is frequently used among the DMD patient population and families should be informed about its use. The evidence to support the use of nutraceuticals in patients with DMD is limited (Davidson and Truby 2009).

Short- and medium-term creatine treatment improves muscle strength in patients with muscular dystrophies but not in metabolic myopathies (Kley et al. 2007; Tarnopolsky et al. 2004; 2007). Currently, no recommendations for the use of creatine is established, and in patients with evidence of renal dysfunction it must be discontinued (Bushby et al. 2010a). Creatine supplementation is not effective in SMA (Moore et al. 2016). Although safe, supplemental glutamine does not appear to improve muscle strength or function in DMD children (Mok and Hankard 2011). Other nutraceuticals including l-arginine, green tea extract, leucine (an essential branched-chain amino acid), taurine, protandim, coenzyme $Q_{10}$, vitamin E, fish oil, herbal or botanical agents and others are being used by some parents, but there is no supportive data. Therefore, their use is not recommended by experts (Bushby et al. 2010a, Davis et al. 2015; Davoodi et al. 2012).

Metformin has been used for weight management in obese patients with pediatric NMDs, and has shown positive effects on weight management and reduced metabolic syndrome. Metformin is dosed as low as 425mg daily in younger children and can be increased up to 1 000mg two times daily. The patient must be monitored by an expert dietitian/nutritionist in DMD (Bushby et al. 2010b).

In children with DMD, topiramate has also been used for weight management. However, its use for weight control is controversial (Carter et al. 2005). Prevention of excess weight gain is preferable to severe restriction in the already obese, but the potential muscle loss associated with negative energy balance must be taken into consideration (Griffiths and Edwards 1988).

Supplements to provide more than the dietary recommended intake for vitamin, mineral, protein, or fat should be discouraged. In any case, each child should be evaluated individually on a routine basis, with the goal of following their established growth curves and avoiding inadequate or excessive intake.

**Key points**

- Gastro-intestinal complications are common in patients with NMDs and almost half of patients have at least one gastro-intestinal problem.
- Each part of the gastro-intestinal system may be affected in NMDs. Oropharyngeal and dental problems, gastro-esophageal reflux disease, gastro-intestinal dysmotility, peptic ulcer disease and abdominal pain, bloating, constipation and related problems are common and may make life unbearable for the family and the patient.
- Although gastro-intestinal complications rarely cause life-threatening events, they lower quality of life of the patients and their parents/care givers. Digestive tract symptoms and signs must be investigated in every patient and treated if present.
- Feeding difficulties are frequently seen in children with NMDs, and their prevalence increases with age.
- The presence of feeding and gastro-intestinal problems have a negative effect on nutrient intake and may lead to the development of underfeeding. On the other hand, immobility and weakness may cause obesity.
- The growth of the patients should therefore be monitored carefully to prevent the development of undernutrition or overnutrition.

**Clinical vignette**

A 10-month-old girl with SMA type 1 was referred to our clinic with fever and difficulty in breathing for 7 days. Pneumonia was diagnosed. Her body weight was 6 000g (−2.34 Standard Deviation Score; Z-score), length 69cm (Z-score 0.14), and weight for length (WfL) Z-score −3.26. She was treated appropriately. Feeding difficulty, swallowing dysfunction (aspiration) and growth retardation led to a nasogastric (NG) tube insertion. Tube feeding commenced (100kcal/kg/day) with a standard formula of 1kcal/ml. Two weeks later she was rehospitalized because of pneumonia and underwent tracheostomy.

On follow-up with nasogastric tube, her anthropometric measurements improved and at 22 months of age her weight, length and WfL Z-scores were −1.26, −0.83 and −1.16, respectively. On the same day a gastrostomy tube was placed and she continued to receive 100kcal/kg/day with 1kcal/ml enteral formula. At 30 months of age her weight, height and body mass index (BMI) Z-scores were −0.42, −0.62 and −0.21, respectively. Energy intake was reduced to 90kcal/kg/day. At 3 years of age her weight, height and BMI Z-scores were 1.97, −0.16 and 2.88, respectively, denoting obesity. Her caloric intake reduced to 75kcal/kg/day to prevent more weight gain.

Comment

SMA type 1 children have reduced lean body mass and lower energy expenditure. The caloric intake relative to age-matched recommendations in kcal/kg decreases from infancy to 3 years and there is little increase in caloric need with increasing age. For the patient discussed here, she gained weight progressively and became obese within 6 months. The energy needs of children with SMA are significantly lower than those predicted by standard equations and even modest caloric increases may cause dramatic weight gain. Energy prescription in these children must be guided by indirect calorimetry where available.

# REFERENCES

Abadie V, Couly G (2013) Congenital feeding and swallowing disorders. *Handb Clin Neurol* 113: 1539–1549.

Alshaikh N, Brunklaus A, Davis T, Robb SA, Quinlivan R, Munot P et al. (2016) Vitamin D in cortico-steroid-naïve and corticosteroid-treated Duchenne muscular dystrophy: what dose achieves optimal 25(OH) vitamin D levels? *Arch Dis Child* 101: 957–961.

Archer SK, Garrod R, Hart N, Miller S (2013b). Dysphagia in Duchenne muscular dystrophy assessed objectively by surface electromyography. *Dysphagia* 28: 188–198.

Balasubramaniam R, Sollecito TP, Stoopler ET (2008) Oral health considerations in muscular dystrophies. *Spec Care Dentist* 28: 243–253.

Barohn RJ, Levine EJ, Olson JO, Mendell JR (1988) Gastric hypomotility in Duchenne's muscular dystrophy. *N Engl J Med* 319: 15–18.

Bellini M, Biagi S, Stasi C, Costa F, Mumolo MG, Ricchiuti A et al. (2006) Gastrointestinal manifestations in myotonic muscular dystrophy. *World J Gastroenterol* 12: 1821–1828.

Bianchi ML, Biggar D, Bushby K, Rogol AD, Rutter MM, Tseng B (2011) Endocrine aspects of Duchenne muscular dystrophy. *Neuromuscul Disord* 21: 298–303.

Biggar WD, Harris VA, Eliasoph L, Alman B (2006) Long-term benefits of deflazacort treatment for boys with Duchenne muscular dystrophy in their second decade. *Neuromuscul Disord* 16: 249–255.

Boland BJ, Silbert PL, Groover RV, Wollan PC, Silverstein MD (1996) Skeletal, cardiac, and smooth muscle failure in Duchenne muscular dystrophy. *Pediatr Neurol* 14: 7–12.

Borrelli O, Salvia G, Mancini V, Santoro L, Tagliente F, Romeo EF et al. (2005) Evolution of gastric electrical features and gastric emptying in children with Duchenne and Becker muscular dystrophy. *Am J Gastroenterol* 100: 695–702.

Braegger C, Decsi T, Dias JA, Hartman C, Kolacek S, Koletzko B et al. (2010) Practical approach to paediatric enteral nutrition: a comment by the ESPGHAN committee on nutrition. *J Pediatr Gastroenterol Nutr* 51: 110–122.

Bushby K, Finkel R, Birnkrant DJ, Case LE, Clemens PR, Cripe L et al. (2010a). Diagnosis and management of Duchenne muscular dystrophy, part 1: diagnosis, and pharmacological and psychosocial management. *Lancet Neurol* 9: 77–93.

Bushby K, Finkel R, Birnkrant DJ, Case LE, Clemens PR, Cripe L et al. (2010b). Diagnosis and management of Duchenne muscular dystrophy, part 2: implementation of multidisciplinary care. *Lancet Neurol* 9: 177–189.

Camelo AL, Awad RA, Madrazo A, Aguilar F (1997) Esophageal motility disorders in Mexican patients with Duchenne's muscular dystrophy. *Acta Gastroenterol Latinoam* 27: 119–122.

Carter GT, Yudkowsky MP, Han JJ, McCrory MA (2005) Topiramate for weight reduction in Duchenne muscular dystrophy. *Muscle Nerve* 31: 788–789.

Colombo I, Scoto M, Manzur AY, Robb SA, Maggi L, Gowda V et al. (2015) Congenital myopathies: natural history of a large pediatric cohort. *Neurology* 84: 28–35.

Davidson ZE, Truby H (2009) A review of nutrition in Duchenne muscular dystrophy. *J Hum Nutr Diet* 22: 383–393.

Davidson ZE, Ryan MM, Kornberg AJ, Sinclair K, Cairns A, Walker KZ et al. (2014) Observations of body mass index in Duchenne muscular dystrophy: a longitudinal study. *Eur J Clin Nutr* 68: 892–897.

Davis RH, Godshall BJ, Seffrood E, Marcus M, LaSalle BA, Wong B et al. (2014) Nutritional practices at a glance: spinal muscular atrophy type I nutrition survey findings. *J Child Neurol* 29: 1467–1472.

Davis J, Samuels E, Mullins L (2015) Nutrition Considerations in Duchenne Muscular Dystrophy. *Nutr Clin Pract* 30: 511–521.

Davoodi J, Markert CD, Voelker KA, Hutson SM, Grange RW (2012) Nutrition strategies to improve physical capabilities in Duchenne muscular dystrophy. *Phys Med Rehabil Clin N Am* 23(1): 187–99, xii–xiii. doi: 10.1016/j.pmr.2011.11.010.

Dinan D, Levine MS, Gordon AR, Rubesin SE, Rombeau JL (2003) Gastric wall weakening resulting in separate perforations in a patient with Duchenne's muscular dystrophy. *AJR Am J Roentgenol* 181: 807–808.

Durkin ET, Schroth MK, Helin M, Shaaban AF (2008) Early laparoscopic fundoplication and gastrostomy in infants with spinal muscular atrophy type I. *J Pediatr Surg* 43: 2031–2037.

Elliott SA, Davidson ZE, Davies PS, Truby H (2012) Predicting resting energy expenditure in boys with Duchenne muscular dystrophy. *Eur J Paediatr Neurol* 16: 631–635.

Giordano C, Powell H, Leopizzi M, De Curtis M, Travaglini C, Sebastiani M et al. (2009) Fatal congenital myopathy and gastrointestinal pseudo-obstruction due to POLG1 mutations. *Neurology* 72: 1103–1105.

Griffiths RD, Edwards RH (1988) A new chart for weight control in Duchenne muscular dystrophy. *Arch Dis Child* 63: 1256–1258.

Haensch CA, Wehe J, Jigalin A, Isenmann S (2011) Gastroparesis in myotonic dystrophy 1. *Clin Auton Res* 21: 125–126.

Institute of Medicine of the National Academies (IMMNA) (2002) *Dietary Reference İntakes for Energy, Carbohydrate, Fat, Fatty Acids, Cholesterol, Protein, Fiber, and Amino Acids*. Washington, DC: National Academies Press.

Jones K, Pitceathly RD, Rose MR, McGowan S, Hill M, Badrising UA et al. (2016) Interventions for dysphagia in long-term, progressive muscle disease. *Cochrane Database Syst Rev* 2: CD004303.

Joosten KF, Hulst JM (2011) Malnutrition in pediatric hospital patients: current issues. *Nutrition* 27: 133–137.

Karasick D, Karasick S, Mapp E (1982) Gastrointestinal radiologic manifestations of proximal spinal muscular atrophy (Kugelberg-Welander syndrome). *J Natl Med Assoc* 74: 475–478.

Kawahara H, Tazuke Y, Soh H, Yoneda A, Fukuzawa M (2014) Does laparoscopy-aided gastrostomy placement improve or worsen gastroesophageal reflux in patients with neurological impairment? *J Pediatr Surg* 49: 1742–1745.

Kley RA, Vorgerd M, Tarnopolsky MA (2007) Creatine for treating muscle disorders. *Cochrane Database Syst Rev* CD004760.

Kraus D, Wong BL, Horn PS, Kaul A (2016) Constipation in Duchenne Muscular Dystrophy: Prevalence, Diagnosis, and Treatment. *J Pediatr* 171: 183–188.

Lo Cascio CM, Latshang TD, Kohler M, Fehr T, Bloch KE (2014) Severe metabolic acidosis in adult patients with Duchenne muscular dystrophy. *Respiration* 87: 499–503.

Maggi L, Scoto M, Cirak S, Robb SA, Klein A, Lillis S et al. (2013) Congenital myopathies – clinical features and frequency of individual subtypes diagnosed over a 5-year period in the United Kingdom. *Neuromuscul Disord* 23: 195–205.

Martigne L, Salleron J, Mayer M, Cuisset JM, Carpentier A, Neve V et al. (2011) Natural evolution of weight status in Duchenne muscular dystrophy: a retrospective audit. *Br J Nutr* 105: 1486–1491.

Mehta NM, Newman H, Tarrant S, Graham RJ (2016) Nutritional status and nutrient intake challenges in children with spinal muscular atrophy. *Pediatr Neurol* 57: 80–83.

Messina S, Pane M, De Rose P, Vasta I, Sorleti D, Aloysius A et al. (2008) Feeding problems and malnutrition in spinal muscular atrophy type II. *Neuromuscul Disord* 18: 389–393.

Mizuno T, Komaki H, Sasaki M, Takanoha S, Kuroda K, Kon K et al. (2012) Efficacy and tolerance of gastrostomy feeding in Japanese muscular dystrophy patients. *Brain Dev* 34: 756–762.

Mochizuki H, Miyatake S, Suzuki M, Shigeyama T, Yatabe K, Ogata K et al. (2008) Mental retardation and lifetime events of Duchenne muscular dystrophy in Japan. *Intern Med* 47: 1207–1210.

Mok E, Hankard R (2011) Glutamine supplementation in sick children: is it beneficial? *J Nutr Metab* 2011: 617597.

Mok E, Letellier G, Cuisset JM, Denjean A, Gottrand F, Hankard R (2010) Assessing change in body composition in children with Duchenne muscular dystrophy: anthropometry and bioelectrical impedance analysis versus dual-energy X-ray absorptiometry. *Clin Nutr* 29: 633–638.

Moore GE, Lindenmayer AW, McConchie GA, Ryan MM, Davidson ZE (2016) Describing nutrition in spinal muscular atrophy: A systematic review. *Neuromuscul Disord* 26: 395–404.

Moxley RT III, Ashwal S, Pandya S, Connolly A, Florence J, Mathews K et al. (2005) Practice parameter: corticosteroid treatment of Duchenne dystrophy: report of the Quality Standards Subcommittee of the American Academy of Neurology and the Practice Committee of the Child Neurology Society. *Neurology* 64: 13–20.

Pane M, Vasta I, Messina S, Sorleti D, Aloysius A, Sciarra F et al. (2006) Feeding problems and weight gain in Duchenne muscular dystrophy. *Eur J Paediatr Neurol* 10: 231–236.

Philpot J, Bagnall A, King C, Dubowitz V, Muntoni F (1999) Feeding problems in merosin deficient congenital muscular dystrophy. *Arch Dis Child* 80: 542–547.

Poruk KE, Davis RH, Smart AL, Chisum BS, Lasalle BA, Chan GM et al. (2012) Observational study of caloric and nutrient intake, bone density, and body composition in infants and children with spinal muscular atrophy type I. *Neuromuscul Disord* 22: 966–973.

Ptomey LT, Wittenbrook W (2015) Position of the Academy of Nutrition and Dietetics: nutrition services for individuals with intellectual and developmental disabilities and special health care needs. *J Acad Nutr Diet* 115: 593–608.

Quartier P, Gherardi RK (2013) Juvenile dermatomyositis. *Handb Clin Neurol* 113: 1457–1463.

Ramelli GP, Aloysius A, King C, Davis T, Muntoni F (2007) Gastrostomy placement in paediatric patients with neuromuscular disorders: indications and outcome. *Dev Med Child Neurol* 49: 367–371.

Rönnblom A, Danielsson A (2004) Hereditary muscular diseases and symptoms from the gastrointestinal tract. *Scand J Gastroenterol* 39: 1–4.

Roper H, Quinlivan R, Workshop P, Workshop Participants (2010) Implementation of "the consensus statement for the standard of care in spinal muscular atrophy" when applied to infants with severe type 1 SMA in the UK. *Arch Dis Child* 95: 845–849.

Sejerson T, Bushby K, Excellence T-NENO, TREAT-NMD EU Network of Excellence (2009) Standards of care for Duchenne muscular dystrophy: brief TREAT-NMD recommendations. *Adv Exp Med Biol* 652: 13–21.

Serretti A, Mandelli L (2010) Antidepressants and body weight: a comprehensive review and meta-analysis. *J Clin Psychiatry* 71: 1259–1272.

Skalsky AJ, Dalal PB (2015) Common complications of pediatric neuromuscular disorders. *Phys Med Rehabil Clin N Am* 26: 21–28.

Söderpalm AC, Magnusson P, Ahlander AC, Karlsson J, Kroksmark AK, Tulinius M et al. (2007) Low bone mineral density and decreased bone turnover in Duchenne muscular dystrophy. *Neuromuscul Disord* 17: 919–928.

Sproule DM, Montes J, Montgomery M, Battista V, Koenigsberger D, Shen W et al. (2009) Increased fat mass and high incidence of overweight despite low body mass index in patients with spinal muscular atrophy. *Neuromuscul Disord* 19: 391–396.

Sproule DM, Hasnain R, Koenigsberger D, Montgomery M, De Vivo DC, Kaufmann P (2012) Age at disease onset predicts likelihood and rapidity of growth failure among infants and young children with spinal muscular atrophy types 1 and 2. *J Child Neurol* 27: 845–851.

Tabbers MM, DiLorenzo C, Berger MY, Faure C, Langendam MW, Nurko S et al. (2014) Evaluation and treatment of functional constipation in infants and children: evidence-based recommendations from ESPGHAN and NASPGHAN. *J Pediatr Gastroenterol Nutr* 58: 258–274.

Tarnopolsky MA (2007) Clinical use of creatine in neuromuscular and neurometabolic disorders. *Subcell Biochem* 46: 183–204.

Tarnopolsky MA, Mahoney DJ, Vajsar J, Rodriguez C, Doherty TJ, Roy BD et al. (2004) Creatine monohydrate enhances strength and body composition in Duchenne muscular dystrophy. *Neurology* 62: 1771–1777.

Terzi N, Prigent H, Lejaille M, Falaize L, Annane D, Orlikowski D et al. (2010) Impact of tracheostomy on swallowing performance in Duchenne muscular dystrophy. *Neuromuscul Disord* 20: 493–498.

Thomson M, Rao P, Rawat D, Wenzl TG (2011) Percutaneous endoscopic gastrostomy and gastro-ocsophageal reflux in neurologically impaired children. *World J Gastroenterol* 17: 191–196.

Tinggaard J, Aksglaede L, Sørensen K, Mouritsen A, Wohlfahrt-Veje C, Hagen CP et al. (2014) The 2014 Danish references from birth to 20 years for height, weight and body mass index. *Acta Paediatr* 103: 214–224.

Toporowska-Kowalska E, Gębora-Kowalska B, Jabłoński J, Fendler W, Wąsowska-Królikowska K (2011) Influence of percutaneous endoscopic gastrostomy on gastro-oesophageal reflux evaluated by multiple intraluminal impedance in children with neurological impairment. *Dev Med Child Neurol* 53: 938–943.

Toussaint M, Davidson Z, Bouvoie V, Evenepoel N, Haan J, Soudon P (2016) Dysphagia in Duchenne muscular dystrophy: practical recommendations to guide management. *Disabil Rehabil* 38: 2052–2062.

van den Engel-Hoek L, de Groot IJ, Erasmus CE (2016) Comment on "Nutrition Considerations in Duchenne Muscular Dystrophy". *Nutr Clin Pract* 31: 273.

van den Engel-Hoek L, de Groot IJM, de Swart BJM, Erasmus CE (2015) Feeding and swallowing disorders in pediatric neuromuscular diseases: an overview. *J Neuromuscul Dis* 2: 357–369.

van den Engel-Hoek L, Erasmus CE, Hendriks JC, Geurts AC, Klein WM, Pillen S et al. (2013) Oral muscles are progressively affected in Duchenne muscular dystrophy: implications for dysphagia treatment. *J Neurol* 260: 1295–1303.

Vandenplas Y, Rudolph CD, Di Lorenzo C, Hassall E, Liptak G et al. (2009) Pediatric gastroesophageal reflux clinical practice guidelines: joint recommendations of the North American Society for Pediatric

Gastroenterology, Hepatology, and Nutrition (NASPGHAN) and the European Society for Pediatric Gastroenterology, Hepatology, and Nutrition (ESPGHAN). *J Pediatr Gastroenterol Nutr* 49: 498–547. doi: doi.10.1097/MPG.0b013e3181b7f563.

Wallace KL, Middleton S, Cook IJ (2000) Development and validation of a self-report symptom inventory to assess the severity of oral-pharyngeal dysphagia. *Gastroenterology* 118: 678–687.

Wang CH, Finkel RS, Bertini ES, Schroth M, Simonds A, Wong B et al. (2007) Consensus statement for standard of care in spinal muscular atrophy. *J Child Neurol* 22: 1027–1049.

Wang CH, Bonnemann CG, Rutkowski A, Sejersen T, Bellini J, Battista V et al. (2010) Consensus statement on standard of care for congenital muscular dystrophies. *J Child Neurol* 25: 1559–1581.

Wang CH, Dowling JJ, North K, Schroth MK, Sejersen T, Shapiro F et al. (2012) Consensus statement on standard of care for congenital myopathies. *J Child Neurol* 27: 363–382.

Wiskin AE, Johnson MJ, Leaf AA, Wootton SA, Beattie RM (2015) How to use: nutritional assessment in children. *Arch Dis Child Educ Pract Ed* 100: 204–209.

Yuan N, Wang CH, Trela A, Albanese CT (2007) Laparoscopic Nissen fundoplication during gastrostomy tube placement and noninvasive ventilation may improve survival in type I and severe type II spinal muscular atrophy. *J Child Neurol* 22: 727–731.

# Section 7
## Cardiac Management

# 27
# CARDIAC MANAGEMENT IN CHILDREN WITH NEUROMUSCULAR DISORDERS

*Karim Wahbi*

## Introduction

This chapter will focus on cardiac involvement in myopathies, and more particularly on their clinical management (diagnosis and treatment). Cardiac involvement is present in a majority of myopathies, especially in paediatric myopathies. This can be explained by the great similarities between striated skeletal and cardiac muscles. For myopathies of genetic origin, most mutations result in abnormal protein expression in both tissues.

CARDIOMYOPATHY PATTERNS

Cardiac involvement may include abnormalities of the cardiac muscle (myocardial abnormalities), generally predominating in the left ventricle, but not exclusively, since the right ventricle and both atria may also be involved and/or abnormalities of the electrical system presenting conduction defects, supraventricular or ventricular arrhythmia.

Cardiomyopathies are generally classified according to the anatomical and functional abnormalities present in the left ventricle. In myopathies, left ventricular dilatation or hypertrophy (asymmetric, predominating at the septal level or symmetric, generally concentric) can be observed (Fig. 27.1). Some patients may also present with left ventricular non-compaction characterised by deep trabeculations in the ventricular wall that are in direct communication with the ventricular chamber (morphological studies show a two-layered myocardium with a non-compacted inner layer and compacted outer layer). Predominant right ventricular involvement may also be observed. Functional properties of the ventricles may also be present, resulting in an impaired contractility (hypokinetic myocardium) and systolic function (mostly quantified by ventricular ejection fraction) and/or abnormalities of the diastolic properties. Both systolic and diastolic abnormalities can result in clinical signs of heart failure.

Electrical abnormalities may be related to a primary involvement of the electrical system and are frequently in this case the first manifestation of cardiac involvement, which may precede myocardial abnormalities. Arrhythmias may also emerge as a complication of advanced myocardial involvement. For example, atrial fibrillation or ventricular arrhythmias

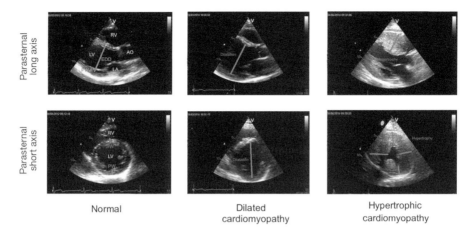

**Fig. 27.1.** Echocardiography patterns of dilated and hypertrophic cardiomyopathy.

may occur in patients with severe left ventricular dysfunction as a result of atrial and ventricular remodelling with fibrosis.

Extremely different patterns of cardiomyopathies may be observed in patients with neuromuscular diseases with several possible combinations of myocardial and electrical abnormalities and several degrees of severity and ages of onset.

Symptoms may differ according to age. The most frequent are dyspnoea, palpitations, lethargy, syncope, and lightheadedness. Clinical presentations are frequently atypical, particularly in the youngest patients, and can appear late in the course of disease.

CARDIAC PROGNOSIS IN MYOPATHIES AND CLINICAL RELEVANCE OF PREVENTIVE MEASURES

While the functional consequences of muscular diseases may be major and represent the most obvious clinical manifestations, cardiac involvement remains frequently asymptomatic until late in the course of the disease. Heart failure symptoms, syncope, palpitations, frequently occur at a stage where myocardial abnormalities are advanced and treatments frequently less efficient. Severe cardiac events (sometimes sudden cardiac death) may represent the first clinical event.

Epidemiological studies show that cardiac complications and respiratory failure represent the two most frequent causes of death in patients with myopathies. These complications may occur in young patients and result in a reduction of life expectancy in this population. The two most frequent modes of cardiac death in patients with myopathies are terminal heart failure, generally due to major left ventricular systolic dysfunction, and sudden death, the underlying mechanisms of which may be major conduction defects (mostly complete atrioventricular blocks) or sustained ventricular tachyarrhythmias (ventricular tachycardia and fibrillation).

The impact of cardiac involvement on survival represents a strong rationale for systematic cardiac screenings, even in asymptomatic patients, which allow an earlier diagnosis of cardiac abnormalities and the use of preventive and curative treatments. In several diseases, the use of preventive measures have proven efficacy on overall survival, prevention of sudden death and significant delay in the development of terminal heart failure. These points will be discussed in sections of the chapter dedicated to disease-specific management. Heart failure prevention relies mostly of specific medications such as angiotensin-converting enzyme inhibitors or beta-adrenergic blockers. The prevention of sudden death frequently requires the implantation of cardiac devices: pacemakers for conduction system disease and cardiac defibrillators (ICDs) for ventricular tachyarrhythmias (ICDs can also treat conduction defects).

TOOLS USED TO DIAGNOSE CARDIOMYOPATHY IN PATIENTS WITH MYOPATHIES

Cardiac evaluation should focus on the diagnosis of myocardial and electrical disease. At the initial diagnosis, an electrocardiogram (ECG) and an echocardiography should be performed in any patient with a myopathy. These two simple and non-invasive examinations provide a global overview of potential cardiac involvement. ECG can identify most of the conduction defects and permanent arrhythmias. Echocardiography can identify most myocardial structural and functional abnormalities. Left ventricular ejection measured by echocardiography remains the standard criterion for the evaluation of heart failure prognosis.

Additional and more accurate myocardial assessments may be useful for early diagnosis and sometimes a better risk stratification in patients with myopathies. Cardiac magnetic resonance imaging (MRI) allows a better characterisation of ventricular diameters, segmental and global contractility (ejection fraction or more accurate parameters such myocardial strain). It can also identify myocardial tissue abnormalities, especially fibrosis which can be detected by late gadolinium enhancement in the myocardial wall or quantified by new techniques such as T1 mapping. One limitation of cardiac MRI in children, besides its availability, is that it may require the use of general anaesthesia, mainly in the youngest.

Several echocardiography techniques have been developed to improve the sensitivity of myocardial contractility assessment and this is based on the evaluation of myocardial deformation. The most frequently used is Speckle tracking, which allows the measurement of myocardial strain, a parameter used to assess the intrinsic contractile properties of the ventricles. The long-term prognostic value of these techniques in cardiomyopathies remains to be demonstrated in large cohorts.

The assessment of arrhythmias may require in-depth investigations, particularly in diseases at high risk for sudden death. Holter-ECG has a better sensitivity than ECG for the diagnosis of arrhythmias, which are in a majority of cases paroxysmal. Electrophysiological study (EPS) is an invasive procedure that allows intracardiac measurement of conduction time intervals and the assessment of susceptibility to ventricular arrhythmias using ventricular stimulation. EPS can be useful in some diseases to clarify indications for cardiac devices such as pacemakers of defibrillators, but relatively scarcely used in paediatric patients.

ADULT-VERSUS PAEDIATRIC-ONSET DISEASES

Within the paediatric population, it is important to distinguish patients with an early-onset of a disease that predominantly affects adults from those suffering from a predominantly paediatric disease.

A majority of adult-onset muscle diseases (and very similarly adult-onset cardiomy-opathies without muscular involvement such as sarcomeric hypertrophic cardiomyopathy) with potential cardiac involvement may have cardiac paediatric presentations. For example, supraventricular arrhythmias may represent the first clinical sign of an "adult-onset" laminopathies or myotonic dystrophy type 1. More severe events such as syncopal blocks or ventricular tachycardia, cardiac arrest or even sudden death may also be the first manifestation of the disease. This has important implications in terms of prevention of potentially life-threatening events for familial screening in young relatives of adults presenting with these diseases. For instance, when a laminopathy is diagnosed in an adult patient, the assessment of the risk of sudden death in the patient's children is a major issue, even if they are asymptomatic. As the youngest age at which severe cardiac events have been reported in inherited myopathies is 10 years, first cardiac screening is generally recommended at this age.

For diseases with a predominantly paediatric presentation the situation is different. In this case, cardiac investigations are necessary at the moment of diagnosis and thereafter according to the initial results and to the general level of risk associated with the disease. This is for instance the case for congenital laminopathies. Contrary to the adult-onset form of the disease, congenital laminopathies may be associated with severe cardiac involvement before the age of 5 years. This example highlights the fact that for several genes, the severity of mutations may underlie a paediatric- or adult-onset of muscular and/or cardiac manifestations. This is also the case for *DMD* (dystrophin: Duchenne vs. Becker) or *TTN* (titin: congenital muscular dystrophy vs. limb-girdle muscular dystrophy and/or dilated cardiomyopathy), in which there is frequently a continuum in the ages of onset and the severity. While the age at onset of a cardiomyopathy may differ in these cases for the same gene, the patterns are generally very similar.

THE FUTURE

Neurologists and cardiologists in charge of the management of paediatric myopathies must take into consideration the fact that patients who will reach adult age will probably develop specific complications that were previously overlooked or unknown. The clinical course of these diseases, and especially of cardiomyopathies, has indeed changed for several years (less sudden deaths, more heart failure) and will continue to change with the improvement of global, multidisciplinary strategies of care, which have contributed to prolong survival. In terms of cardiac prevention, early treatments and follow-ups, these aspects will need to be taken into consideration, very similarly to what happened with repaired congenital heart diseases.

**Duchenne muscular dystrophy and other dystrophinopathies**

Dystrophinopathies encompass a group of conditions caused by mutations in *DMD*, the gene encoding dystrophin. A wide majority of patients diagnosed with dystrophinopathies in childhood or adolescence have Duchenne muscular dystrophy (DMD), but some others may have early-onset Becker muscular dystrophy, which usually develops in early adulthood, or are female carriers of the mutation. This section will present the clinical aspects of DMD cardiomyopathy. For patients with Becker muscular dystrophy or female carriers, the pattern, natural history, and management of cardiomyopathy are very similar to those of DMD.

GENETICS AND PATHOPHYSIOLOGY

DMD is the most common muscular disease, affecting 1 in every 3 500 boys (Mendell and Lloyd-Puryear 2013), caused by out-of-frame mutations in the dystrophin gene associated with absence of dystrophin expression (Koenig et al. 1987; Dent et al. 2005). Dystrophin is a rod-shaped cytoplasmic protein connecting the extracellular matrix, the cellular contractile apparatus and the dystroglycan complex plays a vital role in membrane stability (transmission of forces generated by the sarcomeric contraction to the extracellular matrix) and signalling. In cardiomyocytes, the absence of dystrophin results in membrane damage secondary to contractions, which in turn results in a cascade of events including increased calcium influx into the cell, abnormalities of voltage-gated $Ca^{++}$ channels, overproduction of nitric oxide, and mitochondrial dysfunction.

CARDIOMYOPATHY PATTERN, NATURAL HISTORY AND PROGNOSIS

DMD cardiomyopathy is characterised by left ventricular dilatation, whose development is generally preceded by wall motion abnormalities, left ventricular systolic dysfunction and fibrosis predominating in the postero-basal wall (Nigro et al. 1990) – the reasons for a predominant involvement of this myocardial region are unknown. Pathological examination of the heart also shows fibrosis of the conduction system (Nomura and Hizawa 1982). Conduction system disease may be present and, exceptionally, may lead to the development of complete atrioventricular blocks requiring permanent pacing (Takano et al. 1997). Supraventricular and ventricular arrhythmias can be observed, mainly when systolic function is impaired, but not exclusively. Their incidence is not well documented, nor is the incidence of sudden cardiac death, which occurs mostly in patients with severe impairment of left ventricular function. Sinus tachycardia is frequently observed with heart rates >100bpm in a high proportion of patients and has been linked to abnormal autonomic nervous system activity (Yotsukura et al. 1995).

The prevalence of cardiac abnormalities increases with age. Dilated cardiomyopathy is relatively uncommon before the age of 10 years and then its prevalence increases progressively and reaches up to 80% after 18 years (Corrado et al. 2002). Milder myocardial abnormalities are observed in almost all patients, including left ventricular fibrosis, segmental wall motion abnormalities, and moderate alterations of left ventricular systolic function. These milder abnormalities have been observed in 25% of boys at 6 years of age (Corrado et al. 2002). Heart failure symptoms generally occur late in the course of the disease when ventricular function is severely impaired. Heart failure diagnosis can be challenging with regards to the loss of motor capacity and the frequent association of respiratory involvement.

With improved respiratory support, spinal stabilization surgery, and steroids, patients' life expectancies have increased to the early 30s and cardiomyopathy has emerged as the leading cause of death (Eagle et al. 2002). To date information on the causes of death and accurate description of cardiac causes in large cohorts is still lacking.

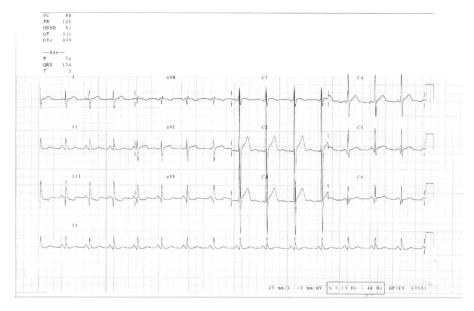

**Fig. 27.2.** Typical electrocardiogram of a patient with Duchenne muscular dystrophy. Tall R waves and increased R/S amplitude in right precordial leads (C1–C3), Q waves.

DIAGNOSIS

Current guidelines from experts in the field of neuromuscular diseases recommend performing the initial cardiac evaluation with an ECG and an echography at the time of diagnosis of DMD and then every 2 years until 10 years of age and yearly after (Bushby et al. 2010).

The ECG is abnormal in almost all patients with DMD, even in patients aged less than 10 years without dilated cardiomyopathy. There is a very uniform pattern that associates tall R waves and increased R/S amplitude in leads V1–V2, Q waves in the infero-lateral leads, incomplete right bundle branch block, and less frequently short PR intervals (Thrush et al. 2009; Perloff et al. 1967) (Fig. 27.2). QRS abnormalities have been linked to the predominant fibrosis in the postero-basal wall.

Echocardiography remains the criterion standard for the detection of myocardial disease regarding its safety, easy access, and cost–effectiveness. In DMD, left ventricular ejection fraction remains the parameter that is the most strongly correlated to long-term prognosis and on which most decisions for treatment should be based. However, its interpretation may be challenging, particularly in teenage patients with scoliosis, chest deformation, and respiratory disease (Corrado et al. 2002).

Holter-ECG is systematically performed in patients with palpitations, lightheadedness, premature atrial or ventricular beats on the ECG, or left ventricular dysfunction.

Cardiac MRI is of potential interest in DMD for myocardial tissue characterisation, particularly the identification of myocardial fibrosis with late gadolinium enhancement, and for a more accurate measurement of ventricular dimensions and function than echography. Late gadolinium enhancement has been shown to increase with age and to be correlated with a decline in left ventricular systolic function (Hor et al. 2013; Tandon et al. 2015); however, its prognostic value, particularly for the prediction of severe heart failure, has not yet been determined. Besides, acquisitions may be hardly feasible in young patients (requiring sedation) and in older patients with severe skeletal and respiratory involvement.

Sera biomarkers, including natriuretic peptides (BNP, NT-pro-BNP) have been poorly correlated to myocardial involvement in DMD, and their ability to improve the early screening of cardiac involvement has been assumed to be low due to the specific haemodynamic regimen of the disease secondary to loss of skeletal muscle function (Kawakubo et al. 2010).

Echo deformation imaging, particularly Speckle tracking, is a promising technique in DMD. However, its ability to improve the early detection of left ventricular contractility abnormalities and the prediction of long-term prognosis needs to be addressed in prospective studies with large cohorts.

TREATMENT

There are few clinical studies, especially few randomised trials, supporting guideline recommendations. Additionally, many observational studies have only included small patient cohorts and have been limited to single centres. Angiotensin-converting enzyme inhibitors (ACEI) are frequently prescribed in patients with DMD before left ventricular dysfunction is detected, generally before 10 years of age, in order to delay its occurrence. The use of this preventive approach is supported by the results of a randomised trial, which showed that the initiation of perindopril at a median age of 10 years in DMD patients with a normal left ventricular function was associated with a lower incidence of systolic dysfunction (left ventricular ejection fraction <45%) at 5 years (Duboc et al. 2005) and an improved overall survival at 10 years (Duboc et al. 2007) (Fig. 27.3).

Beta-adrenergic blockers are indicated for the treatment of left ventricular dysfunction, heart failure, ventricular arrhythmias, or elevated heart rate, particularly in patients with palpitations. Their efficacy in primary prevention in association with ACE inhibitors (ACEIs) remains unknown. Several clinical studies in this preventive indication suggested a potential benefit; however, they included small populations and were not randomised, and were mostly retrospective (Rhodes et al. 2008; Kajimoto et al. 2006; Viollet et al. 2012). Several ongoing randomised studies will provide important information on this indication.

Mineralocorticoid receptor antagonists are an important treatment of heart failure treatment in patients with left ventricular dysfunction. A single randomised study with eplerenone in DMD patients with normal left ventricular ejection fraction suggested a possible benefit by reducing the decline of left ventricular contractility on MRI (circumferential strain) at 1 year (Raman et al. 2015). Additional studies are warranted to confirm the promising results of this study.

Glucocorticoids are currently recommended in patients with DMD who are 5 years of age or older since they have been shown to prolong ambulation and improve pulmonary function (Angelini 2007). Retrospective studies in DMD suggest that steroids improve left ventricular function, reduce the risk of developing heart failure, and improve the long-term prognosis (Schram et al. 2013). However, the results of several of these observational studies may have been influenced by more frequent treatment with ACEIs in the groups on steroids

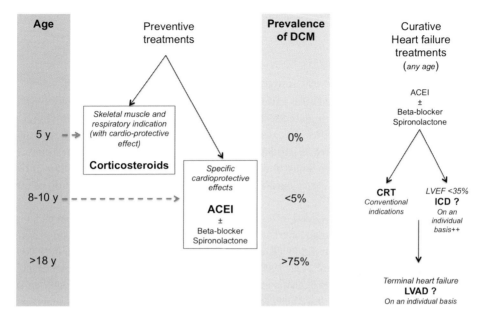

**Fig. 27.3.** Algorithm for preventive and curative treatment for patients with Duchenne muscular dystrophy. DCM: dilated cardiomyopathy; ACEI: angiotensin-converting enzyme inhibitors; CRT: cardiac resynchronisation therapy; LVEF: left ventricular ejection fraction; ICD: implantable cardiac defibrillators; LVAD: left ventricular assist device.

and by the inclusion of selected patients who had the best long-term tolerance of steroids. Additionally, results from studies in animal models of the disease suggest that prednisone may increase fibrosis and have a deleterious effect on ventricular function (Bauer et al. 2008; Janssen et al. 2014). Prospective studies are warranted to reach a conclusion on the cardiac effect of steroids.

Implantable cardiac defibrillators are generally discussed in other dilated cardiomyopathies when the left ventricular ejection fraction is severely impaired (ejection fraction <30–35%) for the prevention of sudden death related to ventricular tachyarrhythmias (Priori et al. 2015). Indications for prophylactic device implantations remain unclear in patients with DMD as there is a lack of data on the risk of sudden death in this very specific population and the apparently low risk for ventricular tachyarrhythmias on existing studies. Decisions for ICDs should probably be taken on an individual basis, after discussion with the families, and take into consideration life expectancy, especially in patients with respiratory failure, the degree of ventricular dysfunction and fibrosis, and the potentially high risk of complications associated with ICD placement in patients with denutrition or severe kyphoscoliosis.

Cardiac transplantation is generally not discussed in patients with DMD with terminal heart failure due to the severity of muscular involvement and respiratory insufficiency. Mechanical circulatory support using left ventricular assist devices has been used in few patients with DMD and could represent an alternative to transplantation, but should probably be restricted to very selected patients, particularly when heart failure appears early in the course of the disease and is associated with few other comorbidities (Ponikowski et al. 2016; Rose et al. 2001).

## Myotonic dystrophy type 1

CARDIOMYOPATHY PATTERN, NATURAL HISTORY AND PROGNOSIS

Cardiac involvement in paediatric patients presenting with myotonic dystrophy type 1 (DM1) includes conduction defects, supraventricular and ventricular arrhythmias, while myocardial abnormalities are exceptional and generally very mild. All these manifestations have been reported in patients aged up to 18 years, in congenital or infantile forms of the disease, but also sometimes as the first, early, manifestation of adult-onset form of the disease (in this case a cardiac event represents the first manifestation of the disease).

Very few studies have provided information on cardiac abnormalities in young patients with DM1 referred for systematic cardiac workup. In a series of cases, conduction system disease has been observed on the ECGs of two out of three patients with congenital DM1 aged under 18 years (Forsberg et al. 1990). A series of 11 cases with cardiac arrhythmias, including events with major prognostic implications such as syncopal sustained ventricular tachycardia or cardiac arrest have been reported (Bassez et al. 2004). Sustained supraventricular tachyarrhythmias have also been described, revealed by palpitations or lightheadedness. These arrhythmias were triggered in several cases by exercise in patients with very mild muscular involvement. The youngest reported age for the occurrence of such cardiac events is 10 years.

A Danish nationwide epidemiological study has assessed the standardised indexed ratio (SIR) between patients with myotonic dystrophy and the general population for a diagnosis of cardiac disease including cardiomyopathy, heart failure, conduction disorders, arrhythmias and implantation of pacemaker, or implantable cardioverter defibrillator. Patients with myotonic dystrophy had a significantly higher risk than others and the standardised indexed ratio was the highest in younger groups, particularly in patients aged 0 to 19 years (SIR = 19.4; 95% confidence intervals = 4.92–52.7) (Lund et al. 2014).

DIAGNOSIS AND FOLLOW-UP

In patients with a genetic or clinical diagnosis of DM1, cardiac evaluations should be carried out at diagnosis, after the age of 10 years, including ECG, echocardiography and Holter-ECG. These examinations should be repeated during follow-up with time intervals depending on the initial findings. In patients practicing sport, exercise testing should be performed, especially in patients with symptoms such as palpitations or dizziness, for the diagnosis of arrhythmias exclusively triggered in this context, which can be otherwise overlooked.

In children of patients with DM1 without clinical signs of the disease, systematic cardiac evaluations should be performed after the age of 10 years for the screening of potentially asymptomatic abnormalities on the ECG or the echocardiography. In individuals with significant abnormalities, genetic testing can be performed to identify mutation carriers and propose tailored strategies for follow-up and treatment.

TREATMENT

In patients with conduction system disease, prophylactic pacing can be discussed on an individual basis, according to the general context, age, symptoms and conduction parameters, particularly if the invasive electrophysiological study shows infrahissian conduction abnormalities (His to ventricle interval >70ms).

The management of supraventricular and ventricular arrhythmias should follow the recommendations for the general population. Class I anti-arrhythmic drugs should be avoided whenever possible due to their potential pro-arrhythmic effect at the ventricular level.

## Congenital muscular dystrophy

Congenital muscular dystrophy encompasses various diseases with very different cardiac patterns, ranging from an absence of abnormalities to myocardial involvement or severe electrical abnormalities.

All patients with congenital muscular dystrophies should undergo cardiac screening at diagnosis. The initial evaluation may help with diagnosis of the type of congenital muscular dystrophy, provides reference values for follow-up, and assists follow-up planning. With respect to ventricular function, left ventricular ejection fraction below 50% should be considered abnormal in patients with congenital muscular dystrophy. Since worsening of ventricular dysfunction is observed in a majority of patients, prompt medical treatment should be initiated even in patients with mild ventricular systolic dysfunction.

LAMINOPATHIES

Congenital muscular dystrophy due to *LMNA* mutations represents the group with the highest risk of developing cardiac disease among congenital muscular dystrophies and more widely among paediatric-onset myopathies. Cardiac manifestations can occur before 1 year of age. Conduction system disease and supraventricular or ventricular ectopics represent the first manifestation of the disease in most cases. Later, patients may have supraventricular arrhythmias such as atrial fibrillation. Conduction defects tend to progress over time and some patients may develop severe, complete atrioventricular blocks. Involvement of the left and right ventricles is frequent and may be revealed by left and/or right-sided heart failure with frequently atypical presentations such as nausea, diarrhoea, and ascites (Makri et al. 2009). Sudden cardiac death has been reported in several patients in relation to severe ventricular arrhythmias or complete atrioventricular blocks.

In primary prevention of sudden death, the use of a cardioverter defibrillator should be discussed in patients with cardiac symptoms, such as syncope or palpitations, conduction defects requiring a pacemaker, left ventricular dysfunction, or significant functional or morphological right ventricular abnormalities. Since the number of reported patients remains low, the risk factors for sudden death have not been clearly identified. An implantable cardioverter defibrillator is feasible in young patients but remains technically difficult especially in patients with extreme thinness or major deformities of the chest wall. Indications should be carefully examined on an individual basis.

In patients with supraventricular arrhythmias, patients should be treated with anticoagulants to prevent thromboembolic complications. However, anticoagulant therapy is difficult in patients with congenital muscular dystrophies, particularly in young children and in patients who could fall and are exposed to haemorrhagic complications.

## Congenital muscular dystrophy type 1A

Left ventricular dysfunction has been reported in approximately one-third of patients with congenital muscular dystrophy type 1A (merosin-deficient congenital muscular dystrophy/ MCD1A) (Jones et al. 2001). The majority of patients did not complain of any symptoms. However, severe heart failure has also been reported in both children and adults (Gilhuis et al. 2002). The main issue in patients with MDC1A is the early detection and treatment of myocardial dysfunction. The prevention of heart failure, which for some patients may develop a long time after the initial diagnosis of the disease, should include an early diagnosis of contractility abnormalities and the prompt initiation of cardiac treatments such as ACE inhibitors.

### DYSTROGLYCANOPATHIES

Myocardial involvement is frequent in patients with dystroglycanopathies. Dilated cardiomyopathy has been frequently reported in patients with mutations in the *FKRP* gene before the age of 5 years (Kefi et al. 2008; Louhichi et al. 2004) as well as in patients with Fukuyama congenital muscular dystrophy in the second decade of life (Nakanishi et al. 2006). Patients with other dystroglycanopathies, such as Walker–Warburg syndrome and muscle–eye–brain disease, should be considered at risk of developing similar complications because they share a similar pathway with an abnormal dystroglycan glycosylation. Severe arrhythmias have not been reported in these patients, except in advanced left ventricular dysfunction. The main issue in patients with dystroglycanopathies is the early detection and treatment of myocardial dysfunction with heart failure medications.

### OTHER CONGENITAL MUSCULAR DYSTROPHIES

Patients with COL6 diseases, such as Ulrich congenital muscular dystrophy and Bethlem myopathy, do not appear to have an increased risk of cardiac involvement (Merlini et al. 2008). Primary cardiac involvement has not been reported in patients with *SEPN1* mutations. However, patients with severe respiratory failure can develop cor pulmonale, right heart failure, and pulmonary hypertension.

## Congenital myopathies

In a majority of cases, congenital myopathies spare the cardiac muscle. No cardiomyopathy has been reported to date in patients with congenital myopathies with mutations in the following genes (when taking into account only the well documented and genetically proven cases): *NEB* (nebulin), *ACTA 1* (skeletal muscle alpha-actin), *TPM2* (beta tropomyosin), *TPM3* (alpha tropomyosin), *TNNT1* (troponin T slow), *CLF2* (cofilin), *KBTBD13*, *KLHL40* (*KBTBD5)*, *MTM1* (myotubularin), *DNM2* (dynamin 2) and *BIN1* (amphiphysin 2).

However, cardiac involvement has been reported with *TTN* and *MYH7* mutations. Homozygous titin deletion in the exons encoding the C-terminal M-line region, causing a frameshift downstream of the titin kinase domain and protein truncation, may result in early fatal dilated or non-compaction cardiomyopathy with heart failure (Carmignac et al. 2007). Homozygous mutations in *MYH7* (slow/beta cardiac myosin heavy chain) may result in the development of myosin storage myopathy with cardiomyopathy, generally left ventricular non-compaction with systolic dysfunction and sometimes conduction system disease (Tajsharghi et al. 2007a; 2007b; Fiorillo et al. 2016).

## Mitochondrial diseases

MITOCHONDRIAL CARDIOMYOPATHY: PREVALENCE, PATTERNS AND PROGNOSIS

Mitochondrial diseases represent a very complex and heterogeneous group of diseases. Cardiac involvement is very frequent, with a prevalence of up to 50% in paediatric cohorts (Darin et al. 2001; Debray et al. 2007; Scaglia et al. 2004). Cardiomyopathy may remain subclinical for years and therefore routine assessment is recommended. It has been reported similarly in both mitochondrial and nuclear gene mutations. It can be present in neonatal (e.g. Leigh [Finsterer at al., 2008], Person [Schiff et al. 2011], or other syndromes [Silvestri et al. 1994]) and infantile and childhood presentations (Marjorie et al. 1981; Igal et al. 1997). Compared with others, patients with cardiomyopathy have an earlier age at onset (33 months *vs.* 40 months) and a substantially increased morbidity (82% *vs.* 5%)(Scaglia et al. 2004). Heart failure may represent the primary cause of death in this population or a complication with significant influence on vital prognosis in the setting of a multi-systemic disease.

Cardiomyopathy may include myocardial involvement and/or electrical abnormalities. Hypertrophic and dilated cardiomyopathies are the most frequent manifestations, but left ventricular non-compaction may also be observed. Hypertrophic cardiomyopathy is concentric, involving all ventricular walls. Left ventricular dysfunction may be present at diagnosis in patients with hypertrophic cardiomyopathy or develop secondarily after the progressive increase of left ventricular mass over years. Electrical abnormalities are more frequently observed in mtDNA disorders (Sembrano et al. 1997; Santorelli et al. 1997) and may include conduction defects, supraventricular and less frequently ventricular arrhythmias, and Wolff–Parkinson–White syndrome (Towbin 2006). Autonomic dysfunction may play a role in bradycardia or tachycardia, and may be diagnosed as postural orthostatic tachycardia syndrome (Kanjwal et al. 2010).

The clinical presentations and patterns vary from one gene, and from one syndrome, to another. It is extremely difficult to give a global overview of all potential abnormalities for each group of disease. The two groups with the most specific patterns and outcomes are patients with MELAS and mtDNA single large-scale deletions. In patients with MELAS (80% with the m.3243A>G mutation), including those with the complete MELAS syndrome and others, hypertrophic cardiomyopathy and Wolff–Parkinson–White syndrome are the most frequent clinical features and patients are at risk for systolic heart failure with impaired myocardial contractility and reduced ventricular ejection fraction. In patients with large-scale deletions mtDNA, especially those with Kearns-Sayre syndrome (KSS), conduction defects are extremely frequent and severe (and are part of the definition of KSS) with a majority of patients developing complete atrioventricular blocks, which represent a potential cause of sudden death.

It is noteworthy to mention that, aside from the chronic involvement of the heart by the disease, rapid alterations of myocardial systolic function may be observed when patients have metabolic crisis. A recovery of myocardial function with normalisation of left ventricular ejection fraction may be observed after the crisis.

DIAGNOSIS

At initial diagnosis, patients should be systematically investigated even in the absence of any symptom. ECG and echocardiogram are the most useful examinations in this context. Holter-ECG may be indicated for the diagnosis of paroxysmal conduction defects or arrhythmias in patients with symptoms such as palpitations or lightheadedness, with an abnormal ECG, or systemically in high-risk patients especially those with Kearns-Sayre syndrome. Cardiac workup should be repeated during follow-up with regards to the possible progression of abnormalities, even in asymptomatic patients, probably every year or every two years according to initial findings, to the genetic findings, and the global severity of the disease.

TREATMENT

No treatment has proven efficacy yet for mitochondrial cardiomyopathy, and especially no benefit at the cardiac level has been associated with antioxidant vitamins/factors such as coenzyme $Q_{10}$, alpha-lipoic acid, vitamin C, or vitamin E. Arginine perfusions, which may be proposed to MELAS patients with stroke-like episodes and/or mitochondrial crisis, have not shown any effect on left ventricular function in this context. A treatment with arginine should, however, probably be attempted in this context with regards to the extreme severity of the natural clinical course.

Cardiac management relies mainly on conventional cardiac therapies for heart failure and sudden death prevention. Patients with clinical signs or symptoms of heart failure or left ventricular systolic dysfunction should be treated with heart failure therapies. The use of these treatments in these patients remains empirical in the absence of controlled studies. Of these, ACE inhibitors and beta-blockers should be used as a first-line treatment. Indications of other heart failure treatments such as loop diuretics, aldosterone antagonists, ivabradine or resynchronisation therapy should be similar as for the general population.

Prophylactic permanent pacing should be proposed to patients with high risk of sudden death due to major conduction defect, particularly those with mtDNA single large-scale deletions who present with any conduction defect on the ECG. Indications for implantable cardiac defibrillators (ICD) have not been defined in patients with mitochondrial disease. ICDs should be discussed for patients with severe left ventricular systolic dysfunction (left ventricular ejection fraction <35%), particularly when the global severity of the disease is otherwise relatively mild with a life expectancy of more than 1 year.

**Glycogen storage diseases**

A majority of glycogen storage myopathies are associated with cardiac involvement, which is often extremely severe. Newborn infants, infants or teenagers may present with dilated or hypertrophic cardiomyopathy and left ventricular systolic dysfunction leading to heart failure or less frequently with ventricular tachyarrhythmias or severe conduction defects and die suddenly. It is difficult to describe in detail cardiac manifestations of all muscular glycogen storage diseases (GSDs). This paragraph will focus on infantile Pompe disease because of its severity and the availability of a curative treatment and provide a global overview of the other diseases at risk for cardiomyopathy.

INFANTILE POMPE DISEASE

Infantile Pompe disease, with less than 1% residual activity of the lysosomal enzyme acid α-glucosidase, manifests in the first months of life and, if left untreated, causes death within 1 year. It manifests as hypertrophic cardiomyopathy as a result of glycogen accumulation with severe impairment of left ventricular systolic function and subsequent severe heart failure.

Echocardiogram shows a major concentric ventricular hypertrophy, with outflow tract and/or mid-ventricular obstruction and impaired ejection fraction in some patients. The ECG shows high voltages, diffuse repolarisation disturbances, and frequently a short PR interval (Gillette et al. 1974; Ansong et al. 2006).

Various studies have shown that enzyme replacement therapy with recombinant human α-glucosidase contributes to reducing ventricular mass and improving ventricular function (Lin et al. 1987; Martiniuk et al. 1998; Meikle et al. 1999), with the first effects being potentially detected within a few weeks (Winkel et al. 2003; 2004; Van den Hout et al. 2000). These studies showed a prominent effect on the heart and a significant benefit on survival.

In attenuated forms of the disease, with residual α-glucosidase activity, which can affect teenagers, the heart is sporadically affected with generally milder hypertrophy and preserved systolic function (Hirschhorn and Reuser 2001; Winkel et al. 2005; Kostera-Pruszczyk et al. 2006).

OTHER DISEASES

In infantile forms of phosphofructokinase deficiency (GSD VII – Tarui disease, *PFK-M*) patients may present with dilated cardiomyopathy and heart failure (Amit et al. 1992). In phosphoglucomutase 1 deficiency (GSD XIV, *PGM1*), dilated cardiomyopathy and heart failure have been reported in patients aged 8 to 15 years, of whom one died suddenly (Tegtmeyer et al. 2014). In muscle glycogen synthase deficiency (*GYS1*), left ventricular hypertrophy has been identified in a majority of patients (patients aged 10, 11 years) and sudden cardiac arrest in one (Kollberg et al. 2007). In debrancher enzyme deficiency (GSD III – Cori disease), concentric hypertrophy is extremely prevalent and may precede skeletal myopathy which generally manifests in adults. In congenital and infantile forms of glycogen branching enzyme deficiency (GSD IV – Andersen disease), dilated cardiomyopathy and heart failure may be present (Servidei et al. 1987). In ubiquitine ligase deficiency (*RBCK1*), truncating mutations in both alleles may manifest as dilated cardiomyopathy and heart failure in adolescents, potentially requiring cardiac transplantation (two cases in patients aged 13 and 14) (Nilsson et al. 2013). In phosphorylase kinase deficiency (*PRKAG2*), infants may present with hypertrophic cardiomyopathy and systolic dysfunction potentially causing death (Akman et al. 2007). *PRKAG2* mutation may be associated with secondary phosphorylase b kinase deficiency (Servidei et al. 1988; Regalado et al. 1999).

## Muscle lipid diseases

Most muscle lipid diseases with congenital or infantile onset are associated with dilated or hypertrophic cardiomyopathy and/or ventricular tachyarrhythmias or severe conduction defects. These cardiomyopathies represent a frequent cause of sudden death or death due to heart failure. This paragraph gives a global overview of several diseases associated with a particularly high morbidity.

In childhood-onset forms of primary carnitine deficiency (*OCTN2*), dilated cardiomyopathy and heart failure are present in the first years of life and can be efficiently treated with L-carnitine supplementation (Tripp et al. 1981). In neutral lipid storage disease with myopathy (NLSDM; adipocyte triglyceride lipase deficiency, *PNPLA2*), neonates and infants may present with dilated cardiomyopathy (Igal et al. 1997). In neonatal forms of multiple acyl-CoA dehydrogenation deficiency (MADD; Electron transfer flavoprotein A or B, *EFTA*, *EFTB*), lipid myocardial infiltration with left ventricular hypertrophy, dilatation and systolic dysfunction have been reported; a 6-month-old child died suddenly (Singla et al. 2008). In carnitine palmitoyltransferase II deficiency (CPT II; *CPT2*), cardiomyopathies with ventricular arrhythmias and conduction defects with a high risk of sudden death have been reported in neonatal presentations (Bonnefont et al. 1999), while in infantile forms heart involvement is present in about half of all cases, occurring either as dilated and hypertrophic cardiomyopathy that may spontaneously recover, or as arrhythmias and conduction disorders (Demaugre et al. 1991). In severe early-onset cardiac and multi-organ failure forms of very-long-chain acyl-CoA dehydrogenase deficiency (VLCAD) deficiency, patients typically present in the first months of life with hypertrophic or dilated cardiomyopathy, ventricular tachycardia and fibrillation, and atrioventricular block (Bonnet et al. 1999). The morbidity resulting from cardiomyopathy is severe; however, cardiac dysfunction may be reversible with early intensive supportive care and diet modification. In long-chain 3-hydroxyacyl-coa dehydrogenase deficiency (LCHAD), hypertrophic or dilated cardiomyopathies and conduction system disease may also be present (Tyni and Pihko 1999). In lipin-1 deficiency (*LPIN1*), dilated cardiomyopathy and severe heart failure have been reported; one patient aged 33 months died suddenly (Schönfelder et al. 2011). In patients with short-chain acyl-CoA dehydrogenase deficiency (SCADD) defect, left ventricular dysfunction has been reported (Amendt et al. 1987).

## Juveline dermatomyositis

CHARACTERISTICS AND PREVALENCE OF CARDIAC ABNORMALITIES

Data on cardiac involvement in juvenile dermatomyositis remain scarce. Small case series suggest that cardiac abnormalities may be present, but generally asymptomatic and not severe. In asymptomatic patients, case control studies have shown evidence of diastolic dysfunction (E/Ea ratio) in 22% of patients after a median of 17 years from disease onset and mild impairment of systolic function assessed with deformation echography (long axis strain) with normal left ventricular ejection fraction (Schwartz et al. 2014). These abnormalities have been correlated with high long-term organ damage scores and high skin disease activity. In the same cohort, heart rate variability was lower in patients than comparison groups assessed by Holter-ECG (Barth et al. 2016), which may indicate autonomic dysfunction, a marker of cardiac prognosis in the general population. Pericarditis with tamponade and ventricular tachycardia have also been described in case reports (Karaca et al. 2006; Jindal et al. 2012).

The long-term impact of these echocardiographic abnormalities remains unclear. To date, no study has suggested that patients may develop major cardiac adverse events or have an impaired prognosis due to cardiac involvement. Changes of echocardiography may be recognised even when patients are in clinical remission (Schwartz et al. 2014).

MANAGEMENT

Cardiac evaluation by ECG and echocardiography is recommended at diagnosis for all patients and should be repeated in patients with high risk of cardiac involvement: hypertension, high disease activity 1 year after diagnosis, long-term high corticosteroid burden or chronic ongoing active disease (Schwartz et al. 2014). There is, however, insufficient evidence to advise on frequency and duration of monitoring. It is noteworthy that prolonged steroid therapy exposes patients to hypertension and other long-term cardiovascular complications.

**Summary**

Cardiac involvement is present in a majority of paediatric myopathies and may present as myocardial abnormalities, generally predominating in the left ventricle and/or electrical system disease including conduction defects, supraventricular and/or ventricular arrhythmias. A range of patterns may be observed from one disease to another with respect to the combinations of myocardial and electrical abnormalities, degrees of severity, and ages at onset. Heart failure or arrhythmias represent frequent causes of death in paediatric myopathies. In many cases, cardiac involvement remains asymptomatic until late in the course of the disease with symptoms occurring at an advanced stage where treatments are less efficient. Therefore, cardiac workup should be systematically performed at initial diagnosis and repeated during follow-up. Early diagnosis and preventive treatments, including heart failure medications, pacemaker and implantable defibrillator have significantly improved life expectancy. These changes have resulted in significant prolongation and modification of the history of the cardiac diseases, with some previously unknown complications potentially emerging in adulthood that neurologists and cardiologists should anticipate and be prepared to prevent.

**Key points**
• Cardiac involvement is present in a majority of paediatric myopathies.
• Cardiomyopathies in myocardial abnormalities and/or electrical system disease may potentially result in heart failure and arrhythmias, which represent two frequent causes of death.
• Cardiomyopathy pattern, clinical course and prognosis differ from one disease to another.

- Cardiac workup should be systematically performed at initial diagnosis and repeated during follow-up.
- Heart failure treatments have proven efficacy to improve vital prognosis, especially in DMD.

### Clinical vignette

A 10-year-old male patient is referred to your clinic for the management of DMD, diagnosed and genetically confirmed at the age of 3 years. He is currently treated with steroids (deflazacort). His last cardiac workup was carried out two years ago and was considered normal with a left ventricular ejection fraction of 60%.

WHAT IS YOUR PLAN FOR THE SCREENING AND TREATMENT OF DUCHENNE MUSCULAR DYSTROPHY-RELATED CARDIOMYOPATHY?

Heart failure is a leading cause of death in patients with this condition in adolescence or in early adulthood. The age of 10 years is a milestone for cardiac involvement since the prevalence of dilated cardiomyopathy is very low before this age, increases progressively thereafter and reaches up to 80% in adulthood. Heart failure treatments, especially angiotensin-converting enzyme (ACE) inhibitors, have proven efficacy to prevent the development of dilated cardiomyopathy and reduce long-term total mortality.

In this patient, ECG and echocardiogram should be performed and repeated on a yearly basis to allow an early diagnosis of dilated cardiomyopathy and prompt reinforcement of heart failure treatment. ACE inhibitors should be initiated, in addition to deflazacort, regardless of his cardiac workup, and beta-blockade or aldosterone antagonists should be discussed due to the presence of the impaired left ventricular ejection fraction.

This observation highlights the importance of early diagnosis and preventive treatments, with potential implications on long-term vital prognosis.

## REFERENCES

Akman HO, Sampayo JN, Ross FA, Scott JW, Wilson G, Benson L et al. (2007) Fatal infantile cardiac glycogenosis with phosphorylase kinase deficiency and a mutation in the gamma2-subunit of AMP-activated protein kinase. *Pediatr Res* 62: 499–504.

Amendt BA, Greene C, Sweetman L, Cloherty J, Shih V, Moon A et al. (1987) Short-chain acyl-coenzyme A dehydrogenase deficiency. Clinical and biochemical studies in two patients. *J Clin Invest* 79: 1303–1309.

Amit R, Bashan N, Abarbanel JM, Shapira Y, Sofer S, Moses S (1992) Fatal familial infantile glycogen storage disease: multisystem phosphofructokinase deficiency. *Muscle Nerve* 15: 455–458.

Angelini C (2007) The role of corticosteroids in muscular dystrophy: a critical appraisal. *Muscle Nerve* 36: 424–435.

Ansong AK, Li JS, Nozik-Grayck E, Ing R, Kravitz RM, Idriss SF et al. (2006) Electrocardiographic response to enzyme replacement therapy for Pompe disease. *Genet Med* 8: 297–301.

Barth Z, Nomeland Witczak B, Schwartz T, Gjesdal K, Flatø B, Koller A et al. (2016) In juvenile dermatomyositis, heart rate variability is reduced, and associated with both cardiac dysfunction and markers of inflammation: a cross-sectional study median 13.5 years after symptom onset. *Rheumatology (Oxford)* 55: 535–543.

Bassez G, Lazarus A, Desguerre I, Varin J, Laforét P, Bécane HM, Meune C et al. (2004) Severe cardiac arrhythmias in young patients with myotonic dystrophy type 1. *Neurology* 63(10): 1939–1941. doi.10.1212/01.wnl.0000144343.91136.cf.

Bauer R, Macgowan GA, Blain A, Bushby K, Straub V (2008) Steroid treatment causes deterioration of myocardial function in the {delta}-sarcoglycan-deficient mouse model for dilated cardiomyopathy. *Cardiovasc Res* 79: 652–661.

Bonnefont JP, Demaugre F, Prip-Buus C, Saudubray JM, Brivet M, Abadi N et al. (1999) Carnitine palmito-yltransferase deficiencies. *Mol Genet Metab* 68: 424–440.

Bonnet D, Martin D, Villain E, Jouvet P, Rabier D, Brivet M et al. (1999) Arrhythmias and conduction defects as presenting symptoms of fatty acid oxidation disorders in children. *Circulation* 100: 2248–2253.

Bushby K, Finkel R, Birnkrant DJ, Case LE, Clemens PR, Cripe L et al. (2010) Diagnosis and management of Duchenne muscular dystrophy, part 1: diagnosis, and pharmacological and psychosocial management. *Lancet Neurol* 9: 77–93.

Carmignac V, Salih MA, Quijano-Roy S, Marchand S, Al Rayess MM, Mukhtar MM et al. (2007) C-terminal titin deletions cause a novel early-onset myopathy with fatal cardiomyopathy. *Ann Neurol* 61: 340–351.

Corrado G, Lissoni A, Beretta S, Terenghi L, Tadeo G, Foglia-Manzillo G et al. (2002) Prognostic value of electrocardiograms, ventricular late potentials, ventricular arrhythmias, and left ventricular systolic dys-function in patients with Duchenne muscular dystrophy. *Am J Cardiol* 89: 838–841.

Darin N, Oldfors A, Moslemi AR, Holme E, Tulinius M (2001) The incidence of mitochondrial encephalo-myopathies in childhood: clinical features and morphological, biochemical, and DNA abnormalities. *Ann Neurol* 49(3): 377–783.

Debray F-G, Lambert M, Chevalier I, Robitaille Y, Decarie JC, Shoubridge EA et al. (2007) Long-term outcome and clinical spectrum of 73 pediatric patients with mitochondrial diseases. *Pediatrics* 119: 722–733.

Dent KM, Dunn DM, von Niederhausern AC, Aoyagi AT, Kerr L, Bromberg MB et al. (2005) Improved molecular diagnosis of dystrophinopathies in an unselected clinical cohort. *Am J Med Genet A* 134: 295–298.

Demaugre F, Bonnefont JP, Colonna M, Cepanec C, Leroux JP, Saudubray JM (1991) Infantile form of carni-tine palmitoyltransferase II deficiency with hepatomuscular symptoms and sudden death. Physiopatho-logical approach to carnitine palmitoyltransferase II deficiencies. *J Clin Invest* 87: 859–864.

Duboc D, Meune C, Lerebours G, Devaux JY, Vaksmann G, Bécane HM (2005) Effect of perindopril on the onset and progression of left ventricular dysfunction in Duchenne muscular dystrophy. *J Am Coll Cardiol* 45: 855–857.

Duboc D, Meune C, Pierre B, Wahbi K, Eymard B, Toutain A et al. (2007) Perindopril preventive treatment on mortality in Duchenne muscular dystrophy: 10 years' follow-up. *Am Heart J* 154: 596–602.

Eagle M, Baudouin SV, Chandler C, Giddings DR, Bullock R, Bushby K (2002) Survival in Duchenne muscular dystrophy: improvements in life expectancy since 1967 and the impact of home nocturnal ventilation. *Neuromuscul Disord* 12: 926–929.

Fiorillo C, Astrea G, Savarese M, Cassandrini D, Brisca G, Trucco F et al. (2016) MYH7-related myopathies: clinical, histopathological and imaging findings in a cohort of Italian patients. *Orphanet J Rare Dis* 11: 91.

Finsterer J (2008) Leigh and Leigh-like syndrome in children and adults. *Pediatr Neurol* 39: 223–235.

Forsberg H, Olofsson BO, Eriksson A, Andersson S (1990) Cardiac involvement in congenital myotonic dystrophy. *Br Heart J* 63: 119–121.

Gilhuis HJ, ten Donkelaar HJ, Tanke RB, Vingerhoets DM, Zwarts MJ, Verrips A Gabreëls FJ (2002) Non-muscular involvement in merosin-negative congenital muscular dystrophy. *Pediatr Neurol* 26(1): 30–36.

Gillette PC, Nihill MR, Singer DB (1974) Electrophysiological mechanism of the short PR interval in Pompe disease. *Am J Dis Child* 128: 622–626.

Hirschhorn R, Reuser AJJ (2001) Glycogen Storage Disease Type II. In Scriver CR, Beaudet AL, Sly WS, Valle D (eds) *The Metabolic and Molecular Bases of Inherited Disease*, 8th eds. New York: McGraw-Hill, pp. 3389–3420.

Hor KN, Taylor MD, Al-Khalidi HR, Cripe LH, Raman SV, Jefferies JL et al. (2013) Prevalence and distri-bution of late gadolinium enhancement in a large population of patients with Duchenne muscular dystrophy: effect of age and left ventricular systolic function. *J Cardiovasc Magn Reson* 15: 107.

Igal RA, Rhoads JM, Coleman RA (1997) Neutral lipid storage disease with fatty liver and cholestasis. *J Pediatr Gastroenterol Nutr* 25: 541–547.

Janssen PM, Murray JD, Schill KE, Rastogi N, Schultz EJ, Tran T et al. (2014) Prednisolone attenuates improvement of cardiac and skeletal contractile function and histopathology by lisinopril and spirono-lactone in the mdx mouse model of Duchenne muscular dystrophy. *PLoS One* 9: e88360.

Jindal G, Singh S, Suri D, Rawat A, Rohit M (2012) Recurrent ventricular tachycardia in a child with juvenile dermatomyositis – an unusual association. *Int J Rheum Dis* 15: e26–e27.

Jones KJ, Morgan G, Johnston H, Tobias V, Ouvrier RA, Wilkinson I et al. (2001) The expanding phenotype of laminin alpha2 chain (merosin) abnormalities: case series and review. *J Med Genet* 38: 649–657.

Kanjwal K, Karabin B, Kanjwal Y, Saeed B, Grubb BP (2010) Autonomic dysfunction presenting as orthostatic intolerance in patients suffering from mitochondrial cytopathy. *Clin Cardiol* 33: 626–629.

Kajimoto H, Ishigaki K, Okumura K, Tomimatsu H, Nakazawa M, Saito K et al. (2006) Beta-blocker therapy for cardiac dysfunction in patients with muscular dystrophy. *Circ J* 70: 991–994.

Karaca NE, Aksu G, Yeniay BS, Kutukculer N (2006) Juvenile dermatomyositis with a rare and remarkable complication: sinus bradycardia. *Rheumatol Int* 27: 179–182.

Kawakubo M et al. (2010) Relationship of natriuretic peptide and transthoracic echocardiographic findings in 135 subjects with muscular dystrophy. *Int J Cardiol* 145: 506–514.

Kefi M, Amouri R, Chabrak S, Mechmeche R, Hentati F (2008) Variable cardiac involvement in Tunisian siblings harboring FKRP gene mutations. *Neuropediatrics* 39: 113–115.

Koenig M, Hoffman EP, Bertelson CJ, Monaco AP, Feener C, Kunkel LM (1987) Complete cloning of the Duchenne muscular dystrophy (DMD) cDNA and preliminary genomic organization of the DMD gene in normal and affected individuals. *Cell* 50: 509–517.

Kollberg G, Tulinius M, Gilljam T, Ostman-Smith I, Forsander G, Jotorp P et al. (2007) Cardiomyopathy and exercise intolerance in muscle glycogen storage disease 0. *N Engl J Med* 357: 1507–1514.

Kostera-Pruszczyk A, Opuchlik A, Lugowska A, Nadaj A, Bojakowski J, Tylki-Szymanska A et al. (2006) Juvenile onset acid maltase deficiency presenting as a rigid spine syndrome. *Neuromuscul Disord* 16: 282–285.

Lin CY, Hwang B, Hsiao KJ, Jin YR (1987) Pompe's disease in Chinese and prenatal diagnosis by determination of alpha-glucosidase activity. *J Inherit Metab Dis* 10: 11–17.

Louhichi N, Triki C, Quijano-Roy S, Richard P, Makri S, Méziou M et al. (2004) New FKRP mutations causing congenital muscular dystrophy associated with mental retardation and central nervous system abnormalities. Identification of a founder mutation in Tunisian families. *Neurogenetics* 5: 27–34.

Lund M, Diaz LJ, Ranthe MF, Petri H, Duno M, Juncker I et al. (2014) Cardiac involvement in myotonic dystrophy: a nationwide cohort study. *Eur Heart J* 35: 2158–2164.

Makri S, Clarke NF, Richard P, Maugenre S, Demay L, Bonne G et al. (2009) Germinal mosaicism for LMNA mimics autosomal recessive congenital muscular dystrophy. *Neuromuscul Disord* 19: 26–28.

Martiniuk F, Chen A, Mack A, Arvanitopoulos E, Chen Y, Rom WN et al. (1998) Carrier frequency for glycogen storage disease type II in New York and estimates of affected individuals born with the disease. *Am J Med Genet* 79: 69–72.

Meikle PJ, Hopwood JJ, Clague AE, Carey WF (1999) Prevalence of lysosomal storage disorders. *JAMA* 281: 249–254.

Merlini L, Martoni E, Grumati P, Sabatelli P, Squarzoni S, Urciuolo A et al. (2008) Autosomal recessive myosclerosis myopathy is a collagen VI disorder. *Neurology* 71: 1245–1253.

Nakanishi T, Sakauchi M, Kaneda Y, Tomimatsu H, Saito K, Nakazawa M et al. (2006) Cardiac involvement in Fukuyama-type congenital muscular dystrophy. *Pediatrics* 117: e1187–e1192.

Nigro G, Comi LI, Politano L, Bain RJ (1990) The incidence and evolution of cardiomyopathy in Duchenne muscular dystrophy. *Int J Cardiol* 26: 271–277.

Nilsson J, Schoser B, Laforet P, Kalev O, Lindberg C, Romero NB et al. (2013) Polyglucosan body myopathy caused by defective ubiquitin ligase RBCK1. *Ann Neurol* 74: 914–919.

Nomura H, Hizawa K (1982) Histopathological study of the conduction system of the heart in Duchenne progressive muscular dystrophy. *Acta Pathol Jpn* 32: 1027–1033.

Mendell JR, Lloyd-Puryear M (2013) Report of MDA muscle disease symposium on newborn screening for Duchenne muscular dystrophy. *Muscle Nerve* 48: 21–26.

Perloff JK, Roberts WC, de Leon AC Jr, O'Doherty D (1967) The distinctive electrocardiogram of Duchenne's progressive muscular dystrophy. An electrocardiographic-pathologic correlative study. *Am J Med* 42: 179–188.

Ponikowski P, Voors AA, Anker SD, Bueno H, Cleland JGF, Coats AJS et al. (2016) 2016 ESC Guidelines for the diagnosis and treatment of acute and chronic heart failure: the Task Force for the diagnosis and treatment of acute and chronic heart failure of the European Society of Cardiology (ESC) Developed with the special contribution of the Heart Failure Association (HFA) of the ESC. *Eur Heart J* 37: 2129–2200.

Priori SG, Blomström-Lundqvist C, Mazzanti A, Blom N, Borggrefe M, Camm J et al. (2015) ESC Guidelines for the management of patients with ventricular arrhythmias and the prevention of sudden cardiac death. *Eur Heart J* 36: 2793–2867.

Raman SV, Hor KN, Mazur W, Halnon NJ, Kissel JT, He X et al. (2015) Eplerenone for early cardiomyopathy in Duchenne muscular dystrophy: a randomised, double-blind, placebo-controlled trial. *Lancet Neurol* 14: 153–161.

Regalado JJ, Rodriguez MM, Ferrer PL (1999) Infantile hypertrophic cardiomyopathy of glycogenosis type IX: isolated cardiac phosphorylase kinase deficiency. *Pediatr Cardiol* 20: 304–307.

Rhodes J, Margossian R, Darras BT, Colan SD, Jenkins KJ, Geva T et al. (2008) Safety and efficacy of carvedilol therapy for patients with dilated cardiomyopathy secondary to muscular dystrophy. *Pediatr Cardiol* 29: 343–351.

Rose EA, Gelijns AC, Moskowitz AJ, Heitjan DF, Stevenson LW, Dembitsky W et al. (2001) Long-term use of a left ventricular assist device for end-stage heart failure. *N Engl J Med* 345: 1435–1443.

Santorelli FM, Tanji K, Shanske S, DiMauro S (1997) Heterogeneous clinical presentation of the mtDNA NARP/T8993G mutation. *Neurology* 49: 270–273.

Scaglia F, Towbin JA, Craigen WJ, Belmont JW, Smith EO, Neish SR et al. (2004) Clinical spectrum, morbidity, and mortality in 113 pediatric patients with mitochondrial disease. *Pediatrics* 114: 925–931.

Schiff M, Ogier de Baulny H, Lombès A (2011) Neonatal cardiomyopathies and metabolic crises due to oxidative phosphorylation defects. *Semin Fetal Neonatal Med* 16: 216–221.

Schönfelder J, Brocke K, Winkler U, Flössel U, Geiger K, von der Hagen M et al. (2011) A case of sudden cardiac death in a patient with LPIN1 gene mutation. *Neuropediatrics* 42: 118. doi: doi.10.1055/s-0031-1274090.

Schram G, Fournier A, Leduc H, Dahdah N, Therien J, Vanasse M et al. (2013) All-cause mortality and cardiovascular outcomes with prophylactic steroid therapy in Duchenne muscular dystrophy. *J Am Coll Cardiol* 61: 948–954.

Schwartz T, Sanner H, Gjesdal O, Flatø B, Sjaastad I (2014) In juvenile dermatomyositis, cardiac systolic dysfunction is present after long-term follow-up and is predicted by sustained early skin activity. *Ann Rheum Dis* 73: 1805–1810.

Seifert BL, Snyder MS, Klein AA, O'Loughlin JE, Magid MS, Engle MA (1992) Development of obstruction to ventricular outflow and impairment of inflow in glycogen storage disease of the heart: serial echocardiographic studies from birth to death at 6 months. *Am Heart J* 123: 239–242.

Sembrano E, Barthlen GM, Wallace S, Lamm C (1997) Polysomnographic findings in a patient with the mitochondrial encephalomyopathy NARP. *Neurology* 49: 1714–1717.

Servidei S, Riepe RE, Langston C, Tani LY, Bricker JT, Crisp-Lindgren N et al. (1987) Severe cardiopathy in branching enzyme deficiency. *J Pediatr* 111: 51–56.

Servidei S, Metlay LA, Chodosh J, DiMauro S (1988) Fatal infantile cardiopathy caused by phosphorylase b kinase deficiency. *J Pediatr* 113: 82–85.

Silvestri G, Santorelli FM, Shanske S, Whitley CB, Schimmenti LA, Smith SA et al. (1994) A new mtDNA mutation in the tRNA(Leu(UUR)) gene associated with maternally inherited cardiomyopathy. *Hum Mutat* 3: 37–43.

Singla M, Guzman G, Griffin AJ, Bharati S (2008) Cardiomyopathy in multiple Acyl-CoA dehydrogenase deficiency: a clinico-pathological correlation and review of literature. *Pediatr Cardiol* 29: 446–451.

Slaughter MS, Rogers JG, Milano CA, Russell SD, Conte JV, Feldman D et al. (2009) Advanced heart failure treated with continuous-flow left ventricular assist device. *N Engl J Med* 361: 2241–2251.

Tajsharghi H, Oldfors A, Swash M (2007a) Myosin storage myopathy with cardiomyopathy. *Neuromuscul Disord* 17: 725.

Tajsharghi H, Oldfors A, Macleod DP, Swash M (2007b) Homozygous mutation in MYH7 in myosin storage myopathy and cardiomyopathy. *Neurology* 68: 962.

Takano N, Honke K, Hasui M, Ohno I, Takemura H (1997) [A case of pacemaker implantation for complete atrioventricular block associated with Duchenne muscular dystrophy]. *No To Hattatsu* 29: 476–480.

Tandon A, Villa CR, Hor KN, Jefferies JL, Gao Z, Towbin JA et al. (2015) Myocardial fibrosis burden predicts left ventricular ejection fraction and is associated with age and steroid treatment duration in Duchenne muscular dystrophy. *J Am Heart Assoc* 4:e001338.

Tegtmeyer LC, Rust S, van Scherpenzeel M, Ng BG, Losfeld ME, Timal S et al. (2014) Multiple phenotypes in phosphoglucomutase 1 deficiency. *N Engl J Med* 370: 533–542.

Towbin J (2006) Mitochondrial cardiology. In DiMauro S, Hirano M, Schon EA (eds) *Mitochondrial Medicine*. Abingdon: Informa Healthcare, pp. 75–104.

Thrush PT, Allen HD, Viollet L, Mendell JR (2009) Re-examination of the electrocardiogram in boys with Duchenne muscular dystrophy and correlation with its dilated cardiomyopathy. *Am J Cardiol* 103: 262–265.

Tripp ME, Katcher ML, Peters HA, Gilbert EF, Arya S, Hodach RJ et al. (1981) Systemic carnitine deficiency presenting as familial endocardial fibroelastosis: a treatable cardiomyopathy. *N Engl J Med* 305(7):385–390.

Tyni T, Pihko H (1999) Long-chain 3-hydroxyacyl-CoA dehydrogenase deficiency. *Acta Paediatr* 88: 237–245.

Van den Hout H, Reuser AJ, Vulto AG, Loonen MCB, Cromme-Dijkhuis A, Van der Ploeg AT (2000) Recombinant human alpha-glucosidase from rabbit milk in Pompe patients. *Lancet* 356: 397–398.

Viollet L, Thrush PT, Flanigan KM, Mendell JR, Allen HD (2012) Effects of angiotensin-converting enzyme inhibitors and/or beta blockers on the cardiomyopathy in Duchenne muscular dystrophy. *Am J Cardiol* 110: 98–102.

Winkel LP, Kamphoven JH, van den Hout HJ, Severijnen LA, van Doorn PA, Reuser AJ et al. (2003) Morphological changes in muscle tissue of patients with infantile Pompe's disease receiving enzyme replacement therapy. *Muscle Nerve* 27: 743–751.

Winkel LP, Van den Hout JM, Kamphoven JH, Disseldorp JA, Remmerswaal M, Arts WF et al. (2004) Enzyme replacement therapy in late-onset Pompe's disease: a three-year follow-up. *Ann Neurol* 55: 495–502.

Winkel LPF, Hagemans MLC, van Doorn PA, Loonen MC, Hop WJ, Reuser AJ et al. (2005) The natural course of non-classic Pompe's disease; a review of 225 published cases. *J Neurol* 252: 875–884.

Yotsukura M, Sasaki K, Kachi E, Sasaki A, Ishihara T, Ishikawa K (1995) Circadian rhythm and variability of heart rate in Duchenne-type progressive muscular dystrophy. *Am J Cardiol* 76: 947–951.

# Section 8

## Psychosocial Aspects

# 28
## COGNITIVE, BEHAVIORAL AND PSYCHOSOCIAL ASPECTS OF GROWING UP WITH A NEUROMUSCULAR DISEASE

*Sam Geuens*

**Introduction**

Children with neuromuscular diseases (NMDs) seem to have a higher risk of developing cognitive, behavioral or psychopathological difficulties. Some of these difficulties seem inherent to the neuromuscular disorders, other are not. NMDs can influence different domains of a child's life and development and while growing up, those children have to face a lot of difficulties compared with healthy peers. This struggle can induce behavior that is not easy to cope with for their caregivers. A multidisciplinary approach is recommended in order to prevent, recognize and manage the difficulties that come on the path of a child growing up into adulthood.

When a child is diagnosed with an NMD, the first and greatest concerns are related to muscle strength, motor development and physical symptoms. Motor problems are often the first visible symptoms and the reason for referral to a medical center. However, a neuromuscular disease can also cause a broad variety of comorbid problems in cognitive, psychiatric, psychosocial or emotional development and functioning. Some of these comorbid symptoms are presumed to be induced by the same genetic defects that cause the neuromuscular problems and are often considered to be a part of the disease. Cognitive delay in patients with Duchenne muscular dystrophy (DMD), for example, had already been described by Duchenne de Boulogne by 1868 (Emery and Muntoni 2003). Yet, not much is known about the impact of those genetic defects on brain development and often a great heterogeneity in severity of symptoms is seen among patients with the same genetic mutations. These underlying neurobiological mechanisms are still poorly understood.

Other comorbid symptoms in patients with NMDs cannot be clearly linked to specific syndromes and occur in great variety independently from genotype. These symptoms can be considered as secondary symptoms induced by the impact of neuromuscular disability on a child's development and functioning in daily life. These symptoms are often more subtle and difficult to detect in the early stages. They appear during the developmental stages of a child growing up into adulthood.

This chapter will describe some cognitive and behavioral aspects that can occur in NMDs in children. However, there is a great variety of symptoms and a lot of the causal mechanisms are not yet understood. During the past two decades, scientific interest has grown and some characteristics have been identified. In some NMDs this evidence is more comprehensive than in others. Myotonic dystrophy type 1 (DM1) and DMD will be used as examples in this chapter, but the approach is applicable to other and rarer neuromuscular disorders such as congenital myopathies, spinal muscular atrophy, Friedreich ataxia, etc. Every child is unique and deserves a customized approach. Knowledge about the specific factors of the underlying neuromuscular pathology should be integrated in the developmental and contextual story of the child in order to interpret behavior and eventually explain difficulties.

**Developmental and behavioral aspects**

Children with motor disabilities are often more vulnerable in their development than other children. While growing up, they have to face a lot of difficulties compared with healthy peers. This struggle can induce behavior that is not easy to cope with for their caregivers. Boys and girls with neuromuscular diseases also need to be nurtured like typically developing children, but the challenges are more difficult and there can be a complex interaction between disability, disease-specific factors, environment and medical treatment. In general, there is a consensus that children with neuromuscular disease are more at risk of developing behavioral and psychological problems.

In myotonic dystrophy type 1 (DM1), for example, behavioral problems are often mentioned, even in the earliest studies. Steyaert et al. (1997) and Goossens et al. (2000) estimated the prevalence of psychiatric disorders in DM1 patients as between 56.6% and 63%, based on Child Behavior Checklist-reports (CBCL). Besides the internal problems, defined by the CBCL by anxious-depressed, withdrawn-depressed or somatic symptoms (40%), attention-deficit–hyperactivity disorder (ADHD) was the most frequent disorder in 30% of the participants. Other authors found conduct disorders (Echenne et al. 2008) or autism spectrum disorders (Ekström et al. 2009) as most frequent comorbidity. There is consensus that anxiety problems and sleep problems are common in the DM1 population (Goossens et al. 2000; Quera et al. 2006). Finally, school problems are frequently reported in DM1 children (69–86.6%). Writing, reading and spelling problems are mainly noticed, even in children without intellectual disability (Cohen et al. 2006; Douniol et al. 2009).

An increased risk of developing behavioral problems is also documented in children with DMD. Leibowitz and Dubowitz (1981) described emotional disturbance in 36.6% (n = 52) of boys with DMD. Subsequent studies showed more specification in behavioral and emotional difficulties. For example, those boys tend to suffer more than healthy peers from feelings of anxiety (Banihani et al. 2015; Pangalila et al. 2015) or problems with psychosocial functioning (Donders and Taneja 2009; Hendriksen et al. 2009). Those findings are mainly based on proxy report questionnaires, but other studies have used more specific diagnostic methods to investigate psychiatric comorbidity in DMD. For instance, several studies report a higher prevalence of autism spectrum disorder (ASD) in boys with DMD compared with the general population. In a review Snow et al. (2013) concluded that there is strong support for a proposed link between DMD and ASD. One in three boys with DMD tend to score higher on ASD screening assessments, but eventually they do not all meet sufficient criteria for formal psychiatric diagnosis. Boys with DMD seem to display more autism-like behavior than healthy boys of their age. More recently, Colombo et al. (2017) confirmed this finding in a study about young children with DMD. These children exhibit a higher prevalence of ASD and intellectual disorder and a higher rate on the CBCL Internalizing Problems scale than would be expected in the general population (Colombo et al. 2017). Also, symptoms of ADHD are frequently linked to DMD. Most of the studies investigating this comorbidity used parental questionnaires, and prevalence of ADHD in DMD boys was estimated between 11.7% and 33% (Hendriksen and Vles 2008; Colombo et al. 2017). Other behavioral problems reported in DMD are obsessive-compulsive problems which occur in about 4% of boys with DMD (Hendriksen and Vles 2008).

Both DM1 and DMD are examples of NMDs where the genetic deficit seems to influence the development of the child, resulting in behavioral and psychiatric comorbidities. In other NMDs, such as spinal muscular atrophy (SMA), facioscapulohumeral dystrophy (FSHD), Friedreich ataxia (FA) or Becker muscular dystrophy (BMD), the impact of the gene mutations on neurocognitive functioning is less clear. Studies investigating this impact are scarce and those disorders seem to have a less clear impact on psychosocial development of children. However, children with NMDs in general seem to be vulnerable for psychological difficulties and can be at risk of developing social, behavioral and emotional problems. Awareness and screening for those problems is very important to prevent or recognize psychologic pathology at an early stage. The following section will describe some important factors for a child with a neuromuscular disease growing up into adulthood.

DEVELOPMENTAL STAGES

A child's development exists in different stages in different domains. Every stage is characterized by its own developmental challenges. If the child has fully completed one step, it can grow to the following stage. Eventually the child will grow into adulthood with a minimal risk of developing disturbing issues. This is a multidimensional and individual process and every child has his/her own path to follow, but eventually all adults will have passed the same developmental steps. The developmental psychologist Erikson (1964) distinguished different psychosocial steps in his theory (Table 28.1). If a task cannot be fulfilled by a child, the child is at risk for a developmental crisis that can have an impact in later stages in his/her life.

Children with a neuromuscular disease are more vulnerable to not being able to complete those psychosocial stages, as illustrated in Table 28.1. For example, these children can experience more problems with achieving autonomy in their early childhood due to motor impairment. This can lead to dependency, not being able to explore and accept their own limitations, lower self-esteem and eventually difficulties with identity and separation from parents in their puberty. This issue can be identified in a lot of young adults with NMDs.

**TABLE 28.1**

Psychosocial developmental stages and risk and recommendations in children with neuromuscular diseases

| Age | Erikson's psychosocial stages[a] | Risks | Recommendations |
|---|---|---|---|
| 0–1 year | Basic trust versus mistrust | Pain, long hospitalizations, intensive medical care, being uncomfortable, etc., can interfere with this first and important psychosocial stage where children must gain confidence that the world is safe. Mistrust occurs when parents are obstructed in giving warm, responsive care to their child. | Let parents be parents and let them be with their child as much as possible. Guide parents in how to comfort or take care of their child, even when intensive medical care is needed. Encourage skin-on-skin contact. |
| 1–3 years | Autonomy versus shame and doubt | Motor skills are important for the child to explore the world and learn how to choose and decide for themselves. Reasonable free choice should be permitted. Motor impairment can inhibit this feeling of choice and induce shame and doubt. | Stimulate the exploration of the world, even when motor functions are limited. Bring the world to the child if needed. Give the child as much as mobility as possible. Give the child the possibility to make mistakes. Overprotection can also be harmful. |
| 3–6 years | Initiative versus guilt | Through play children experiment with human characteristics and which kind of person they can become. They learn social and emotional behavior by this make-believe play. When obstructed by motor impairment or by isolation from other children, they cannot develop this sense of ambition and responsibility (taking initiative). When too much self-control is demanded, this can lead to overcontrol and feelings of guilt. | Stimulate fantasy play, make-believe play and contact with other children. Facilitate the opportunities to experiment with different human roles. Don't expect too much of a child, be understanding for their frustrations and feelings of anxiety or doubt. |
| 6–11 years | Industry versus diffusion | By working with others (e.g. at school), children develop the capacity to work and cooperate. They learn they can be successful in their own process of growth. Inferiority develops when negative experiences at home, at school, or with peers, lead to feelings of incompetence. | Give goals that are within the range of their capacities. Have realistic expectations. Stimulate working together with other children and going to school. Help them to cope with negative experiences. |

Continued

**TABLE 28.1**

Continued

| | | |
|---|---|---|
| Adolescence | Identity versus identity confusion | Adolescents try to find out who they are and what place they have in society. They separate from parents and experiment with values and what kind of person they want to be. Identity confusion can occur when teenagers don't find a realistic role in society. | Invest in a relationship of trust.<br>Learn them how to speak about difficult subjects.<br>Give them the opportunity to experiment and make mistakes within realistic boundaries.<br>Give them a lot of understanding and prevent feelings of loneliness. |
| Young adulthood | Intimacy versus isolation | Young adults work on establishing intimate ties to others. When they are unsure of their own identity and body, this process can become more complex. Earlier disappointments can obstruct the formation of new relationships and lead to isolation | Create the openness to talk about relationships, sexuality and their own development.<br>Stimulate them to seek help for their own doubts or fears if needed.<br>Reassure them they are as valuable as everyone. |

[a] Berk (2004)

Professionals should be aware of those vulnerabilities and try to prevent developmental stagnation. They can do this by stimulating the acts that lead to the fulfilling of the psychosocial stage: giving a child independency by mobility, providing parents with nurturing guidance, stimulating social participation, helping a child reaching normal goals at school despite his/her physical limitations, etc.

PARENTING

It is always devastating news for parents when their child is diagnosed with a neuromuscular disease. Suddenly, their perspectives on the future and their dreams vanish and what remains is uncertainty. Parents will react with their own coping skills, but it is recommended that psychological support is provided from the beginning. This support can start as parental counseling during the difficult time around the diagnosis and can grow into guidance throughout the following years, providing the parents with parenting advice. Often, parents find it difficult to know how to react to the behavior of their child with a neuromuscular disease. They can have many questions through the different developmental stages of their child. A healthcare professional specializing in children and youngsters with NMDs can provide psycho-education about the development of children, the way to nurture them and the vulnerabilities that come along with a specific disease. It is important that the behavior of a child is interpreted in a right way to know how to react on it. A child will learn from the reaction of their environment and if this is not adequate, it can lead to developmental consequences in later stages. For example, it is a natural reaction for parents and other caregivers to compensate for a child's motor loss. They want to make sure the child is feeling happy and this can lead to material and emotional pampering or a "laissez-faire" parenting style. This is no problem and can be comforting during a short period, but it can be problematic if it lasts longer during the child's development, interfering with several developmental tasks. Another example is when parents want to protect their child by not telling them the truth about their medical condition. This is very understandable, but eventually this can harm the child's development of their own identity. A healthcare professional, such as a pediatric psychologist, can advise parents from the beginning how to nurture a child with a neuromuscular disease and how to deal with both the primary or secondary behavioral consequences of the disease. By doing so, prevention of psychopathology can become a goal.

## School

School is a very important place for a child as they spend a lot of time there. Children do not only achieve academic knowledge and skills in school. It is also a place where they can grow up among peers and where they are stimulated to practice social, emotional and relational skills. Their world gets bigger by going to school and it protects them from isolation and understimulation. This is the case for every child and, thus, also for children with NMDs. Often, young children with a neuromuscular disease struggle to attend school on a regular basis and there are a lot of different reasons for this: not every school is adapted to children with limited motor functions, those children are more vulnerable to infections and are therefore more hospitalized or at home, parents want to protect them as long as they can, not every school is confident enough to have a child with complex needs in their school, children are not motivated to go to school, etc. Despite the fact that those reasons are truly understandable, a joint effort should be made by parents, healthcare professionals and schools to maximize the amount of education a child can get. Even a child with a neuromuscular disease should go to school as much as possible or at least get education in other ways. There will be more difficulties complicating this process that there are with healthy children. Those difficulties can be practical, emotional or medical, but a joint plan should be made by all caregivers in order to overcome those difficulties and give the child the chance to develop together with their peers.

All three domains described (developmental stages, parenting and going to school) get more complex when there is comorbidity of motor limitations and cognitive or learning problems. As mentioned before, some NMDs can give rise to comorbid problems in cognitive and neuropsychological functioning. These aspects will be discussed in the next section.

**Cognitive and neuropsychological functioning**
Understanding the complex dyad between neuromuscular and neuropsychological (dys-) functioning is difficult, but it should be considered for every child with an NMD. In some cases, there will be no visible cognitive or neuropsychological impairment but screening for it is certainly meaningful. Some difficulties only appear during the later stages and can be considered as growing into deficit: there always has been a vulnerability for this dysfunction, but it only becomes a problem at a later age when more complex behavior or functioning is expected from the child. An example of this can be dyscalculia which does not appear before a child is confronted with mathematics in elementary school. Other, less concrete difficulties that only appear in the later stages of development are problems with executive functioning, for example. Knowing which children are vulnerable for which problems makes it possible to screen from the beginning or to diagnose them at an early stage and to implement early interventions if necessary. To do so, it is important to be aware of the impact of NMDs on cognitive and neuropsychological functioning. Below, we will discuss some aspects of this impact.

Intelligence is probably the best documented domain in cognitive research in children with NMDs, but evidence and consensus in some populations is more exhaustive than in others and a critical interpretation of the results is recommended. In myotonic dystrophy type 1 (DM1), for example, most studies do not include children with the congenital form, although they are most affected. In six studies carried out between 2004 and 2015, a mean full-scale IQ (FSIQ) of 67.6 was found. This is the lower limit of a range that Douniol et al. (2009) obtained in a meta-review based on seven studies. According to this review, children with DM1 can be divided into two groups: children with a normal intelligence normally distributed around a mean IQ of 91 (standard deviation = 13) and children with a mild intellectual disability normally distributed around a mean IQ of 58 (standard deviation = 9). However, this analysis is based on a small sample of children (N = 36).

Several studies suggest that verbal IQ is significantly higher than performance IQ in children with DM1 (Angeard et al. 2011; Douniol et al. 2012). This seems to be the case in DM1 patients with an IQ below average, but not in children with an intellectual disability (IQ <70) (Douniol et al. 2009). More evidence exists regarding the negative correlation between the number of CTG-repeats and FSIQ. When there was inheritance from mother's side, the CTG-repeats were higher and the FSIQ was lower (Steyaert et al. 1997; Goossens et al. 2000; Angeard et al. 2007; Douniol et al. 2009). Some studies also report a progressive cognitive decline in some children with DM1 (Echenne et al. 2008).

The same heterogeneity range of cognitive capacities is seen in intelligence research in boys with DMD. In 1968 Cohen et al. estimated the prevalence of intellectual disability among DMD patients about 21% based on IQ estimations done by proxy reports. Future research has confirmed and nuanced the increased prevalence of intellectual disability in a DMD population compared to the general population. A lot of studies used psychometric measures in order to investigate the impact of DMD on intellectual functioning taking into account the possible impact of disease severity, reduced educational and social opportunities and muscle degeneration (and the implications for IQ-tests). There is a consensus that boys with DMD are more at risk of developing intellectual disability compared to the general population, measured with full-scale IQ (FIQ). Studies investigating the difference between verbal IQ (VIQ) and performance IQ (PIQ) often suggest that those with DMD tend to perform more poorly on the verbal than on the performance measures of intelligence testing (Pane et al. 2012; Banihani et al. 2015). In a meta-analysis conducted by Cotton et al. (2001), data from 32 studies between 1960 and 1999 regarding FIQ, VIQ and PIQ from 1 146 males with DMD was analyzed. They confirmed the consensus that boys with DMD tend to score 1 standard deviation below the mean IQ of a healthy population. There seems to be a link with mutations in the dystrophin gene, expression of dystrophin isoforms in the brain and cognitive abilities. Moreover, boys with a mutation in the last third exons of the dystrophin gene (e.g. Dp71) are more at risk of developing an intellectual disability (Ricotti et al. 2016). But the relation between genotype and phenotype is not fully understood and Cotton et al. (2001) emphasized the complexity behind the full-scale IQ and recommended a broader neuropsychological approach to identify specific subgroups of cognitive deficits.

This is an important message and during the last 15 years more research has focused on the identification of specific neuropsychological profiles in DMD, DM1 and other NMDs in children. The only consensus, however, is the conclusion that there is a great heterogeneity among patients and specific profiles do not seem to suit all patients. Depending on the chosen methodology or neuropsychological tests, different conclusions can be made. Yet, there seem to be some underlying vulnerabilities among children with the same neuromuscular disease. Examples of these disease-specific risks are an impaired verbal working memory and less expressive speech in boys with DMD (Snow et al. 2013), cognitive fatigue (Douniol et al. 2012) and impaired working memory in DM1 (Angeard et al. 2007; Wozniak et al. 2013), executive and memory and visuospatial deficits in patients with Friedreich ataxia (Mantovan et al. 2006).

The challenge, however, is that not all symptoms described above appear in every patient and that some patients may show additional neuropsychological symptoms which are not empirically demonstrated in large groups. It is recommended that healthcare professionals and caregivers are aware of the neuropsychological vulnerabilities and risks of a certain neuromuscular disease, but also maintain an open approach to the unique functioning of the child. Measurements of intelligence are widely used for this and can provide important information about the general functioning of the child. Indeed, the intellectual level of functioning can give an overall view on the cognitive development of a child compared to their peers, but it is necessary to be careful in using a full-scale IQ, verbal (VIQ) or performance (PIQ) intelligence quotient to explain behavior or to predict school functioning at a later age. These IQs can be a predictor for future academic achievement, but the true potential of a child can never be caught in just one measurement or number. Especially for children with NMDs, the values of the different IQ-scales need to be put into perspective. Most cognitive tests measuring intelligence in children use tasks where motor speed and functioning are expected. Children with less motor control will score lower on these tasks, which can look like they have less potential for the cognitive function the task is supposed to measure. This should be taken into account when the results are being interpreted. Furthermore, the lack of consensus in empirical studies about neuropsychological profiles in NMDs demonstrates the great heterogeneity between children, but is also a sign of the discrepancy between different neuropsychological functions in one individual child. Therefore, it is recommended that conclusions are not only based on rough and general scales such as intelligence scales, but are supplemented with the results of specific neuropsychological tasks, and all results are combined into a neuropsychological profile with the strengths and weaknesses of this individual child. Doing so, the full potential of the child will be acknowledged and advice or interventions can be based on the strengths of a child, but taking into account the weaknesses and potential pitfalls.

**Conclusions**

Despite their physical impairment, children with NMDs are children who want to grow up and explore the world. However, having motor limitations can complicate the psychosocial, emotional and cognitive development of those children. These children tend to have a greater vulnerability for developing psychological problems. Stimulating them, and giving them the chances to complete their psychosocial developmental stages, should be a goal in an attempt to prevent psychological or behavioral problems at a later age. This can be a difficult process as some NMDs directly cause psychopathology in children. A multidisciplinary approach is recommended and guidance for parents as well as schools should be provided. More scientific research is also needed to identify specific factors that influence the developmental trajectories in children with NMDs.

**Key points**
- Be aware of the fact that a neuromuscular disease does not only affect motor functioning, but also has a great impact on other domains of a child's development.
- Behavior is a complex interaction of disease-specific vulnerabilities, developmental stages and contextual and child factors.
- Be aware of the different psychosocial stages of a child and make interventions to stimulate the completion of each stage.
- Make efforts to prevent developmental stagnation in the later stages of child's life.
- Provide psycho-education and guidance for parents and other caregivers.
- Stimulate children to go to school or get as much as education as possible.

- Screen for disease-specific cognitive and neuropsychological deficits.
- Use specific neuropsychological tests to measure specific functions rather than only using rough, general scales such as intelligence quotients.
- Construct a profile of the cognitive strengths and weaknesses of each individual child to provide customized advice.

**Clinical vignette**

A 14-year-old boy with DM1 was referred to our center with episodes of epileptic-like behavior. During those episodes the boy seemed absent, was not responsive and seemed less conscious. After a few minutes, this disappeared and after some rest, he could continue his activities. An electroencephalogram (EEG) and a neurologic examination could not objective signs of epilepsy. This behavior never happened at home or when the parents were nearby, but always in school or in new situations (such as a summer camp). The parents reported that the boy was more stressed lately. He attended a special school, but he was assigned to some new and more challenging tasks. Because of his age he had also been moved to an older group in his soccer team and at summer camp. His parents found that he had been less happy and more withdrawn during the past few months.

We conducted a neuropsychological examination and had several interviews with the boy, the parents and the school. The boy has lower intellectual capacities (total IQ of 54), but he had a very discrepant neuropsychological profile. The processing of verbal information was really difficult for him, but when visual information was given, he could process this really well, even higher than expected based on his IQ. We concluded that this boy was trying to cope with some difficulties or stressful events in his life on his own, which was completely healthy for his psychosocial developmental stage. He did not want to rely on his parents or other adults anymore for help, but he had not the cognitive capacity to invent new coping strategies or verbalize difficulties when the situation became too complex. In those moments, he blocked and had a psychosomatic reaction.

We gave him, his parents and school staff psycho-education on this. Based on his strong visual information processing skills, we designed other coping strategies for him and trained him to foresee such situations, recognize his stress and to signal this to the people in his environment. This gave him more control over the situation and he had only a few episodes during the following weeks, but none of them as intense as before. The episodes disappeared when he was moving on to other developmental tasks.

REFERENCES

Angeard N, Gargiulo M, Jacquette A, Radvanyi H, Eymard B, Héron D (2007) Cognitive profile in childhood myotonic dystrophy type 1: is there a global impairment? *Neuromuscul Disord* 17: 451–458.

Angeard N, Jacquette A, Gargiulo M, Radvanyi H, Moutier S, Eymard B et al. (2011) A new window on neurocognitive dysfunction in the childhood form of myotonic dystrophy type 1 (DM1). *Neuromuscul Disord* 21: 468–476.

Banihani R, Smile S, Yoon G, Dupuis A, Mosleh M, Snider A et al. (2015) Cognitive and neurobehavioral profile in boys with Duchenne muscular dystrophy. *J Child Neurol* 30: 1472–1482.

Berk LE (2004) *Development Through the Lifespan*, 3rd edn. Boston: Pearson.

Cohen HJ, Molnar GE, Taft LT (1968) The genetic relationship of progressive muscular dystrophy (Duchenne type) and mental retardation. *Dev Med Child Neurol* 10: 754–765.

Cohen D, Plaza M, Angeard N, Lanthier-Gazzano O, Baraud P, Riviére J (2006) Reading and spelling impairments in children and adolescents with infantile myotonic dystrophy. *J Neurolingistics* 6(19): 455–465. doi: 10.1016/j.jneuroling.2006.03.007.

Colombo P, Nobile M, Tesei A, Civati F, Gandossini S, Mani E et al. (2017) Assessing mental health in boys with Duchenne muscular dystrophy : emotional, behavioural and neurodevelopmental profile in an Italian clinical sample. *Eur J Paediatr Neurol* 21: 639–647.

Cotton S, Voudouris NJ, Greenwood KM (2001) Intelligence and Duchenne muscular dystrophy: full-scale, verbal, and performance intelligence quotients. *Dev Med Child Neurol* 43: 497–501.

Donders J, Taneja C (2009) Neurobehavioral characteristics of children with Duchenne muscular dystrophy. *Child Neuropsychol* 15: 295–304.

Douniol M, Jacquette A, Guilé JM, Tanguy ML, Angeard N, Héron D et al. (2009) Psychiatric and cognitive phenotype in children and adolescents with myotonic dystrophy. *Eur Child Adolesc Psychiatry* 18: 705–715.

Douniol M, Jacquette A, Cohen D, Bodeau N, Rachidi L, Angeard N et al. (2012) Psychiatric and cognitive phenotype of childhood myotonic dystrophy type 1. *Dev Med Child Neurol* 54: 905–911.

Echenne B, Rideau A, Roubertie A, Sébire G, Rivier F, Lemieux B (2008) Myotonic dystrophy type I in childhood Long-term evolution in patients surviving the neonatal period. *Eur J Paediatr Neurol* 12: 210–223.

Ekström A B, Hakenäs-Plate L, Mar T, Wentz E (2009) Cognition and adaptive skills in myotonic dystrophy type 1: a study of 55 individuals with congenital and childhood forms. *Dev Med Child Neurol* 51: 982–990.

Emery E, Muntoni F (2003) *Duchenne Muscular Dystrophy*. Oxford: Oxford University Press.

Erikson EH (1964) *Insight and Responsibility*. New York: Norton.

Goossens E, Steyaert J, De Die-Smulders C, Willekens D, Fryns JP (2000) Emotional and behavioral profile and child psychiatric diagnosis in the childhood type of myotonic dystrophy. *Genet Couns* 11: 317–327.

Hendriksen JGM, Vles JSH (2008) Neuropsychiatric disorders in males with duchenne muscular dystrophy: frequency rate of attention-deficit hyperactivity disorder (ADHD), autism spectrum disorder, and obsessive – compulsive disorder. *J Child Neurol* 23: 477–481.

Hendriksen JG, Poysky JT, Schrans DG, Schouten EG, Aldenkamp AP, Vles JS (2009) Psychosocial adjustment in males with Duchenne muscular dystrophy: psychometric properties and clinical utility of a parent-report questionnaire. *J Pediatr Psychol* 34: 69–78.

Leibowitz D, Dubowitz V (1981) Intellect and behaviour in Duchenne muscular dystrophy. *Dev Med Child Neurol* 23: 577–590.

Mantovan MC, Martinuzzi A, Squarzanti F, Bolla A, Silvestri I, Liessi G et al. (2006) Exploring mental status in Friedreich's ataxia: a combined neuropsychological, behavioral and neuroimaging study. *Eur J Neurol* 13: 827–835.

Pane M, Lombardo ME, Alfieri P, D'Amico A, Bianco F, Vasco G et al. (2012) Attention deficit hyperactivity disorder and cognitive function in Duchenne muscular dystrophy: phenotype-genotype correlation. *J Pediatr* 161: 705–9.e1.

Pangalila RF, van den Bos GA, Bartels B, Bergen M, Stam HJ, Roebroeck ME (2015) Prevalence of fatigue, pain, and affective disorders in adults with duchenne muscular dystrophy and their associations with quality of life. *Arch Phys Med Rehabil* 96: 1242–1247.

Quera Salva MA, Blumen M, Jacquette A, Durand MC, Andre S, De Villiers M et al. (2006) Sleep disorders in childhood-onset myotonic dystrophy type 1. *Neuromuscul Disord* 16: 564–570.

Ricotti V, Mandy WPL, Scoto M, Pane M, Deconinck N, Messina S et al. (2016) Neurodevelopmental, emotional, and behavioural problems in Duchenne muscular dystrophy in relation to underlying dystrophin gene mutations. *Dev Med Child Neurol* 58: 77–84.

Snow WM, Anderson JE, Jakobson LS (2013) Neuropsychological and neurobehavioral functioning in Duchenne muscular dystrophy: a review. *Neurosci Biobehav Rev* 37: 743–752.

Steyaert J, Umans S, Willekens D, Legius E, Pijkels E, de Die-Smulders C et al. (1997) A study of the cognitive and psychological profile in 16 children with congenital or juvenile myotonic dystrophy. *Clin Genet* 52: 135–141.

Wozniak JR, Mueller BA, Bell CJ, Muetzel RL, Lim KO, Day JW (2013) Diffusion tensor imaging reveals widespread white matter abnormalities in children and adolescents with myotonic dystrophy type 1. *J Neurol* 260: 1122–1131.

# 29
# TRANSITION TO ADULTHOOD

*Ros Quinlivan*

## Introduction

The aim of this chapter will be to define the term "transition" and to discuss the importance of transition planning for young people with neuromuscular disease (NMD). Transition is an important concept, when planned carefully, it has the potential to reduce morbidity and improve quality of life in later life by preparing the young person to take responsibility for their health. This chapter will predominantly focus on transition planning in the context of Duchenne muscular dystrophy (DMD) as it is the most common neuromuscular condition seen in children; however, the issues raised in this discussion will be relevant for all young people with neuromuscular disease.

It might be argued that if paediatricians were willing to assume lifelong responsibility for co-managing patients with complex long-term conditions, there should be no need for transition services (Schor 2015). This might be especially true for patients with rare neuromuscular disease since many adult medical teams lack experience in managing this relatively new population of young adults. Such a model may seem pragmatic, and in fact, may be the preferred option for many centres; however, it makes no attempt to equip the young adult with the necessary skills required to take responsibility for their own healthcare. In the long term this approach may lead to negative psychosocial and health consequences for the individual concerned.

It is important that healthcare professionals recognise the unique development needs of adolescents, teenagers, and young adults (aged 10–25 years). The goal of effective transition should be to ensure success in empowering and equipping the young person with the necessary skills to manage their own healthcare confidently and successfully. Much of the research into the impact of transition has been undertaken in specific adolescent populations; for example, such as those with diabetes or cystic fibrosis. The long-term health economic effects of transition have not been studied extensively in people with neuromuscular disease, although there have been a small number of surveys based upon service-user satisfaction and psychosocial wellbeing in DMD which will be discussed later. In addition, there is a need to change the culture within adult health and social services to accommodate the complex medical and psychosocial needs of young adults with neuromuscular diseases who have highly specific and complex health and psychosocial needs. This may require reorganisation of several specialist services (for example: neurology, cardiology, respiratory, gastroenterology) into a single location for efficient delivery of coordinated, pro-active, holistic, multi-disciplinary care that is more convenient for the patient.

**What is transition?**

Blum et al. (1993) defined the term transition as "the purposeful planned movement of adolescents and young adults with chronic health conditions from a child centred to adult oriented healthcare system". Adulthood should not be considered as a developmental stage that is age specific, but rather as a "social construct with no readily definable markers" (Blum et al. 1993). The development of high-level executive function is not correlated with age but rather with brain growth and development, which continues into young adulthood after physical growth has stopped, usually to the early to mid-20s (Giedd et al. 2008).

The World Health Organization (WHO) identifies adolescence as a critical time in a person's lifespan. It is a period of development from 10 to 19 years of age where there are rapid changes in both physical and sexual development. A sense of identity develops and in the later adolescent years there is progression to financial and social independence. The physical determinants of adolescent growth are universal but the length and defining features of this stage in development will vary between individuals, cultures and socio-economic groups (WHO 2014).

Adolescents should not be considered the same as young adults, although they may be physically and mentally more mature than children, they are generally not capable of understanding complex concepts or anticipating the consequences of their behaviour. They do not understand or appreciate the degree of control that they have, or can have, over decision making. This makes them more likely to undertake high-risk activities and may potentially make them more vulnerable to exploitation (WHO 2014).

Attitudes to life and the behavioural patterns that develop during adolescence can have a long-lasting effect on health; for example. adopting unhealthy eating patterns and a sedentary lifestyle can potentially have adverse health consequences later in life leading to obesity, type 2 diabetes and cardiovascular disease. Adolescents identify strongly with their peer group and this can pose significant psychological issues for the young person who has a chronic long-term condition or disability since they may perceive themselves and be perceived by others as "different". The drive to be "normal" and "not different" is profoundly strong and overrides all other concerns which may lead to denial of the underlying health condition and poor compliance with treatment. Thus, it is not surprising that health outcomes are poorest for teenagers and young adults with certain chronic conditions compared with any other age group; for example, poor long-term follow-up for young adult survivors in childhood cancer (Szalda et al. 2016), and compliance with treatment is poor in individuals diagnosed with type 1 diabetes in adolescence, leading to avoidable unplanned hospital admissions (Lotstein et al. 2013).

Thus, ensuring that young people with chronic long-term conditions are equipped with the knowledge and skills to enable them to develop a positive approach towards managing their condition is essential and will not only have lifelong beneficial consequences for the individual but also potentially significant economic benefits for the society.

As already mentioned, psychosocial health is another important aspect to consider during adolescent development. The peak age at onset of a psychiatric disorder in the population is 14 years of age (Giedd et al. 2008). Mental health disorders, such as anxiety and depression frequently begin in adolescence and are likely to have a detrimental impact on an individual's ability to self-manage their disease. Furthermore, the frequency of both anxiety and depressive illness is higher in young people with chronic long-term conditions (Pinquart and Shen 2011).

In an unpublished two-part study to review the effect of transition arrangements at our hospital, a questionnaire was sent to 1 385 young adults aged 16–25 years with a chronic neurological condition (Pattni and Quinlivan, unpublished work 2016). The underlying diagnoses of those surveyed included: neuromuscular disease, inherited metabolic disease, multiple sclerosis and epilepsy. The response rate was 24%, of those who responded, 60% felt that their condition had prevented their ambitions from being achieved, 24% reported not participating in work or education, 73% reported depression and/or anxiety and 83% reported that their condition had a significant impact on their social life, home life and hobbies, 50% of the respondents were still living with their parents.

In a paediatric setting, the medical care of children with long-term conditions is patient- and family-centred. On the other hand, in adult services there is a shift in paradigm where the patient is expected to demonstrate autonomy and assume responsibility for their own health. This is a major change, not only for the patient, but also for the parents who have previously been at the centre of their child's healthcare. Transition planning, therefore, needs to support parents to "let go and take a back seat" in their son or daughter's future medical care. The second part of Pattni's unpublished study showed how difficult this can be for parents of boys with DMD who experienced a deep sense of loss when their son transitioned to adult services. They mourned the loss of the paediatric team that they had known for many years and the peer support they received from other parents in the service. They reported feeling that just at a time when their son was becoming more vulnerable, they were losing the support that they felt they needed. They also articulated the feeling of loss of a healthy son, to quote one parent: "just as he should be flying the nest, he has become more dependent". From the point of view of the young man with DMD there was a significant feeling of helplessness expressed, leading to passivity and anxiety about managing their healthcare for example: "I let my mum open all my letters and deal with my appointments", "I leave it to my parents to tell the doctor about my medication, I would be afraid of making a mistake". "I am worried that the new team will not recognise when I am unwell". Thus, transition planning for young men with DMD should focus upon developing self-confidence and an understanding of their condition to empower them for the future.

## Changing natural history in neuromuscular disease

The natural history of many neuromuscular diseases has changed substantially in recent years due to improved survival following the introduction of non-invasive ventilation (NIV). In Canada, for example, the number of children using NIV has risen sharply in recent years and 5-year survival for children with chronic respiratory failure treated with NIV is 95%; of the children reported in this cohort, 47% had an underlying neuromuscular diagnosis (McDougall et al. 2013). Prior to the use of NIV, transition for children with neu-romuscular disease was not considered a priority, young people with severe and progressive neuromuscular disorders, such as DMD, died in adolescence or early adulthood. At a time of increasing vulnerability associated with reaching what was the end-stage of their disease, it was neither considered appropriate nor in the patient's best interests to transfer care to a new medical team. However, following the widespread use of NIV in recent years there has been a marked epidemiological change leading to a rapidly expanding cohort of young adults with rare neuromuscular diseases. In DMD, for example, mean survival has increased from 19.9 years to 30 years (Eagle et al. 2007), with some adults surviving into their fifth decade (Saito et al. 2017 and Rahbek et al. 2005), and in Canada there are now more chil-dren leaving the home ventilation service and transitioning to adult healthcare than there are children joining the service (McDougall et al. 2013). Improvements in multi-disciplinary management and including the development of international care standards (Birnkrant et al. 2018a; 2018b; 2018c), early treatment of cardiomyopathy with angiotensin converting enzyme inhibitors (ACEI), beta blockers and the use of corticosteroids will almost certainly extend life further for people with DMD, indeed some clinicians are reporting a greater number of adults than children living with DMD in their country (Rahbek et al. 2005).

A major impact of these improvements in healthcare is a relatively new and expanding population of young people who have not been adequately prepared for adulthood. One feature unique to many young adults with neuromuscular disease is the severe degree of physical impairment and, in some cases, intellectual impairment which bring significant psychosocial challenges. These severely impaired young people are wholly dependent on others (either parents or carers) for all of their day to day physical and personal needs, such as feeding, dressing and toileting. This has a great potential to impact on the ability of the individual to develop independence, as is the norm during adolescence. Thus, the concept of independent self-management is not necessarily possible for the young person with a neuromuscular disorder such as DMD. Some authors have suggested that, instead of focus-ing on independence in these individuals, the concept of "shared management" should be promoted where there is a gradual shift in responsibility from parents and service providers to the young person. This approach stresses the importance of "interdependence" using the concept of "do it on my own with support", in order to promote the young person's inde-pendence while still acknowledging their need for support (Gall et al. 2006; Hamdani et al. 2015).

At the time of diagnosis, the parents of a child with DMD may have been informed that their son had a life-limiting condition. As a consequence, when their son reaches adoles-cence there are few expectations that he will lead an independent existence in adulthood; thus, aspirations for higher education or work may not have been considered by the individ-ual, their parents or school teachers. Given the significant improvement in life-expectancy now being reported, there needs to be change in professional, parental and individual perceptions that DMD is a "chronic long-term condition" rather than a "life-limiting and terminal disease" (Schrans et al. 2013).

In 2009, a report on the transition experiences of men living with DMD was prepared for the UK Department of Health by David Abbott and gave uncomfortable insights into the lives of adults living with DMD (Abbott et al. 2012). The study surveyed the opinions of 40 affected men and revealed that one-third of them spent all day at home and did not go to school, college or work. Thirty-seven of the respondents described their overall experience of service provision as "problematic" with variable access to specialised services. Only 50% had access to a social worker and the provision of "care packages" was variable. Physical care was provided for most of the men by their parents, which was deemed likely to interfere with their ability to develop proper adult relationships.

There has been a disappointing lack of progress since Abbot's report in 2009; in 2015 a European survey of adults with DMD published by Rodger et al. (2015) showed that one-third of the respondents living in the UK did not regularly attend hospital appointments for essential cardiac and respiratory monitoring and a proportion were not attending any specialist follow-up. This compared unfavourably with children with DMD living in the UK where almost 100% of respondents reported regular attendance at hospital appointments. The study identified considerable variation between European countries; in the UK for example, 93% adult of men with DMD were still living with parents, compared with Denmark where 61% were either living independently or with a partner. None of the UK respondents were employed, compared with 17% of those living in Germany. In Germany 49% were in higher education compared with only 25% in the UK. In the UK, almost one-third of respondents did not leave their house in a whole week (Rodger et al. 2015). It could be argued, that earlier and more effective transition planning would improve these outcomes where transition goals can be set for the young person with DMD.

### Delivering a transition service

Numerous policy documents and guidelines on transition have been published by professional bodies whose role is to either deliver or commission healthcare many of which are accessible free on line (see Websites section), for example:

• American Academy of Pediatrics;
• Canadian Pediatric Society;
• Care Quality Commission (CQC) (UK);
• National Institute for Clinical Excellence (NICE) (UK);
• Royal College of Pediatrics and Child Health (UK);
• Society of Adolescent Health and Medicine (USA and Canada).

In 2016, in the UK, the National Institute of Clinical Evidence (NICE) published a transition guideline which all healthcare providers in the UK have a duty to follow (Singh et al. 2016). However, recent research suggests that, despite legal and health frameworks, transition care for DMD is highly diverse and sometimes lacking, although positive transition experiences were characterised by forward planning and long-standing relationships between the family and healthcare professionals (Rodger et al. 2012).

The transition process should begin in early adolescence and there needs to be an understanding that it is not simply an action that entails handing care over to the adult team at a fixed point in time. The neuromuscular team should initiate discussions with the child and their parents about a transition plan when the child is about 12 years of age, certainly this should happen no later than 14 years of age. At an early stage, information should be provided about the adult team, the place where care will be transferred to and the approximate age when this will happen. Skills that should be developed during this time include communication (including an understanding of confidentiality issues), decision making, self-care (with and without support) and self-advocacy. To facilitate this process, a key worker/transition co-ordinator should be allocated to support the young person and their family during this time. The young person should be included in all discussions and aspects of decision making during clinic appointments and should be made to feel as though they are an equal partner in the process. Enabling the young person to make his or her own decisions and setting small goals between clinic appointments will help to foster a sense of control and independence.

Psychosocial support is very important and should be available throughout this time with access to a clinical psychologist if required. Supervised peer support and mentoring, where appropriate, from an older patient may also be beneficial. Young people want to be included in service design and it is important that their views are listened to when developing transition services.

Ensuring close links between the paediatric and adult services is essential for seamless transfer of care to take place. This is especially important to prevent the young person from falling between gaps in service provision. A transition clinic, where the young person can be seen jointly by both the paediatric and adult teams ensures good communication between teams and encourages the use of shared protocols. The timing of transfer to the adult service should be shared and agreed by all parties, maintaining a flexible approach is essential, depending upon the "transition readiness" of the young person to transfer care.

As already discussed, there is good evidence for an increase in morbidity and mortality following the transfer from paediatric to adult services. In my own adult service, I have encountered young people with DMD who do not comply with essential and life-saving treatment such as NIV and cardiac medications and who undertake in risky behaviours such as acute alcohol binging resulting in emergency hospital admission. Transition, being a gradual process of empowerment, should equip young people with the skills and knowledge necessary to manage their own healthcare in both paediatric and adult services to improve long-term outcomes and patient experience and thus prevent these situations from occurring. It is important that the transition program developed is holistic in order to address the medical, psychosocial and vocational needs of the young person.

Ready, Steady, Go is a transition pathway/ plan described by Nagra et al. (2015). It is suitable for children from the age of 11 years and can be adapted to the individual needs of the service (Figs. 29.1 and 29.2). The key principle of "ready, steady go" is to empower the young person to manage their own healthcare confidently and successfully and includes the following goals: healthy lifestyle, including diet and sexual health; educational and vocational issues that realistically meet expectations; psychosocial issues; and developing the understanding of the concept of transition.

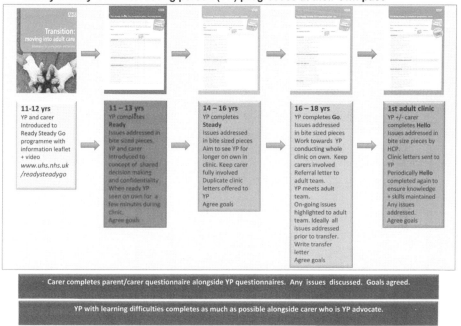

**Fig. 29.1.** The Ready, Steady, Go programme. Reprinted from Nagra (2015) with permission from BMJ Publishing Group Ltd.

"Parent Project Muscular Dystrophy (PPMD)" is an international DMD charity that has undertaken pioneering work to look specifically at transition issues affecting boys with DMD. Following a series of interviews, they identified six success factors for adolescents and young adults with DMD (Schrans et al. 2013):

> social and physical support leads to independence, the importance of setting goals and reaching them in an inventive way, daily activities give satisfaction, acceptance, coping and optimism are vital, access to good medical and psychosocial information is vital, continuity of care during transition to adulthood is vital.

A workshop of invited experts was then convened to work on these identified themes in more detail and a Delphi technique was adopted to determine opinions on six key areas called "fact sheets", these included: taboo subjects such as end of life, sexuality, dependence on others, being a burden and continual loss of expectation. Thinking about transition early with an emphasis on teaching the skills required for independence and developing goals was emphasised. Important concepts specific for this population included coping with DMD, including the roles of various healthcare professionals and parents, and dealing with "watershed" moments such as the initiation of nocturnal ventilation, transition to adult services, scoliosis surgery and life-threatening pneumonia (Schrans et al. 2013). Although this

# The Ready Steady Go transition programme - Getting Ready

NHS

Ready Steady Go programme

The medical and nursing team aim to support you as you grow up and help you gradually develop the confidence and skills to take charge of your own healthcare.

Filling in this questionnaire will help the team create a programme to suit you.
**Please answer all questions that are relevant to you and ask if you are unsure.**

Name:                                    Date:

| Knowledge and skills | Yes | I would like some extra advice/help with this | Comment |
|---|---|---|---|
| **KNOWLEDGE** | | | |
| I can describe my condition | | | |
| I know when to take my medications, names, doses, how often, etc | | | |
| I know who's in the medical and nursing team. | | | |
| I understand the differences between paediatric and adult health care | | | |
| I know about resources that offer support for young people with my condition | | | |
| **SELF ADVOCACY (speaking up for yourself)** | | | |
| I feel ready to start preparing to be seen alone for part of the clinic visit in the future | | | |
| I ask my own questions in clinic | | | |
| I have heard and know about 'Ask 3 Questions' | | | |
| **HEALTH AND LIFESTYLE** | | | |
| I understand it is important to exercise for my general health and condition | | | |
| I understand the risks of alcohol, drugs and smoking to my health | | | |
| I understand what appropriate eating means for my general health | | | |
| I am aware that my condition can affect how I develop e.g. puberty | | | |
| I know where and how I can access information about sexual health | | | |

# The Ready Steady Go transition programme - Getting Ready

| Knowledge and skills | Yes | I would like some extra advice/help with this | Comment |
|---|---|---|---|
| **DAILY LIVING** | | | |
| I can look after myself at home in terms of dressing and bathing/showering etc | | | |
| I can make my own snacks/meals | | | |
| I am able to be away from home overnight. | | | |
| **SCHOOL AND YOUR FUTURE** | | | |
| I am managing at school e.g. getting to and around school, school work, PE, friends, etc | | | |
| I know what I want to do when I leave school | | | |
| **LEISURE** | | | |
| I can use public transport and access my local community, e.g. shops, leisure centre, cinema | | | |
| I see my friends outside school hours | | | |
| **MANAGING YOUR EMOTIONS** | | | |
| I know how to deal with unwelcome comments/ bullying | | | |
| I know someone I can talk to when I feel sad/ fed-up | | | |
| I know how to deal with emotions such as anger or anxiety | | | |
| I am happy with life | | | |
| **TRANSFER TO ADULT CARE** | | | |
| I understand the meaning of 'transition' and transfer of information about me | | | |

Please list anything else you would like help or advice with:

_____

_____

_____

Thank you

**Fig. 29.2.** Getting ready. Reprinted from Nagra (2015) with permission from BMJ Publishing Group Ltd.

work focussed on transition for DMD, these "success factors" could be transferable to other young people with severe neuromuscular disorders and the goals could be incorporated into a "ready, steady, go" transition pathway which could form a framework for professionals looking after young people with neuromuscular disease.

Transition outcomes can and should be monitored including treatment compliance, autonomy including knowledge about their condition, medication and self-management. Social satisfaction, parental satisfaction and psychological behavioural outcomes should also be assessed using quality of life measures.

**Ensuring adult services are suitable for adult neuromuscular patients**

So far, this discussion has focussed on the role of paediatric services in delivering an effective transition pathway. However, given that brain development continues into early adulthood, the transition process should continue until 25 years of age and, thus, does not end at the point of transfer to adult services. Adult services need to offer a flexible approach and an accessible environment that is "young person friendly". It is important that clinical teams use language that is easily understood by the young person. Utilising charities, expert patients and peer support groups as mentors can be very helpful and should be encouraged. Specific care and attention will be needed for the young person with learning disability and/ or autism, both of which are common in patients with DMD. Our own experience has shown that DMD adults with learning difficulties occurred in more than 50% of those with premature death and this experience has also been reported by other groups (Mochizuki et al. 2008 and Anderson et al. 2002) suggesting that this group of DMD patients have a worse prognosis. An assessment of "capacity" for decision making may be needed and where the young person is deemed to "lack capacity" then parents/ carers may need "power or attorney" to make decisions on behalf of the young adult. Safeguarding concerns may need to be raised and a patient advocate appointed if parents and carers do not appear to cooperate in the best interests of the young person with learning difficulties.

Adult neuromuscular services have been reported to be fragmented with poor communication between hospital specialists and primary care physicians and there is a lack of access to specialised therapists and allied health professionals (Rodger et al. 2012; Hill and Phillips 2006; Nijman et al. 2013). For the young adult with a complex neuromuscular disease, this leads to a significant change in which healthcare is delivered compared with paediatric services which are generally very well coordinated.

Fragmented care with limited access to specialist services has been shown to substantially increase the number of avoidable acute hospital admissions, many of which are prolonged and may involve admission to intensive care (Quinlivan et al. 2014). Acute hospital admissions are burdensome for neuromuscular patients and pose a significant economic burden for healthcare providers; in the UK, the cost of unplanned emergency admissions for neuromuscular patients has been estimated to be in the region of £28 million per year (Muscular Dystrophy Campaign 2011 web page, link in references).

Given that international standards of care for DMD (Bushby et al. 2018a, 2018b, 2018c) stress the importance of coordinated multi-disciplinary care, and there is a rapidly growing new population of young DMD adults with highly complex medical needs, it is important that healthcare providers review the way services are provided. In the early 1980s a new cohort of young adults with cystic fibrosis were surviving to adulthood and it was deemed necessary to develop the first UK adult cystic fibrosis centre in Manchester in 1982 (Webb et al. 2010). That first small cohort has since become a much larger population, and there are now 24 centres looking after adults with cystic fibrosis in the UK where care is coordinated, multi-disciplinary, and provided in accessible units.

Along the same lines, at our hospital, we recently developed a specialised unit to provide coordinated care for people with complex neuromuscular diseases (Quinlivan et al. 2014). A major reason for this change was that young adults with DMD reported difficulty in attending multiple hospital appointments to see various specialists which they found fatiguing. Furthermore, there was a lack of essential equipment such as hoists. Since most neuromuscular disease is associated with respiratory insufficiency requiring regular sleep studies, why not provide all aspects of medical and therapy care around the sleep study admission? We obtained charitable funding to build a small in-patient unit comprising six beds in an adapted environment called the Neuromuscular Complex Care Centre (NMCCC). A young person with DMD was involved in the design of the unit. We developed a business case to include consultant neurology, respiratory, cardiology and gastroenterology sessions together with allied health professionals in clinical psychology, speech and language therapy, physiotherapy, dietetics and occupational therapy. The professionals meet weekly at a multi-disciplinary team meeting, thus substantially improving communication between specialties. After the first 2 years in operation, more than 50% of the patients who had been admitted reported a reduction in acute unplanned admissions and 90% reported improved management with better co-ordination of care (Nastasi et al. 2016).

To improve our transition service for young adults we developed a "young person steering committee" which included young people as committee members. At their suggestion, we organised "a young person's open day" for peer support, information about our services and information on relevant topics such as: "going to university with a disability", "applying for disabled student grants", "living independently", "driving" etc. Following this we developed a young person's support group led by a clinical psychologist; the group meet on a Saturday and one of the goals is to improve social participation.

**Summary**

Transition is a process of moving from childhood to becoming an independent adult who is confident in the ability to self-manage their own health. Transition planning should start early, by 11–12 years, and continue up to 25 years and is important to ensure the long-term health and psychosocial wellbeing of the individual. A flexible approach is essential, taking into account the developmental and cultural background of the young person. A key worker should be allocated to support the young person, set goals and provide psychosocial support. Parents should be given support to "let go and take a back seat" in their son or daughter's healthcare. There should be close working with adult teams including a joint clinic and shared protocols across adult and paediatric centres to ensure consistency and a seamless approach. For young adults with learning disability, an assessment of capacity to make decisions should be undertaken. In this situation parents may need "power of attorney" to make decisions.

Adult services for young adults with neuromuscular disease need to be developed so that complex multi-disciplinary care can be streamlined and carefully coordinated. Peer support and mentoring by another patient can be particularly helpful and can be supported by charitable organisations.

## Key points
- Transition planning should start by 11–14 years of age.
- A key worker should be allocated.
- Consider developing a healthcare passport.
- The young person should be involved in healthcare planning and treated as an equal partner.
- There should be close links between health, education and social care.
- There should be a flexible approach when planning the time of transfer to adult services.
- There should be shared protocols with the adult service.
- There should be an opportunity to meet the adult healthcare team before transfer to prevent the young person "slipping through the net".
- There should be peer support and psychological support for the young person.
- The adult services should pay attention to environment making it young "person friendly" and accessible.

## Clinical vignette
Mohammed has DMD and has just transferred to adult services at 17.5 years of age. A transition plan was first discussed with him and his parents when he was 11 years old. He was introduced to Ruth, his transition co-ordinator, who prepared a transition plan and set small goals to help him develop decision making skills after each appointment. At 14 years of age he enrolled for "Takin' charge" – a two year transition programme developed by the Action Duchenne charity designed to help boys with DMD understand their condition and develop assertive skills so that they can make decisions. This included opportunities to attend mentoring workshops run by older men with DMD. During his last few years in the paediatric service he met the adult physician on a few occasions. Discussions included living independently, learning to drive, applying for jobs or university and how to apply for grants.

## Websites
American Academy of Pediatrics: https://pediatrics.aappublications.org/content/pediatrics/128/1/182.full.pdf
Canadian Pediatric Society: https://www.cps.ca/en/documents/position/transition-youth-special-needs
Care Quality commission (CQC): Children's transition to adult health services https://www.cqc.org.uk/sites/default/files/CQC_Transition%20Report.pdf
Got transition: http://www.gottransition.org/
National Institute for Clinical Excellence (NICE): https://www.nice.org.uk/guidance/ng43
National Collaborative Workforce on Disability: http://www.ncwd-youth.info/
Royal College of Nursing: https://www.rcn.org.uk/library/subject-guides/children-and-young-people-transition-to-adult-services
Royal College of Pediatrics and Child Health: https://www.rcpch.ac.uk/topic/transition-adult
Parent Project Muscular Dystrophy: https://www.parentprojectmd.org/

## REFERENCES

Abbott D, Carpenter J, Bushby K (2012) Transition to adulthood for young men with Duchenne muscular dystrophy: research from the UK. *Neuromuscul Disord* 22: 445–446.

Anderson JL, Head SI, Rae C, Morley J (2002) Brain function in Duchenne muscular dystrophy. *Brain* 125: 4–13.

Birnkrant D, Bushby K, Bann CM, Apkon SD, Blackwell A, Brumbaugh D et al. (2018) Diagnosis and management of Duchenne muscular dystrophy, part 1: diagnosis, and neuromuscular, rehabilitation, endocrine, and gastrointestinal and nutritional management. *Lancet Neurol* 17(3): 251–67.

Birnkrant DJ, Bushby K, Bann CM, Alman BA, Apkon SD, Blackwell A et al. (2018) Diagnosis and management of Duchenne muscular dystrophy, part 2: respiratory, cardiac, bone health, and orthopaedic management. *Lancet Neurol* 17(4): 347–61.

Birnkrant DJ, Bushby K, Bann CM, Apkon SD, Blackwell A, Colvin MK et al. (2018) Diagnosis and management of Duchenne muscular dystrophy, part 3: primary care, emergency management, psychosocial care, and transitions of care across the lifespan. *Lancet Neurol* 17(5): 445–55.

Blum RW, Garell D, Hodgman CH, Jorissen TW, Okinow NA, Orr DP et al. (1993) Transition from child-centered to adult health-care systems for adolescents with chronic conditions. A position paper of the Society for Adolescent Medicine. *J Adolesc Health* 14: 570–576.

Eagle M, Bourke J, Bullock R, Gibson M, Mehta J, Giddings D et al. (2007) Managing Duchenne muscular dystrophy – the additive effect of spinal surgery and home nocturnal ventilation in improving survival. *Neuromuscul Disord* 17: 470–475.

Gall C, Kingsnorth S, Healy H (2006) Growing up ready: a shared management approach. *Phys Occup Ther Pediatr* 26: 47–62.

Giedd J, Blumenthal J, Jeffries, N et al. (1999). Brain development during childhood and adolescence: a longitudinal MRI study. *Nat Neurosci* 2(10) 861–863.

Hamdani Y, Mistry B, Gibson BE (2015) Transitioning to adulthood with a progressive condition: best practice assumptions and individual experiences of young men with Duchenne muscular dystrophy. *Disabil Rehabil* 37: 1144–1151.

Hill ME, Phillips MF (2006) Service provision for adults with long-term disability: a review of services for adults with chronic neuromuscular conditions in the United Kingdom. *Neuromuscul Disord* 16: 107–112.

Lotstein DS, Seid M, Klingensmith G, Case D, Lawrence JM, Pihoker C et al. (2013) Transition from pediatric to adult care for youth diagnosed with type 1 diabetes in adolescence. *Pediatrics* 131:e1062–e1070.

McDougall CM, Adderley RJ, Wensley DF, Seear MD (2013) Long-term ventilation in children: longitudinal trends and outcomes. *Arch Dis Child* 98: 660–665.

Mochizuki H, Miyatake S, Suzuki M, Shigeyama T, Yatabe K, Ogata K et al. (2008) Mental retardation and lifetime events of Duchenne muscular dystrophy in Japan. *Intern Med* 47: 1207–1210.

Muscular Dystrophy UK (2011) Invest to save: Improving services and reducing costs. https://www.musculardystrophyuk.org/assets/0002/4945/Muscular_Dystrophy_Campaign_Invest_to_Save_Report.pdf

Nagra A, McGinnity PM, Davis N, Salmon AP (2015) Implementing transition: Ready Steady Go. *Arch Dis Child Educ Pract Ed* 100: 313–320.

Nastasi L, Desikan M, Turner C, Parton M, Morrow J, Carr A et al. (2016) Quality of care in the first Neuromuscular Complex Care Centre in the UK from the patients' perspective. *Neuromuscul Disord* 26:S206.

Nijman JL, Groenen AM, Horemans AM, Delnoij DM (2013) Quality of hospital care for neuromuscular disorders from the patients' perspective. *Neuromuscul Disord* 23: 279–282.

Paus T, Keshavan M, Giedd JN (2008) Why do many psychiatric disorders emerge during adolescence? *Nat Rev Neurosci* 9: 947–957.

Pinquart M, Shen Y (2011) Depressive symptoms in children and adolescents with chronic physical illness: an updated meta-analysis. *J Pediatr Psychol* 36: 375–384.

Quinlivan R, Matthews E, Hanna MG (2014) Innovative care model for patients with complex muscle diseases. *Curr Opin Neurol* 27: 607–613.

Rahbek J, Werge B, Madsen A, Marquardt J, Steffensen BF, Jeppesen J (2005) Adult life with Duchenne muscular dystrophy: observations among an emerging and unforeseen patient population. *Pediatr Rehabil* 8: 17–28.

Rodger S, Steffensen BF, Lochmüller H (2012) Transition from childhood to adulthood in Duchenne muscular dystrophy (DMD) *Orph J Rare Dis* 7(Suppl 2): A8.

Rodger S, Woods KL, Bladen CL, Stringer A, Vry J, Gramsch K et al. (2015) Adult care for Duchenne muscular dystrophy in the UK. *J Neurol* 262: 629–641.

Saito T, Kawai M, Kimura E, Ogata K, Takahashi T, Kobayashi M et al. (2017) Study of Duchenne muscular dystrophy long-term survivors aged 40 years and older living in specialized institutions in Japan. *Neuromuscul Disord* 27: 107–114.

Schor EL (2015) Transition: changing old habits. *Pediatrics* 135: 958–960.

Schrans DG, Abbott D, Peay HL, Pangalila RF, Vroom E, Goemans N et al. (2013) Transition in Duchenne muscular dystrophy: An expert meeting report and description of transition needs in an emergent patient population: (Parent Project Muscular Dystrophy Transition Expert Meeting 17–18 June 2011, Amsterdam, The Netherlands). *Neuromuscul Disord* 23: 283–286.

Singh S, Anderson B, Liabo K, Ganeshamoorthy T, on behalf of the guideline committee (2016) Supporting young people in their transition to adults' services: summary of NICE guidance. *BMJ* 353: i2225.

Szalda D, Pierce L, Hobbie W, Ginsberg JP, Brumley L, Wasik M et al. (2016) Engagement and experience with cancer-related follow-up care among young adult survivors of childhood cancer after transfer to adult care. *J Cancer Surviv* 10: 342–350.

Webb AK, Dudley-Southern R, Jones AM (2010) Development of a modern adult cystic fibrosis centre in Manchester. *J R Soc Med* 103(Suppl 1): S15–S19.

WHO (2014) *Health for the world's adolescents. A second chance in the second decade.* Geneva: World Health Organization. www.who.int/adolescent/second-decade.

# 30
# SEXUAL HEALTH NEEDS IN PATIENTS WITH NEUROMUSCULAR DISORDERS

*Laurent Servais*

## Introduction

Sexuality is undeniably a key factor of human quality of life. The World Health Organization views sexuality as an integral component of the human experience and provides a holistic definition of sexuality as the integration of somatic, emotional, intellectual and social aspects of sexual beings in positive ways to enrich and enhance personality, communication, and love (World Health Organization 1975). Sexual expression relies on an intricate connection of functional anatomical and physiological systems, cognition and emotions. In contrast with other neurological conditions, literature is scarce in regard to sexuality and neuromuscular disorders.

## Current knowledge

Indeed, prior studies have given insight into the sexual experience of patients in palliative care (Vitrano et al. 2011) and in various neurological conditions such as multiple sclerosis (Bronner et al. 2010), epilepsy (Mölleken et al. 2010), Parkinson disease (Wielinski et al. 2010), intellectual disability (Servais 2006) or post-stroke sequellae (Schmitz and Finkelstein 2010). Similarly, sexual health needs in serious non-neurological conditions such as cancer or cardiovascular disease (Günzler et al. 2010), or in more benign conditions such as sleep apnoea (Reishtein et al. 2010) or fibromyalgia (Orellana et al. 2009) have been reported.

In contrast, published studies covering sexuality in the field of neuromuscular disorders are very sparse. A Danish survey conducted in 65 adult Duchenne muscular dystrophy (DMD) patients has reported the importance of romantic and sexual life in this population (Rahbek et al. 2005). Previously, a French study conducted in ventilated DMD patients indicated that 80% of them were not satisfied with their sexual lives (Raphaël et al. 2002).

The sexual problems encountered in Charcot–Marie–Tooth patients has also received limited interest (Vinci et al. 2007; Bird et al. 1994). In patients with amyotrophic lateral sclerosis, a significant decrease in sexual activity and satisfaction after disease onset was reported (Bird et al. 1994).

Pregnancy and obstetric management (Argov et al. 2009), regarded as sexual health needs, have infrequently been addressed for patients with facioscapulohumeral dystrophy

(Ciafaloni et al. 2006), spinal muscular atrophy (SMA) (Rudnik et al. 1992; Carter et al. 1994; Pugh et al. 2009; Buettner 2003; Yim et al. 2003; Flunt et al. 2009), autoimmune myasthenia (Almeida et al. 2010), myotonic dystrophy (Rudnik-Schöneborn and Zerres 2004; Rudnik-Schöneborn et al. 2006), congenital myasthenia (Servais et al. 2013), or Pompe disease (Perniconi et al. 2016).

Erectile dysfunction has been reported as a potential complication of hypogonadism in myotonic dystrophy type 1 (Peric et al. 2013).

In a complete review covering sexual dysfunction and neurological disorders (Rees et al. 2007), the only neuromuscular disorders discussed were Guillain–Barré syndrome with residual disability, recessively inherited type II congenital sensory neuropathy and familial dysautonomia. These three conditions are more likely to have sexual dysfunction.

**Factors affecting sexual health needs**

Potential implications of neuromuscular disorders on sexuality have a great diversity, influenced more by the age at onset of the disorders than by the specificity of the phenotype. Some diseases may become symptomatic at birth or few months after, such as SMA type 1 or 2, and hinder movements from the early beginning of life. Others may develop when the patient is already married and has children. This explains the large range of interaction between physical impairment and sexuality. As an intermediate between these two extremes, DMD develops in childhood, and loss of ambulation with progressive significant weakness of the upper limbs appears during early puberty. Central nervous involvement in some patients may also cause specific issues in comparison with typically intelligent, but physically disabled, teenagers with SMA or congenital myopathy.

Sexual development, seen in a broader sense, is intimately linked to bonding and human relations. It occupies an important place in the life of adolescents with neuromuscular diseases, who are faced with challenges and limitations, from diminished social opportunities to decreased or absent sexual activity. Sexual problems are usually not included in the diagnostic workup or in standard care. However, open talk with teenage patients has revealed that sexually related issues constitute a major concern.

In our experience, the potential impact of a patient's disease on his/her sexuality is strongly dependant of the age at onset of symptoms. In this view, three patterns of interaction may be described: (1) diseases occurring early in life, before or rapidly after walking acquisition, such as SMA type 2; (2) disease with progressive loss of ambulation before adulthood, such as DMD; (3) adult-onset disease, such as myotonic dystrophy type 1.

**The point of view of neuromuscular disorder patients**

From the open talk during the consultation, it appears that expectancies towards affective life and sexuality in SMA occurred early in life, and were not restricted by the consciousness of the disability. Patients described their adolescent expectancies as marriage, complete sexual life and pregnancy. Their needs thus mostly relate to receiving advice for safely seeking partners, especially with regard to online dating. Our experience is that young men could be quite emotionally vulnerable and may be subject to internet abuse when looking for girlfriends, who would be accepting of their disabilities, on internet dating sites. Since the loss of, sometimes huge, amounts of money may cause shame and feelings of guilt, it is rarely spontaneously reported. Another need expressed by some young patients is related to the physical possibility of intercourse in the context of spinal and hip surgery.

There is no published data about sexual expectancies or sexual health needs in these patients, except for some reported pregnancies (Rudnik et al. 1992; Carter et al. 1994; Pugh et al. 2009; Buettner 2003; Yim et al. 2003; Flunt et al. 2009). Indeed, pregnancies have been reported in SMA type 3 and even in SMA type 2 patients where vital capacity was as low as 0.34L (Rudnik et al. 1992). In the majority of patients, pregnancy itself does not lead to clinical deterioration, but bulbar symptoms and acute general weakness may occur in the postpartum period.

To some extent, cerebral palsy (CP) can be compared to SMA type 2, since cerebral palsy has early onset of symptoms that can lead to severe disability. In patients with cerebral palsy, affective and sexual activity is frequent although less than in the rest of the population (Wiegerink et al. 2010). However, the comparison between cerebral palsy and SMA type 2 is not completely valid since, approximately, only the 20% most severe disabled patients with cerebral palsy (Rosenbaum et al. 2002) present a functional deficit comparable to that which is observed in SMA type 2. In addition, cerebral palsy also leads to lower limbs spasticity and more frequently to sphincter problems.

### Sexual health needs for Duchenne muscular dystrophy patients

DMD constitutes the most frequent neuromuscular disorder in children and in adolescents. Symptoms occur before the age of 5, the patient loses ambulation during his early adolescence and subsequently the use of his upper limbs when they have already experienced manual masturbation. DMD patients admit that unmet challenges in their sexual life significantly interfere with their quality of life, such as the loss of the ability to masturbate.

It is frequently presumed that sexual activity of adolescent patients with chronic conditions follows a curve of decline. However, a French survey conducted in 7 936 12–25-year-old students even suggested that adolescents with chronic medical conditions are more likely to have ever experienced sexual intercourse than typically developing adolescents (Choquet et al. 1997). In contrast, one pilot study conducted in 40 neuromuscular patients noticed that in general, neuromuscular disorders with an onset in childhood or adolescence and relatively rapid progression result in severe physical limitations that interfere with psychosocial and psychosexual development (Anderson et al. 1983).

DMD is the condition for which sexual expectancies have been partially studied in young adults (Rahbek et al. 2005; Raphaël et al. 2002). From these two papers, it appears that most of the adults with DMD, despite heavy immobilisation, are still capable of functioning in a variety of activities that are associated with normal life. They are not satisfied with their sexual life in 80% of cases, have had sexual experiences in 49% of cases and used prostitution in 25% of cases. Moreover the majority of them report a painful need for love (Rahbek et al. 2005). Our personal experience is in line with these data. In addition, some patients require the prescription of tadalafil or sidelafil, which require cardiac evaluation given the high incidence of cardiomyopathy in this population. DMD patients may also be at risk of internet abuse, and through open discussion with patients, it is not uncommon to learn that they were solicited to send money abroad to girls they had never met, but with whom they have chatted online for some weeks. Another point which is much more frequently and clearly expressed by patients is the delayed of puberty due to steroid use.

### Sexual health needs for myotonic dystrophy 1 patients

Myotonic dystrophy type 1 is the most prevalent muscular disorder in adulthood. It is associated with central nervous system involvement and with a peculiar neuropsychological profile (Sistiaga et al. 2010). It is also associated with endocrine dysfunction, such as hypogonadism. Erectile dysfunction is frequent in this population, as reported in the literature and in our personal experience (Peric et al. 2013).

### Counselling

The need for sexual counselling for neuromuscular patients is a real and not futile issue, and we must take into consideration this counselling to overcome the physical limitations imposed by the evolution of the disease. An important aim is to increase awareness of the range of expressions of human sexuality so that the individual or couple increase the options available to them, and thereby increase sexual satisfaction.

Taking the opportunity of having private talks with patients after the age of 15 years and progressively asking questions about sexual expectation and need is generally greatly appreciated by patients, and may help to consider questions and issues that the patient will never dare to talk about at first, and certainly not in front of their parents.

In conclusion, the sexual health needs of patients with neuromuscular disorders vary broadly. Some of them are probably not directly related with their disease, whilst some others obviously are. They significantly interfere with patient's quality of life and we believe that they should be identified during follow-up consultations in all patients, in order to help them to verbalise and to initiate the search of potential solutions. A holistic approach of neuromuscular disorders should include all aspects of life including sexual well-being.

### Key points
- The pattern, the level and the age at onset of disability cause a broad range of affective and sexual need in patients with neuromuscular diseases.
- Physicians must give the patient chances to openly discuss their sexual needs, in order to propose social or medical solutions when available.

## REFERENCES

Almeida C, Coutinho E, Moreira D, Santos E, Aguiar J (2010) Myasthenia gravis and pregnancy: anaesthetic management – a series of cases. *Eur J Anaesthesiol* 27: 985–990.
Anderson F, Bardach JL (1983) Sexuality and neuromuscular disease: a pilot study. *Int Rehabil Med* 5: 21–26.
Argov Z, de Visser M (2009) What we do not know about pregnancy in hereditary neuromuscular disorders. *Neuromuscul Disord* 19: 675–679.

Bird TD, Lipe HP, Crabtree LD (1994) Impotence associated with the Charcot-Marie-Tooth syndrome. *Eur Neurol* 34: 155–157.

Bronner G, Elran E, Golomb J, Korczyn AD (2010) Female sexuality in multiple sclerosis: the multidimensional nature of the problem and the intervention. *Acta Neurol Scand* 121: 289–301.

Buettner AU (2003) Anaesthesia for caesarean section in a patient with spinal muscular atrophy. *Anaesth Intensive Care* 31: 92–94.

Carter GT, Bonekat HW, Milio L (1994) Successful pregnancies in the presence of spinal muscular atrophy: two case reports. *Arch Phys Med Rehabil* 75: 229–231.

Choquet M, Du Pasquier Fediaevsky L, Manfredi R (1997) Sexual behavior among adolescents reporting chronic conditions: a French national survey. *J Adolesc Health* 20: 62–67.

Ciafaloni E, Pressman EK, Loi AM, Smirnow AM, Guntrum DJ, Dilek N et al. (2006) Pregnancy and birth outcomes in women with facioscapulohumeral muscular dystrophy. *Neurology* 67: 1887–1889.

Flunt D, Andreadis N, Menadue C, Welsh AW (2009) Clinical commentary: obstetric and respiratory management of pregnancy with severe spinal muscular atrophy. *Obstet Gynecol Int* 2009: 942301.

Günzler C, Kriston L, Agyemang A, Riemann D, Berner MM, SPARK-Studiengruppe (2010) [Sexual dysfunction and its consequences in patients with cardiovascular diseases]. *Herz* 35: 410–419.

Mölleken D, Richter-Appelt H, Stodieck S, Bengner T (2010) Influence of personality on sexual quality of life in epilepsy. *Epileptic Disord* 12: 125–132.

Orellana C, Gratacós J, Galisteo C, Larrosa M (2009) Sexual dysfunction in patients with fibromyalgia. *Curr Rheumatol Rep* 11: 437–442.

Peric S, Nisic T, Milicev M, Basta I, Marjanovic I, Peric M et al. (2013) Hypogonadism and erectile dysfunction in myotonic dystrophy type 1. *Acta Myologica* 32: 106–109.

Perniconi B, Vauthier-Brouzes D, Morélot-Panzini C, Dommergues M, Nizard J, Taouagh N et al. (2016) Multidisciplinary care allowing uneventful vaginal delivery in a woman with Pompe disease. *Neuromuscul Disord* 26: 610–613.

Pugh CP, Healey SK, Crane JM, Young D (2000) Successful pregnancy and spinal muscular atrophy. *Obstet Gynecol* 95: 1034.

Rahbek J, Werge B, Madsen A, Marquardt J, Steffensen BF, Jeppesen J (2005) Adult life with Duchenne muscular dystrophy: observations among an emerging and unforeseen patient population. *Pediatr Rehabil* 8: 17–28.

Raphaël JC, Dazord A, Jaillard P, Andronikof-Sanglade A, Benony H, Kovess V, Charpak Y, Auriant I (2002) [Assessment of quality of life for home ventilated patients with Duchenne muscular dystrophy]. *Rev Neurol (Paris)* 158: 453–460.

Rees PM, Fowler CJ, Maas CP (2007) Sexual function in men and women with neurological disorders. *Lancet* 369: 512–525.

Reishtein JL, Maislin G, Weaver TE, Multisite Study group (2010) Outcome of CPAP treatment on intimate and sexual relationships in men with obstructive sleep apnea. *J Clin Sleep Med* 6: 221–226.

Rosenbaum PL, Walter SD, Hanna SE, Palisano RJ, Russell DJ, Raina P et al. (2002) Prognosis for gross motor function in cerebral palsy: creation of motor development curves. *JAMA* 288: 1357–1363.

Rudnik-Schöneborn S, Zerres K, Ignatius J, Rietschel M (1992) Pregnancy and spinal muscular atrophy. *J Neurol* 239: 26–30.

Rudnik-Schöneborn S, Zerres K (2004) Outcome in pregnancies complicated by myotonic dystrophy: a study of 31 patients and review of the literature. *Eur J Obstet Gynecol Reprod Biol* 114: 44–53.

Rudnik-Schöneborn S, Schneider-Gold C, Raabe U, Kress W, Zerres K, Schoser BG (2006) Outcome and effect of pregnancy in myotonic dystrophy type 2. *Neurology* 66: 579–580.

Schmitz MA, Finkelstein M (2010) Perspectives on poststroke sexual issues and rehabilitation needs. *Top Stroke Rehabil* 17: 204–213.

Servais L (2006) Sexual health care in persons with intellectual disabilities. *Ment Retard Dev Disabil Res Rev* 12: 48–56.

Servais L, Baudoin H, Zehrouni K, Richard P, Sternberg D, Fournier E et al. (2013) Pregnancy in congenital myasthenic syndrome. *J Neurol* 260: 815–819.

Sistiaga A, Urreta I, Jodar M, Cobo AM, Emparanza J, Otaegui D et al. (2010) Cognitive/personality pattern and triplet expansion size in adult myotonic dystrophy type 1 (DM1): CTG repeats, cognition and personality in DM1. *Psychol Med* 40: 487–495.

Vinci P, Gargiulo P, Navarro-Cremades F (2007) Sexuality in Charcot-Marie-Tooth disease. *Eura Medicophys* 43: 295–296.

Vitrano V, Catania V, Mercadante S (2011) Sexuality in patients with advanced cancer: a prospective study in a population admitted to an acute pain relief and palliative care unit. *Am J Hosp Palliat Care* 28: 198–202.

Wiegerink DJ, Stam HJ, Gorter JW, Cohen-Kettenis PT, Roebroeck ME, Transition Research Group South-west Netherlands (2010) Development of romantic relationships and sexual activity in young adults with cerebral palsy: a longitudinal study. *Arch Phys Med Rehabil* 91: 1423–1428.

Wielinski CL, Varpness SC, Erickson-Davis C, Paraschos AJ, Parashos SA (2010) Sexual and relationship satisfaction among persons with young-onset Parkinson's disease. *J Sex Med* 7: 1438–1444.

World Health Organization (1975) Education and treatment in human sexuality: the training of health professionals. *WHO Tech Rep Ser* 572: 6.

Yim R, Kirschner K, Murphy E, Parson J, Winslow C (2003) Successful pregnancy in a patient with spinal muscular atrophy and severe kyphoscoliosis. *Am J Phys Med Rehabil* 82: 222–225.

# INDEX

Tables and figures are designated with a lower case, italicised *t* and *f* respectively.

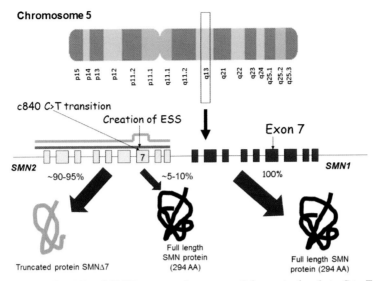

**Fig. 6.1.** Diagram of *SMN1* and *SMN2* genes on chromosome 5 demonstrating that a C-to-T transition at position 6 of *SMN2* creates an exonic splicing suppressor (ESS), which then leads to skipping of exon 7 during transcription, resulting in the production of truncated nonfunctional SMN protein. AA: amino acids. Reprinted from Darras et al. (2015) with permission from Elsevier.

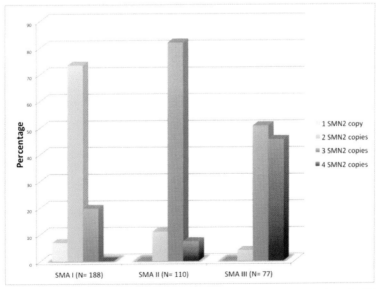

**Fig. 6.2.** Frequency of patients with SMA types I, II and III and *SMN2* copy numbers. In SMA type I, 80% of patients had 1 or 2 copies of *SMN2*; in SMA type II, 82% of patients had 3 copies of *SMN2*; and in SMA type III, 96% of patients carried 3 or 4 *SMN2* copies. Adapted from Feldkötter et al. (2002) with permission from Elsevier.

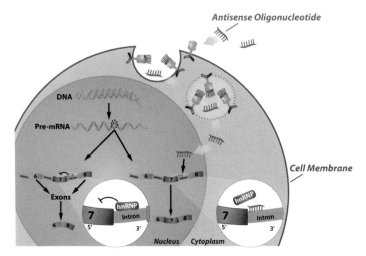

**Fig. 6.3.** Mechanism of action for SMN antisense oligonucleotide (ASO). ASOs enter the cytoplasm of the cells by endocytosis, and enter the nucleus where they bind to the *SMN2* pre-mRNA, displacing protein hnRNP which normally suppresses splicing of exon 7. This action enhances exon 7 inclusion and results in the production of full-length SMN protein. Courtesy of Frank Bennett, PhD, Ionis Pharmaceuticals, Carlsbad, CA, USA.

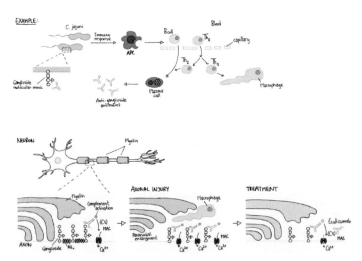

**Fig. 8.1.** The pathogenesis of Guillain–Barré syndrome (GBS). Several studies have demonstrated that anti-GM1 and anti-GQ1b autoantibodies bind to gangliosides of peripheral nerve and neuromuscular junctions, and anti-GD1a antibodies bind to the nodes of Ranvier, paranodal myelin and neuromuscular junction. This binding allows complement activation that leads to the disruption of voltage-gated sodium channel ($Na_v$) clusters, and the formation of the membrane attack complex, which in turn causes axonal intracellular calcium influx and subsequent injury. The nodal disturbed architecture and the axonal injury typically attract macrophages that find their way between the axon and myelin sheet. Complement inhibition could theoretically stop an important step of the pathogenesis at place in GBS. Eculizumab, an anti-C5 monoclonal antibody that is licensed for the treatment for paroxystic hemoglobinuria is currently being tested in two randomized, blinded, placebo-controlled trials in adults. The trigger mechanism (a molecular mimic of gangliosides) that leads to the production of anti-gangliosides in GBS is well described in the case of *Campylobacter jejuni* infection but only convincingly in the case of acute motor axonal neuropathy (AMAN).

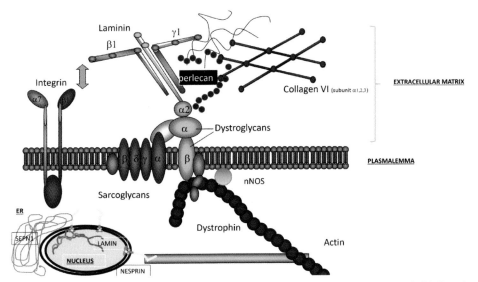

**Fig. 10.1.** Representation of the cellular localisation of the proteins involved in CMDs, DMD/BMD and LGMD. Most genetic defects causing CMD and the milder LGMD affect proteins of plasma membrane–extracellular matrix interface. The three α-chains of Collagen VI, a major component of the extracellular matrix, associate with the basal lamina. Laminin α2 interacts with the α-dystroglycan complex, which is also located in the extracellular matrix, linking the extracellular matrix with the dystrophin-associated glycoprotein (DAG) complex, the sarcoglycans and dystrophin, the latter being involved in Duchenne/Becker dystrophinopathies. A smaller proportion of muscular dystrophies *s* is caused by mutations in genes encoding intracellular proteins, such as Lamin A/C and Nesprin located at the inner nuclear membrane or encoding proteins of the endoplasmatic reticulum such as Selenoprotein1.

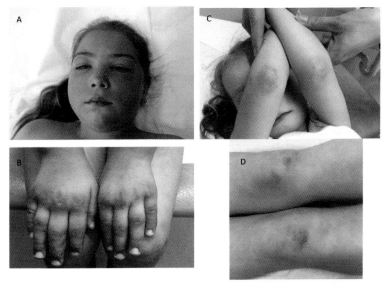

**Fig. 19.1.** Heliotrope discoloration and violaceous suffusion with edema of the upper eyelids in a girl with acute dermatomyositis. Erythematous, scaly rash in a malar distribution (**A**); Gottron papules: symmetrical, scaly, erythematous papules over the metacarpophalangeal and interphalangeal joints of the hands (**B**); Gottron papules on the elbows (**C**) and knees (**D**).

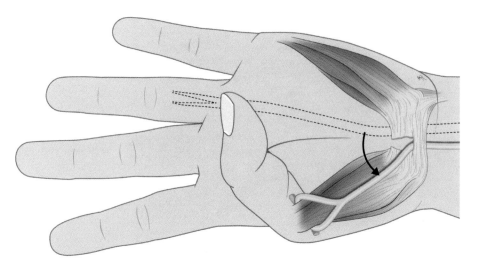

**Fig. 23.1.** Michelinakis and Vourexakis described a technique using the proximal part of the flexor retinaculum as a fulcrum for the flexor tendon of the fourth finger. Illustration by Myrthe Boijmans, www.myrtheboymans.nl.

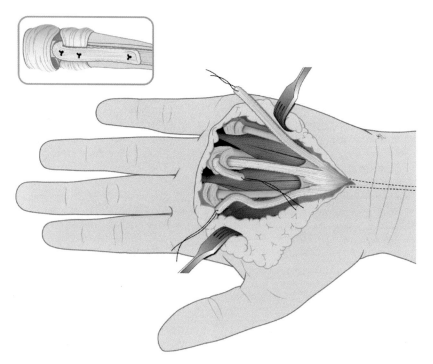

**Fig. 23.2.** Transfer of the palmaris longus tendon, prolonged with palmar aponeurosis and looped around the A1 flexor pulley, was described by Ochiai et al. in 1992. This technique avoids the need for a free tendon graft. PL = palmaris longus. Illustration by Myrthe Boijmans, www.myrtheboymans.nl.

# Other titles from Mac Keith Press www.mackeith.co.uk

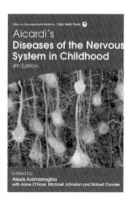

## Aicardi's Diseases of the Nervous System in Childhood, 4th Edition
Alexis Arzimanoglou, Anne O'Hare, Michael V Johnston and Robert Ouvrier (Editors)

*Clinics in Developmental Medicine*
2018 ▪ 1524pp ▪ softback ▪ 978-1-909962-80-4

This fourth edition retains the patient-focussed, clinical approach of its predecessors. The international team of editors and contributors has honoured the request of the late Jean Aicardi, that his book remain 'resolutely clinical', which distinguishes *Diseases of the Nervous System in Childhood* from other texts in the field. New edition completely updated and revised and now in full colour.

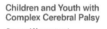
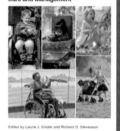

## Children and Youth with Complex Cerebral Palsy: Care and Management
Laurie J. Glader and Richard D. Stevenson (Editors)

*A practical guide from Mac Keith Press*
2019 ▪ 404pp ▪ softback ▪ 978-1-909962-98-9

This is the first practical guide to explore management of the many medical comorbidities that children with complex CP face, including orthopaedics, mobility needs, cognition and sensory impairment, difficult behaviours, respiratory complications and nutrition, amongst others. Uniquely, contributors include children and parents, providing applied wisdom for family-centred care. Clinical Care Tools are provided to help guide clinicians and include a Medical Review Supplement, Equipment and Services Checklist and an ICF-Based Care: Goals and Management Form.

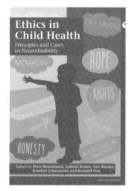

## Ethics in Child Health: Principles and Cases in Neurodisability
Peter L. Rosenbaum, Gabriel M. Ronen, Eric Racine, Jennifer Johannesen and Bernard Dan (Editors)

*A practical guide from Mac Keith Press*
2016 ▪ 396pp ▪ softback ▪ 978-1-909962-63-7

This book explores the ethical dimensions of issues that have either been ignored or not recognised. Each chapter is built around an illustrative scenario and discusses how ethical principles can be utilised to inform decision-making. 'Themes for Discussion' at the end of each chapter will help professionals and policy makers put practical ethical thinking at the heart of care.

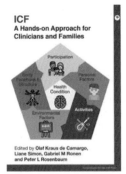

## ICF: A Hands-on Approach for Clinicians and Families
Olaf Kraus de Camargo, Liane Simon, Gabriel M. Ronen and Peter L. Rosenbaum (Editors)

*A practical guide from Mac Keith Press*
2019 ▪ 192pp ▪ softback ▪ 978-1-911612-04-9

This accessible handbook introduces the World Health Organisation's International Classification of Functioning, Disability and Health (ICF) to professionals working with children with disabilities and their families. It contains an overview of the elements of the ICF but focusses on practical applications, including how the ICF framework can be used with children, families and carers to formulate health and management goals.

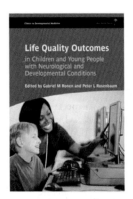

## Life Quality Outcomes in Children and Young People with Neurological and Developmental Conditions
Gabriel M. Ronen and Peter L. Rosenbaum (Editors)

*Clinics in Developmental Medicine*
2013 ▪ 394pp ▪ hardback ▪ 978-1-908316-58-5

Healthcare professionals need to understand their patients' views of their condition and its effects on their health and well-being. This book builds on the World Health Organization's concepts of 'health', 'functioning' and 'quality of life' for young people with neurodisabilities: it emphasises the importance of engaging with patients in the identification of both treatment goals and their evaluation. Uniquely, it enables healthcare professionals to find critically reviewed outcomes-related information.

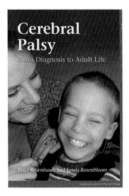

## Cerebral Palsy: From Diagnosis to Adult Life
Peter L. Rosenbaum and Lewis Rosenbloom (Editors)

*A practical guide from Mac Keith Press*
2012 ▪ 224pp ▪ softback ▪ 978-1-908316-50-9

This book has been designed to provide readers with an understanding of cerebral palsy as a developmental as well as a neurological condition. It details the nature of cerebral palsy, its causes and its clinical manifestations. Using clear, accessible language (supported by an extensive glossary) the authors have blended current science with metaphor to explain the biomedical underpinnings of cerebral palsy.

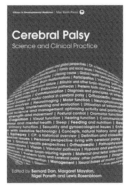

## Cerebral Palsy: Science and Clinical Practice
Bernard Dan, Margaret Mayston, Nigel Paneth and Lewis Rosenbloom (Editors)

*Clinics in Developmental Medicine*
2015 ▪ 648pp ▪ hardback ▪ 978-1-909962-38-5

This landmark title considers all aspects of cerebral palsy from the causes to clinical problems and their implications for individuals. An international team of experts present a wide range of person-centred assessment approaches, including clinical evaluation, measurement scales, neuroimaging and gait analysis. The perspective of the book spans the lifelong course of cerebral palsy, taking into account worldwide differences in socio-economic and cultural factors. Full integrated colour, with extensive cross-referencing make this a highly attractive and useful reference.

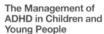
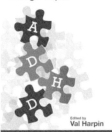

## The Management of ADHD in Children and Young People
Val Harpin (Editor)

*A practical guide from Mac Keith Press*
2017 ▪ 292pp ▪ softback ▪ 978-1-909962-72-9

This book is an accessible and practical guide on all aspects of assessment of children and young people with Attention Deficit Hyperactivity Disorder (ADHD) and how they can be managed successfully. The multi-professional team of authors discusses referral, assessment and diagnosis, psychological management, pharmacological management, and co-existing conditions, as well as ADHD in the school setting. New research on girls with ADHD is also featured. Case scenarios are included that bring these topics to life.

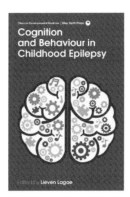

## Cognition and Behaviour in Childhood Epilepsy
Lieven Lagae (Editor)

*Clinics in Developmental Medicine*
2017 ▪ 186pp ▪ hardback ▪ 978-1-909962-87-3

For many parents, cognitive and behavioral comorbidities, such as ADHD, autism and intellectual disability, are the real burden of childhood epilepsy. This title offers concrete guidance and treatment strategies for childhood epilepsy in general, and for the comorbidities associated with each epilepsy syndrome and their pathophysiology. The book is written by experts in the field with an important clinical experience, while chapters by clinical neuropsychologists provide a strong theoretical background.

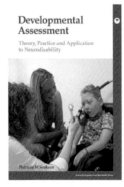

## Developmental Assessment: Theory, Practice and Application to Neurodisability
Patricia M. Sonksen

*A practical guide from Mac Keith Press*
2016 ▪ 384pp ▪ softback ▪ 978-1-909962-56-9
£39.95 / €56.50 / $65.00

This handbook presents a new approach to assessing development in preschool children that can be applied across the developmental spectrum. The reader is taught how to confirm whether development is typical, and if it is not, is signposted to the likely nature and severity of the impairments with a plan of action. The author uses numerous case vignettes from her 40 years' experience to bring to life her approach with clear summary key points and helpful illustrations.

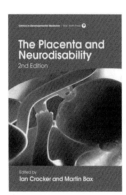

## The Placenta and Neurodisability, 2nd Edition
Ian Crocker and Martin Bax (Editors)

*Clinics in Developmental Medicine*
2015 ▪ 176pp ▪ hardback ▪ 978-1-909962-53-8
£50.00 / €67.50 / $80.00

This comprehensive and authoritative book discusses the critical role of the utero-placenta in neurodisability, both at term and preterm. It examines aspects of fetal compromise and possible cerebro-protective interventions, recent evidence on fetal growth and mental illness, as well as cerebro-therapeutics. Throughout the book, information from the basic sciences is placed within the clinical context.

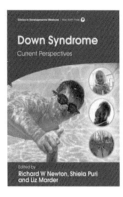

## Down Syndrome: Current Perspectives
Richard W. Newton, Shiela Puri and Liz Marder (Editors)

*Clinics in Developmental Medicine*
2015 ▪ 320pp ▪ hardback ▪ 978-1-909962-47-7
£95.00 / €128.30 / $150.00

Down syndrome remains the most common recognisable form of intellectual disability. The challenge for doctors today is how to capture the rapidly expanding body of scientific knowledge and devise models of care to meet the needs of individuals and their families. *Down Syndrome: Current Perspectives* provides doctors and other health professionals with the information they need to address the challenges that can present in the management of this syndrome.